Electrical Installations in Hazardous Areas

Electrical Installations in Hazardous Areas

Eur Ing *Alan McMillan* C Eng FIEE FInstMC

BUTTERWORTH
HEINEMANN

Butterworth-Heinemann
Linacre House, Jordan Hill, Oxford OX2 8DP
225 Wildwood Avenue, Woburn, MA 01801-2041
A division of Reed Educational and Professional Publishing Ltd

A member of the Reed Elsevier plc group

OXFORD BOSTON JOHANNESBURG
MELBOURNE NEW DELHI SINGAPORE

First published 1998

British Library Cataloguing in Publication Data
A catalogue record for this book is available from the British Library

Library of Congress Cataloguing in Publication Data
A catalogue record for this book is available from the Library of Congress

ISBN 0 7506 3768 4

Typeset by Laser Words, Madras, India
Printed and bound in Great Britain by
Biddles Ltd, Guildford and King's Lynn

Contents

Preface

The technology of application of electrical equipment in explosive atmospheres is very old, dating almost from the original application of electricity to apparatus other than lighting. From its origins it has been developed in most industrialized countries with the United Kingdom, Germany and the United Sates of America being in the vanguard. As the world moves closer together this technology has, like all others, been coordinated so that its detail will be the same in all countries, principally to allow free marketing around the world. This has led to more detailed standard requirements particularly in the case of apparatus construction.

In the UK the considerable standardization of technology is defined in more than 30 published standards (some national, some European and some international). While this is basically good, in that it details what is necessary and thus makes the achievement of safety easier in principle, it has drawbacks in that there is considerable complication which can cause confusion. Despite the longevity of the technology I can find no serious attempt in the UK to produce a freely published volume, such as this, which brings together the entire technology under one roof, as it were. This fact, together with the pivotal role played by the UK in development through the British Standards Institution, which brought together all the necessary expertise to produce the necessary technical standards, the Safety in Mines Research Establishment (now the Health and Safety Laboratory of the Health and Safety Executive) and the Electrical Research Association (now ERA Technology), organizations that carried out much of the research work necessary to permit the current standards to exist and the large contribution made by UK industry, led me to write this volume.

The field can be divided into three facets:

1. The determination of the likelihood and the areas contaminated or likely to be contaminated by explosive atmospheres produced by fuels such as gas, vapour, mist, dust or a combination of these. This is still the least researched of the areas of this technology, principally because there are so many variations, in particular circumstances occurring in practical locations.
2. The construction of electrical equipment so that it is unlikely to become an ignition source. This has been heavily researched in many countries because, unlike area classification, it is relatively specific and lends itself more readily to specification.
3. The installation, operation, maintenance and inspection of electrical equipment. This again is heavily influenced by the circumstances

occurring at particular situations and is thus not as easily specified as equipment construction. It is, however, more specifiable than 1 above.

In writing this book I have tried to address all three facets of the technology and, rather than reproducing all the content of standards and codes, I have been selective in discussing most of the principal requirements therein, while at the same time trying to explain the reasoning which led to their inclusion. Therefore, when applying the technology it will be necessary to address the appropriate standards and codes in all cases but this book will, by provision of the background reasoning, make those documents more understandable. In addition, by developing practical examples of their use, it will assist in their application.

This field is not one for inexperienced engineers and technologists and thus must be approached with care. In addition there are many local conditions which can vary the advice given here and those involved need to be aware of this and have sufficient expertise to determine conditions under which additional requirements are necessary and those, much less common, where relaxations are possible. The onus is, of course, always on the occupier of a location to be able to justify what is done on safety grounds and it is hoped that this book will assist in this activity.

The contents here relate to the situation in the UK but differences in Europe and other countries are not great and its content should be useful elsewhere.

Finally, unlike the situation historically existing, where this technology was often applied in isolation, it is now important to recognize that it can only be applied as a part of an overall safety strategy. That is not to say that its requirements can be ignored if they adversely affect other safety features but rather that, if such is the case, an alternative approach to achievement of its requirements should be sought. It should always be remembered that electrical installations in explosive atmospheres should only exist where necessary (i.e., where they can be fully justified).

Alan McMillan

1

Introduction

Where combustible or flammable materials are stored or processed there is, in most circumstances, a possibility of their leaking or otherwise having the ability to produce what may be described as an explosive atmosphere in conjunction with the oxygen present in air. This is true for gases, vapours, mists and dusts and, as electricity is widely used in industries and other places where such explosive atmospheres can occur, the propensity of electrical energy to create sparking or hot surfaces presents a possibility that the explosive atmospheres may be ignited with resultant fire or explosion. This hazard has been recognized for many decades – almost since the use of electricity was introduced into mining and other industries – and the precautions taken to overcome this problem date back, in their basic inception, to the turn of the twentieth century and before.

There is no way in which explosions can be totally prevented in industries where explosive atmospheres can occur as all human endeavour is fallible but it is necessary to develop our operations to a degree where such explosions are so rare that their risk is far outweighed by the benefits of the processes in which they may occur. Such balance is evident in the coalmining industry where the overall risks associated with working underground, where explosions are one constituent, have been seen as justifiable on the basis of society's need for fuel. It is true that the risks are minimized as far as possible but only to a level consistent with the need to win coal and accidents still occur. It remains true, however, that the risk of these accidents has been reduced to a level acceptable to our society and particularly those working in the industry. That is not to say that when a risk is identified by an incident nothing is done. We always learn from these and invariably they result in changes to our operating systems and equipment in order to minimize the risk of a repeat. Notwithstanding all of our efforts, however, accidents of significant proportion still occur with a degree of regularity which causes us all concern.

1.1 Examples of historic incidents

The following are examples of the more significant incidents occurring in the UK and, although they were not necessarily caused by electricity, there is in at least one of the cases a suspicion of electrical initiation and electricity, as has already been indicated, is seen as an obvious igniting agent.

Senghennyd colliery – 1913

An underground firedamp (methane) explosion caused a roof fall which cut off over 400 miners from a shaft in a burning section of the colliery. Most of them died from the resulting suffocation.

Flixborough – 1974

A modification to a process plant, said by the accident report not to have been properly considered, was identified as causing a major release of flammable gas resulting in an immense aerial explosion. Loss of life on the plant was mercifully low (probably because it was Saturday) but damage to the plant and surrounding residential and other properties was significant.

Piper Alpha – 1988

This oil platform was effectively destroyed by a gas explosion which resulted from a major release of gas suggested to be due to erroneous process operation. The initial and subsequent explosions and fire effectively prevented controlled evacuation of the platform and heavy loss of life was caused.

Texaco Pembroke refinery – 1994

A major vapour explosion occurred leading to a major fire which was extremely difficult to extinguish. The refinery burned for a considerable time with consequent adverse effects on the local environment. Casualties were light but the refinery suffered considerable damage.

The above examples clearly demonstrate the dangers present, particularly in locations where escape of personnel is difficult and it is essential, therefore, that all involved have an understanding of the technology used to minimize the risk of explosion.

1.2 Technological approach

The objective of the technology associated with the use of electrical equipment in potentially explosive atmospheres is to reduce the risk of an explosion to an acceptable level. To have an explosion three elements are necessary – namely fuel, oxygen and a source of ignition (see Fig. 1.1). Oxygen is present in air to a sufficient extent to support combustion and cannot normally be excluded, which leaves only the fuel and ignition sources as elements to which influence can be applied. This has formed

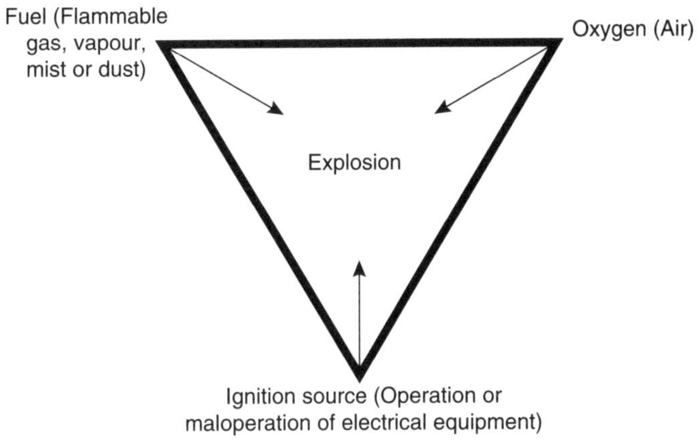

Fig. 1.1 The explosion triangle

the basis for technology since the turn of the twentieth century when the problem was first identified in the mining industry. While in other areas of risk the approach is often based much more heavily on statistical analysis than is the case here, the approach in respect of explosive atmospheres is well established and accepted, having been in use since the early 1900s. The presence of many subjective areas which make statistical analysis difficult have also limited the statistical approach although there have been many attempts to apply such an approach. Thus current and foreseeable future technology is based upon that currently used, and there is no indication of a radical change to readdress the technology on a statistical basis as is done, for example, in the nuclear industry.

A typical attempt to analyse the statistical level of security achieved in relation to gas, vapour and mist releases is that in a paper by W.A. Hicks and K.J. Brown at the 1971 Institution of Electrical Engineers Conference[1] which identified the risk of ignition as between 10^{-5} and 10^{-14}. Many others however have produced different figures as the assumptions made in respect of the subjective elements of the technology vary.

The technology is currently based upon the identification of the risk of an explosive atmosphere being present in a particular place coupled with the identification of the likelihood of electrical equipment within the explosive atmosphere malfunctioning in a way which would cause it to become a source of ignition coincident with the presence of that explosive atmosphere. The objectives are not just to identify these coincidences but to utilize the information so obtained to influence the design of particular process plants and similar operational situations in a way so as to minimize the risk of creation of an explosive atmosphere, and hence the risk of an explosion due to electrical installations. To this end, the generality of the approach is to seek out situations where an explosive atmosphere is normally present of necessity due to the process involved, situations where the likelihood of its presence is high and situations where the likelihood is of its presence is low but identifiable. In this scenario catastrophe does not play a part and although it is necessary to plan for catastrophe such plans are by and large outside the scope of this technology. In addition this technology should not be used in isolation but as part of an overall safety strategy for a location where the problem occurs.

Having identified the possible presence of an Explosive Atmosphere it is then the part of technology to identify those electrical installations which really need to be present rather than those which convenience would make desirable, and ensure that these are protected in a way which makes the overall risk of an explosion sufficiently low.

1.3 History of development

The use of electrical equipment in explosive atmospheres was originally the province of the mining industry and, although the technology was used in surface industry, significant developments in this latter area are more contemporary being to a large extent post war. While the present approach is to minimize the chance of a release of flammable material, or where a release occurs to minimize the build up of the material in the atmosphere, it is probably somewhat surprising that in early coal production the method used to deal with releases of methane (firedamp) was to deliberately burn off the explosive atmosphere. This was done by a specifically designated miner called the 'firelighter'. The method used took advantage of the fact that methane is lighter than air (relative density is around 0.55) and thus methane/air mixtures collected preferentially near the roof of the workings. Warning was given by changes in colour of the flames of the lamps used by miners and the workings were then cleared. A torch was inserted into the methane air cloud, igniting it and burning off the methane. The technique fell into disrepute for obvious reasons and was replaced by the introduction of the use of ventilation to restrict the possibility of explosive atmospheres forming and the employment of a safety lamp (Fig. 1.2) to minimize the risk of ignition.

The introduction of electricity in the latter part of the nineteenth century and the early part of the twentieth century led to significant other risks being identified. Initially electricity was utilized for lighting and motive force. The lighting was typically provided by incandescent filament lamps, none of the more sophisticated lamps having been developed at the time, and the motive force usually by either dc or wound rotor ac machines which were initially typical of the motors available. Both lighting and machines required control equipment (often as simple as a switch) but this equipment also introduced risks associated with hot surfaces and sparks, together with the possibility of the presence of both methane and coal dust.

The solutions to these problems in relation to gas, vapour and mist releases were developed in both the UK and Germany along very similar lines and in very similar time scales. In Germany the organization principally involved was what is now known as the Berggewerkschaftlichen

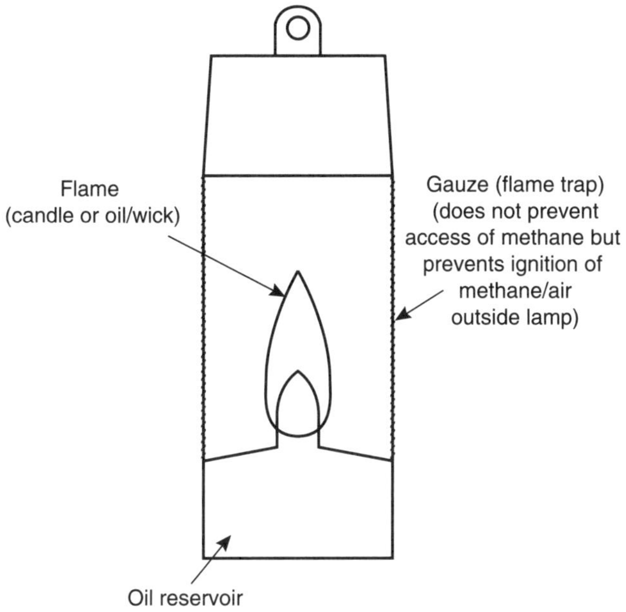

Fig. 1.2 Principle of Davy Lamp

Versuchsstrecke (BVS) and Dr. Ing. Carl Beyling of that organization was awarded the Gold Medal of the UK Institution of Mining Engineers in 1938 for his work in this area. In the UK a similar but governmental organization had significant involvement in similar developments. This is now as the Health and Safety Laboratory of the Health and Safety Executive but is better known by its earlier title of the Safety in Mines Research Establishment.

The initial technique for protection of electrical equipment was what we now know as flameproof enclosure and intended for high-power electrical equipment where the level of electrical energy necessary for equipment operation was always sufficient to initiate ignition if released in a spark or as heat. This was well developed as early as 1905 and was rapidly followed by a second technique, now known as the intrinsically safe circuit. This second technique was developed for mine signalling systems and relied upon the fact that intelligence could be transmitted by very small amounts of electrical energy which, if released, was not sufficient to ignite any expected explosive atmosphere. The advantage of this latter technique was in the flexibility which it offered as large heavy protective enclosures were not necessary.

Initially these two techniques were developed for the mining industry where methane was the most sensitive flammable material present but as the techniques began to be applied to surface industry two significant differences in approach became rapidly apparent. First it was recognized that releases of flammable material were normally from installed equipment and more predictable in quantity and frequency, and second the recognition that far from dealing with one gas and one dust, as in mining, surface industry was dealing with a myriad of different materials each with its own characteristics. This recognition led to development of the technique of area classification to define the risks of explosive atmospheres occurring in specific locations and the development of additional types of protection to more readily reflect the varying levels of hazard which could be identified. It is these two factors that led to the current UK and international industrial practice which this book seeks to describe.

1.4 UK legislation

The basic historic UK legislation covering the use of electrical equipment in explosive atmospheres is that included in the Electricity Regulations[2] of the Factories Acts[3]. Regulation 27 of these regulations states:

> All conductors and apparatus exposed to the weather, wet, corrosion, inflammable surroundings or explosive atmosphere, or used in any process or for any special purpose other than for lighting or power, shall be so constructed or protected, and such special precautions shall be taken as may be necessary adequately to prevent danger in view of such exposure or use.

This regulation clearly states the objective to be achieved but does not define the method of its achievement. While one may be concerned at this, its intent is to allow the widest possible range of approaches to the achievement of the required level of security and thus to give the maximum freedom of operation to industry, while at the same time, laying upon that industry the requirement to achieve an adequate level of security in its operation.

Regulation 27 remained in force, even after the enactment of the Health and Safety at Work Act 1974[4], until replaced by Regulation 6 of the 1989 Electricity at Work Regulations[5]. Regulation 6 states:

> Electrical equipment which may reasonably foreseeably be exposed to:-
>
> (a) mechanical damage;
> (b) the effects of weather, natural hazards, temperature or pressure;
> (c) the effects of wet, dirty, dusty or corrosive conditions; or
> (d) any flammable or explosive substance, including dusts, vapours or gases,
>
> shall be of such construction or as necessary protected as to prevent, so far as is reasonably practible, danger arising from such exposure.

The tenor of this new regulation, now current, is very much the same as its predecessor. The objective to be achieved is specified and within that objective maximum freedom is given to industry in methods of its achievement.

The above method of legislating, while common in the UK, contrasts significantly with legislation in countries such as Germany where legislation tends to be more specific, giving much more detail in respect of the precautions to be adopted. There is, however, little or no evidence available to suggest that one or the other approach produces a better result as far as safety is concerned. Thus, the UK approach has much to commend it providing as it does maximum flexibility but, conversely, practitioners in the UK must be fully competent to deal with the flexibility permitted.

In respect of dusts, a further regulation exists in the Factories Acts[3] which reflects the different nature of such materials, in that when a dust is released it does not disperse as is the case with gases, vapours and mists but settles and forms a layer which can be re-formed as a cloud at any time by any sort of physical intervention. The regulation in question is Regulation 31(1) which states:

> When, in connection with any grinding, sieving, or other process giving rise to dust, there may escape dust of such a character and to such an extent as to be liable to explode on ignition, all practicable steps shall be taken to prevent such an explosion by enclosure of the plant used in the process, and by removal or prevention of accumulation of any dust that may escape in spite of the enclosure, and by exclusion or effective enclosure of possible sources of ignition.

While not specifically referring to electrical equipment, this regulation includes it as a possible source of ignition and identifies the method of protection as effective enclosure. This is possible as dust is nothing like as penetrative as gas, vapour or mist and can effectively be excluded with much less difficulty.

To underpin these regulations and give guidance, many British Standards and Codes containing details of acceptable methods of compliance and third-party certification facilities have been developed to give purchasers of electrical equipment confidence. These certification schemes do not, however, extend to installation and use.

In the past, when equipment construction Standards were limited and lacked detail, a great deal of expertise was necessary within the certification bodies as it was they who had to interpret what general statements within Standards actually meant. Thus, it was not surprising that the certification body in the UK was associated with the Health and Safety Executive and the Safety in Mines Research Establishment organizations which made great contributions to the more detailed technological base currently available.

Now, with much more detailed requirements, this relationship, while remaining useful, is no longer necessary. The contribution of organizations such as the Safety in Mines Research Establishment, and the Electrical Research Association (now ERA Technology Ltd), the latter through its industry sponsored project work, to the detail existing in current Standards and Codes cannot however be overstated.

In addition to the above organizations, which were principally associated with the construction of equipment, a great deal of work was done by industry in general and organizations such as The Institute of Petroleum which produced a model code of safe practice[6] for the oil industry. Industry, unlike the governmental organizations, concentrated much of its work on the matters associated with how hazardous areas were formed and matters associated with installation and maintenance. Individual companies also made significant contributions and, as an example of this, the RoSPA/ICI Code of Practice[7] covering use of electrical equipment in explosive atmospheres in the chemical industry is probably one of the finest documents of its type ever produced.

1.5 European legislation

With the accession of the UK to the EU it became subject to EU legislation in this field. The first such legislation produced was the Explosive Atmospheres Directive 1975[8]. This Directive was limited to equipment for gas, vapour and mist risks and was what is described as an optional Directive, solely concerned with barriers to trade. It did not dictate what must be used in explosive atmospheres but merely identified equipment which could not be defined by individual member states as unsuitable for use in their country. The Directive referred to all constituent parts of electrical installations capable of use in potentially explosive atmospheres, other than mines and its Article 4 set the scene as follows:

> Member States may not, on grounds of safety requirements for the design and manufacture of electrical equipment for use in Potentially Explosive Atmosphere, prohibit the sale or free movement or the use, for its proper purpose of the electrical equipment (covered by the Directive)

While this clearly prevented individual member countries from insisting that all equipment used must comply with individual national requirements, it did not prevent equipment complying with national requirements from use in addition to that complying with the Directive even though these could differ.

The 1975 Directive also had to define what was required of equipment to comply with it, and this led to considerable emphasis on the work of the European Committee for Electrical Standardization (CENELEC)[9] which produced a range of very detailed Standards describing the construction of suitable electrical equipment (the EN 50 - - - range of European Standards). These Standards were then given legal status by being referred to in Supplementary Directives[10] or the EU Journal[12]. To ensure that equipment did indeed comply the basic Directive recognized the Distinctive Community Mark (Fig. 1.3) which could only be affixed to equipment in compliance with the Standards referred to in the Supplementary arrangements and required that this compliance be attested by a Certificate of Conformity or Inspection Certificate issued by an approved body. The Certificate of Conformity was for equipment which complied with one of the recognized

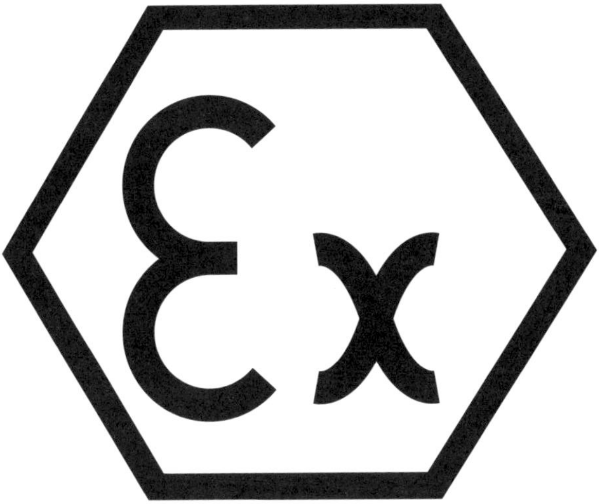

Fig. 1.3 The Distinctive Community Mark

CENELEC Standards referred to in the Supplementary Directives, and the Inspection Certificate for equipment which did not comply but was considered by the approved body to be of at least equivalent safety. In this latter case, however, all of the approved bodies in all member states had to agree on equivalence and thus, although this route allowed some flexibility, it was seldom used due to its expensive and time consuming nature.

The Explosive Atmospheres Directive 1975[8] remained in force until 1996 when it was superseded by a new Directive on the subject[11]. The new Directive followed the EU 'new approach' in which the technical requirements were included within the Directive, rather than by reference to Standards Unlike its predecessor, in this Directive there was a mandatory requirement that after a certain cut-off date all equipment put into use must of necessity comply with it and, unlike its predecessor, included dusts – bringing equipment for use in dust risks into the certification net set up by its predecessor. Article 2 of this Directive states:

> Member States shall take all appropriate measures to ensure that the equipment, protective systems and devices to which this Directive applies may be placed on the market and put into service only if, when properly installed and maintained and used for their intended purpose, they do not endanger the health and safety of persons and, where appropriate, domestic animals or property.

As the essential requirements for health and safety are included in this Directive it effectively excludes all other equipment. The exclusion of non-complying equipment (including that complying with the 1976 Directive) will come into force in on 30 June 2003. European Standards are no longer referred to in the new Directive but will be identified in the EU Journal[12] as acceptable as a means of compliance with the Directive (but not, as before, the only means of compliance). In addition non-electrical equipment and systems have been brought into the scope of the new Directive.

Both of the Directives are brought into effect in Great Britain by the Explosive Atmosphere (Certification) Regulations[13] and in Northern Ireland by similar legislation.

The EU Directives and National Implementation legislation referred to above refer only to the construction of equipment and not to its installation and use which is still a matter for National Law. A Directive[14] is in discussion within the EU, however, which will address matters of installation and use. This Directive is still at a relatively early stage but its implications are far reaching. It formalizes the requirements on employers to identify hazardous areas (with notices), to classify such areas and to consult with and inform employees. It also formalizes the requirement for the use of experts (properly trained and experienced personnel) in the workplace to oversee installations. While much of what is included is correct and is commonsense, it adds a degree of formality not hitherto seen in the UK and thus, when promulgated, may have a significant effect on UK industry. Having said that, much of what is in the proposed Directive is in accordance with the recommendations and guidance in this book and other guides.

1.6 Certification

As has been stated there is no specific requirement for certification in respect of equipment used in hazardous areas in the UK, other than that associated with the EU Directives associated with construction and marketing of equipment and ensuing National Law. Certification has, however, become accepted as the norm, at least in the more hazardous of the affected areas and is an important aspect of the technology. It must be noted however that over the years the vision of certification has changed from that of inspection by a body expert in hazardous area technology, such as the Safety in Mines Research Establishment and its associates, against not very specific standards, to inspection by a competent test laboratory against very detailed standards not requiring anything like the previous level of expertise.

Within the EU there are now some 17 approved bodies for such certification, including the non-EU European and Scandinavian countries with whom the EU has agreements. As far as EU legislation is concerned, these are all equivalent and a certificate from any one of them is sufficient to demonstrate that the equipment satisfies the requirements of the appropriate European Standard. Equipment which is certified by any one of these 17 approved bodies is normally identified by the manufacturer by marking the apparatus with the Distinctive Community Mark in addition to any marking associated with the certification.

The 17 approved bodies are:

Belgium (EU)
Institut Scientifique de Service Public (ISSEP)
Division de colfontaine

Rue Grande 60
B–7340 Paturages

Denmark (EU)
Danmarks Elektriske Materielkontrol (DEMKO)
Lyskær 8
D–2730 Herlev

Germany (EU)
Physikalisch-Technische Bundesanstalt (PTB)
Bundesallee 100
D–38116 Braunschweig

Bergbau-Versuchsstrecke (BVS)
Postfach 14 01 20
Beylingstraße 65
D–44329 Dortmund 14

Spain (EU)
Laboratorio Oficial José María Madariaga (LOM)
Calle Alenza 1 y 2
E–28003 Madrid

France (EU)
Institut National de L'Environnement Industriel et des Risques (INERIS)
Boite Postale N°2
F–60550 Verneuil-en-Halatte

Laboratoire Central des Industries Électriques(LCIE)
Boite Postale N°8
F–92266 Fontenay-aux-Roses

Italy (EU)
Centro Elettrotecnico Sperimentale Italiano (CESI)
Via Rubattino 54
I–20134 Milano

Netherlands (EU)
NV KEMA
Utrechtseweg 310
PO Box 9035
NL–6800 ET Arnhem

Great Britain (EU)
Electrical Equipment Certification Service (EECS)
Health & Safety Executive
Harpur Hill
Buxton
Derbyshire SK17 9JN

Sira Certification Service (SCS)
South Hill
Chislehurst
Kent BR7 5EH

Northern Ireland (EU)
Industrial Science Centre
Department of Economic Development
17 Antrim Road
Lisburn
County Antrim BT2 3AL

Finland (EU)
Technical Research Centre of Finland (VTT)
Automation/Electrotechnical Testing
Otakaari 7B, Espoo
P.O. Box 13051
FIN–02044 VTT

Norway (non-EU)
Norges Elektriske Materiellkontroll (NEMKO)
Postboks 73 Blindern
N–0314 Oslo 3

Austria (EU)
Bundesversuchs-und-Forschungsanstalt Arsenal (BVFA)
Faradaygasse 3
A–1030 Wein Austria

Technischer Überwachungs-Verein Östereich (TÜV-A)
Krugerstrasse 16
A–1015 Wein Austria

Sweden (EU)
Swedish National Testing and Research Institute (SP)
Box 857
S–501 15 Borås Sweden

It will be noted that in the case of the Industrial Science Centre in Northern Ireland no set of initials is given after the title. This is significant as the initials are those which appear on the certificates issued by the approved bodies. The reason for this lies in the slightly unusual nature of the relationship between Great Britain and Northern Ireland in that British legislation in this area does not apply to Northern Ireland, which results in the need for an approved body in Northern Ireland even though that organization has no plans to issue any certificates and it certainly does not at present.

It might also be thought odd that the Safety in Mines Research Establishment or its successor, the Health and Safety Laboratory, is not present despite its long history of expertise in this area. This is because it was part of the British Civil Service (Government Service). The current Government associated body is the Electrical Equipment Certification Service which comes from the same roots and has access to the same expertise as did the Safety in Mines Research Establishment. Some of the listed bodies have logos and these are shown in Fig. 1.4 to assist in their recognition.

The certificates issued by all of these approved bodies have exactly the same format which assists in their usage whatever their source. They identify the equipment certified, together with its certification code

Ex

Electrical Equipment
Certification Service

EECS / BASEEFA

sira
Certification Service

NATIONAL ACCREDITATION OF CERTIFICATION BODIES
Registration Number
011

SCS

Ex

Physical/SCH
Technische
Bundesanstalt

PTB

Fig. 1.4 Typical certification logos

(described later) and the manufacturer. An example of a typical certificate is given in Fig. 1.5. What should be noted is the limit of the certificate. It only specifies the equipment as being in accordance with the detailed construction requirements in the specified Standard and does not address installation which will vary depending upon the country of installation. Therefore care needs to be taken in careful consideration of the way in which equipment is installed, so as to ensure that the safety elements included in its construction are not negated by its method of installation.

The listed approved bodies meet regularly in a working group titled Heads of Test Houses Liaison Committee (HOTL)[15] which was set up by the Commission of the EU. The object of this group is to ensure that all approved bodies use the Standards in the same way and present their certificates in the same way. It is not intended to be a body for the deciding of the meaning of unclear parts of the Standards although it, of necessity becomes involved in such activity. The clarification and interpretation of Standards is for the Standards' writing bodies (CENELEC in this case) but such bodies are by their nature cumbersome and thus queries on Standards

British Approvals Service for Electrical Equipment in Flammable Atmospheres

BASEEFA

1 ***Certificate of Conformity***

2 **BAS No. Ex 96D9999**

3 This certificate is issued for the electrical apparatus:

CONTROL CONSOLE TYPE ABC.123

4 Manufactured and submitted for certification by:

A. MANUFACTURER LTD
of 123 Fore Street, Buxton, SK17 9JK

5 This electrical apparatus and any acceptable variation thereto is specified in the Schedule to this Certificate and the documents therein referred to.

6 BASEEFA being an Approved Certification Body in accordance with Article 14 of the Council Directive of the European Communities of 18 December 1975 (76/117/EEC) certifies that the apparatus has been found to comply with harmonised European Standards:

EN50014 (1977) + Amd 1 to 5
EN50018 (1977) + Amd 1 to 3

and has successfully met the examination and test requirements recorded in confidential Report number:

96(C)9999 dated 27 February 1996

7 The apparatus marking shall include the code:

EEx d IIB T4

8 The manufacturer of the electrical apparatus referred to in this certificate, has the responsibility to ensure that the apparatus conforms to the specification laid down in the Schedule to this certificate and has satisfied routine verifications and tests specified therein.

9 This apparatus may be marked with the Distinctive Community Mark specified in Annex II to the Council Directive of 16 January 1984 (Doc 84/47/EEC). A facsimile of this mark is printed on sheet 1 of this certificate.

File No: EECS 9999/01/001

Sheet 1 of 2

This certificate is granted subject to the general conditions of the Electrical Equipment Certification Service. It does not necessarily indicate that the apparatus may be used in particular industries or circumstances. Representation of equipment as "Certified" is valid only when the number of this certificate is given on the relevant EECS Manufacturing Licence or Verification Certificate.

I M CLEARE
DIRECTOR
27 February 1996

NATIONAL ACCREDITATION OF CERTIFICATION BODIES
Registration Number 020

HSE

Electrical Equipment Certification Service
Health and Safety Executive
Harpur Hill, Buxton, Derbyshire. SK17 9JN. United Kingdom
Tel: 01298 28000 Fax: 01298 28244

Fig. 1.5 Example of equipment certificate

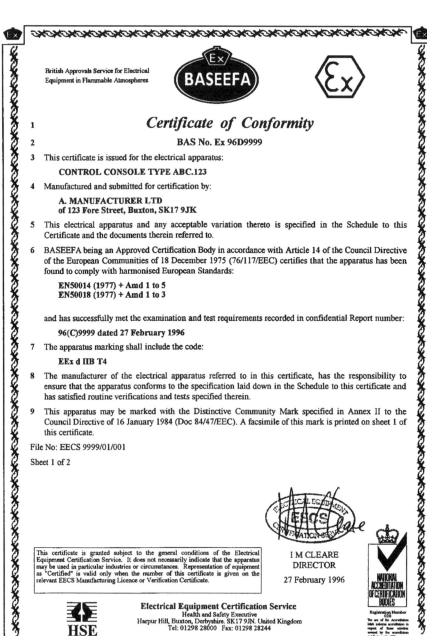

can take considerable time to resolve. Because of the commercial nature of the use of certification HOTL performs a valuable role in providing speedy temporary clarification pending the decision of the Standards writing body and to this end HOTL members notify that body of all temporary clarifications which they have adopted. The Standards writing body may then endorse or override them as it wishes, in its own good time. This does not normally represent any problem for the holder of a certificate based on an HOTL clarification later overturned by the Standards writing body because, unless a prima-facie danger is identified in relation to the HOTL decision, the certificate would be allowed to stand, although members of HOTL would automatically adopt the official clarification as soon as it was available for future certification.

Many of the approved bodies issue certificates to equipment complying with their own or national Standards in addition to equipment complying with the European Standards referred to in the Directive. These are not covered by the Directive and their acceptance is a matter for the individual user. This is likewise true of certificates issued by bodies not approved by the EU even though they may be national bodies and likewise acceptance is a matter for the individual. Where these latter certificates are in relation to the European Standards then it is only the expertise of the non-approved certification body which must be considered but in other cases (e.g, Factory Mutual Research Corporation and Underwriters Laboratories in the USA) the Standards to which the equipment is certified (or listed which is what the activity is called in the USA) differ significantly, and the effect of this must also be considered.

1.7 Certificate and labelling information

There is no real short cut to identification of suitable equipment as the schedules issued with certificates of conformity and inspection certificates contain information which is necessary to the user. These should always be made available to the purchasers of certified equipment and there is a legal obligation upon suppliers to do this insofar as safety is dependent upon such information. There is, however, a standard coding which appears on both certificate and label usually and this is as follows.

Certifying body reference

This appears usually as a set of initials and these are those shown in brackets in Section 1.5 of this chapter (e.g., PTB, LCIE, etc.).

Certificate number

This appears as follows:

Ex 96 D 2 123 (X)

The various parts of this Code have the following meanings:

Ex – explosion protected equipment
96 – the last two digits of the year of issue
D – amendment status of the Standard used for certification
2 – principal method of protection

1 = flameproof or pressurized (see Chapters 10 and 11)
2 = intrinsic safety (see Chapter 13)
3 = increased safety (see Chapter 12)
4 = type N (n) apparatus (see Chapter 14)
5 = special protection (apparatus which does not wholly comply with one of the Standards but is considered as suitable)
6 = battery operated vehicles (usually using more than one type of protection)
7 = oil immersed or powder filled (see Chapter 9)
123 = serial number of certificate within year
X = indicates that there are special (unusual) installation conditions associated with the equipment and these will be specified on the certificate. If U appears instead of X or no suffix, it means that the equipment is considered to be a component and cannot be used unless incorporated in other equipment and further certified

Protection coding

This normally appears in the following form:
EEx d IIC T4
The meaning of these symbols is as follows:

E – indicates that the equipment complies with a European Standard. The symbol will not be present if such is not the case.
Ex – indicates explosion protected equipment
d – indicates the type of protection used

o = oil immersion (see Chapter 9)
p = pressurization (see Chapter 11)
q = powder filling (see Chapter 9)
d = flameproof enclosure (see Chapter 10)
e = increased safety (see Chapter 12)
i = intrinsic safety (see Chapter 13) (Intrinsic safety usually appears with a further suffix, for example ia or ib)
m = encapsulation (see Chapter 9)
n = type n equipment (See Chapter 14); (n sometimes appears as

'N' indicating it is to a UK national Standard and not a European Standard)

IIC – indicates the explosive atmosphere in which the apparatus was tested for spark ignition

IIA – equipment is tested in an ideal mixture of propane and air

IIB – equipment is tested in an ideal mixture of ethylene and air

IIC – equipment is tested in an ideal mixture of hydrogen and air (where the equipment is to a type of protection where sparking is prevented the letter will be omitted and only II will appear as sub-grouping is not necessary)

T4 – indicates the maximum temperature achieved by any ignition capable part of the equipment and indicates that no part of the equipment will exceed

T1 450 °C

T2 300 °C

T3 200 °C

T4 135 °C

T5 100 °C

T6 85 °C

An ambient temperature of 40 °C is assumed unless otherwise stated on the label and certificate

Historically, there have been other methods of coding in Europe and remain different methods in the USA. These are shown in Tables. 1.1 and 1.2. It must however be noted that because of slightly differing information forming the basis for these that the relationship is only approximate.

Table 1.1 Relationship of grouping and classification systems

Current European	Historic GB		German	USA
	Flame proof	Intrinsic Safety		
sub-group IIA	Group II	class 2c	class 1	Group D
sub-group IIB	Group III	class 2d	class 2	Group C
sub-group IIC	Group IV	class 2e and 2f	class 3a and 3n	Group B and A

Notes:

1 UK Flameproof Group IV excludes acetylene which was treated separately.

2 UK intrinsic safety class 2e did not include acetylene, but 2f did.

3 German class 3a excludes acetylene as does USA Group B and UK Class 2e. Acetylene is included in German class 3n, USA Group A and UK Class 2f.

4 In the USA the following Groups are also present: E – Conducting dusts; F – non-Conducting dusts; G – Flour and Grain dust.

5 To add further complexity, USA apparatus is classed as to its intended use. Class A is for gases and vapours, Class B is for dusts and class C is for fibres and flyings.

Table 1.2 Relationship of temperature classification systems

European and UK	German	USA
T1	G1	T1
T2	G2	T2
–	–	T2A (280 °C)
–	–	T2B (260 °C)
–	–	T2C (230 °C)
–	–	T2D (215 °C)
T3	G3	T3
–	–	T3A (180 °C)
–	–	T3B (165 °C)
–	–	T3C (160 °C)
T4	G4	T4
–	–	T4A (120 °C)
T5	G5	T5
T6	–	T6

Note: Prior to the introduction of a separate temperature classification system in the USA temperature classification was associated with the grouping system as follows: Groups A, B and D were given a maximum temperature of 280 °C; Group C was given a maximum temperature of 180 °C; Groups E and F were given a temperature of 200 °C; and Group G a temperature of 165 °C.

1.8 The future of certification

As has been stated, the situation in regard to certification is significantly affected by the 1990 Directive[11] which came into force early in 1996. While this will initially rely on European Standards referred to in the European Journal[12] it is certain that the breadth of the essential requirements contained within the Directive[11] will ultimately be used. As these essential requirements are couched in much more general terms than the Standards, then the approved bodies will have to revert to the expert interpretation of more general requirements much as they did before the advent of the more detailed Standards. The level of expertise of the certification bodies will once again, therefore, become of paramount importance. To this end the HOTL grouping will assume a much greater significance and it is unlikely that it will contain sufficient expertise without introducing industrial expertise into it. How this can be done without making it as cumbersome as a Standards-making body will no doubt become a matter for considerable debate in the not too distant future.

The inclusion of non-electrical equipment for which the level of detailed standardization in this area is much lower will mean that the problem of certification to the requirements contained in the new Directive[11] will be apparent much sooner. Not only will the currently approved bodies not have any detailed Standards but they will probably have only limited expertise in the non-electrical areas covered. As a result of this it is likely that a new set of approved bodies will appear separately from those in the electrical sphere.

Another inclusion in this new Directive is the requirement for a manufacturer or supplier to have a quality management system in most cases and to have that also certified to a set of requirements similar to BS/EN/ISO 9002[16] (although the requirements are again enshrined in the Directive).

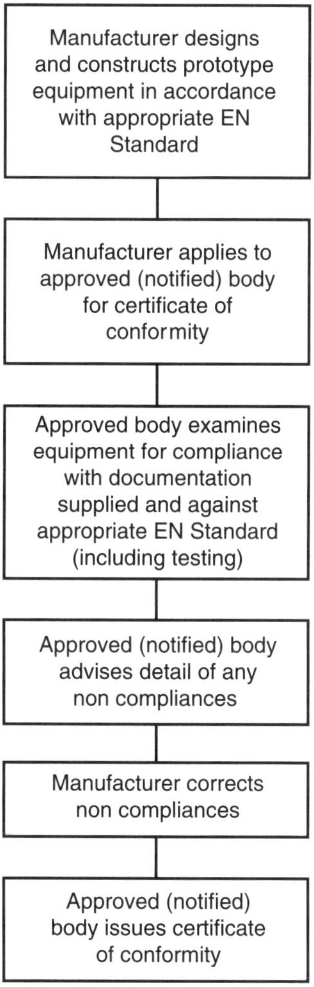

Note: In the UK both approved (notified) bodies require a quality system to be in place at the manufacturers which is certified by a certification body acceptable to them to BS/EN/ISO 9002 (they issue such certificates).

Fig. 1.6(a) Route to certification – Directive 76/117/EEC

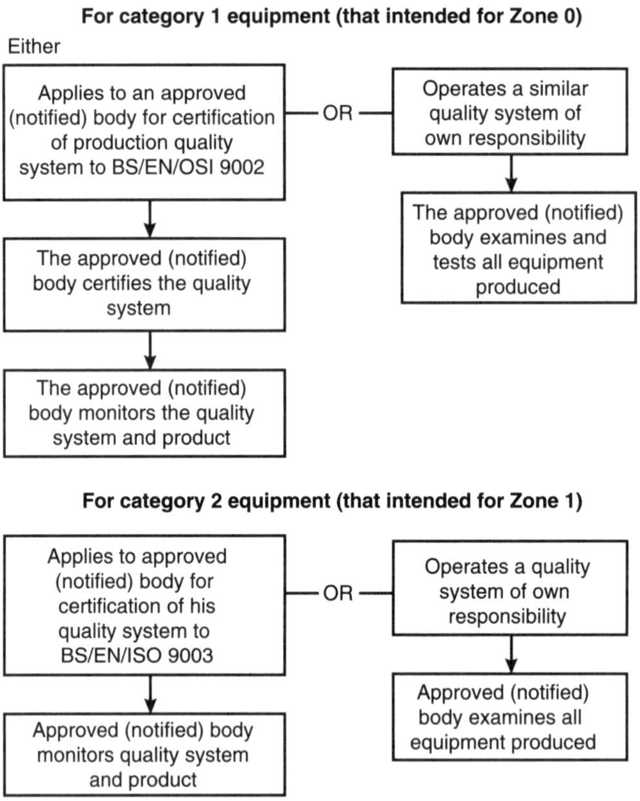
For category 1 equipment (that intended for Zone 0)
Either
Applies to an approved (notified) body for certification of production quality system to BS/EN/OSI 9002
OR
Operates a similar quality system of own responsibility
The approved (notified) body examines and tests all equipment produced
The approved (notified) body certifies the quality system
The approved (notified) body monitors the quality system and product
For category 2 equipment (that intended for Zone 1)
Applies to approved (notified) body for certification of his quality system to BS/EN/ISO 9003
OR
Operates a quality system of own responsibility
Approved (notified) body examines all equipment produced
Approved (notified) body monitors quality system and product

Fig. 1.6(b) Route to certification – Directive 94/9/EC

This will give more confidence to the user that purchases will accurately reflect the certification but, as the quality management requirements are again extremely subjective, it will cause considerable interpretive problems and is a further need for an expanded HOTL. The route to certification under the new Directive is given in Fig. 1.6a. When the manufacturer has obtained a type certificate for a product, using the system in Fig. 1.6a in accordance with the appropriate EN Standard or the essential requirements of the Directive, the steps illustrated by Fig. 1.6b are followed in respect of category 1 and category 2 equipment. (For category 3 equipment (intended for Zone 2) no certification by an approved (notified) body is necessary. The manufacturer confirms compliance by declaration and application of CE Mark.)

References

1 Hicks, W. F and Brown, K. J (1971). Assessment of explosion probability for intrinsically safe apparatus. (IEE Conference on electrical safety in hazardous environments – 16–18 March).

2 The Electricity (Factories Act) Special Regulations 1908 and 1944
3 The Factories Act 1961
4 The Health and Safety at Work Act 1974
5 Electricity at Work Regulations 1989
6 Institute of Petroleum Area Classification Code for Petroleum Installations (1990).
7 RoSPA/ICI Engineering Codes and Regulations Electrical Installations in Flammable Atmospheres (1973). Group C (Electrical), Volume 1.5.
8 76/117/EEC (1975). Council Directive (on the approximation of the laws of Member States concerning electrical equipment for use in potentially explosive atmospheres). 18 December, 1975.
9 Comité Europèen de Normalization Electrique (CENELEC), Rue de Stassart 35, B–1050 Brussels.
10 Directives supplementary to 76/117/EEC: Council Directive 79/196/EEC; Commission Directive 84/47/EEC; Commission Directive 88/571/EEC; Council Directive 90/487/EEC.
11 94/9/EC (1994). Directive of the European Parliament and Council on the approximation of the laws of Member States concerning equipment and protective systems intended for use in potentially explosive atmospheres. 23 March.
12 Official Journal of the European Communities.
13 The Electrical Equipment for Explosive Atmospheres (Certification) Regulations 1990.
14 6430/92 EN. Proposal for a Council Directive concerning minimum requirements for improving the safety and health and protection of workers in potentially explosive atmospheres (Draft document).
15 HOTL is a working party set up and funded by the Commission comprising the heads of all Approved (Notified) Bodies and representatives of Directorate General III and Directorate General V of the Commission.
16 BS/EN/ISO 9002: (1994) Quality Systems – Specification for production, installation and servicing.

— 2 —

Area classification

Philosophy, objectives and procedures

The basic objective of area classification (be it for gas, vapour, mist or dust risks) is to identify the possibility of an explosive atmosphere existing in a given location and, more importantly, to influence the design of any plant or facility to minimize such risks. To this end, it is a tool to be used together with the operational requirements in the design of any plant, process or facility, and the result will invariably be a compromise between convenience of operation and security against explosion. This balance must take account of certain situations which are generally not permissible, such as the continuous presence of an explosive atmosphere in an unrestricted area, and the limits which are placed on the acceptability of any situation where an explosive atmosphere may be present. This chapter seeks to identify the principles upon which area classification is based to achieve these objectives, the part played in area classification by those involved in design or operation of plants and locations where explosive atmosphere may be present, and the procedures which need to be undertaken in the identification of hazardous areas.

2.1 Basic properties of flammable and combustible materials

The materials with which we are concerned are gases, vapour mists and dusts. Each of these materials behaves in a different way and this affects the classification process.

2.1.1 Flammable gases

A gas is a material whose normal state at ambient temperatures and pressures is as a vapour. These materials cannot be liquidized at ambient temperature by pressure alone and must also be cooled. Therefore, they are not likely to be present in the form of liquid and, if they are, they will rapidly vaporize once released. Area classification is a measure of the area contaminated by their release and is not likely to be greatly influenced by an residual effect due to their continued presence after the release ceases, provided there is sufficient ventilation for their removal.

There are several features of primary importance in respect of gases which determine the approach which is adopted in respect of electrical installations with which they may come into contact. These are:

Relative density in respect of air and determines how the gas will disperse when no other influences are present (e.g., gas released at high speed will disperse in a manner governed by the energy of release rather than by the effects of wind and density;

Minimum ignition energy, the minimum energy released as an arc or spark which will ignite the most easily ignitable mixture of the gas and air;

Maximum experimental safe gap defines the burning characteristics of the ideal gas/air mixture (which may differ from the most easily ignitable mixture) insofar as its ability to burn through small gaps is concerned;

Ignition temperature, the minimum temperature at which the ideal gas/air mixture will spontaneously ignite.

As soon as it is released a gas will mix with air, either by the energy of its own rapidity of release or turbulent air movement. Where the release of a gas is at low velocity and the air movement is small (as in badly ventilated buildings) mixing is not as efficient and the mixture will vary from place to place giving large and unpredictable hazardous areas.

2.1.2 Flammable vapours

Flammable vapours are very similar to gases in that they are in the vapour phase. The difference is that they can be liquefied by pressure alone and thus are more easily liquefied. A flammable vapour may be only the vapour which exists because of a flammable liquid; as all such liquids have vapour pressures (partial pressures in air) at temperatures well below their boiling points and once the percentage of vapour in air created by the vapour pressure exceeds the lower explosive limit, an explosive atmosphere can exist even though the release is a liquid.

The explosive atmosphere created by a vapour release will have a significantly varying persistence time after cessation of a release. If it is released as a vapour or as a liquid which has a boiling point significantly lower than ambient temperature then the persistence will be low, whereas if it is released from a liquid surface and the liquid boiling point is above ambient temperature then it will be high. The formation of an explosive atmosphere is caused by the mixing of the vapour with air and the criteria are as described for gas, as are the parameters which have primary importance.

2.1.3 Flammable mists

This is an entirely different situation to that which exists in the case of gases and vapours. A mist is created by release at high pressure (mists have been formed by pressures as low as 2×10^5 N/m^2 gauge) in such a way that very fine particles (droplets) of liquid are produced. (Mists can form explosive atmospheres in mixture with air even if the liquid forming them is considered not to have sufficient vapour pressure to form an explosive atmosphere.) These particles will recombine to form a liquid much more readily than gas or vapour, but if very finely divided the mist has a significant existence time and the particles will remain in suspension in air for a long period. Much less is known about the performance of mists in air but they are normally treated in the same way as gases and vapours for the purpose of area classification.

2.1.4 Flammable liquids

This is something of a misnomer as liquid does not burn. Flammable liquid indicates a liquid which, at normal ambient temperature and pressure or the temperature and pressure at which it is handled or stored, has a vapour pressure (partial pressure) sufficient to liberate enough vapour to form an explosive atmosphere.

2.1.5 Combustible dusts

A combustible dust is a dust which will burn when mixed with air or which, in layer form, will burn if ignited. It should not be confused with an explosive. These need to be treated in a different way to gases, vapours and mists in that, while a release is normally in cloud form, once released the dust will not disperse as will the gas/vapour or mist but will initially form a cloud and then settle as a dust layer. Once released only housekeeping can affect the persistence of clouds by disturbed layers.

The important parameters for dust are different from those used for gases and vapours and are as follows:

Cloud ignition energy, the minimum energy which is required in the form of an arc or spark to ignite a gas cloud;

Cloud ignition temperature, the minimum temperature at which an ideal mixture of the dust in suspension with air will ignite. This can depend on particle size;

Layer ignition temperature, the minimum temperature at which a layer of the dust of specific thickness will ignite and burn;

Particle size, the size of particle from which a dust is formed and which have an effect on its ignition capability.

2.2 Basis of area classification

Area classification is based upon those situations which can occur in practical plant and factory operation which produce an explosive atmosphere with a degree of regularity and which requires consideration of the introduction of equipment that may become an ignition source. It does not seek to address the possibility of explosions which occur in catastrophic failure conditions which, by and large, are not easily predictable. It must be remembered, however, that a procedure to deal with catastrophe is necessary even though that procedure does not form part of the area classification process and the requirements which that process engenders.

There are basically three situations which can predictably occur in any operation of in which flammable materials are involved. First, a situation in which an explosive atmosphere is present for long periods or always as a result of operational necessity. Typical of such situations are the interiors of process vessels or equipment processing gases, vapours mists or dusts where air is also present, the interiors of stock tanks where liquids, gases or vapours are present with air, silos and mills where dust and air are both present, etc.

Second, a situation in which explosive atmospheres occur regularly in normal operation of the plant or process. Typical of such situations are those surrounding rotating seals on machines which are the subject of wear, manual loading points on such things as vessels where gases, vapours, mists and dusts are loaded, powder bag loading points, paint spraying facilities, etc.

Third, a situation in which explosive atmospheres occur rarely and normally result from failure of equipment or procedures. Typical of such situations are the failure of a gasketted joint in a process pipe releasing a gas, vapour, mist or liquid, the overflowing of a vessel due to failure of process control functions releasing a liquid, powder handling rooms where dust deposits can form and then be agitated into clouds, etc.

2.3 General approach to area classification

Modern area classification is based, unlike its more historical predecessor described in BS/CP 1003[1], upon identification of individual sources of hazard and their result. BS/CP 1003 was based upon a general appraisal of the areas at risk and identification of the hazard from this general appraisal. This led to variation in application by different organizations which is some cases led to over classification where entire plants were classified as having high level of risk and, more worryingly, underclassification where inadequately protected electrical equipment was installed. Older, already classified, plants need therefore to be reasessed in accordance with modern thinking if they were originally classified in this generalized way.

Identification of sources of hazard is formalized in respect of gases, vapours and mists in BS 5345, Part 2[2] and although no such formal identification exists for dusts in BS 6467 Part 2[3] the document likely to succeed it (EC 1241-3[4]) contains a similar form of identification. Therefore sources of release can be categorized, be they gas, vapour, mist or dust.

BS EN 60079-10

2.4 Classification of sources of release

Sources of release are now classified using the following basis:

Continuous grade of release

This a point or location from which a flammable gas, flammable vapour, flammable mist or combustible dust may be released continuously or for long periods into the atmosphere, so that an explosive atmosphere could be formed during the period of release;

Primary grade of release

This is a point or location from which a flammable gas, flammable vapour, flammable mist or combustible dust may be released periodically or occasionally in normal operation into the atmosphere, so that an explosive atmosphere could be formed during the period of release;

Secondary grade of release

This is a point or location from which a flammable gas, flammable vapour, flammable mist or combustible dust is not expected to be released in normal operation, but at which release may be expected infrequently and for short periods or where dust layers form to an extent such that if disturbed an explosive atmosphere would be formed.

The three release levels listed above are the basic elements contributing to the identification of the grade of any particular source of release. One company code[5] did introduce numerical guidance in 1973. This guidance never achieved sufficient support to be included in any national or international Standards or Codes. It has nonetheless been widely used since its inception and, given its intent to identify a division between types of release to assist in their identification rather than be a strict numerical division, has become generally accepted if used with care.

What is identified is the following:

Continuous grade release is a release which is present for more than 1000 hours per year (more than 10 per cent of the year approx);

Primary grade release is a release which is present for between 10 and 1000 hours per year (between 0.1 per cent and 10 per cent of the year approx);

Secondary grade release is a release which is present for less than 10 hours per year (less than 0.1 per cent of the year).

The reason why these figures need to be treated with care is that they are very general. In a given circumstance, for example, a rotating seal may only leak once in, say, 3 years according to records in a particular plant and there would be a desire to identify it as a secondary grade source of release from that information. The generality is, however, that it may just be accidental in the particular set of circumstances surrounding that case at that particular time and if a different period of 3 years was chosen, releases would be seen to be much more frequent. Therefore, the general case which defines it as a primary grade of release needs to be used in all circumstances, unless a very high level of confidence exists the circumstances of the particular situation are such as to justify a differing approach in that case. Such a situation is expected to be very rare indeed and so the general case, as identified in this book, should be used in all but very few circumstances. Should sufficient confidence exist, however, an alternative approach is clearly acceptable but a full justification must be produced in all such cases.

2.5 Hazardous zonal classification

Having identified the types of release which we expect it is then possible to identify the risk of the presence of an explosive atmosphere in a given area. This is determined by the likelihood of release, the nature of the release and the ventilation in the area of release. Clearly, with the exception of releases inside vessels, the persistence of explosive atmospheres is determined to a significant extent by such things as the level of ventilation at the location of the release and the characteristics of dispersion of the flammable material. It is necessary to define the risk of the presence of an explosive atmosphere in some way which is related to the source of release and these other parameters.

2.5.1 Gases, vapours and mists

The methods of defining a risk of the presence of an explosive atmosphere for gases, vapours and mists are highly developed and such areas are divided into three levels.

Zone 0

Zone 0 is a zone in which an explosive gas, vapour, mist/air mixture (explosive atmosphere) is continuously present or present for long periods.

Zone 1

Zone 1 is a zone in which an explosive gas, vapour, mist/air mixture (explosive atmosphere) is likely to occur in normal operation.

Zone 2

Zone 2 is a zone in which an explosive gas, vapour, mist/air mixture (explosive atmosphere) is not likely to occur in normal operation and, if it occurs, it will only exist for a short time.

These definitions are given in BS 5345 part 2[2] and similar ones with the same intended meaning, can be found in many documents. The current reference to places where explosive atmosphere can occur specifies them as zones but the term is no different in meaning to more historic references to areas. Many countries have national area classification systems, either historic or current, which are related to the now internationally recognized system described above and as shown in Table 2.1.

Table 2.1 Relationships between national area classification systems

IEC/CENELEC/GB (Note 1)	German (Note 2)	French (Note 3)	USA
Zone 0	Special area in Ex order	Division 1	Division 1
Zone 1	Normal area in Ex order	Division 1	Division 1
Zone 2	Hazardous area not within Ex order	Division 2	Division 2

Notes:
1 Although not specifically naming them it is clear that Germany historically operated the three-level risk system. The IEC/CENELEC/GB system is now used.
2 France historically has merged Zone 0 and 1 to form a single Division 1. It now uses the IEC/CENELEC/GB system.
3 The USA has historically operated in the same way as France but has recently begun to use the IEC/CENELEC/GB three-Zone system.

2.5.2 Dusts

In respect of dusts the situation is more fluid. The degree of formality is less than that for gases and vapours and has only been effectively addressed in the UK and internationally in the last 15–20 years. Within the UK, hazardous areas caused by dusts are currently defined in a different way to those caused by gases, vapours and mists.

Zone Z

Zone Z is a zone in which a combustible dust is, or may be, present as a cloud during normal processing, handling or cleaning operations in sufficient quantity result in an explosible concentration of combustible dust in mixture with air (explosive atmosphere).

Zone Y

Areas not classified as Zone Z in which accumulations or layers of combustible dust may be present under abnormal conditions and give rise to ignitable mixtures of dust and air (explosive atmosphere) are designated as Zone Y.

These definitions, which are similar to those appearing in BS 6467, Part 2[3] and other documents, are on the face of it very different to those for gases, not least because only two Zones exist as a result of the exclusion from the scope of BS 6467, Part 2[3] of the interior of dust handling equipment. Taking this fact into account, however, the differences are not as great as would initially seem the case and, allowing for the differences in performance of released dust from that of released gas, vapour or mist, there appears to be an easily identified relationship between Zone 1 and Zone Z and likewise between Zone 2 and Zone Y.

These definitions in respect of dusts will be replaced in the near future by three new definitions in IEC 1241-3[4] which is an international document and thus will bring the definitions for dust hazardous areas up to the same status as those for gases, vapours and mists.

Zone 20

Zone 20 is a Zone in which combustible dust, as a cloud, is present continuously or frequently, during normal operation, in sufficient quantity to be capable of producing an explosible concentration of combustible dust in mixture with air (explosive atmosphere), and/or where layers of dust of uncontrollable and excessive thickness can be formed. An example of this Zone is the inside of processing equipment.

Zone 21

Zone 21 is a Zone not classified as Zone 20 in which combustible dust, as a cloud, is likely to occur during normal operation in sufficient quantities to be capable of producing an explosible concentration of combustible dust in mixture with air (explosive atmosphere). Examples of these areas are given as those immediately surrounding powder filling or discharging sites.

Zone 22

Zone 22 is a Zone not classified as Zone 21 in which a combustible dust, as a cloud, can occur infrequently, and persist only for a short period, or in which accumulations or layers of combustible dust can give rise to an explosive concentration of combustible dust in mixture with air (explosive atmosphere). Examples of this are given typically as areas of mills where dust released from leaks can settle and give rise to dust layers which can be agitated into a cloud by physical shocks or air turbulence.

These newer definitions show a much clearer relationship to the zonal definitions for gases, vapours and mists while still drawing attention to the differences which exist. Typical of these are the ability of dust to settle and persist even in well-ventilated locations and its ability to burn as a layer in addition to its dangers as a cloud. The general approach has historically been to attempt, in Zones 21 and 22 (Zones Z and Y) to limit dust layers to less than 5 mm thickness and electrical equipment is designed assuming a 5 mm thickness of dust (See BS 6467, Part 2[3] and IEC 1241-3[4]). The latter of these two documents also identifies 1 mm as the thickness of the layer of dust above which an explosive atmosphere is possible. The legal requirements in the UK in regard to housekeeping (see Chapter 1) need to take these two figures into account and ensure that the layers allowed to accumulate do not infringe these limits for a particular classification.

2.5.3 Relationship between sources of release and Zones

In the case of gases, vapours and mists where ventilation is good, for example outdoor situations, there is a clear relationship between the grade of release and the zonal classification which is as follows: continuous grade of release gives rise to a Zone 0; primary grade of release gives rise to a Zone 1; secondary grade of release gives rise to a Zone 2. This relationship, however, ceases to be true as soon as any of the parameters change. A primary grade source of release may, for instance, only give rise to a Zone 2 if special local ventilation is applied to effectively dilute the release to below its explosive concentration at the point of leakage. Likewise, a secondary grade source of release may give rise to a Zone 1 if local ventilation is restricted.

In relation to dusts, the situation is much more tenuous as the formation of layers is not really Zone specific and the classification depends much more upon human intervention as housekeeping is a significant contributor to the situation.

2.6 Collection of information

In order to carry out a formal area classification exercise it is necessary to first collect information on both the flammable material and the methods utilized to contain it and the local ventilation conditions need to be identified.

2.6.1 Information on fuels (gases, vapours and mists)

Taking the situation in respect of gases, vapours and mists, the following information in respect of the flammable materials is necessary as a minimum.

The *flashpoint*; the temperature at which sufficient vapour is released from a liquid to allow the production of an explosive atmosphere above its surface. Below this temperature the gas or vapour and air mixture is not normally ignitable although a mist may still be capable of forming an explosive atmosphere below this temperature.

The *ignition temperature*; the minimum temperature at atmospheric pressure necessary to ignite an ideal mixture of the flammable gas or vapour in air. This determines the limit of maximum temperature of equipment permitted within the hazardous area.

The *flammable range*; the range of percentage mixtures of the flammable gas or vapour with air between which ignition is possible at atmospheric pressure. The lower flammable limit is normally the important one as it determines the extent of the explosive atmosphere. Figure 2.1 shows typical flammable range and sensitivity information.

The *gas/vapour density*; normally quoted as relative to air which is assumed as for the flashpoint. This parameter has an effect upon the dispersion of the flammable gas or vapour insofar as it may be lighter or heavier than air and may also be necessary if calculation is necessary.

The *boiling point*; the temperature at which a flammable liquid will boil at atmospheric pressure. If it is below the actual temperature at the point of release then the released liquid will vaporize quickly.

The *molecular weight*; this information is necessary in case calculation is required.

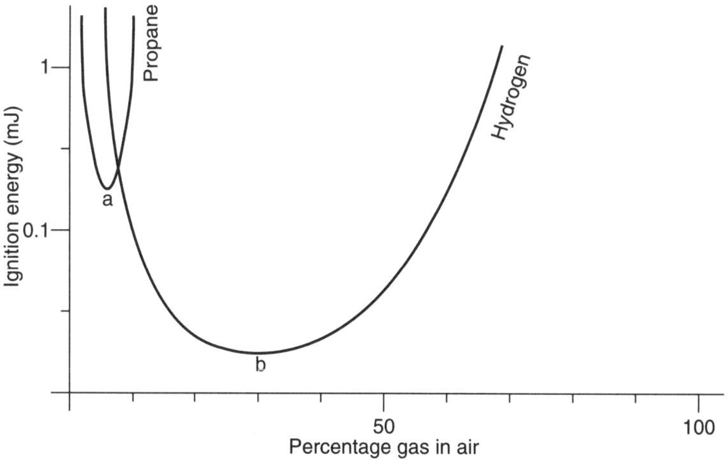

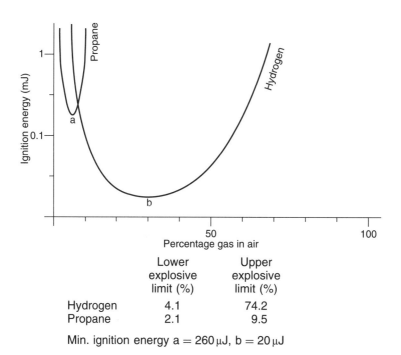

	Lower explosive limit (%)	Upper explosive limit (%)
Hydrogen	4.1	74.2
Propane	2.1	9.5

Min. ignition energy a = 260 μJ, b = 20 μJ

Fig. 2.1 Typical ignition characteristics

The *latent heat of vaporization*; information again necessary in case calculation is required.

The *heat capacity*; information is necessary in case calculation is required.

The *sub-group*; unnecessary for the purposes of area classification but, as explained in later chapters, is important in the selection of electrical equipment for installation. All electrical equipment for surface industry is Group II equipment but some is given a sub-group which relates to its possible use. These sub-groups are described in detail later but are IIA, IIB and IIC. Gases and vapours are associated with these sub-groups to permit selection of appropriate equipment. Dusts are not so specifically related to sub-groups but, as these sub-groups specify the maximum energy which apparatus may release in an arc or spark, they can be used to identify apparatus suitable for specific dust risks. The sub-grouping system is referred to in Chapter 1 and in later chapters.

The *surface temperature class*; a classification system related to the maximum temperature achieved by electrical equipment and gases and vapours are associated with these temperature classes on the basis of their ignition temperatures. The temperature classification system is intended for use with gases and vapours but, although dusts are not so specifically associated with these classes, they specify the maximum temperature which surfaces may reach and, as such, can be used to identify apparatus suitable for particular dust risks. This system is referred to in Chapter 1 and later chapters.

Figure 2.2 is a typical blank form used to collect the necessary information on the above parameters.

2.6.2 Information on fuels (dusts)

For dusts, the requirements are different. It is advisable to exclude dust from equipment which might spark, but both layers of dust which form on apparatus and dust clouds may be ignited by temperature. While it is possible for dusts to be ignited by sparks or arcs this is, because of the dust exclusion from the interior of apparatus, an uncommon problem and, when it occurs, it is dealt with as described in later chapters. The following information is thus important.

The *dust cloud ignition temperature*; the minimum temperature at atmospheric pressure at which an ideal cloud of dust can be ignited.

The *dust layer ignition temperature*; the minimum ignition temperature of a 5 mm layer of dust at atmospheric pressure.

The *temperature class*; again an equipment matter, but dusts are associated with this classification as described earlier to permit selection of appropriate equipment.

The *conductivity of dust*; a dust with a resistivity of less than 10^3 Ωm is considered as a conducting dust, as opposed to other dusts which are considered as non-conducting. This has an influence on the choice of electrical equipment and its installation.

Description of Material	Properties of flammable materials – Gas/Vapour/Liquid									
	Flash point °C	Initial Boiling Point °C	Auto-Ignition Temp °C	Gas/ Vapour Density Air = 1	Gas/ Vapour Density	Flamm Range % Vol	Mol. Wt.	Lt. Ht. of Vap. Kj/Kg	Heat. Cap. Kj/Kg/K	Group/ T Class BS 5345

Fig. 2.2 Form for collection of information on gases, vapours and mists

The *decomposition products of dust*; it is also necessary to know if flammable gases or vapours are produced by the decomposition of dust at temperatures below their ignition temperatures as this can have a significant adverse effect upon the situation.

Figure 2.3 is a typical blank form which may be used to collect this information.

2.6.3 Information on process conditions

Having collected the necessary information on the parameters of the fuel (gas, vapour, mist or dust) itself it is necessary, in order to carry out an area classification exercise, to identify the way in which the fuel (gas, vapour, liquid or dust) is contained and the likelihood of its release, and thus the formation of an explosive atmosphere. Typical examples of such information follow.

The *containment type*; is the way in which the flammable material is contained where possible releases may occur. A typical example may be pipe flanges.

The *location*; the location of the particular containment on the plant or process site is necessary. A typical location may be, for example, in the tank farm above tank 'X'.

The *process material*; material handled within the containment and thus forming the possibly leaking fuel. This gives a direct reference to the previously gathered information on the fuel.

The *process conditions*; conditions, for example, of temperature and pressure at the point of possible release are necessary as these will have an effect upon the quantity released and the possibility of its ignition. Although a material may have a flashpoint which is above ambient temperature it may ignite if released at high temperature.

The *description of containment*; the detail of containment is necessary to determine the leakage possible. If the containment is a pipe flange then the type of gasket becomes important.

From the above information the grade of the possible source of hazard can be established, together with the extent of any hazardous area produced. A typical method for carrying out this exercise is a List of Equipment for Area Classification (LEAC) Table of which an example is given in Fig. 2.4. This also includes the appropriate Group (IIA, IIB or IIC) for any electrical equipment and similarly the temperature class (T1–T6) appropriate and becomes the basic record of the area classification exercise.

2.7 Procedures

Area classification is not simply intended to identify hazardous areas on process plants and in similar areas where design has already been completed using only operational and economic factors as influence, but to

Description of Materials	Properties of flammable materials – Dust						
	Is Dust Cloud Flammable (2)		Dust Cloud Ignition Temp. (°C) (3)	Dust Layer Ignition Temp. (°C) (4)	Are Flammable Vapours Evolved During Decomposition (5)	Is Dust Conducting (6)	Apparatus Temp. Class (T1–T6) (7)
	At Environment Temp. <110°C	At Environment Temp. >110°C					

Fig. 2.3 Form for collection of information on dusts

Equip. No.	Title	Location	Process Materials Handled	Conditions (Temp. & Pressure)	Description of Process Material Containment (Eg. Closed System, Vents, Seals, Drains)	Source of Hazard SH0, SH1, SH2 OR Non-Haz	Horizontal Dist. (m) from source to:-		Apparatus Group/ Temp Class	Remarks
							Zone 1/ Zone 2 Boundary	Zone 2 Non-Haz Boundary		

Fig. 2.4 List of equipment for area classification (LEAC)

be part of the design process and to significantly affect the design process in order to minimize the explosion risks. This means that hazardous areas should be eliminated as far as is possible, leaving only those which are absolutely necessary and introduce only an acceptable level of risk. To this end, area classification should begin on a process plant, for example as soon as process-line diagrams are available and should be constantly refined throughout the design process, influencing all stages of process design. The following is typical of the type of argument which is addressed in the progress to a final area classification.

Is the quantity of flammable material small? In some places, such as laboratories, only small amounts of flammable material are normally present and the operation of these areas is such that security against explosion can be produced by other methods (e.g., utilization of the continuous presence of trained staff together with special operating procedures). In such circumstances area classification may not be appropriate. These cases will, however, be few and the objective is to achieve the required level of security by other means. It is necessary to act with extreme caution when selecting such areas. Where an alternative to area classification cannot be justified and significant amounts of flammable material can be identified as present, a further question must be asked.

Can the flammable material be released? If the flammable material cannot be released in such a way that it can mix with air (either inside a process vessel or externally) then an explosive atmosphere cannot be formed and a hazardous area cannot exist. This is, however, very unlikely and it is usual that where such materials exist some form of release will usually be present (an exception to this rule is where, for example, an all-welded pipeline passes through an area in which case a release within the scope of area classification will not be considered).

How does the release occur? If release is possible within the range of releases associated with area classification it then becomes necessary to determine the nature of release. (Is it, for example, from the free surface of a liquid in contact with air, due to a pipe joint failure or due to a moving seal all of which are examples of releases within the scope of area classification.) The identification of the type of release will allow it to be graded as described earlier in this chapter.

Having identified the release as to its grade (continuous, primary or secondary) it is then necessary to determine if the Grade can be reduced (e.g., primary to secondary, etc.). The objective should be to produce the smallest number of releases of the lowest aggregate grade possible taking account of practical operational considerations. There is a balance here in that the product has to remain saleable in general or its manufacture becomes pointless. Such an argument does give a little flexibility but cannot be used to allow a coach and horses to be driven through the general approach given in this guide as there comes a point where, on safety grounds, the manufacturing or other activity becomes unacceptable. Large unconfined Zones 0 and Zones 1 are not, for example, generally acceptable whatever the operational justification. It should also be remembered that those who carry out the area classification procedures carry a personal responsibility in addition to the corporate responsibility carried by their organization. Decisions which introduce hazards which are considered to be unacceptable, either because of a later incident or identification as such during third-party inspections will be placed at the door of those who make them in addition to their organizations.

Typical examples of methods of reducing or removing sources of hazard are: blanketing a vessel vapour space with inert gas which reduces the source of hazard produced by the liquid surface to secondary grade from continuous grade as, provided the blanketing has sufficient integrity, its failure is abnormal. (This does not affect the grade of release constituted by any atmospheric vent.); the use of all-welded pipe instead of gaskets or screwed connections which removes the possibility of leakage; and dilution with copious quantities of air at the point of release so that the mixture of released flammable material and air is below the lower explosive limit at the point of release. (It is recognized that there must, in these circumstances, be a very small area of explosive atmosphere at the actual point of release but its volume will be negligible.)

What is the rate of release? Having optimized the types of release in order to minimize both their number and severity it is then necessary to quantify the amount of explosive atmosphere which will be formed by each release. To do this it is necessary to quantify the amount of flammable material which can be released and this is normally done by identifying the rate of release from each source. For outdoor circumstances an equilibrium will be reached in its mixing with air and an extent of explosive atmosphere resulting can be identified. This is not the primary objective, however, which is to minimize the release by improvements to design of containment and therefore to minimize the extent of any hazardous area and risk. Typical of such improvements are: the use of spirally supported gaskets instead of Standard CAF* gaskets or similar gaskets. The former will not break in a transverse direction and the results of a piece of gasket being blown out of the joint is removed. Retained '(o)' rings have a similar effect although in this case transverse cracking not likely with spirally supported gaskets must be considered; and throttle bushes on rotating seals which serve to limit the amount of flammable material released on abnormal failure of the seal, although not in the case of a failure which is considered as normal operation and, therefore, a primary grade source of release. The application of the above will result in a sensible area classification which is not unduly onerous but, at the same time, is fully objective.

The activity of area classification involves the classic sources of release which are, in general, fixed such as pipes, pumps and vessels but is not limited to these. In many operations it is necessary to transport flammable materials around process areas and working sites and the exercise must also take account of such activities, particularly with respect to the transport

*Term normally used to describe an unsupported gasket historically made from compressed Asbestos Fibre.

containment and the methods of its loading and discharging. In addition, the physical structures involved must be considered. While, for example, a solid wall may be an effective barrier to the transmission of an explosive atmosphere, any door which it contains will have to be considered as a source of hazard as it communicates with the area on the other side of such a wall. This is particularly important when considering boundary walls as it is not generally acceptable to communicate an explosive atmosphere on to neighbouring sites and any accident which relates to such an activity is likely to be seen as the responsibility of the creator of the explosive atmosphere. Figures 2.5 and 2.6 show the area classification procedure described here in tabular form.

2.8 Personnel involved

The area classification procedure can have a significant effect on the design of a particular process, notwithstanding the effect which its results have on the acceptability of the process. Its importance cannot be overrated and it must form one of the prime parts of the design process. This is not only true from a safety point of view but corrections to a process after design and construction are complete can be very expensive and can even challenge the viability of a particular activity resulting in waste of investment. For this reason, it is necessary that area classification be seen by those involved as fundamental to the design process and the seniority of those involved should reflect this. To this end, the area classification procedure should start as soon as possible after the inception of the design process and be carried out by a group formally constituted as follows.

The *Project manager/works manager*; the presence of whom on the area classification team gives the necessary seniority to ensure the credibility of the exercise. The project engineer or works manager should chair the group and, while it is recognized that these senior people may delegate the duty of area classification, it is stressed that the seniority of the person to whom the duty is delegated must be sufficient to ensure the credibility of the exercise and he or she must be seen as the representative of the project engineer or works manager.

The *Process engineer*; usually a chemical engineer, is an important part of the group as he or she will be expert on the performance of the process materials and their chemical properties. It may be that their involvement is primarily in the early part of the exercise but he or she should be available throughout.

The *Mechanical/machines engineer*; is necessary to discussions on the mechanical properties of the containment and the practicability of any necessary or advisable modifications. He or she will, or via associates, also have access to the detail of any special process machinery intended to be used in the process. The importance of the mechanical aspects of containment cannot be overstressed.

The *Safety Officer*; to advise on the wider aspects of safety so that, for example, a release acceptable for area classification purposes but not on

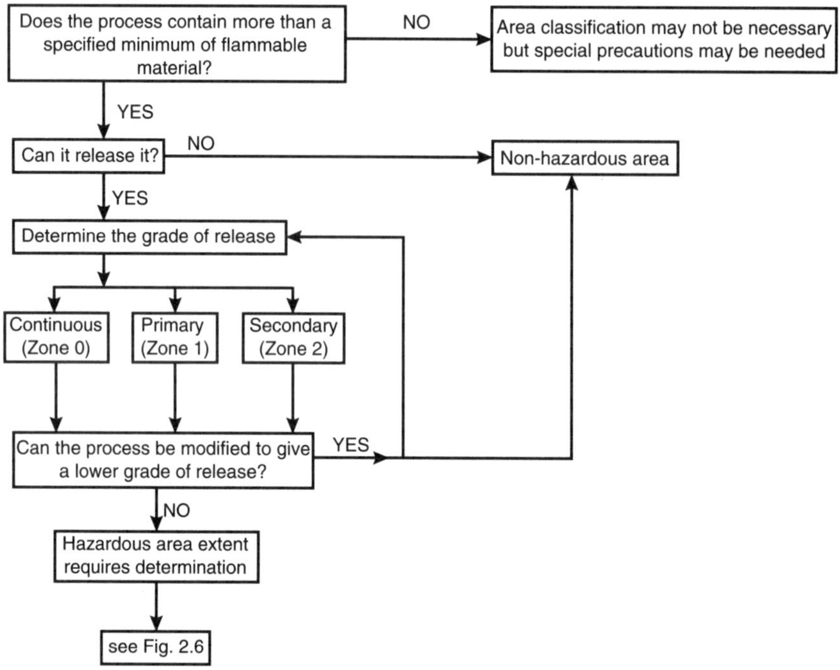

Fig. 2.5 Area classification procedure for explosive atmospheres

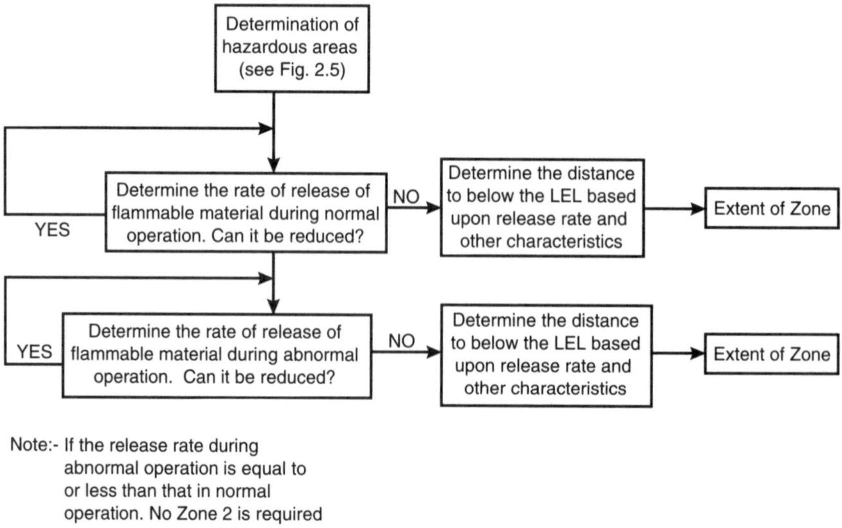

Fig. 2.6 Extent of hazardous areas

grounds of toxicity is not countenanced. The safety officer will also have the overall responsibility for safety on the site where the process is eventually located and it is therefore essential that he or she finds the results of the area classification acceptable.

Electrical/instrument engineer; although in the future area classification will form the basis for the selection of all equipment, both mechanical and electrical, it has only been the latter which has historically been formally associated with the technique. Therefore, the role of the electrical/instrument engineer has been, and will continue to be, to advise on the limitations of electrical installation in classified areas and the reliability of electrical installations, as these can have an effect upon the possibility of release of flammable material and its severity. As almost all process activities are effected by electrical drives, illuminated by electric light and monitored by electrical instrumentation, the area classification, in defining what electrical installations are possible, has a fundamental effect on the process and its design.

Site representative; any process or activity has to be carried out on a particular site. It is necessary, therefore, to have a representative of site management on the group to identify particular facets on the chosen site during the design process so that final construction and use will be trouble free. This is no less true of the area classification exercise.

2.9 Results of area classification and frequency of repeats

The area classification exercise carried out by the above group should, as already identified be commenced as soon as possible during the design process and continually refined until construction is complete. Its results should be recorded on LEAC sheets and form a dossier, together with all necessary supporting information which should be accessible to or given into the custody of those who have to manage the operation of the process. As soon as possible after commencement of operation, and certainly within one year, the area classification should be reviewed in relation to practical operating experience and after that regular reviews should be undertaken. The frequency of such reviews should be determined on the basis of experience but in no case should the period between reviews be more than two years. The period to be used will depend upon operating experience and, if it is found that each review results in significant area classification changes then the review period should be shortened. Likewise, if no changes are found the period can be elongated up to the two-year limit. Any change in process or equipment on the site should result in an immediate area classification review.

References

1 BS/CP 1003 Electrical Apparatus and Associated Equipment for use in Explosive Atmospheres other than Mining Applications: Part 1 (1964). Choice Installation and Maintenance of

Flameproof and Intrinsically Safe Equipment; Part 2 (1966). Methods of Meeting the Explosion Hazard other than by Use of Flameproof and Intrinsically Safe Equipment; Part 3 (1967). Division 2 Areas.

2 BS 5345 Selection, Installation and Maintenance of Electrical Apparatus for use in Potentially Explosive Atmospheres (other than mining operations or explosives processing and manufacture). Part 2 (1983). Classification of hazardous areas.

3 IEC 1241-3 Electrical apparatus with protection by enclosure for use in the presence of combustible dusts Part 2 (1988). Guide to Selection, Installation and Maintenance.

4 BSI 94/213454 Draft IEC Publication IEC 1241–3. Electrical Apparatus for use in the presence of Combustible Dust. Part 3. Classification of areas where combustible dusts are or may be present

5 RoSPA/ICI Engineering Codes and Regulations, Electrical Installation in Flammable Atmosphere (1973). Group C (Electrical), Volume 1.5.

6 CAF Term normally used to describe an unsupported gasket, historically made from compressed asbestos fibre.

— 3 —

Area classification practice for gases, vapours and mists in freely ventilated situations

Introduction

In Chapter 2 the mechanizms associated with area classification, together with the constitution of teams to carry it out, and the detail of information necessary to produce an area classification were examined. This chapter will now look at the actual production of an area classification for a particular works or plant. This will be based upon the information produced as a result of the execution of the exercises envisaged in Chapter 2 and available knowledge of the performance of flammable gases, vapours and mists when released into an atmosphere or other area where sufficient oxygen exists to support combustion.

A tremendous amount of research work has been carried out in a relatively coordinated way on the production of methods of protection of electrical equipment intended for use in explosive atmospheres. The same cannot, unfortunately, be said of work carried out in respect of area classification which has been less intensive and more fragmented. This is recognized in BS 5345, Part 2[1] which attempted to describe the detail of area classification but, while describing excellently all of the facets of area classification and the procedures necessary for its execution, the code[1] was forced to direct its readers to other industrial and similar codes[2,3] for the detail of extents of hazardous areas. This situation was made necessary because of the diversity of view of those involved in area classification which has lead, and continues to lead, to differences in the treatment of hazardous area definition in different industries and sometimes in different companies.

The reassuring thing in all of this is that adoption of almost any published industry code will produce an acceptably secure area classification if its application is by personnel knowledgeable in the business of area classification, operating without undue commercial pressures and with access to full information of the operations carried out at the site being classified and the flammable materials involved. It must be remembered, however, that each industry or company code is based upon a particular approach to area classification and these approaches may vary between codes. Extreme care is therefore necessary if a particular plant is classified using information from more than one code. For this reason, the objective of this chapter is to examine the background philosophy of area classification and provide examples of extents of hazardous areas based upon that philosophy, and its execution and additional information given in this chapter. Account is also taken of the possibility of using the mathematical formulae given in Chapter 4 and these formulae are used in producing many of the examples given in this chapter.

3.1 Containment of flammable materials

Flammable materials may be contained in a variety of ways in a process plant; the most obvious way being as a gas or vapour usually at some elevated pressures which are necessary either to transport it or for some other process reason. Such circumstances are the most easily dealt with as the construction of an explosive atmosphere is by mixing of the gas or vapour with air and the definition of explosive limits is by volume mixture. Therefore, it is merely a question of determination of the release rate and the mechanism by which the gas or vapour is mixed with air which, in freely ventilated areas, is usually by virtue of its own motion or by wind effects. There are several other ways in which a flammable material may exist and this makes the area classification exercise much more complicated.

3.1.1 Effects of storage conditions

The flammable material, may for instance, be contained at high pressure and, therefore what at normal ambient pressure would be a vapour is actually stored as a liquid. When such a liquid is released, the pressure falls and vaporization takes place. This of course is typically the way in which a refrigerator works and a study of this identifies the necessity of heat input to effect vaporization (latent heat of vaporization). As the liquid vaporizes there will be a loss of temperature until the temperature of the liquid falls to its boiling point. At this point, vaporization will cease until external heat is added. In such circumstances there will be an immediate evaporation of a percentage of the liquid followed by further, slower evaporation when the residual liquid reaches a heat source. This percentage needs to be defined; a possible calculative method is given in Chapter 4.

The flammable material may be contained at a pressure below its boiling point and this may be thought to indicate that it will not produce much vapour on initial release. This is not wholly true as the release orifice may be such as to support the formation of mists which are finely divided liquid particles and perform in a similar manner to vapours as far as formation of explosive atmospheres are concerned. With small orifices it can be shown that significant mist formation is possible at gauge pressures as low as $2 \times 10^5\ \mathrm{N/m^2}$ while with larger orifices this is less likely although even in these latter circumstances some part of the liquid release may be released as a mist. In addition, the liquid may even be below its flashpoint at the point of release and the mist may still be capable of being ignited if appropriately mixed with air. Another typical method by which a mist may be produced is where a flammable vapour is contained as a liquid at pressure. The turbulence created by pressure reduction coupled with vaporization, which has already been described, will cause the production of some mist in addition to the vapour at the point of release. This must also be taken into account.

There is also the containment of a flammable liquid above its flashpoint but below its boiling point. There is little flammable vapour produced on liquid release and therefore, jet formation is possible. Such jets, unless contained, can travel significant distances before striking the ground or an obstruction and where they cease to travel a pool will be formed. This pool will be controlled in size either by ground contours or by the evaporation rate of the material and significant hazardous areas can be produced some distance from the source of leakage, in addition to which there is the risk that the liquid jet may come into contact with a hot surface which will exacerbate the situation. All of these matters must be considered.

3.1.2 Effect of sunlight on storage vessels

A further problem exists where flammable liquids are contained for significant periods and the containment is in direct sunlight. Typical of such cases is the normal stock tank. There is considerable evidence that in such circumstances significant solar gain can occur and the mixture of vapour and air in the tank above the liquid can adopt a temperature significantly above ambient, encouraging evaporation. This may cause liquids with flashpoints above ambient which would not otherwise be considered to be flammable materials to become so and may cause some flammable materials to reach their boiling points. These matters also require to be taken into account.

3.1.3 Oxygen enrichment

Finally, it must be remembered that area classification is based upon the mixture of a flammable gas, vapour or mist with air at atmospheric pressure. In addition, the technology is based upon mixtures of flammable materials with air. Conditions necessary for ignition vary, particularly with increased levels of oxygen such as which occur in oxidation processes and equipment which is considered suitable for use in explosive atmospheres, assuming as it does atmospheric pressure and air, may not be suitable for use in such circumstances. Where such situations arise the area classification evaluation must take account of them, and they must be identified as special to ensure that those involved in the selection of equipment for such areas are aware of the possibility that normally protected equipment may not be suitable and the resultant necessity to exclude it and select only equipment which has been shown to be suitable for the specific environment.

3.1.4 General consideration of release

Taking account of the above it is necessary to consider all points from which flammable material may be released and to identify areas contaminated by those releases appropriately. Historically this has been done by a generalized method of area classification but since 1970 the more exact source of hazard method of area classification which is considerably more objective has come to the fore and the examples given in this chapter are based on this latter method.

3.2 Generalized method of area classification

The generalized method of area classification is the method which has been historically used. The knowledge of the performance of plant gained over many years has now, however permitted a more precise method, known as the source of hazard method. That does not mean that the generalized method may not be used but it has become less popular as its correct application often gives more extensive hazardous areas than those which actually exist. This increases the costs of operation of a given plant and sometimes leads to conflict due to the perceived extent of areas of high hazard (Zones 0 and 1) by regulatory bodies and others as being excessively large which, as one of the principal objectives of area classification is to influence plant design, leads to excessive expenditure. Occasionally if not carefully executed it can also lead to certain hazardous areas not being adequately identified which leads to unnecessary danger.

The generalized method of area classification does not require each source of hazard to be uniquely identified but that a judgment be made on the basis of the presence of flammable materials in a particular area, together with a general identification of types of process equipment which are known to leak. This requires a set of basic yardsticks against which such judgments may be made.

3.2.1 Generalized zonal classification specification

Zone 0

Zone 0 is an area (Zone) which includes the interiors of closed or ventilated vessels containing flammable liquids or vapours and air. Clearly this only applies to the vapour spaces of closed or ventilated tanks containing flammable liquids but as these tanks usually have a varying quantity of liquid within them, the Zone 0 extends to the lowest liquid level possible.

A Zone 0 will also occur in the vapour space of an open-topped tank containing a flammable liquid. All other places where flammable gas or vapours normally released will also be Zone 0.

Zone 1

Zone 1 is any area containing vessels, pumps, compressors, pipes fittings and similar items of equipment which may be considered to leak in normal operation (e.g., with some degree of regularity) and any area containing such things as relief valves, vents and similar devices which are designed to release flammable gases, vapours and liquids in normal operation will be classified as Zone 1.

Areas containing sample points which are not specially designed to prevent release in normal operation are in Zone 1. In the case of sample points the Zone 1 can, however, be limited to the immediate location of the sample point particularly if sampling is manual.

Finally, areas where releases are so rare as not to be assumed to occur in normal operation will also be identified as Zone 1 if ventilation is restricted. Such areas include both indoor areas and other areas where, as a result of any form of containment or airflow restriction, ventilation is considered to be restricted.

Zone 2

An area containing vessels, pumps, compressors and similar equipment which are so well maintained that leaks can be assumed only to occur very rarely (in abnormal operation) and relief valves which only operate very rarely (abnormally) will be classified as Zone 2. The vents associated with such things as bursting discs will also normally give rise to Zone 2 in areas in which they occur. In all these cases the Zone 2 classification is only acceptable provided that the areas in question are freely ventilated, that is, the equivalent of a normal outdoor situation, so that the released vapour is rapidly dispersed. Less well-ventilated zones in these Zones 2, such as pits and trenches, will be defined as Zone 1.

As a result of the danger to personnel carrying out sampling, sampling points are normally designed to ensure that any area into which personnel access for sampling purposes are Zone 2.

3.2.2 Generalized extents of zones

The extents of the zones produced by this approach tend to be arbitrary and large. The interiors of vessels are well defined but when the less hazardous areas – such as Zone 1 and particularly Zone 2 – are considered, entire locations have to be classified, particularly in the case of Zone 2 where it is not unknown for an entire plant to be classified.

The Generalized method if properly used must, however, be accepted as valid as it over, rather than under, classifies. Regrettably, there is ample scope for incorrect use and, in addition, the areas designated as Zone 1 and Zone 2 often become larger than would be acceptable if the source of hazard method were used. This can cause considerable loss of credibility when identified by third parties and the generalized method is now seldom used except for very congested parts of plant and, even here, it is only used as an adjunct to the source of hazard method.

3.3 The source of hazard method of area classification

The source of hazard method of area classification was introduced progressively from around 1970 onwards. The generalized method described in Section 3.2 had been used extensively before that time and there was growing concern in industry that the hazardous areas being described by that method were too large to represent the true picture. This was particularly true in the case of Zone 1 which covered significant areas and in doing so led to questions being asked in respect of free access of plant personnel to this zone (the frequency of release of flammables in Zone 1 is significant and as a significant number of flammables can be toxic or asphyxiant, exposure of personnel may not be considered acceptable). This and the cost implication led to many pressures being applied to restrict the size of these hazardous areas. The use of the generalized method was found not to lend itself to doing this without introducing significant risk and attempts to achieve the required reduction led to a bewildering variation of conclusions which threatened the confidence which was placed in area classification.

These problems led to a much closer examination of the technology of area classification which, in turn, led to the development of the source of hazard method. This method is very different to the generalized method in that each source of release and the mode of release at that point, have to be identified. Release quantities and dispersal criteria have to be identified and from this information the extent of a hazardous area emanating from a particular release determined. The method of determination of this extent is partly by the use of mathematical approaches similar to those explained in Chapter 4, although these are to a degree inexact, as witnessed by the failure of those involved to agree a single mathematical approach, and partly by experimental evidence and observation. Although there is still some controversy regarding these it is noticeable that most of the approaches published give relatively similar results and smaller hazardous areas than was the case with the generalized method. In addition, there is no evidence in over 25 years of use of the source of hazard method that the results achieved have increased the risk of explosion where the technique has been properly applied.

While the source of hazard method identifies each source of release and the hazardous area created by it, there is still the problem of multiple sources in the same or close locations. It is clearly not likely that all of the sources of release will release at the same time but in multiple cases some may, and the extent of any hazardous area so produced requires to be identified. In the case of secondary grade sources of release the release is so infrequent that it is unlikely that such sources need to be in any way added, but the same cannot be true of primary grade sources of release which release much more frequently. In such cases it is necessary to take account of simultaneous release. Clearly in the case of many such sources of hazard it would be unreasonable to assume that all released simultaneously and therefore some sort of guide is necessary. Table 3.1 gives a method of calculating total release from multiple sources of release when deciding upon ventilation requirements for indoor areas, but clearly it can also be applied with some confidence to multiple sources of release in any situation. It was first published in 1973 in the RoSPA/ICI Code[2].

Table 3.1 Simultaneous release from sources of hazard

Number of sources of hazard 1	Number releasing simultaneously
1	1
2	2
3–5	3
6–9	4
10–13	5
14–18	6
19–23	7
24–28	8
29–33	9
34–39	10
40–45	11
46–51	12

Another difference brought about by the source of hazard approach is the clear identification for the first time that Zone 1 as not automatically surrounded by Zone 2. While this was also true in the generalized method this fact tended to be obscured by the generality and it became common belief that Zone 1 was always surrounded by Zone 2. The source of hazard method automatically dispersed that misunderstanding as to have a hazardous area it is first necessary to identify a source of release which creates it. Therefore, a leak would have to be identified as possibly behaving in two distinctly different ways to produce both a Zone 1 and a Zone 2. This of course leads to another fact that was not before clearly identified and that fact is that a single source of leakage can behave in different ways in different circumstances. When a source of hazard is identified under the source of hazard method it is necessary to identify if that source can behave in more than one way and then to identify the hazardous area created by each of the possible methods of operation.

3.3.1 Types of release

In any process there are typical releases which fall into categories and to which most normally encountered releases will fall. The following are typical of these.

Release of gas or vapour under pressure

Most processes put gases and vapours under pressure to transport them from place to place, to maintain them in a stable state or for such reasons as injection into process vessels or similar functions. The release velocity of any gas or vapour under pressure can be shown to be high and normally at the speed of sound in the gas or vapour in question. This velocity is so high that the gas or vapour will mix with air due to its own turbulence and prevailing wind conditions will have little or no effect in outdoor situations. This will remain true unless the jet of gas or vapour meets an obstruction in which case velocity is likely to dramatically reduce and the wind become the prime dispersant. Indoors or in less well-ventilated situations, unless special precautions are taken, dispersion is into a limited amount of air and there is a cumulative effect which can contaminate the whole indoor or shielded area and so special precautions are often necessary. These can include the extensive use of local extract ventilation and it is often advantageous to ensure that gases and vapours under pressure are excluded as far as possible from areas where ventilation is restricted.

Release of liquids under pressure

Liquids contained under pressure will often release as a jet and hazardous areas may be defined in part by the distance travelled by such jets. Vaporization at the point of release will be minimal provided the liquid is below its boiling point at atmospheric pressure. Therefore, the principal source of vapour is evaporation from the surface of the pool which is created by the jet of liquid. Due to the distances travelled it is often wise to fit any possible leak source with a baffle to prevent the jet from forming which limits the location of the pool. The size of the pool can also be limited by design of its location which leads to bunding. At any significant pressure (it is hard to be specific as both leak geometry and pressure play a part) there is also the possibility of the formation of mists which are finely divided liquid particles. These behave like a gas or vapour and, provided the liquid has a flashpoint, ignition of mists of liquids below their flashpoints is possible. Therefore, where mists can occur flashpoint ceases to be a dividing criterion.

Release of liquefied gases and vapours

Where gases and vapours are maintained as liquid by pressure or a combination of pressure and temperature, release will usually result in instant vaporization of some of the release. The remainder remains liquid until it can obtain sufficient heat energy to transform itself in to a gas or vapour. There will be a hazardous area due to the immediately formed gas or vapour and, in addition the liquid pool scenario will hold. In addition, the vaporization will create some mist due to the turbulence created and the resulting situation is very complex indeed.

Unpressurized releases

In many containers, such as stock tanks, road tankers, paint vats, etc. there will be an explosive atmosphere in the vapour space caused by the vapour released by liquids above their flashpoints and below their boiling points. In normal circumstances these vapours will be relatively heavy and will not exit the vapour space of the container in any significant quantity while equilibrium is maintained. Such containments are, however, frequently filled and that operation expels the flammable material into the surrounding area causing a hazardous area.

Communication between physical locations

A hazardous area may often be contained by a wall or similar blocking device which effectively defines a zonal limit. In these circumstances it is necessary to consider any opening in the blocking wall, such as a door or cable trunk, as these can act as conduits to transfer the explosive atmosphere from one area to another. The only effective way to do this is to consider any such opening as a source of hazard in the remote area and act accordingly.

Pressurized gases and reagents

In many cases gases or reagents used above their flashpoints will be present in or taken into particular areas for purposes such as analysis. While having no direct relation to the process, these flammable materials can equally be identified as sources of hazard and must be treated accordingly. The problem here is that if they have not been identified in the construction of the plant, they may be more significantly sensitive than the process materials and the equipment chosen for the plant may not be suitable for them.

While the source of hazard method of area classification requires each source of hazard and its resulting hazardous area to be identified there are some generalizations which may be used to simplify the area classification activity, and although these often give excessive hazardous areas they are

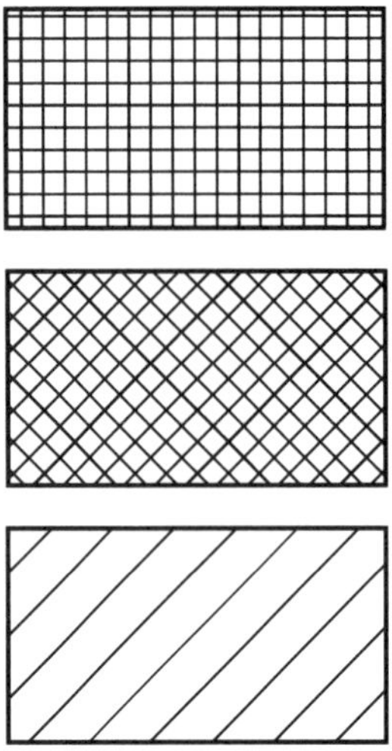

Fig. 3.1 Identification of zones

much more objective than those created by the generalized method and can offer a significant saving in both time and money without endangering security.

The nomenclature used to describe the various grades of hazardous area are shown in Fig. 3.1.

3.3.2 Releases from pipe joints

There are five principal methods of joining two pipes: namely welding; gasketting; use of compression (olive) glands; use of 'o' rings; and screwing. Welded joints effectively make the two sections of pipe one continuous section and if properly carried out and checked, are not considered to constitute a source of release as far as area classification is concerned. This does not mean that welds never rupture but the frequency of such ruptures is so low that it can be neglected as far as area classification is concerned. None of the other types of joint is considered to be sufficiently unreliable to release in normal operation (excepting where human intervention is likely – see special circumstances) if properly chosen and executed and pipe joints in general are not considered as producing any primary grade sources of release and generally constitute Zone 2. They are, however, considered eminently capable of producing secondary grade sources of release and the mechanism for this is different in each case. A screwed joint is likely to produce leakage up its threads and relatively small quantities of released material at relatively low velocities. In this case wind dispersion is the norm. A typical compression joint will produce a small-line release up its olive and, like the screwed joint release, velocities are likely to be relatively low due to the construction of the joint. An 'o' ring seal will only produce leaks if it cracks. As it is located in a recess there is little chance of blowout and the leak geometry will be a crack in the ring. In this case release velocities may be high due to the lack of any modifying elements in the joint. Finally, the gasket is the most usual pipe joint and here there are two possibilities. A normal Compressed Asbestos Fibre (CAF) gasket is retained by pressure alone and at all but very low pressures blowout of part of the gasket must be considered giving rise to a fairly large orifice. The size of the blowout is normally related to the positioning of bolts on the flange and a typical size can be quoted. To prevent such blowouts it is possible to use a spirally supported gasket, which is a gasket fabricated of similar material but with a spiral metal support wound within it. While this effectively prevents blowouts there is still the possibility of leaks between the pipe flanges and the gasket due to joint stress or relaxation. As gaskets are usually used on larger pipes this will be larger than is the case for compression fittings.

The above reflects the situation for pipe joints where routine or regular breakage is not considered a possibility. Where such breakage is likely it is normally because of human intervention due to such activities as the spading-off of pipes for removal of process equipment and similar activities to give sufficient confidence to allow entry of such things as vessels where the possibility of leakage of flammable cannot be countenanced because of other problems such as toxicity. In carrying out the exercise of spading-off, human intervention in the close proximity of the flange is necessary and the possibility of leakage of flammable materials is increased and must be taken into account. Well over 50 per cent of flammable materials are toxic at much lower levels than their lower explosive limit and the creation of a significant explosive atmosphere in an area where personnel are likely to be present at the time of creation is not acceptable. The procedures for breaking pipes in such circumstances must take account of that fact and the removal of flammable materials from the pipe before such activity is necessary. This should dictate the breaking procedure and the procedure adopted before the break activity itself. Such procedures should eliminate the possibility of significant explosive atmospheres occurring at the time of breakage of the joint.

While this is the case for toxic materials it should also dictate the procedure for all joint breakages as it would result in so then no significant explosive atmosphere at the time of joint breakage. It is, however, prudent to acknowledge that such procedures are fallible and to take account of this, a nominal Zone 1 of 1 m radius around the joint should be identified. It is stressed that this will only apply to joint breaking which takes place on a relatively regular basis (e.g., possibly more than once a month on average) as less regular actions will result only in Zone 2 which is taken care of by the random leak scenarios dealt with in this chapter.

Taking the above considerations into account it is possible to define typical leaks which will cover most normal situations and simplify the area classification process. In the following examples and tables the figures used are as follows:

CAF[6] gasket

Release aperture $4 \times 10^{-5}\,m^2$ (25 mm × 1.6 mm)
Release velocity high (unimpeded) or low (impeded)
This aperture is based upon a piece of gasket being ejected from a joint between two fixing bolts. The dimension is chosen to cover all but small bore pipes where it may be pessimistic.

Spirally supported gasket

Release aperture $2.5 \times 10^{-6}\,m^2$ (50 mm × 0.05 mm)
Release velocity high (unimpeded) or low (impeded)
This aperture is based upon relaxation of the joint as parts of the gasket cannot be ejected. Again, it is sized to be valid for all but small bore pipes where it may be restrictive.

'o' Ring

Release aperture $10^{-6}\,m^2$ (1 mm × 1 mm)
Release velocity high (unimpeded) or low (impeded)
Here release aperture is based upon a crack in the 'o' ring.

Compression joint

Release aperture $10^{-6}\,m^2$ (0.1 mm × 10 mm)
Release velocity low (impeded)
This is based on a relaxation in the metal/metal of a compression joint and will be of low velocity as its path is labyrinthine around the olive.

Screwed joint

Release aperture $5 \times 10^{-7}\,m^2$ (small and labyrinthine)
Release velocity low (impeded)
Release is based upon exit via the threads of the joint.

While being, to a degree, arbitrary the above figures are fairly conservative and thus have a low likelihood of being smaller than what actually happens in practice. The hazardous areas produced by their use is likely to be larger in the vast majority of cases to that which actually occurs in practice. It must be stressed that if local knowledge provides more accurate figures for the particular situation then, if larger, these should be used. Likewise, although the release velocities are given as high for gaskets and 'o' rings any obstruction either within the leak orifice after its smallest point or close to it will significantly reduce that velocity and unless such obstructions can confidently be ruled out dispersion by the wind should always be considered.

3.3.3 Typical extents of Zone 2 from pipe joint releases

Gas or vapour release

The hazardous area typically created by a gas or vapour release is given in Fig. 3.2 and values for its extent for both high velocity and low velocity

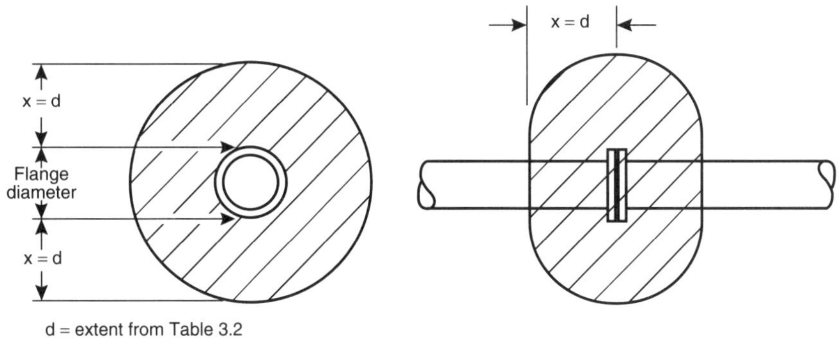

Fig. 3.2 Extent of Zone 2 (relative density 0.7 to 1.3)

Table 3.2 Extent of hazardous area – gas release

Pressure 10^5 N/m^2	Extent of hazardous area in metres			
	1	2	3	4
1.35	3.0	1.0	0.5	0.5
1.7	3.5	1.0	0.5	0.5
2.0	4.5	1.0	1.0	0.5
3.0	5.5	1.5	1.0	1.0
5.0	7.0	2.0	1.0	1.0
10.0	9.5	2.5	1.5	1.0
20.0	13.5	3.5	2.5	1.5
30.0	16.5	4.5	3.0	2.0
50.0	21.5	5.5	3.5	2.5
100.0	31.5	8.5	5.0	3.5

Notes:
1 Release from CAF gasket
2 Release from spirally supported gasket
3 Release from 'o' ring or compression joint with olive.
4 Release from screwed joint

releases are given in Table 3.2. These figures, based on the calculations in Chapter 4 are considered as a worst case scenario and will occasionally be larger than would be expected in practice. They may be reduced when suitable evidence can be produced to justify such a reduction. They are basically radial distances from the outside of the pipe and only apply to gases and vapours of similar density to air (0.7 to 1.3 relative to air). When the relative density of the gas or vapour is outside these limits there is a gravitational effect due to the difference and this will change the geometry of the hazardous area as shown in Fig. 3.3 and 3.4. There is also the effect of proximity to the ground where air movement is less than in elevated

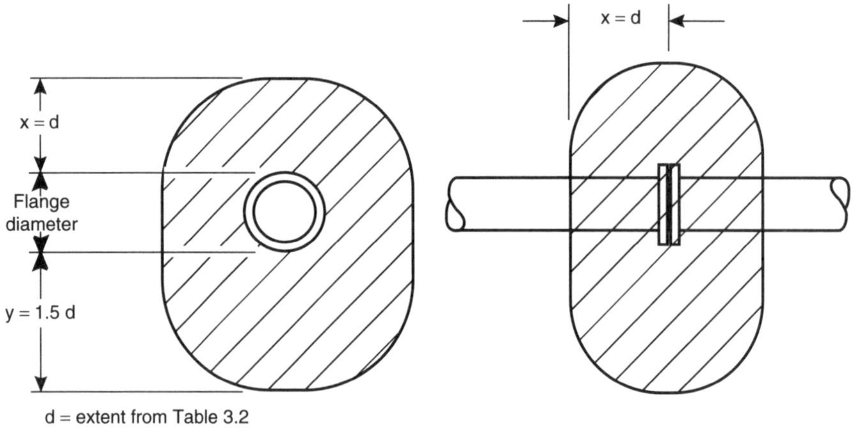

Fig. 3.3 Extent of Zone 2 (relative density >1.3)

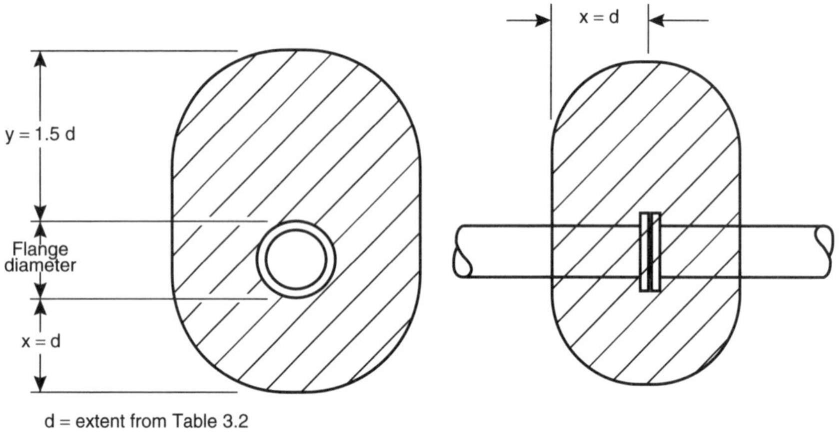

Fig. 3.4 Extent of Zone 2 (relative density <0.7)

circumstances and these effects are shown in Fig. 3.5. When determining the extent of a hazardous area in a particular case all of these effects need to be taken into account.

Liquid releases

When a liquid which is released there is a further problem with the possibility of the formation of liquid jets which can travel significant distances before they strike the ground, and the formation of pools of liquid from which vapour escapes when the liquid strikes the ground. For this reason, it is preferable to place a baffle on the joint to prevent the formation of jets and then to control the formation of any pool to limit the size of any hazardous are a which results. This type of action will typically produce a

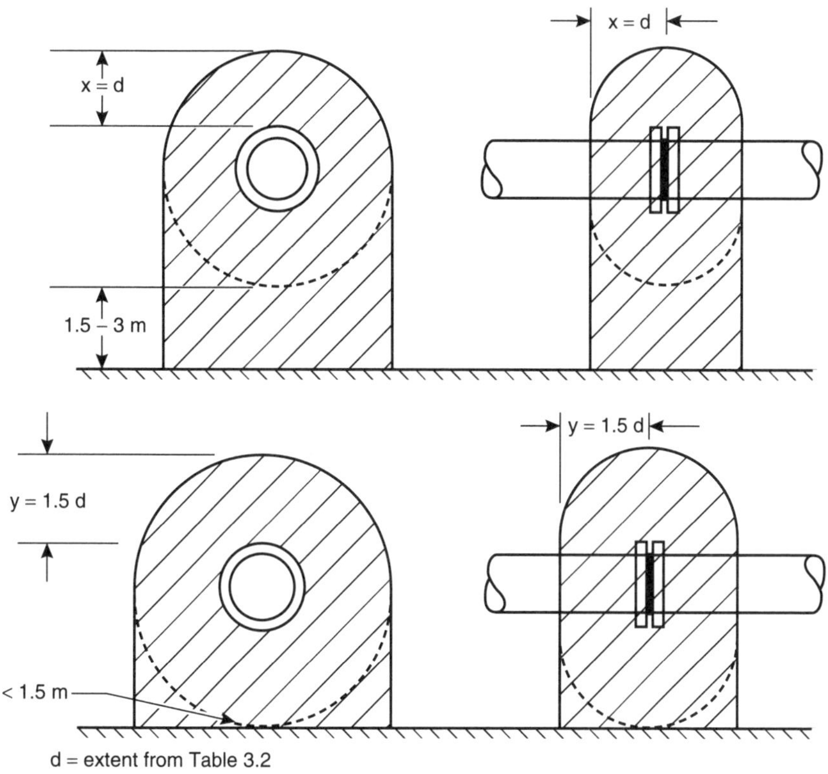

Fig. 3.5 Effect of proximity to ground, walls, etc

pool of known, controlled dimensions under the pipe unless the liquid is collected by containment local to the pipe and transferred to a safe disposal point. If it is not deliberately contained, the pool will grow until the rate of vaporization from its surface is equal to the rate of leakage from the leak. The size of the pool will be determined by the rate of leakage and the temperature of the liquid as the nearer the temperature is to the boiling point the more rapid the vaporization. Therefore, the nearer the temperature approaches the boiling point, the smaller will be the pool. Conversely, the hazardous area around the pool will become larger as the boiling point is approached as the rate of vaporization will increase. Tables 3.3, 3.4, 3.5 and 3.6 describe the pool size created by a leak from one of the types of joint failure described above, at various pressures upstream of the leak. The pool will develop symmetrically on a flat surface but any slope will cause distortion of its shape and thus the dimension of any hazardous area created. In cases where the dimensions of the pool are determined by containment (the preferred method of dealing with pools) the containment must be such that it will contain the maximum volume expected to leak from the pipe in any one incident. Clearly, therefore, the preferred method would be to shroud the joint to prevent the formation of jets and then to collect the

Table 3.3 Areas of pools formed by leaks from CAF gaskets at various pressures

Liquid release pressure	Area of pool when liquid vapour pressure is the following percentage of atmospheric pressure in m^2				
N/m^2	<10%	25%	50%	75%	>90%
1×10^4	207	83	42	28	23
3×10^4	399	160	80	53	44
1×10^5	765	306	173	102	85
3×10^5	1515	606	303	202	168
1×10^6	2767	1107	553	369	307
3×10^6	5192	2077	1040	692	577
1×10^7	9702	3881	1920	1293	1078

Table 3.4 Areas of pools produced by liquid leaks from spirally supported gaskets at various pressures

Liquid release pressure	Area of pool when liquid vapour pressure is the following percentage of atmospheric pressure in m^2				
N/m^2	<10%	25%	50%	75%	>90%
1×10^4	12.0	4.0	2.0	1.5	1.0
3×10^4	21.0	8.0	3.5	2.5	2.0
1×10^5	41.0	16.5	7.5	5.0	3.5
3×10^5	70.0	28.0	13.0	9.0	6.5
1×10^6	144.0	62.0	29.0	19.0	15.0
3×10^6	249.0	113.0	53.0	33.0	28.0
1×10^7	506.0	243.0	115.0	72.0	60.0

liquid leaking as near to the pipe as possible from where it can be diverted to a collection and disposal system.

The hazardous area created around a pool depends upon the geometry of the pool and the proximity of the pool temperature to the boiling point of the flammable material. Typical extents of this hazardous area are given in Table 3.7. This table is based upon the partial pressure developed by the flammable material which affects the effective lower explosive limit of the mixture leaving the pool edge after which it is diluted by wind turbulence as a line source. The tables are based upon the fact that the mixture leaving the pool edge carries a saturated level of the flammable material and should be acceptable for all shapes of pool. The wind speed used is 2 m/sec. Speeds

Table 3.5 Areas of pools formed by leaks from joints using 'o' rings or compression joints with olives at various pressures

Liquid release pressure	Area of pool when liquid vapour pressure is the following percentage of atmospheric pressure in m^2				
N/m^2	<10%	25%	50%	75%	>90%
1×10^4	4.5	1.5	0.5	0.5	0.3
3×10^4	16.0	5.5	2.5	1.5	1.5
1×10^5	20.0	7.0	3.5	2.0	2.0
3×10^5	40.0	15.0	7.0	4.5	4.0
1×10^6	74.0	30.0	14.0	9.0	7.0
3×10^6	147.0	63.0	30.0	20.0	16.0
1×10^7	307.0	139.0	65.0	44.0	34.0

Table 3.6 Areas of pools formed by leaks from screwed joints at various pressures

Liquid release pressure	Area of pool when liquid vapour pressure is the following percentage of atmospheric pressure in m^2				
N/m^2	<10%	25%	50%	75%	>90%
1×10^4	2.0	0.6	0.3	0.2	0.2
3×10^4	4.5	1.5	1.0	0.5	0.5
1×10^5	9.0	3.0	1.5	1.0	0.5
3×10^5	19.0	7.0	3.5	2.0	1.0
1×10^6	35.0	14.0	6.0	4.0	3.0
3×10^6	70.0	28.0	13.0	8.0	6.5
1×10^7	137.0	55.0	23.0	15.0	12.0

used in Europe vary between 0. 5 and 2 m/sec. but, as will be seen from the equations in Chapter 4 relating to pools, the difference which changes in wind speed make within this range is not great and airflow remains turbulent.

Releases of liquid as mist

In addition to this there is the possibility of mist formation and unless this can be totally excluded, a conclusion difficult to reach, the only valid assumption is that some or all of the liquid release vaporizes at its boiling

Table 3.7 Extent of hazardous areas above and beyond pool limits

Pool area	Extent of hazardous area above and beyond pools when liquid vapour pressure is the following percentage of atmospheric pressure in m				
m^2	<10%	25%	50%	75%	>90%
0.1	0.04	0.1	0.2	0.3	0.4
0.3	0.07	0.2	0.4	0.5	0.7
1.0	0.1	0.3	0.6	1.0	1.0
3.0	0.2	0.5	1.0	1.5	2.0
10.0	0.4	0.8	2.0	2.5	3.0
30.0	0.6	1.5	3.0	4.5	5.5
100.0	1.0	2.5	5.0	7.5	9.0
300.0	2.0	5.0	10.0	15.0	18.0
1000.0	3.0	7.5	15.0	23.0	27.0
3000.0	4.5	12.0	23.0	34.0	41.0
10 000.0	7.5	19.0	38.0	56.0	68.0

point and determine a hazardous area around the source of release on that basis. In order to do this two factors are very important, the first being the release pressure, and the second being the leak orifice geometry. In the case of small orifices and high pressure, all of the liquid may form the mist and in the case of larger orifices and low pressure, only a small part of the liquid (if any) may be released as a mist. The determination of the hazardous area due to the mist should always assume low release velocity and wind dispersion. As there are so many unknowns in this set of circumstances the low velocity model is the worst case. Table 3.8 lists typical hazardous areas created by mists, taking some account of the above but it must be stated that the account taken is, to a degree, arbitrary as there is little evidence upon which to make an accurate determination. The figures are, however, felt to be on the restrictive side. Again, the figure for wind speed taken is 2 m/sec.

Figures 3.6 and 3.7 give guidance upon which to determine the hazardous area due to a liquid leak using the information in Tables 3.3 to 3.8. The unification of the two separate hazardous areas (i.e., mist and pool related) is to take account of any vaporization from the jet which forms the pool before it reaches the ground. It must be noted that the pool will form with its centre at the point at which the jet reaches the ground in normal circumstances and the horizontal distance travelled by the jet will cause considerable extension of the hazardous area. All of the above represents worst case figures in normal conditions and more detailed knowledge of any particular set of circumstances may allow a reduction of the size of the hazardous area or changes to its geometry.

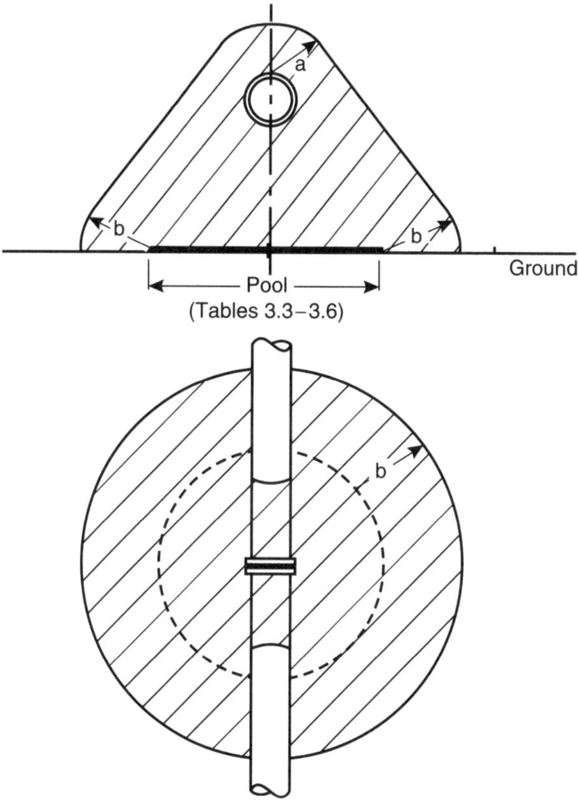

Fig. 3.6 Composite effects of liquid released below its boiling point. a = Table 3.8, b = Table 3.7. *Note*: The area due to mist (Table 3.8) should be adjusted in accordance with Fig. 3.5 where appropriate

Material contained as liquid by pressure and/or temperature

The final situation occurs when the containment of the flammable material contains a material kept liquid by pressure or pressure and temperature. In these circumstances there will be immediate vaporization on release due to the reduction in pressure and this will result in a vapour at the point of release and, because of the turbulence resulting from the vaporization, some mist also. Again, this mist is not definable and the only way to treat the situation is to make an assumption as to the quantity of the flammable material which forms a mist, in addition to that which vaporizes at the point of release. The liquid remaining after vaporization has taken place may be assumed to reach the ground (as this is the worst case scenario) but it will rapidly vaporize and it can be assumed that no pool of any size will form. This assumption can be made because when vaporization at the orifice has taken place, the heat demands of such vaporization have reduced the flammable material to a temperature below its boiling point due to the extraction of heat to support the vaporization activity. At this

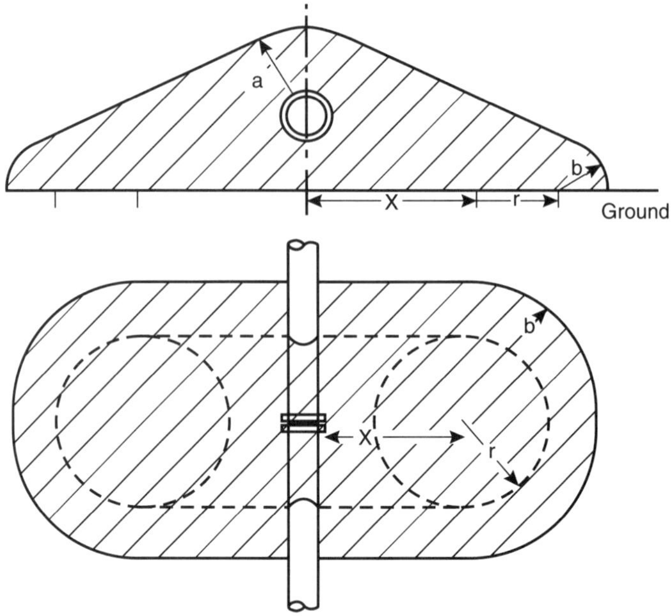

a = Greater of distance created by jet trajectory or Table 3.8 (for jet trajectory see Chapter 4)
b = Extent of hazardous areas beyond pool edge (Table 3.7)
r = Radius or half crosswind distance of pool (from Tables 3.3 to 3.6)
X = Maximum distance travelled by jet before it reaches ground (see Chapter 4)

Fig. 3.7 Effects of liquid jets on hazardous areas

point significant vaporization will cease until another source of heat is available and that source is assumed to be the heat capacity of the ground. It is possible to calculate how much will vaporize and the remainder is the amount which will reach the ground as a liquid. The hazardous area produced by the liquid in transit will be small due to its velocity, but should be treated as it is for liquid release where the liquid is below its boiling point (i.e., by the joining of the hazardous area around the leak with the hazardous area created by vaporization at ground level which can be assumed to be a ground-level point source).

Table 3.9 gives worst case figures for the hazardous area created by the ground-level point source and the hazardous area around the leak will generally be in accordance with Table 3.2, based upon the amount of flammable material which evaporates immediately on release assuming a vapour with a relative density of greater than 1.3. In addition, the extent of any hazardous area around the leak source must be increased by a factor equivalent to that necessary to allow for a doubling of the amount vaporizing at the leak source to accommodate any mist being formed by the effects of possible vaporization in the leak path, unless this can be ruled

Table 3.8 Hazardous areas due to mist formation

Release pressure N/m^2	Extent of hazardous area around leak in m^2			
	CAF gasket	Spirally supported gasket	'o' ring and olive joint	Screwed joint
1×10^4	2.0	1.0	1.0	1.0
3×10^4	2.0	1.5	1.5	1.0
1×10^5	3.0	2.0	2.0	1.0
3×10^5	5.5	3.0	3.0	2.0
1×10^6	8.0	4.5	3.5	2.5
3×10^6	15.5	6.0	5.0	3.5
1×10^7	21.5	8.0	7.0	5.0

Note: The formation of mists was based on the following assumptions for the purposes of this table:

CAF Gaskets:
5% below 10^5 N/m^2
10% between 10^5 N/m^2 and 10^6 N/m^2
20% above 10^6 N/m^2
Spirally supported gaskets
40% up to 10^5 N/m^2
100% above 10^5 N/m^2
'o' Rings, olives and screwed joints:
100% in all cases

Table 3.9 Hazardous areas based upon vaporization of liquid leaking above its boiling point

Release pressure N/m^2	Extent of hazardous area due to vaporization at leaking joints in m^2			
	CAF gasket	Spirally supported gasket	'o' ring and olive joint	Screwed joint
1×10^5	22.0	5.0	4.0	2.0
3×10^5	30.0	6.5	4.0	2.5
1×10^6	41.0	9.0	5.5	2.5
3×10^6	55.0	12.0	7.5	5.0
1×10^7	77.0	17.0	10.0	7.0

Note: These distances are based upon a liquid leak where all of the liquid vaporizes immediately outside the leak path.

out in particular circumstances (e.g., pressures above 10^5N/m^2 coupled with short uncomplicated orifices – a situation difficult to guarantee in general). This corresponds to an increase in the extent of the hazardous area by approximately 1.5. The composite hazardous area produced is shown in Fig. 3.8.

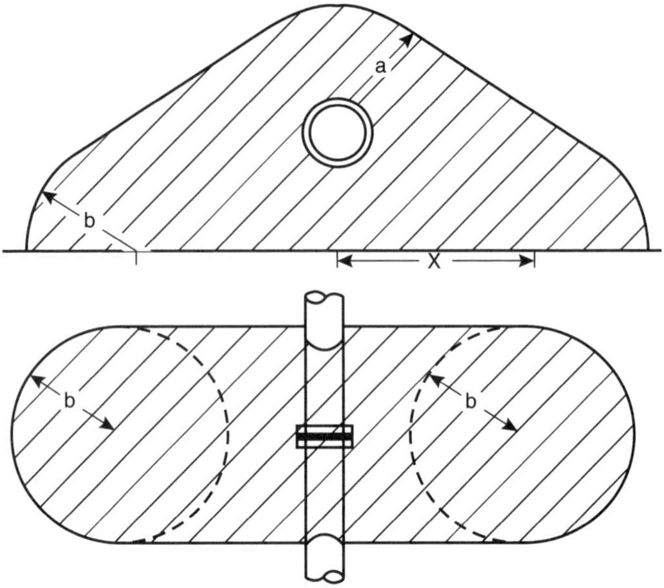

a = Table 3.9 or maximum jet trajectory (Chapter 4)
b = Table 3.10
X = Distance travelled by jet before striking ground (Chapter 4)

Fig. 3.8 Liquid release above boiling point

Table 3.10 Hazardous areas at ground level from liquid leaking above its boiling point and reaching the ground

Release pressure N/m^2	Extent of hazardous area from leaks of liquid above its atmospheric boiling point which vaporizes on contact with the ground m^2			
	CAF gasket	Spirally supported gasket	'o' ring and olive joint	Screwed joint
1×10^5	29.0	6.5	3.0	2.0
3×10^5	40.0	8.5	5.5	3.5
1×10^6	55.0	14.0	7.5	5.0
3×10^6	74.0	18.5	10.0	9.5
1×10^7	104.0	26.0	13.5	9.5

Note: These figures are based upon 90% of the release reaching the ground and 10% being vaporized in transit.

3.3.4 Special pipe joint circumstances

Sections 3.3.1 to 3.3.3 attempt to describe the hazardous areas created by leaks from pipe joints in a variety of circumstances in the normal course of events. There may be specific conditions existing in particular circumstances which may vary these figures in either direction (particular leaks could be smaller or air movement could be restricted by surrounding plant) and at the changeover points for the three scenarios described here the *actual* situation will vary from those described. Any such circumstances should be identified and allowances made for them in the area classification process. Finally, there is the problem of hazardous areas created by human intervention such as spading activities which is dealt with earlier in Section 3.3.1.

3.3.5 Releases from moving seals

Sections 3.3.2 to 3.3.4 dealt with static seals such as those relating to the sealing of pipe joints and similar situations. In addition to these, there are seals which have to cope with maintenance of their sealing characteristics where the parts between which sealing is necessary are moving relative to one another. Typical of these are the seals achieved at the operating shafts of valves, compressors and pumps, and such seals take the form of packed glands which form a friction seal, or other mechanical sealing means which normally rely to a much greater extent upon the sealing surfaces being wetted during operation. The important difference between these types of seal and the static seals used in pipe joints and similar circumstances is that these seals are subjected to wear in operation due to the moving parts with which they are associated and this gives rise to a risk of release in normal operation; a situation not normally present in the previous cases discussed. Because of this, the types of seal are chosen to reflect the function which they perform with extreme care and the following is normally the case.

Valve seals

Valve seals are normally of the packed-gland type in the case of both rotary valves and direct-acting valves where the valve strokes in a linear direction. This means that the valve almost always has some flexible sealing medium (either an 'o' ring or some similar packing material) which is in intimate contact with both the fixed and moving parts of the valve. The rate of wear on this is what determines the surrounding hazardous areas, in that if a single valve is present and this is only operated rarely then the likelihood of leakage in normal operation is so small as to be insignificant. If, however, the valve is operated regularly as part of the process operation then the situation is very different and much more regular leakage of the valve seal must be considered. Likewise, if several valves are located locally to one another the possibility of one of them leaking is similarly greater and, even if they are only operated rarely, it must be assumed that release of flammable material into the location in which they are installed is more regular and occurs in normal operation. For these reasons valve leakages, other than those associated with their piping connections which are dealt with in Sections 3.3.2 to 3.3.4, should be dealt with as follows:

Single rarely operated valve
No Zone 1 is created. Zone 2 is as for a spirally supported gasketted pipe joint as it is unlikely that part of the gasket could be ejected from the gland but wear is expected to be greater than would be the case for an 'o' ring joint due to the movement generated by operation of the valve (see Section 3.3.2).

Multiple Rarely Operated Valves
Zone 1 is sized as for a Zone 2 from the single rarely operated valves on the extremities of the group. The Zone 2 is synonymous with the Zone 1.

Single Regularly Operated Valves
Zone 1 of 1 m around the seal is chosen to take account of progressive wear during operation. Zone 2 is as for a single rarely operated valve.

Multiple Regularly operated valves
Zone 1 is determined on the basis of Table 3.1 or for multiple rarely operated valves, whichever is larger. Zone 2 is synonymous with Zone 1.

Rotating seals

When pumps and rotary compressors are considered it is clear that the facility for seal wear is great and, because the seals are necessarily wetted by the fluid being compressed or pumped, there is some leakage of flammable material in normal operation. For any type of seal used the amount of fluid released in normal operation is such that no realistic Zone 1 will be created by leakage, due to its liquid nature and slow vaporization where it is released as a liquid below its atmospheric boiling point. This is not true, however, where gas is released or liquid is released above its atmospheric boiling point. In such cases, a small hazardous area will be created around the seal and to allow for this a Zone 1 of 1 m radius should be delineated around the seal. The basic criteria for rotating seals is as follows:

Pump with packed gland or mechanical seal where leakage is of liquid below its boiling point
There is no Zone 1. Zone 2 is produced on the basis of a spirally supported gasket from Tables 3.4, 3.7 and 3.8. The ground proximity to the leak should also be taken into account (see Figs. 3.3 and 3.4).

Pump with packed gland or mechanical seal where leakage is of liquid above its atmospheric pressure boiling point
Zone 1 of 1 m radius is present. Zone 2 is produced on the basis of spirally supported gaskets from Tables 3.9 and 3.10. The ground proximity to the leak should also be taken into account (see Figs. 3.3 and 3.4).

Pump with packed gland or mechanical seal where leakage is of compressed gas
Zone 1 of 1 m radius is present. Zone 2 should be taken from Table 3.2 for a spirally supported gasket. Account should also be taken of the proximity of the ground to the leak (see Figs. 3.3 and 3.4).

While it is clearly possible to utilize packed gland type seals for all of the above situations it is recommended that mechanical seals are used, particularly in the case of gases and liquids above their atmospheric-pressure boiling points, because of their enhanced performance in respect of wear. Throttle bushes are also recommended in these cases to give added confidence in maximum-leak rates. Although it is less likely that concentrations of rotating pumps and compressors will occur to the extent that hazardous areas will be modified as discussed in the case of valves, it is necessary to identify this situation if it occurs and treat the hazardous areas created as for valves.

Moving reciprocating seals

Reciprocating compressors and pumps present a slightly different situation as the leakage around their pistons is into a crankcase or the chamber behind the piston. In cases where the crankcase is ventilated the hazardous area is created at the ventilation exit which may be in a different location, rather than at the location of compression. Therefore, apart from the hazardous areas created by piping in the compressor location, a further hazardous area may be created elsewhere. Where the leakage concerned is in normal operation, a Zone 1 of 1 m radius around the point where the leakage reaches the atmosphere is sufficient but, for abnormal circumstances the releases from the compressor moving seals, both at the point of normal exhaust to atmosphere and local to the seal itself should be considered as those for a spirally supported gasket (see Table 3.2). As a result of the compressor duty, this type of consideration will result in significant hazardous areas.

3.4 Other practical well-ventilated situations

The previous sections have discussed the performance of leaking flammable materials from the more classic leak sources such as pipe flanges and pump/compressor seals, but there are many particular situations which require specific consideration.

3.4.1 The fixed roof vented stock tank

This type of tank is extremely common on most process plant for the storage of flammable materials which are normally liquid. Most of these are in well-ventilated outdoor areas and commonly have free vents to allow escape of vapour during filling and entry of air during emptying. They do, however, exhibit a particular problem in that when in direct sunlight solar gain can occur, particularly in their vapour space and temperatures higher than the typical ambient maximum of 32 °C can occur. The extent of this solar gain is nowhere directly specified but a figure of 47.5 °C for small tanks is specified in one company code and the HSE Booklet, HS(G)50[4] defines Flammable Liquids as those with flashpoints up to 55 °C. It is prudent to take the latter for the basis of discussion of explosive atmospheres around stock tanks of this type and not to store any flammable liquid with a boiling point below 55 °C in such tanks. These tanks are normally bunded to contain spillages of the contained flammable liquids in cases of gross overfilling or leakage and the bund-in effect determines the extent of the pool of flammable liquid. This, of course, may not be true in cases where a bund encompasses several tanks and normal pool dimension determination applies.

There are two normal situations which apply. These are the situation within the tank and the situation outside the tank when normal filling and emptying operations are carried out. In addition, there is always the possibility that in abnormal circumstances the tank will be overfilled resulting in flammable liquid being present in the bund. This abnormal situation also takes account of any flange leakage, etc., in the proximity of the bund. To ensure that the bund is effective its nearest point to the tank should always be more than 1 m so that liquid leakages from the tank always fall into the bund (leakages due to overfilling or flange leakage local to the tank will normally be at a pressure close to the liquid head pressure of the tank – if this is not so, the bund should be designed accordingly). The bund should also be capable of containing the entire tank contents with a safety factor (say 1.1). Making these assumptions, the area classification for the tank and its surrounding areas is as shown in Fig. 3.9.

Zone 0 Because of the regular emptying action, air is constantly being drawn into the tank vapour space and mixed with vapour. It is likely, therefore, that somewhere in that vapour space an explosive atmosphere

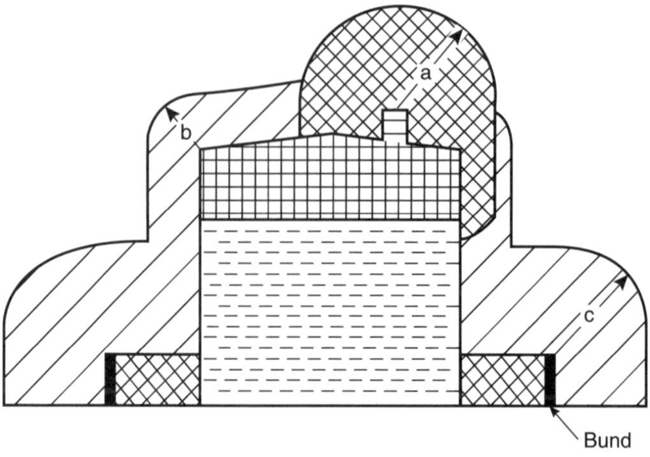

Fig. 3.9 Fixed roof stock tank. a = 3 m, b = 1.5 m, c = 2.5 m

will exist normally and as the actual part of the vapour space cannot be defined, the entire vapour space must be classified as Zone 0.

Zone 1 In addition to the drawing in of air in the emptying cycle, the filling cycle will exhaust a mixture of flammable vapour and air from the vent and, as this flammable vapour is almost certain to be heavier than air, an explosive atmosphere will form around the vent. This will tend to travel downwards and outwards along the tank top possibly overlapping the edges of the tank. The liquid pool in the bund, in abnormal circumstances, will give off vapour into the bund which, unless very large and shallow, will form a containment impeding the dispersal of the vapour. It is likely that the interior of the bund will also be Zone 1 due to this impeded dispersal.

Zone 2 If the tank is overfilled, flammable liquid will exit the vent, travel down the sides of the tank and collect in the bund. There will be vaporization from the outside of the tank and from the surface of the pool which will create a Zone 2 around the tank and beyond the bund wall. A Zone 2 will also be produced by leakage from the tank and associated pipework but this will be contained within the Zone 2, caused by overfilling.

Limitations and other considerations

In producing Fig. 3.9, a tank of some 250 m^3 capacity has been used and no pumps or other pressurizing devices have been considered as present within the bund. The water drainage facilities necessarily associated with the bund have also not been considered as they are assumed not to transmit flammable liquid or vapour from the bund. Their design should achieve this in any properly designed installation but if it does not then such possibilities must be considered in area classification.

In conditions where solar gain brings the contained flammable liquid near to its boiling point, consideration should be given to providing a cover to prevent direct sunlight from striking the tank. This has the effect of removing solar gain and reducing internal tank maximum temperatures to around 32 °C with corresponding reduction in the range of liquids considered as flammable liquids. Such action can, however, have an adverse effect on the external hazardous areas created. If the cover is flat, then the area under the cover will all become Zone 1 with a 1 m distance laterally from the edge of the cover and a similar radial distance from any vents in the top of the cover. A cover with sides is not recommended as this could severely adversely affect the ventilation in the area between the tank top and the cover with the result, at the worst, of creating a Zone 0 in that space, particularly if there are no top vents in the cover to create a chimney effect.

3.4.2 The floating roof tank

These tanks are different to fixed roof tanks in that the tank roof is supported by the liquid within the tank and moves up and down with the level of

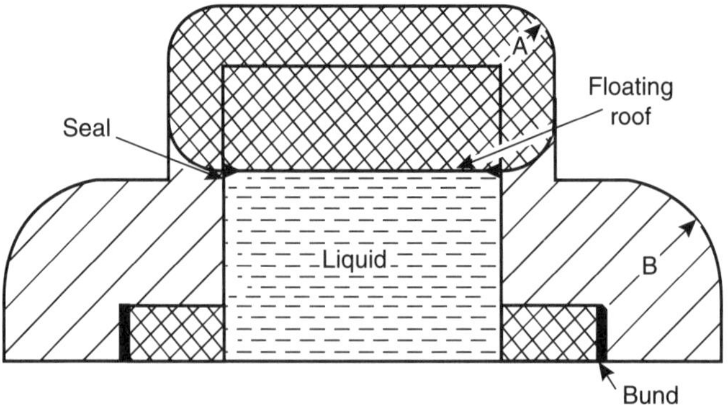

Fig. 3.10 Floating roof stock tank. A = 1.5 m, B = 2.5 m

liquid. A seal is provided between the moving roof and the walls of the tank and vapour can only be present in this situation where it, or small quantities of liquid, pass that seal. This, of course, is either a situation of 'normal operation' or, in cases where the amount of liquid passing the seal normally gives sufficient vapour to create an explosive atmosphere, a continuous situation. There is also the possibility of the walls of the tank which are above the roof restricting dispersion and causing the explosive atmosphere to persist. This effect will be exacerbated where a cover is fitted to protect the top of the tank roof from the environment. The result of this is shown in Fig. 3.10 and is basically as follows:

Zone 0 does not exist within the tank, unlike the fixed roof case as the roof is in intimate contact with the stored liquid. Provided the space in the tank above the roof is unimpeded, the retention of flammable vapour will not be sufficient to create a Zone 0 in this space and, therefore some advantage over fixed roof tanks is apparent.

The interior of the tank above the tank roof will be Zone 1 and this will extend for 1.5 m above and laterally from the edges of the tank. As the vapour is generally heavier than air the Zone 1 can be expected to extend further down the sides of the tank accordingly. In abnormal circumstances the behaviour of the tank will be similar to a fixed roof tank in that liquid will overflow into the bund. As in the case of the fixed roof tank a pool will form in the bund and the vapour space above that pool will contain an explosive atmosphere. Because of the likely interference of the bund wall with ventilation, there will be persistence within the bund and the interior vapour space will be Zone 1.

As in the case of the fixed roof tank there is the abnormal possibility of overflow of liquid into the bund and to allow for this a Zone 2 of 1.5 m from the top of the tank and around its sides will be present. This will not show where the Zone 1 exists as it has a similar extent and is thus masked. A Zone 2 will also exist from the bund limits for a vertical and horizontal distance of 2.5 m, as for the fixed roof tank.

Limitations and other considerations

As for the fixed roof tank, a tank of some 250 m^3 capacity has been considered with no pumps or similar equipment being contained within the bund. Again, drainage devices are assumed not to transmit flammable liquid out of the bund. The effects of a cover will also be similar to those which occur with the fixed roof tank although in this case it is more likely that a cover will be present in view of the construction of the tank.

3.4.3 Tanks containing gas, vapour or liquefied vapours

These tanks are normally sealed as the gas, vapour or liquid will be under pressure. Leaks from these should be treated as for leaks from pipe and similar joints as, even if it is liquid which is released, it will rapidly vaporize. Such tanks may, however, be bunded to take care of massive releases which, although outside the scope of area classification (e.g., catastrophic) may need to be taken care of. If such bunds are used then, even if the releases are secondary grade (abnormal) the bunds may create conditions where the explosive atmosphere persists within them and their interiors, as for liquid storage tanks, should be considered as Zone 1.

For low pressure storage, such as is the case with gasholders, water seals are often used. Where this is the case the possibility of gas exiting through the liquid must be considered if the pressure inside the holder is too high, or venting at pressure relief valves where these are provided to prevent overpressurizing. In such circumstances the following area classification may be appropriate and is shown diagrammatically in Fig. 3.11. There should be no Zone 0 either inside or, in the proximity of, the storage holder as, if this were so (particularly within the holder), it would be tantamount to storing and delivering an explosive atmosphere to a process and, in any event, the liquid sealing arrangements should be such as to achieve the same conditions as in a floating roof tank. It is highly likely that release at pressure relief valves to a limited extent will occur in normal operation. This limited release will give rise to a Zone 1 but as the pressure will be very low, the Zone 1 will be of limited size. A figure of 3 m is suggested as adequate to cover this eventuality.

In abnormal circumstances, overpressurizing due to overfilling the tank will cause significantly more release at the pressure relief valve and, in addition, releases at the water seal or seals. The area contaminated in these circumstances will be larger and a hazardous area of 10 m from both of these leakage points is suggested as necessary to cover this eventuality.

Limitations and other considerations

In selecting the above hazardous areas, normal venting is assumed to be from an orifice of around 2 cm^2 at $10^4\,N/m^2$, the passage through the

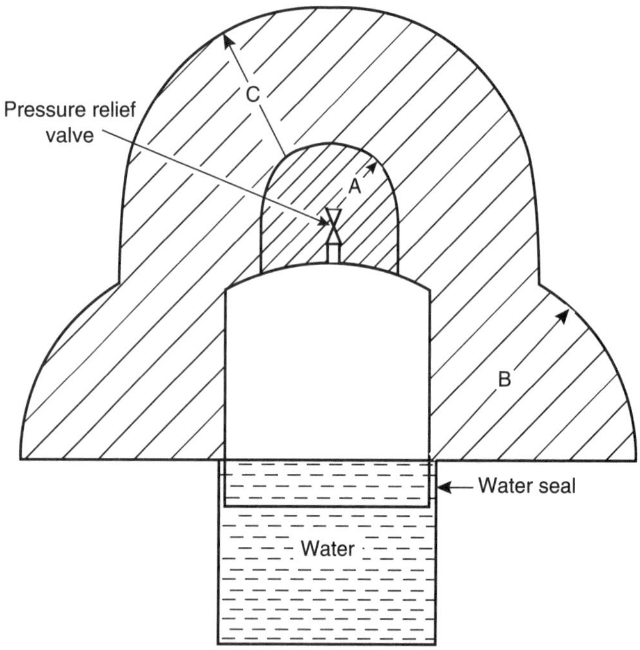

Fig. 3.11 Water sealed gas storage tank. A = 3 m, B = 10 m, C = 7 m

diaphragm or water seal of the pressure relief valve being considered as partial. This is not so in the case of abnormal situations where full passage through the pressure relief valve, or a significant part of the water seal, is considered.

3.4.4 Road and rail tanks for flammable liquids

Liquids are regularly transported by road or rail. In general, the areas through which they pass in transit are not classified because the time for which they dwell in those places is limited which, coupled with the fact that any leakage during transit is abnormal, means that the likelihood of a given area being contaminated with an explosive atmosphere is so low that area classification is not relevant. While the above is generally true, care must be taken in this regard because in areas where transport tanks dwell for significant times, or where a large number of such tanks are stationary for a considerable time, area classification may be relevant. In general, the division between where area classification is or is not necessary is taken to be the division between places such as general car parks – where tanks may reside overnight together with other transporters – and locations specifically designated for tank parking such as the locality of loading stations on airports, etc.

The results of this approach is that it is not generally considered as necessary to area classify such places as parking areas where general public access is available, but it becomes necessary in the case of parking areas on sites where the materials are used and are designated specifically for such tanks. Typical of these are railway sidings dedicated to the marshalling of tanks, specific areas of dockyards again dedicated to location of tanks prior to loading or unloading, and similar locations in process plant areas. This generalization is not, however, always valid as there may be places where many tankers regularly park and in such cases the division described above becomes harder to justify. Due to the uncontrolled nature of such parking places it is not possible to use classic area classification and so the presence of the driver becomes critical. Routes and parking procedures need to be determined to minimize the number of tankers parked in any one location for significant periods, to reduce the need for overnight parking and to ensure that when the vehicle is left there is no evidence of leakage, all of which will reduce the risk to an acceptable level. There are many government regulations in this area, typical of which are The Dangerous Substances (Conveyance by Road in Road Tankers and Tank Containers) Regulations 1981[5] which should be consulted in this regard.

Wherever tankers are loaded, off-loaded/discharged or parked when loaded in significant numbers there is little justification for not applying the normal area classification procedures, and the tank and its contents form a source of release in these circumstances unless particular sources of release are prevented (i.e., the source of release from tank vents may be removed by an extraction system which will prevent any hazardous area being formed apart from in the immediate vicinity of the vent, but in such circumstances the vent exhaust needs consideration). In addition tanker bays used for unloading only will be different from those used for loading since there is little or no release from vents.

Tankers containing unpressurized flammable liquids below their boiling point

These tankers are normally of mostly welded construction and thus the only sources of release which generally need to be considered are the following: releases from any joints for pipework connection, etc.; releases from vents due to loading; and releases from flexible pipes used to connect the tanker to fixed plant.

The area classification around the tanker resulting from the tanker itself and its immediate coupling (not the fixed plant in the loading area which must be dealt with additionally) will be as follows.

Zone 0 The interior of the tanker.

Zone 1 When a tanker is loaded or unloaded there is always the danger of a small leak of liquid during coupling or uncoupling. To allow for this, which is a primary grade source of release a Zone 1 needs to be defined around the coupling points. The size of this is, to a degree, arbitrary due

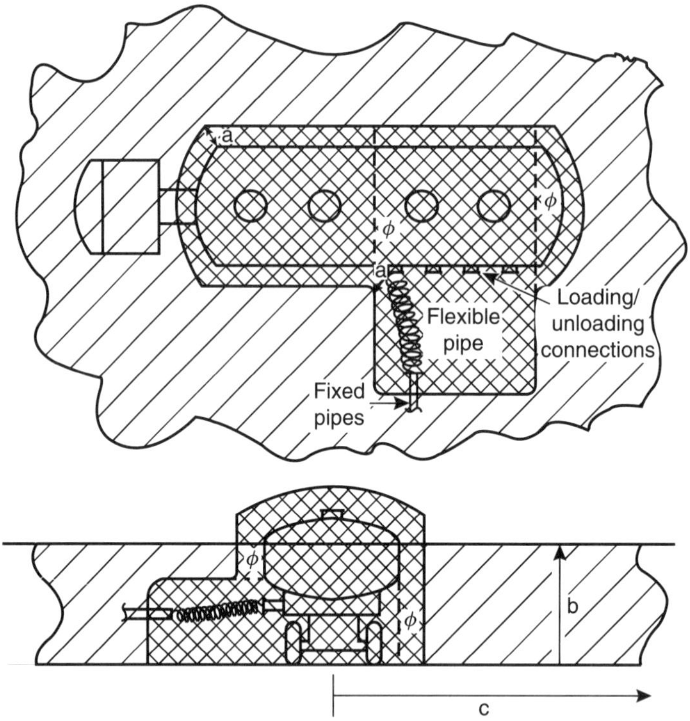

a = 1.5 m
b = } These depend upon the characteristics of the pool formed by
c = } any liquid release
ϕ = Limit of Zone 1 for off-loading operation

Fig. 3.12 Loading and off-loading of road/rail tankers

to the lack of knowledge in regard to the amount of such a manually introduced leak but it is not likely to be large and a Zone 1 of 1.5 m above and around the source of leakage projected down to the ground (as shown in Fig. 3.12) should cover all eventualities. The downward projection takes account of the fact that the vapour is likely to be heavier than air. In the case of tanker off-loading the hazardous area defined due to the vents will not exist, and in this case the extent of the Zone 1 due to the coupling will be defined by the dotted lines in Fig. 3.12. This Zone 1 extends right under the tanker to take account of the restricted ventilation there due to the presence of the tanker.

A third primary grade source of release exists in the flexible pipes used to couple tankers which are subjected to regular movement and failure in normal operation can result. Such failure is likely to take the form of a small crack and, as the pressure is low (being usually the tank head pressure), release in these circumstances. For this reason it is considered as appropriate to limit the Zone 1 produced to a distance of 1.5 m above and around the flexible coupling projected vertically down to the ground.

Zone 2 This will result due to abnormal circumstances, the first of which will occur if the tanker is overfilled. In these circumstances the liquid will, as in the case of a fixed tank, flow out of the vents and down the sides of the tank, ultimately forming a pool on the ground. The Zone 2 produced above and around the tank by this event will be no larger than the Zone 1 produced by vapour release and the resulting Zone 2 will be invisible in the case of the loading of road/rail tankers but, as it is due to abnormal circumstances, it cannot be presumed not to exist in the unloading scenario. Therefore a 1.5 m Zone 2 above and around the tank will be present in all circumstances and will be projected vertically down to the ground. The pool of flammable liquid formed on the ground will grow until it is either contained or until its vaporization rate is equal to the release rate of liquid from the tank (see Chapter 4). The hazardous area created by this pool will be Zone 2 and will be sized as given in Table 3.7.

A second source of release in abnormal circumstances will be that occurring when a flexible connecting pipe actually ruptures. In this circumstance it is not expected that total rupture will take place due to the sort of reinforcement provided in such connecting pipes and, therefore, a similar release to that occurring with rupture of a CAF gasket is considered to be a fair model. Again, the release of liquid will form a pool and the dimensions of this pool can be determined from Table 3.3. The extent of the hazardous area around the pool so formed can then be determined from Table 3.7. As the pressure will be low in these cases it is unlikely that any mist will form and the Zone 2 around the connecting pipe will be minimal. This is academic as a Zone 1 of 1.5 m has already been declared and this will encompass any small Zone 2 around the connecting pipe.

Finally, it is highly unlikely that solar gain will occur in road/rail tankers unless they are parked for long periods in direct sunlight immediately prior to unloading. Provided care is taken in this regard only liquids with flash-points below 32 °C need be considered.

Road or rail tankers containing gases under pressure or liquefied gases and vapours

Road or rail tankers which contain gases or vapours under pressure, or liquefied gases or vapours which will of course be also under pressure, will behave as any other vessel in such circumstances. The mechanisms of release will be principally as follows: liquid, gas or vapour leakages due to coupling and uncoupling; liquid, gas or vapour leakages due to failure of valve actuator failure; liquid, gas or vapour leakages due to failure of fixed pipe joints; and liquid, gas or vapour leakage due to failure of flexible couplings.

These leaks normally give rise to the following hazardous areas. The interior of the tank should be considered as Zone 0 as, even though it is less likely that air will enter, there is always the possibility that the tank will regularly be empty and, rather than try to define and control such periods, it is better to assume Zone 0. Such an assumption will not normally be unnecessarily restrictive.

Zone 1 will result from one of three scenarios which give rise to primary grade sources of release, two due to failure and one due to manual intervention. Of the two due to failure, the first is the valve stem or actuator and the Zone 1 deriving from this source should be based upon the normal Zone 1 which results from a regularly operated valve and which is appropriate in this case. Therefore, a Zone 1 will be assumed to exist above and around the valve for 1 m. The second scenario will be a failure in the flexible coupling pipe and here the orifice is expected to be small and so total vaporization can be assumed at the point of release. It is considered that such a release will be similar to that occurring when a screwed joint leaks as, because personnel are involved, it is almost certain that anything larger would be very noticeable and evoke immediate rectification. The Zone 1 produced should be determined from Table 3.9 and that at ground level from Table 3.10. The third primary grade source of release is that which could occur due to manual intervention during coupling or uncoupling but this is expected to be so small that it is covered by the Zone 1 due to flexible pipe failure. If, however, the coupling point is remote from the flexible pipe then it should be surround by a Zone 1 of similar proportions to that produced for the flexible pipe and Tables 3.9 and 3.10 apply.

The Zone 2 areas present will be due to the flexible pipe, couplings and other joints and the valve actuating stem. The valve stem seal can be considered as a spirally-supported gasket for Zone 2 definition purposes and the flexible joint as a CAF gasket rupture and the extent of Zone 2 at joints, couplings and the flexible joint can be derived from Tables 3.9 and 3.10. It must again be emphasized that the above takes account only of the hazardous areas created by the tank itself and its immediate environs. The hazardous area created by fixed plant surrounding the tank must be additionally dealt with.

3.4.5 Oil/water separators

Oil/water separators are open vessels into which a mixture of water and (usually spilled) oils are placed and permitted to dwell for a significant time. The objective of this is to allow the water to separate from the oil so that the one can be disposed of and the other allowed into the normal drains. Theoretically, the vessel will normally contain primarily lower volatility oils as those with higher volatilities will have been subject to significant vaporization before the mixture reaches the separator. Where the majority of the oils used at a particular site are of high volatility this type of oil/water separation is not appropriate and another method should be chosen as the hazardous areas produced by this method would not be acceptable. This gives rise to the following area classifications. The interior of the separator will be Zone 0, but this Zone will not extend beyond the extremities of the separator due to the oils it contains being of low volatility. It would be unwise to use an oil/water separator of this type if the oils were of high volatility and some other approach should be used in those circumstances. Zone 1 occurs in cases where the separator contains oils of a higher volatility than normally and, due to wind action, a hazardous area will exist outside the oil/water separator. In these cases the mix of volatility should be such as to permit the use of the 50 per cent column of Table 3.7, using the area of the separator as the pool size. In cases where a significant number of the oils on the plant – which may be fed to the separator – are of high volatility the >90 per cent line should be used. The hazardous area is shown in Fig. 3.13 for a ground level oil/water separator but if the separator is above ground level, with its base at or around ground level, the Zone 1 merely extends vertically down the separator sides.

Zone 2 occurs in abnormal circumstances, such as after a major release of oil of high volatility where a larger hazardous area will exist around the separator. The extent of this area can be derived from Table 3.7 using the >90 per cent column. As previously stated this area becomes Zone 1 if a significant number of the oils used on the site are of high volatility.

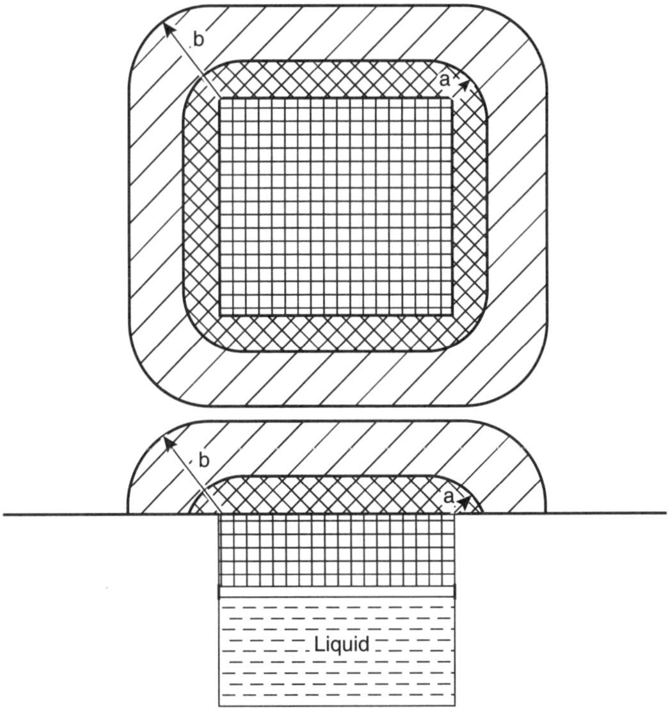

Fig. 3.13 Oil/water separator. a = 50% column of Table 3.7, b =>90% column of Table 3.7

In such cases no Zone 2 exists visibly as its size is synonymous with the Zone 1.

Figure 3.13 is for a ground level oil/water separator but if the ground is at or about the base level of the separator then the Zone 2 is projected vertically down the separator side.

Finally, should the oil/water separator overflow, a pool of mixed oil and water would form. The Zone 2 associated with this pool can be derived using Table 3.7 assuming the highest volatility oil is present. Because water is present and may cause the mixture to be transmitted further than would be the case if only oil were present, it is advisable to mechanically limit the pool size with some sort of containment sized to contain the maximum overflow possible. This containment size should then be used in all circumstances for determination (using Table 3.7) even where the equilibrium pool size is smaller.

3.4.6 Other open vessels

Open vessels will behave in a very similar manner to oil/water separators, except that usually only one flammable material is present. This will give the following hazardous areas.

Zone 0 will be the interior of the vessel.

Zone 1 will be as for an oil/water separator but defined on the basis of the boiling point of the single flammable liquid where appropriate. As before, it is not recommended that open vessels be used where the liquid contained has a boiling point of less than twice the ambient temperature of the location (this effectively means boiling points of more than 65 °C in the UK).

The only situation giving rise to a Zone 2 is the overflow situation and the Zone 2 resulting should be defined as for oil/water separators in this circumstance.

3.4.7 Open drains

Open drainage gullies are often used to collect released flammable liquids so that the dimensions of any pool can be accurately defined, and to provide a route for collection and disposal of such liquids. They do not, unlike oil/water separators, normally contain flammable liquids but may do so in cases of spillage. The presence of such liquids within them is, therefore, either in normal operation or only abnormal and, because they actually drain away the flammable liquid, overflow is abnormal. This leads to the following hazardous areas.

If the flow into the drain is in normal operation the interior of the drain is Zone 0 because of the persistence effect which the containment of the drain

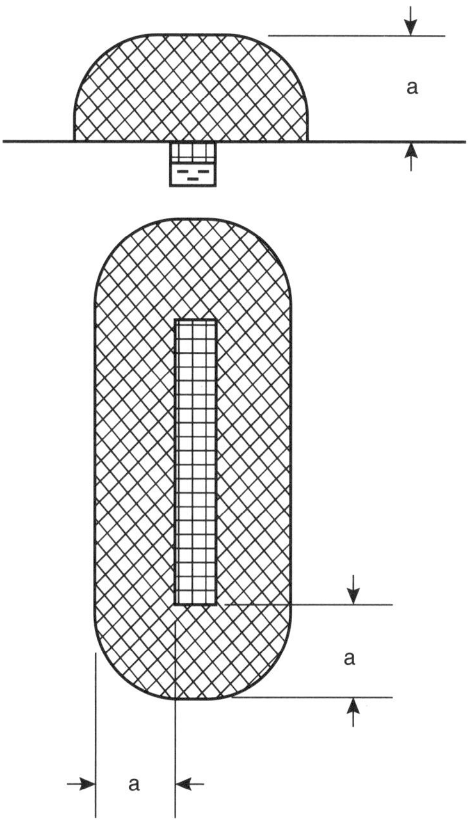

Fig. 3.14 Open drains. a = 1 m

will introduce. In other cases no Zone 0 exists. It would not be considered as acceptable to have a flammable material exhausting into an open drain continuously. If the release into the drain is abnormal, a Zone 0 will still exist within the drain at any point where, because of the geometry of the drain, liquid collects and will become static and persist until it has all evaporated.

Zone 1 occurs where the drain acts as a long narrow pool and the area around it will contain an explosive atmosphere from time to time, due to wind action. A Zone 1 will exist around the drain (as shown in Fig. 3.14) where release into the drain is in either normal or abnormal operation. This is nominally chosen as 1 m which, although to a degree arbitrary, is likely to be larger than any practical distance achieved. Collection of flammable liquids at low spots in the drain are unlikely to affect the extent of the Zone 1 described here. The combination of normal release into the drain coincident with drain blockage could produce an external pool which will grow until the release stops or the evaporation rate exceeds the release rate. A Zone 2 will be produced by this pool in accordance with Table 3.7, the dimensions of the pool being defined by either the containment of the pool where this exists or, where no containment exists by calculation (see Chapter 4).

3.4.8 Trenches

There are two types of trench normally encountered. The first is a trench which contains pipework and there is the possibility of a leak within it due to pipe joints or valve seals, etc. This means that the leak could occur in normal operation (a primary grade release) or only abnormally (a secondary grade source of release). Such trenches should be given the same type of treatment as drains based upon the type of leak and the quantity of flammable material leaking (if the leak is liquid). If the release is of gas or vapour then types of, and the extent of, hazardous areas produced should be those produced by the leak occurring outside the trench but should extend throughout any length of trench between blockages. (It is normal to put deliberate blockages in trenches to prevent transmission of flammable materials from one part of a plant to another.) In these cases the interior of the trench will be Zone 1 even if the release is only abnormal due to the persistence introduced by the trench.

The second type of trench is that which is not intended to contain any flammable materials such as a trench used for a cable route. Such trenches are only important insofar as they may be in areas defined as hazardous areas for another reason. The hazardous area inside the trench will in such cases be as follows:

External Zone 0 – Internal Zone 0
External Zone 1 – Internal Zone 1
External Zone 2 – Internal Zone 1

The hazardous are a within the trench will again exist for the entire length between blockages. The increase in hazard in external Zone 2 is to take account of the persistence occurring within the trench. The above relationship will remain true in the alternative case where flammable liquid leaks into the drain from an external pool. The presumption in the case of liquids is that action is taken in a reasonable time to remove the flammable material from the drain (which is considered as essential).

3.4.9 Sampling points

The problem with sampling points is that most are manual and, apart from the doubtful wisdom of deliberately creating a significant hazardous area by a routing action, there is the problem as the personnel sampling at the sampling point would be within the hazardous area at the time when flammable materials were present. As the majority of flammable materials are also toxic this is not a situation which can be accepted. Sampling arrangements are usually carefully designed to minimize the hazardous area created in normal operation so that the only significant hazardous area occurs in abnormal operation.

Sampling liquids

Any sampling point used for sampling liquids should be so arranged that any spillages occurring during normal sampling are removed immediately. To do this the sampling arrangements should incorporate features which satisfy those achieved by the sampling system shown in Fig. 3.15. The tundish or receptor of spillages below the sampling point should transfer any spillage to a closed storage facility safe disposal system. For liquids of low volatility (it is suggested that these will have atmospheric boiling points of at least four times ambient temperature) the effects of gravity will normally be all that is needed to ensure spillage collection in the tundish, but in other cases it is likely that some form of extract system to draw

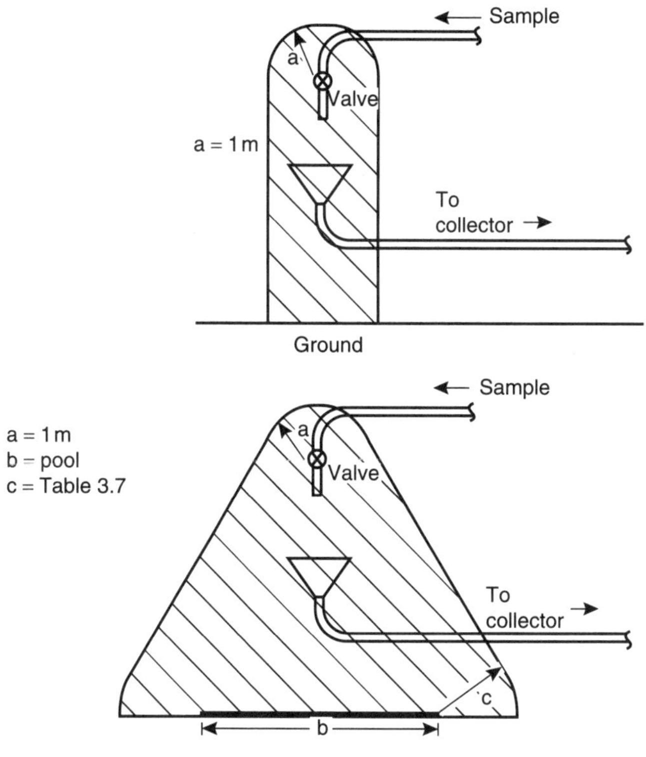

Fig. 3.15 Liquid sampling

spillages into the tundish will be necessary. If these techniques are used the release of flammable material into the atmosphere surrounding the sampling point in normal operation will be minimal and no significant Zone 1 will exist. There will, however, remain the possibility of significant release in abnormal operation due to such things as failure of the sampling valve which will release too much liquid for the tundish to deal with, or blockage of the tundish itself. In both of these cases there will be significant leakage of flammable liquid and possible splashing around the sampling point. This situation will produce a small Zone 2 around the sampling point and a pool below it which will grow until it is contained either physically or by the evaporation rate. It will then create a hazardous area as defined in Table 3.7. The result of this is given in Fig. 3.15 and is as follows.

There are no Zones 0 and 1.

Zone 2 consists of a sphere of 1 m around the sampling point and a pool with surrounding hazardous area below it.

Where the flammable material is not toxic simpler arrangements are possible but not recommended as they will probably create larger hazardous areas, the justification for which is doubtful in view of the ease with which the above arrangements can be used. Details of toxicity for more usual materials is given in HSE Guidance Note EH 40.[6]

Sampling gases and vapours

Sampling gases, vapours and liquefied vapours under pressure can give rise to a hazardous area of significant proportions and cannot be permitted. It is necessary to utilize the closed-in-line sampling system shown in Fig. 3.16

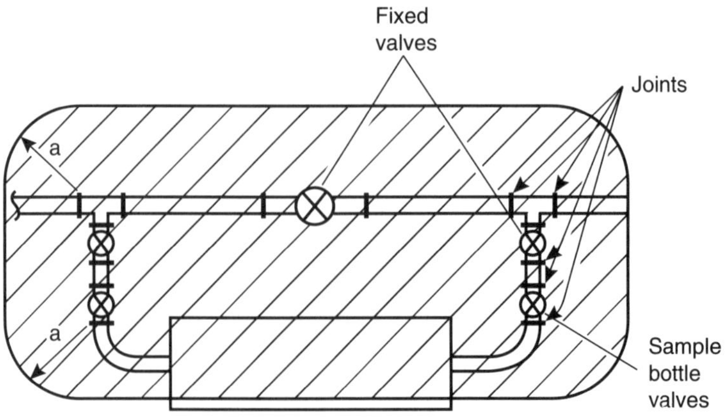

Fig. 3.16 Gas sampling. a = Table 3.2 for appropriate joints. *Note*: Release from value stems assumed less than joints. If this is not so the hazardous area should be adjusted to take account of hazardous areas from column 3 of Table 3.2

and, in some cases, even to allow for the evacuation of the spaces between the sample bottle and fixed valves before disconnection of the sample bottle. This is likely only in the case of liquefied gases as, otherwise, the amount of flammable material stored in this interspace will be small if the system is properly designed. Again the objective is to effectively eliminate any Zone 1 so that only in abnormal operation will a hazardous area be present. These abnormal situations will include valve seal failure, pipe-joint failure and incorrect connection by personnel, the latter of which would be expected to be quickly corrected as the sampling personnel would be present. The hazardous area would, therefore, be most likely from pipe-joint or valve failure, both of which are dealt with in sections 3.5.1 and 3.5.2 and in Table 3.2. The result of this is as follows.

There are no Zones 0 and 1

Zone 2 consists of an area in accordance with line 3 of Table 3.2 around the valve stem and an area in accordance with the appropriate column of Table 3.2 around each joint, as shown in Fig. 3.16.

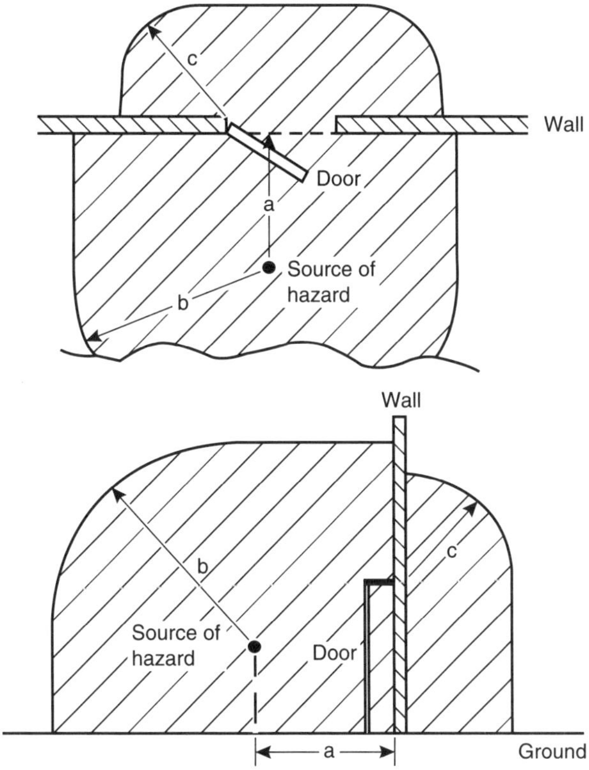

a = Distance of wall from source of hazard
b = Extent of hazardous area ignoring wall
c = b−a

Fig. 3.17 Openings between spaces

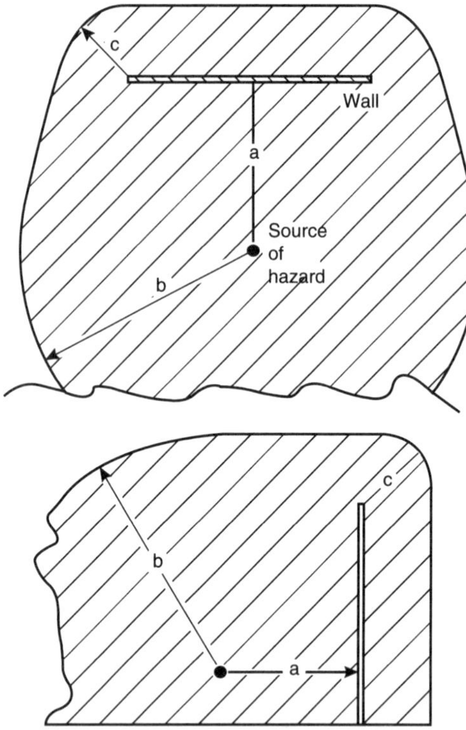

a = Distance of wall from source of hazard
b = Extent of hazardous area ignoring wall
c = b−a

Fig. 3.18 Hazardous areas due to short walls

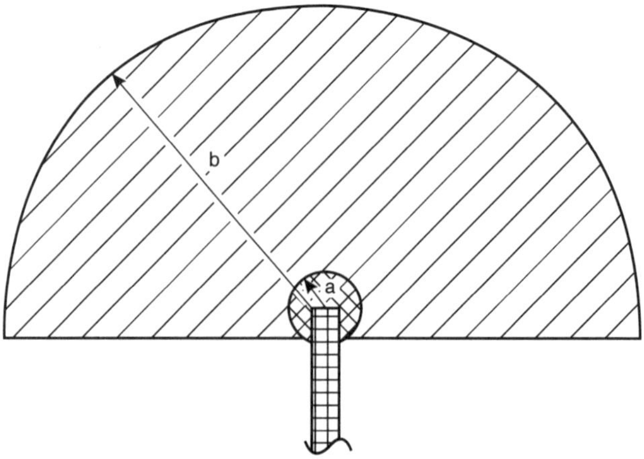

Fig. 3.19 Release at vent. a = 1 m, b = Calculated from Chapter 4 based on jelrelease extent equation and volume of gas/vapour released. *Note*: Where release is from a bursting disc Zone 0 inside vent and Zone 1 immediately surrounding the vent, both become Zone 2

3.4.10 Walls and appertures

Where extents of hazardous areas are defined by a wall which contains a door then the door will become a source of release insofar as the non-hazardous area side of the wall is concerned and will result in a hazardous area as shown in Fig. 3.17. Likewise where a wall is short the hazardous area will extend around it as shown in Fig. 3.18. In both cases the extension is based upon the original extent of the hazardous area and the distance between the source of hazard and the wall.

3.4.11 Vents

Vents normally only operate in abnormal circumstances, such as the opening of a relief valve, or rupture of a bursting disc. In such cases, relatively large amounts of flammable gas or vapour are released via a vent or flare stack if released directly to the surrounding atmosphere. This section only refers to such direct situations as, in other cases, secondary containment is usually the norm and that can be dealt with in accordance with earlier sections of this chapter. The flare is assumed not to be ignited as this possibility exists.

In the case of a bursting disc there will be no release of flammable material in normal operation but in the case of a relief valve a slight leakage through the seat must be considered possible (this does not include the valve-operating stem which should be dealt with separately). In the one case a Zone 1 may be present at the vent exit and in the other not. When the valve opens or the bursting disc ruptures a significant flow of flammable material will occur in both cases but this will only be in abnormal operation. The small amount of release due to valve-seat leakage will drift from the vent outlet but the release due to operation of the valve or rupture of the bursting disc will be a rapid flow. This means that the hazardous area due to the former will be a small sphere as a result of the drift being wind dispersed, while the latter will be a plume because the jet turbulence will be mixing. This gives a rather unusual hazardous area distribution which is shown in Fig. 3.19, with the Zone 2 shown allowing for the wind distortion of the plume and this is as follows.

Zone 0 is within the vent stack but only if a relief valve is used.

Zone 1 a sphere of 1 m around the vent outlet in cases where the relief valve is used.

Zone 2 a hemisphere superimposed upon the top of the vent in all cases and the interior of the vent stack where a bursting disc is used.

References

1 BS 5345 — Selection, Installation and Maintenance of Electrical Apparatus for use in Potentially Explosive Atmospheres (other than mining operations or

	explosives processing and manufacture). Part 2 (1983). Classification of hazardous areas.
2 RoSPA/ICI	Engineering Codes and Regulations, Electrical Installations in Flammable Atmospheres (1973). Group C (Electrical), Volume 1.5.
3 Institute of Petroleum	Model Code of Safe Practice in the Petroleum Industry (1990). Part 15. Area Classification Code for Petroleum Installations.
4 HS (G) 50	Health and Safety Executive Booklet. The Storage of Flammable Liquids in Fixed Tanks (up to 10 000 m^3 total capacity) (1996).
5	The Dangerous Substances (conveyance by road in road tankers and tank containers) Regulations 1981. HMSO (SI 1981/1059).
6 EH 40	Guidance Note from the Health and Safety Executive, Occupational Exposure Limits. (Regularly updated.)

— 4 —

Calculation of release rates and the extents of hazardous areas

Methods for the determination of release rates and the extents of areas of explosive atmosphere (hazardous areas) created by any given leak or leaks have been the subject of much discussion and are recognized as a difficult area of technology. There are several schools of thought and, as a result, it has proved impossible to settle upon a method which has full confidence of all relevant interests. This has resulted in the lack of any nationally or internationally agreed method and so those involved are left to select a procedure acceptable to them from a variety of industry-based and other sectorial codes. Several attempts have been made to include bases for calculative procedures in national and international codes but disagreements as to their accuracy have almost always resulted in a failure to agree on their inclusion. Nonetheless, those involved in the classification of hazardous areas have always had to use some form of estimation/calculation to justify the hazardous areas which they specify in each particular case and it must be remembered that, provided the methods used produce results similar to those recorded in subjective assessment, which has in the past been the only possibility, the use of a limited form of calculation as described in this chapter may be justified. As will be seen this chapter is not concerned with absolute accuracy but merely with a gauging operation and the assumptions made are all aimed at giving overestimates rather than underestimates.

The problem experienced in any method of area classification is the lack of information from experimentation on mixing of releases with air when such releases are accidental rather than deliberate. This causes problems in both the subjective approach to area classification and in proving that the mathematical approach is totally valid.

Most of the mathematics which has existed for some time is based upon calculation of fluid flow from orifices specially designed to ensure the maximum flow for minimum effort (e.g., situations where flow or mixing is required for operational reasons rather than as a result of an unwanted leak). The last serious attempt to produce a mathematical approach was during the production of BS 5345, Part 2[1] (1975–82) and, although a relatively comprehensive set of formulae based upon classical theory and experimentation were proposed, those involved did not feel able to recommend the approach in a national document, principally because of the possibility of misuse by those not sufficiently expert or failure of such people to identify the limitations of such formulae. The approach was, however, used in at least one company code[2] and, in general, gave results which had a reasonable level. confidence and which have since given no indication of inadequacy. The latest international Code, BS/EN 6079-10[3] which is expected to replace BS 5345, Part 2[1] in the relatively near future has, in common with all of its predecessors, failed to effectively approach the determination of outdoor hazardous area extents by mathematical means indicating that doubt still remains although it does contain a basic mathematical relationship. Its subjective approach does, however, give some yardsticks against which mathematically produced solutions can be measured and, as this code has the confidence of most of the world's developed countries, it can serve to support the mathematical approaches included in this chapter. This is helpful as, notwithstanding the difficulty in producing an approach which will satisfy everyone, there remains the necessity to carry out the business of area classification.

For the above reasons the mathematical approaches described in this chapter are included in this book. The use of these mathematical relationships must, however, be carefully approached and only by those sufficiently expert to identify their limitations. There is no evidence that the calculations described do anything but define hazardous areas at least as large as is necessary when expertly used. This is because they are largely based on ideal releases from nozzles rather than the accidental leaks which occur due to failure of such containment elements as glands and gaskets or, in the case of those included in the new IEC document[2], because of the many safety factors added.

The basis for this mathematical approach comes from sources such as Perry[4] and work done by Sutton and Katau based on a combination of fluid dynamics, kinetic theory of gases and practical measurements. Most of these latter formulae were reported in British Standards Institution Draft Document 79/27013[5] in 1979 and constituted the proposal for a calculative approach which was not adopted as earlier described.

4.1 Releases of gas and vapour

The release of gas or vapour from an orifice or nozzle is given by the following equation which is widely accepted:

$$\text{Mass release (G)} = C_d a P\{(\delta M/RT)(2/\delta + 1)^{(\delta+1/\delta-1)}\}^{0.5} \quad \text{kg/s}$$

where G =	mass release	kg/s
C_d =	coefficient of discharge	–
a =	cross-sectional area of leak	m^2
P =	upstream pressure	N/m^2
δ =	ratio of specific heats Cp/Cv	–
M =	molecular weight	–
R =	gas constant (8312)	m/kgMole/ °K
T =	absolute temperature of released	Gas °K

The ratio of specific heats (specific heat at constant pressure divided by the specific heat at constant volume) has a value of around 1.4 or less for the vast majority of flammable gases and vapours as shown by Table 4.1. If we substitute the value 1.4 for δ the mass release equation can be simplified. In addition, the coefficient of discharge C_d has a maximum value of around 0.8 in ideal circumstances allowing further simplification and the final equation becomes:

$$G = 0.006aP(M/t)^{0.5} \qquad \text{kg/s (Equation 4.1)}$$

This equation is, however, only valid if the upstream pressure is greater than a specific multiple of the downstream pressure (atmospheric pressure in our case) which multiple is called the critical pressure ratio. This ratio is given by the following equation:

$$P/P_a = [(\delta + 1)/2]^{\delta/(\delta-1)} \qquad \text{(Equation 4.2)}$$

where P_a = atmospheric pressure $\quad n/m^2$

Using the value of 1.4 for δ the critical ratio is 1.9 and so, rounding up, Equation 4.1 can be assumed to be only valid when the absolute upstream pressure exceeds $2 \times 10^5\,N/m^2$. Where this is not so the effects of atmospheric pressure become significant and the mass release equation becomes:

$$G = C_d a[2\sigma(P - P_a)]^{0.5} \qquad \text{kg/s}$$

where σ = density of gas at atmospheric pressure and release temperature

The density of the gas or vapour can be expressed in terms of the molecular weight and the molar volume ($22.4\,m^3$/kg Mole) and this gives a more recognizable equation as follows:

$$G = 3.95a\{M(P - 10^5/T)^{0.5}\} \qquad \text{kg/s (Equation 4.3)}$$

The results of Equations 4.1 and 4.3 can, if required, be converted into volume release by use of the following equation:

$$\text{Released volume (V)} = V_o\ G\ T/T_oM \qquad m^3/s$$

where V_o = molar volume $\quad$ m3/kg Mole
T_o = melting point of ice $\quad$ (273 °K)

This equation simplifies to the following:

$$V = 0.082GT/M \qquad m^3/s \text{ (Equation 4.4)}$$

Table 4.1 Data for flammable materials for use with electrical equipment (from BS 5345, Part I (1989))

1	2	3	4	5	6	7	8	9	10	11	12	13	14
Flammable material	Formula	Melting point	Boiling point	Relative vapour density	Flash point	Flammable limits				Ignition temperature	Minimum igniting current	T class of suitable apparatus	Apparatus group
						LFL	UFL	LFL	UFL				
		°C	°C		°C	Vol.%	Vol.%	mg/L	mg/L	°C	mA		
acetaldehyde	CH_3CHO	−123	20	1.52	−38	4	57	73	1040	140	–	T4	IIA
acetic acid	CH_3COOH	17	118	2.07	40	5.4	16	100	430	485	–	T1	IIA
acetic anhydride	$(CH_3CO)_2O$	−73	140	3.52	54	2.7	10	–	–	(334)	–	(T2)	IIA
acetone	$(CH_3)_2CO$	−95	56	2.0	−19	2.15	13	60	310	535	–	T1	IIA
acetonitrile	CH_3CN	−45	82	1.42	5	–	4.4	16	–	523	–	T1	IIA
acetyl chloride	CH_3COCI	−112	51	2.7	4	5.0	–	–	–	390	–	T2	IIA
acetylene (see clause **37**)	$CH{\equiv}CH$	−81	−84*	0.9	–	1.5	100	–	–	305	24	T2	IIC
acrylonitrile	$CH_2{=}CHCN$	−82	77	1.83	−5	3	17	65	380	480	–	T1	IIA
allyl alcohol	$CH_2{=}CHCH_2OH$	–	–	–	21	–	–	–	–	–	–	†	IIA
allyl chloride	$CH_2{=}CHCH_2Cl$	−135	45	2.64	−20	3.2	11.2	105	360	485	–	TI	IIA
allylene	$CH_3C{\equiv}CH$	−103	−23	1.38	–	1.7	–	28	–	–	–	T	IIB
ammonia	NH_3	−78	−33	0.59	–	15	28	105	200	630	–	T1	IIA
amphetamine	$C_6H_5CH_2CH(NH_2CH_3$	–	200	4.67	<100	–	–	–	–	–	–	†	IIA
aniline	$C_6H_5NH_2$	−6	184	3.22	75	1.2	8.3	–	–	617	–	T1	(IIA)
benzaldehyde	C_6H_5CHO	−26	179	3.66	65	1.4	–	60	–	190	–	T4	(IIA)
benzene	C_6H_6	−6	80	2.7	−11	1.2	8	39	270	560	–	T1	IIA
blast furance gas	mixture	–	–	–	–	28.0	70.0	–	–	–	–	†	IIA
blue water gas	mixture	–	–	–	–	–	–	–	–	–	–	T1	IIC
1-bromobutane	$CH_3(CH_2)_2CH_2Br$	−112	102	4.72	<21	2.5	–	230	–	265	–	T3	IIA
bromoethane	C_2H_5Br	−119	38	3.75	< −20	6.7	11.3	300	510	510	–	T1	IIA
buta-1,3-diene	$CH_2{=}CHCH{=}CH_2$	−109	−4	1.87	–	2.1	12.5	25	290	430	65	T2	IIA
butane	C_4H_{10}	−138	−1	2.05	−60	1.5	8.5	37	210	365	80	T2	IIA
butanone (ethyl methyl ketone)	$C_2H_5COCH_3$	−86	80	2.48	−1	1.8	11.5	50	350	505	–	T1	IIA

butan-1-ol	$CH_3(CH_2)_2CH_2OH$	−89	118	2.55	29	1.7	9.0	43	350	340	–	T2	IIA
butyl acetate	$CH_3COOCH_2(CH_2)_2CH_3$	−77	127	4.01	22	1.4	8	58	360	370	–	T2	IIA
butyl glycolate (butyl hydroxyacetate)	$HOCH_2COOC_4H_9$	–	356	4.45	61	–	–	–	–	–	–	†	IIB
butyl styrene	$C_6H_5C(CH_2)_3{=}CH_2$	–	–	–	–	–	–	–	–	–	–	†	IIB
butylamine	$C_4H_9NH_2$	−104	63	2.52	−9	–	–	–	–	(312)	–	(T2)	IIA
butyldigol	$CH_3(CH_2)_3OCH_2$-$CH_2OCH_2CH_2OH$	88	231	5.59	78	–	–	–	–	225	–	T3	IIA
butyraldehyde	$CH_3CH_2CH_2CHO$	−97	75	2.48	< −5	1.4	12.5	42	380	230	–	T3	IIA
but-1-ene	$CH_3{=}CHCH_2CH_3$	−185	−6	1.95	–	1.6	10	35	235	385	–	T2	IIA
but-2-ene‡	$CH_3CH{=}CHCH_3$	–	4	1.94	–	1.7	9	–	–	(325)	–	(T2)	IIB
carbon disulphide. (see clause **37**)	CS_2	−112	46	2.64	−20	1.0	60	30	1900	102	–	T5	IIC
carbon monoxide (see **38.2**)	CO	−205	−191	0.97	–	12.5	74.2	145	870	605	90	T1	IIA
chlorobenzene	C_6H_5Cl	45	132	3.88	28	1.3	7.1	60	520	637	–	T1	IIA
1-chlorobutane	$CH_3(CH_2)_2CH_2CI$	−123	78	3.2	<0	1.8	10	65	390	(460)	–	(TI)	IIA
chloroethane (ethyl choloride)	C_2H_5CI	−136	12	2.22	–	3.6	15.4	95	400	510	–	T1	IIA
2-chloroethanol	CH_2CICH_2OH	−70	129	2.78	55	5.0	16	160	540	425	–	T2	IIA
chloroethylene (vinyl chloride)	$CH_2{=}CHCI$	−154	−14	2.15	–	3.8	29.3	95	770	470	–	T1	IIA
chloromethane (methyl chloride)	CH_3CI	−98	−24	1.78	–	10.7	13.4	150	400	652	–	T1	IIA
chloromethyl methyl ether	CH_3OCH_2CI	−103	60	–	–	–	–	–	–	–	–	†	IIA
1-chloropropane (*n*-chloropropane)	C_3H_7CI	−123	37	2.7	−18	2.8	10.7	70	300	(592)	–	(T1)	IIA
2-chloropropane (*iso*-chloropropane)	$(CH_3)_2CHCI$	–	47	2.7	−32	2.6	11.1	–	–	520	–	T1	IIA

(continued overleaf)

Table 4.1 *(continued)*

1	2	3	4	5	6	7	8	9	10	11	12	13	14
Flammable materials	Formula	Melting point	Boiling point	Relative vapour density	Flash point	Flammable limits				Ignition temperature	Minimum igniting current	T class of suitable apparatus	Apparatus group
						LFL	UFL	LFL	UFL				
		°C	°C		°C	Vol.%	Vol.%	mg/L	mg/L	°C	mA		
α-chlorotoluene (benzyl chloride)	$C_6H_5CH_2Cl$	−39	179	4.36	60	1.2	–	55	–	585	–	T1	IIA
1-chloro-2 3-epoxypropane	OCH_2CHCH_2Cl	−57	116	3.30	(40)	–	–	–	–	–	–	†	IIA
coal tar naphtha	Mixture	–	–	–	–	–	–	–	–	272	–	T3	IIA
coke oven gas (see clause **37**)	Mixture	–	–	–	–	–	–	–	–	500	–	T1	
cresol§	$CH_3C_6H_4OH$	11	191	3.73	81	1.1	–	45	–	555	–	T1	IIA
crotonaldehyde	$CH_3CH{=}CHCHO$	−75	102	2.41	13	2.1	15.5	–	–	(230)	–	(T3)	IIB
cumene (*iso*-propylbenzene)	$C_6H_5CH(CH_3)_2$	−97	152	4.13	36	0.88	6.5	–	–	420	–	T2	IIA
cyclobutane	$CH_2(CH_2)_2CH_2$	−91	13	1.93	–	1.8	–	42	–	–	–	†	IIA
cycloheptane	$CH_2(CH_2)_5CH_2$	–	119	3.39	< 21	–	–	–	–	–	–	†	IIA
cyclohexane	$CH_2(CH_2)_4CH_2$	7	81	2.9	−18	1.2	7.8	40	290	259	–	T3	IIA
cyclohexanol	$CH_2(CH_2)_4CHOH$	24	161	3.45	68	1.2	–	–	–	300	–	T2	IIA
cyclohexanone	$CH_2(CH-2)_4CO$	−31	156	3.38	43	1.4	9.4	53	380	419	–	T2	IIA
cyclohexene	$CH_2(CH_2)_4CH{=}CH$	−104	83	2.83	< −20	1.2	–	–	–	(310)	–	(T2)	IIA
cyclohexylamine	$CH_2(CH_2)_4CHNH_2$	−18	134	3.42	32	–	–	–	–	290	–	T3	IIA
cyclopentane	$CH_2(CH_2)_3CH_2$	−93	47	–	−37	–	–	–	–	(380)	–	(T2)	IIA
cyclopropane	$CH_2CH_2CH_2$	−127	−33	1.45	–	2.4	10.4	40	185	495	–	T1	IIA

decahydronaphthalene	$CH_2(CH_2)_3CHCH(CH_2)_3CH_2$	−43	196	4.76	54	0.7	4.9	40	280	260	–	T3	IIA
decane	$C_{10}H_{22}$(approx.)	−30	173	4.9	96	0.8	5.4	–	–	205	–	T3	IIA
dibutyl ether	$(C_4H_9)_2O$	−95	141	4.48	25	1.5	7.6	48	460	185	–	T4	IIB
dichlorobenzene	$C_6H_4Cl_2$	−18	179	5.07	66	2.2	9.2	130	750	(640)	–	(T1)	IIA
1,1-dichloroethane	CH_3CHCl_2	−98	57	3.42	−10	5.6	16	225	660	440	–	T2	IIA
1,2-dichloroethane	CH_2ClCH_2Cl	−36	84	3.42	(5)	6.2	15.9	–	–	(413)	–	(T2)	IIA
(ethylene dichloride)													
1,1-dichloroethylene	$CH_2{=}CCl_2$	–	37	3.4	−18	7.3	16	–	–	(570)	–	(T1)	IIA
(vinylidene chloride)													
1,2-dichlorothylene	$ClCH{=}CHCl$	−122	33	3.55	−10	9.7	12.8	220	650	(440)	–	(T2)	IIA
(1,2-dichloroethene)													
1,2-dichloropropane	$CH_3CHClCH_2Cl$	< −80	96	3.9	15	3.4	14.5	160	690	555	–	T1	IIA
diethyl ether	$(C_2H_5)_2O$	−116	34	2.55	< −20	1.7	36	50	1100	170	75	T4	IIB
diethyl ketone	$C_2H_5COC_2H_5$	–	–	–	(55)	–	–	–	–	–	–	†	IIA
diethyl oxalate	$(COOC_2H_5)_2$	−41	180	5.04	76	–	–	–	–	–	–	†	IIA
diethyl sulphate	$(C_2H_5)_2SO_4$	−25	208	5.31	104	–	–	–	–	–	–	†	IIA
diethylamine	$(C_2H_5)2NH$	−50	56	2.53	< −20	1.7	10.1	50	305	(310)	–	(T2)	IIA
2-diethylaminoethanol	$(C_2H_5)_2NC_2H_4OH$	–	161	4.04	(60)	–	–	–	–	–	–	†	IIA
diethyldichlorosilane	$(C_2H_5)_2SiCl_2$	–	–	–	–	–	–	–	–	–	–	†	IIC
dihexyl ether	$(CH_3(CH_2)_5)_2O$	−43	227	6.43	75	–	–	–	–	185	–	T4	IIA
di-isobutylene	$C_2H_5CH(CH_3)CH(CH_3)C_2H_5$	−106	105	3.87	(2)	–	–	–	–	(305)	–	(T2)	IIA
di-isopropyl ether	$((CH_3)_2CH)_2O$	−86	69	3.52	−28	1.4	21	–	–	(416)	–	(T2)	IIA
dimethyl ether	$(CH_3)_2O$	−141	−25	1.59	–	3.7	27.0	38	520	–	–	†	IIB
dimethylamine	$(CH_3)_2NH$	−92	7	1.55	–	2.8	14.4	52	270	(400)	–	(T2)	IIA
dimethylaniline	$C_6H_3(CH_3)_2NH_2$	2	194	4.17	63	1.2	7.0	60	350	370	–	T2	IIA
dimenthylformamide	$HCON(CH_3)_2$	−61	152	2.51	58	2.2	15.2	–	–	(440)	–	(T2)	IIA
(formdimethylamide)													
1,4-dioxane	$OCH_2CH_2OCH_2CH_2$	10	101	3.03	11	1.9	22.5	70	820	379	–	T2	IIB
1,3-dioxolane	$OCH_2CH_2OCH_2$	−26	74	2.55	(2)	–	–	–	–	–	–	†	IIB
dipentyl ether	$(C_5H_{11})_2O$	−69	170	5.45	(57)	–	–	–	–	170	–	T4	IIA
dipropyl ether	$(C_3H_7)_2O$	122	90	3.53	< 21	–	–	–	–	170	–	T4	IIB
ditertiary butyl	$(CH_3)_3COOC(CH_3)_3$	–	–	–	18	–	–	–	–	170	–	T4	IIB
peroxide													

(continued overleaf)

Table 4.1 *(continued)*

1	2	3	4	5	6	7	8	9	10	11	12	13	14
Flammable materials	Formula	Melting point	Boiling point	Relative vapour density	Flash point	Flammable limits				Ignition temperature	Minimum igniting current	T class of suitable apparatus	Apparatus group
						LFL	UFL	LFL	UFL				
		°C	°C		°C	Vol.%	Vol.%	mg/L	mg/L	°C	mA		
1,2-epoxypropane (propylene oxide) (methyloxirane)	CH_3CHCH_2O	–	–	–	−37	–	–	–	–	–	–	†	IIB
ethane	CH_3CH_3	−183	−87	1.04	–	3.0	15.5	37	195	515	70	T1	IIA
ethanethiol	C_2H_5SH	−148	35	2.11	−20	2.8	18	70	460	295	–	T3	IIA
ethanol (ethyl alcohol)	C_2H_5OH	−144	78	1.59	12	3.3	19	67	290	425	75	T2	IIA
ethanolamine (2-aminoethanol)	$NH_2CH_2CH_2OH$	10	172	2.1	85	–	–	–	–	–	–	†	IIA
2-ethoxyethanol	$C_2H_5OCH_2CH_2OH$	–	135	3.1	95	1.8	15.7	–	–	235	–	T3	IIB
ethoxyethyl acetate	$CH_3COOCH_2CH_2OC_2H_5$	–	156	4.6	47	–	–	–	–	380	–	T2	IIA
ethyl acetate	$CH_3COOCH_2CH_3$	−83	77	3.04	−4	2.1	11.5	75	420	460	–	T1	IIA
ethyl acetoacetate	$CH_3COCH_2COOC_2H_5$	–	180	–	(84)	–	–	–	–	295	–	T3	IIB
ethyl acetylene	$C_2H_5C{\equiv}CH$	–	–	–	–	–	–	–	–	–	–	†	IIB
ethyl acrylate	$CH_2{=}CHCOOC_2H_5$	> −75	100	3.45	9	1.8	–	74	–	–	–	†	IIB
ethyl benzene	$C_2H_5C_6H_5$	−95	135	3.66	15	1.0	6.7	44	–	431	–	T2	IIA
ethyl cyclobutane	$C_2H_5CHCH_2CH_2CH_2$	–	–	2.0	< −16	1.2	7.7	–	–	210	–	T3	IIA
ethyl cyclohexane	$C_2H_5CH(CH_2)_4CH_2$	–	131	3.87	14	0.9	6.6	–	–	262	–	T3	IIA
ethyl cyclopentane	$C_2H_5CH(CH_2)_3CH_2$	–	103	3.4	1	1.1	6.7	–	–	260	–	T3	IIA
ethyl formate	$HCOOCH_2CH_3$	−80	54	2.55	< −20	2.7	16.5	80	500	440	–	T2	IIA
ethyl methacrylate	$CH_2{=}CCH_3COOC_2H_5$	–	240	3.9	(20)	–	–	–	–	–	–	†	IIA
ethyl methyl ether	$CH_3OC_2H_5$	–	8	2.087	–	2.0	10.1	49	255	190	–	T4	IIB

ethyldigol	$C_2H_5O(CH_2)_2O(CH_2)_2OH$	–	202	4.62	94	–	–	–	–	–	–	†	IIA
ethylene	$CH_2{=}CH_2$	−169	−104	0.97	–	2.7	34	31	390	425	45	T2	IIB
ethylenediamine (1,2-diaminoethane)	$NH_2CH_2CH_2NH_2$	8	116	2.07	34	–	–	–	–	385	–	T2	IIA
ethylene oxide (epoxy ethane) (oxirane)	CH_2CH_2O	−112	11	1.52	–	3.7	100	55	1820	440	40	T2	IIB
formaldehyde	$HCHO$	−117	−19	1.03	–	7	73	87	910	424	–	T2	IIB
formic acid	$HCOOH$	–	101	1.6	68	–	–	–	–	(520)	–	(T1)	IIA
2-furaldehyde (furfuraldehyde)	$OCH{=}CHCH{=}CCHO$	–	161	3.3	60	2.1	19.3	–	–	315	–	T2	IIA
furan	$CH{=}CHCH{-}CHO$	–	–	–	60	–	–	–	–	–	–	†	IIA
heptane	C_7H_{16}	−91	98	3.46	−4	1.1	6.7	46	280	215	75	T3	IIA
heptan-1-oI	$C_7H_{15}OH$	−34	176	4.03	60	–	–	–	–	–	–	†	IIA
heptan-2-one (amyl methyl ketone)	$CH_3CO(CH_2)_4CH_3$	−35	151	3.94	(49)	–	–	–	–	–	–	†	IIA
hept-2-ene (2-heptene)	$CH_3(CH_2)_3CH{=}CHCH_3$	–	–	–	<0	–	–	–	–	–	–	†	IIA
hexane	$CH_3(CH_2)_4CH_3$	−95	69	2.97	−21	1.2	7.4	42	265	233	75	T3	IIA
hexan-2-one (butyl methyl ketone)	$CH_3CO(CH_2)_3CH_3$	−56	28	3.46	23	1.2	8	50	330	(530)	–	(T1)	IIA
hydrogen cyanide	HCN	–	26	0.90	−18	5.6	40	–	–	(538)	–	(T1)	IIB
hydrogen sulphide	H_2S	−86	−60	1.19	–	4.3	45.5	60	650	270	–	T3	IIB
hydrogen (see clause **37**)	H_2	−259	−253	0.07	–	4.0	75.6	3.3	64	560	21	T1	IIC
4-hydroxy-4-methylpentan-2-one	$CH_3COCH_2C(CH_3)_2OH$	−47	166	4.0	58	1.8	6.9	–	–	680	–	T1	IIA
isopentane (2-methylbutane)	$(CH_3)_2CHCH_2CH_3$	–	–	–	< −51	–	–	–	–	–	–	†	IIA
isopropyl nitrate	$(CH_3)_2CHONO_2$	–	105	–	20	2	100	–	–	175	–	T4	IIB
iso-octane	$(CH_3)_2CHCH_2C(CH_3)_3$	–	–	–	−12	–	–	–	–	411	–	T2	IIA

(continued overleaf)

Table 4.1 *(continued)*

1	2	3	4	5	6	7	8	9	10	11	12	13	14
Flammable materials	Formula	Melting point	Boiling point	Relative vapour density	Flash point	Flammable limits				Ignition temperature	Minimum igniting current	T class of suitable apparatus	Apparatus group
						LFL	UFL	LFL	UFL				
		°C	°C		°C	Vol.%	Vol.%	mg/L	mg/L	°C	mA		
kerosine	Mixture	–	150	–	38	0.7	5	–	–	210	–	T3	IIA
(*RS*)-*P*-mentha-1,8-diene (dipentene)	$C_{10}H_{16}$	−75	175	4.66	42	0.7	6.1	–	–	237	–	†	IIA
metaldehyde	$(C_2H_4O)_4$	246¶	112*	6.07	36	–	–	–	–	–	–	†	IIA
methane (firedamp) (see **7.4.1**)	CH_4	−182	−161	0.55	–	5	15	–	–	595	85	T1	I
methane(industrial) (see clause **37**)	CH_4	–	–	–	–	–	–	–	–	–	–	T1	IIA
methanol	CH_3OH	−98	65	1.11	11	6.7	36	73	350	455	70	T1	IIA
2-methoxyethanol	$CH_3OCH_2CH_2OH$	−86	124	2.63	39	2.5	14	80	630	285	–	T3	IIB
methyl acetate	CH_3COOCH_3	−99	57	2.56	−10	3.1	16	95	500	475	–	T1	IIA
methyl acetoacetate	$CH_3CO_2CH_2COCH_3$	–	170	4.0	67	–	–	–	–	280	–	T3	IIA
methyl acetylene	$CH_3C{\equiv}CH$	–	−23	1.4	–	1.7	–	–	–	–	–	†	IIB
methyl acrylate	$CH_2{=}CHCOOCH_3$	< −75	80	3.0	−3	2.8	25	100	895	–	–	†	IIB
methyl cyclobutane	$CH_3CHCH_2CH_2CH_2$	–	–	–	–	–	–	–	–	–	–	†	IIA
methyl cyclohexane	$CH_3CH(CH_2)_4CH_2$	−127	101	3.38	−4	1.15	6.7	45	–	260	–	T3	IIA
methyl cyclohexanol	$C_7H_{13}OH$(isomer not stated)	−38	168	3.95	68	–	–	–	–	295	–	T3	IIA
methyl cyclopentane	$CH_3CH(CH_2)_3CH_2$	–	72	2.9	< −7	–	–	–	–	–	–	†	IIA
methyl formate	$HCOOCH_3$	−100	32	2.07	< −20	5	23	120	570	450	–	T1	IIA
methyl methacrylate	$CH_2{=}CCH_3COOCH_3$	–	–	–	(10)	–	–	–	–	–	–	†	IIA
2-methyl propan-1-ol	$(CH_3)_2CHCH_2OH$	−108	107	2.55	–	1.7	10.9	–	–	408	–	(T2)	IIA

(isobutyl alcohol)													
methyl styrene	C_9H^{10}(isomer not stated)	–	172	4.1	57	0.7	–	–	–	(495)	–	(T1)	IIA
methylamine	CH_3NH_2	−92	−6	1.07	–	5	20.7	60	270	430	–	T2	IIA
4-methylpentan-2-one (isobutyl methyl ketone)	$(CH_3)_2CHCH_2COCH_3$	−80	116	3.45	16	1.4	7.5	–	–	(459)	–	(T1)	IIA
morpholine	$OCH_2CH_2NHCH_2CH_2$	−3	128	3.0	(40)	–	–	–	–	(310)	–	(T2)	IIA
naphtha	Mixture	–	35	2.5	−6	0.9	6	–	–	290	–	T3	IIA
naphthalene	$C_{10}H_8$	80	218	4.42	77	0.9	5.9	45	320	528	–	T1	IIA
natural gas	Mixture	–	–	–	–	–	–	–	–	–	–	T1	IIA
nitrobenzene	$C_6H_5NO_2$	6	211	4.25	88	1.8	–	90	–	480	–	T1	IIA
nitroethane	$C_2H_5NO_2$	−90	115	2.58	27	–	–	–	–	410	–	T2	IIB
nitromethane	CH_3NO_2	−29	101	2.11	36	–	–	–	–	415	–	T2	IIA
1-nitropropane	$C_3H_7NO_2$	−108	131	3.06	49	–	–	–	–	420	–	T2	IIB
nonane	C_9H_{20}	−54	151	4.43	30	0.8	5.6	37	300	205	–	T3	IIA
nonanol**	$C_9H_{19}OH$	–	178	4.97	75	0.8	6.1	–	–	–	–	†	IIA
n-hexanol††	$C_6H_{13}OH$	−45	157	3.5	63	1.2	–	–	–	–	–	†	IIA
octaldehyde	$C_7H_{15}CHO$	–	163	4.42	52	–	–	–	–	–	–	†	IIA
octane	$CH_3(CH_2)_6CH_3$	−56	126	3.93	13	1.0	3.2	–	–	210	–	T3	IIA
octanol‡‡	$C_8H_{17}OH$	−16	195	4.5	81	–	–	–	–	–	–	†	IIA
paraformaldehyde	poly(CH_2O)	–	25	–	70	–	–	–	–	300	–	T2	IIB
paraldehyde (2,4,6-trimethyl-1,3,5-trioxane)	$(CH_3CHO)_3$	12	124	4.56	17	1.3	–	70	–	235	–	T3	IIA
pentane (mixed isomers)	C_5H_{12}	−130	36	2.48	< −20	1.4	8.0	41	240	285	73	T3	IIA
pentane-2,4-dione (acetylacetone)	$CH_3COCH_2COCH_3$	−23	140	3.5	34	1.7	–	–	–	340	–	T2	IIA
pentanol(mixed isomers)	$C_5H_{11}OH$	−78	138	3.04	34	1.2	10.5	44	380	300	–	T2	IIA
pentylacetate	$CH_3COOC_5H_1$	−78	147	4.48	25	1.0	7.1	60	550	375	–	T2	IIA
petroleum	Mixture	–	–	–	< −20	–	–	–	–	–	–	T3	IIA
phenol	C_6H_5OH	41	182	3.24	75	–	–	–	–	605	–	T1	IIA

(continued overleaf)

Table 4.1 *(continued)*

1	2	3	4	5	6	7	8	9	10	11	12	13	14
Flammable materials	Formula	Melting point	Boiling point	Relative vapour density	Flash point	Flammable limits				Ignition temperature	Minimum igniting current	T class of suitable apparatus	Apparatus group
						LFL	UFL	LFL	UFL				
		°C	°C		°C	Vol.%	Vol.%	mg/L	mg/L	°C	mA		
propane	$CH_3CH_2CH_3$	−188	−42	1.56	–	2.0	9.5	39	180	470	70	T1	IIA
propanethiol (propyl mercaptan)	C_3H_7SH	–	–	–	–	–	–	–	–	–	–	†	IIB
propan-1-ol (propyl alcohol)	$(CH_3)_2CH_2OH$	−126	97	2.07	15	2.15	13.5	50	340	405	–	T2	IIB
propan-2-ol (isopropyl alcohol)	$(CH_3)_2CHOH$	−86	83	2.07	12	2.0	12	–	–	425	–	T2	IIA
propene	$CH_2{=}CHCH_3$	−185	−48	1.5	–	2.0	11.7	35	210	(455)	–	(T1)	IIA
propylacetate	$CH_3COOCH_2CH_2CH_3$	–	–	–	14	–	–	–	–	–	–	†	IIA
propylamine	$CH_3(CH_2)_2NH_2$	−101	32	2.04	< −20	2.0	10.4	49	260	(320)	–	(T2)	IIA
pyridine	Mixture	−42	115	2.73	17	1.8	12.0	56	350	550	–	T1	IIA
p-cymene	$CH_3C_6H_4CH(CH_3)_2$	−70	177	4.62	47	0.7	5.6	–	–	435	–	T2	IIA
styrene	$C_6H_5CH{=}CH_2$	−31	145	3.6	30	1.1	8.0	45	350	490	–	T1	IIA
tetrafluoroethylene	$CF_2{=}CF_2$	–	–	–	–	–	–	–	–	–	–	†	IIB
tetrahydrofuran	$CH_2(CH_2)_2CH_2O$	−108	64	2.49	−17	2.0	11.8	46	360	224	–	T3	IIB
tetrahydrofurfuryl alcohol	$OCH_2CH_2CH_2CHCH_2OH$	–	178	3.52	70	1.5	9.7	60	410	280	–	T3	IIB

terahydrothiophen	$CH_2(CH_2)_2CH_2S$	–	–	–	–	–	–	–	–	–	–	†	IIA
3a,4,7,7a-tetrahydro-4,7-methanoindene	$CHCH{=}CHCH_2CHCHCH{=}CHCHCH_2$	–	–	–	(32)	–	–	–	–	–	–	†	IIA
thiophene	$CH{=}CHCH{=}CHS$	–	84	2.90	–1	–	–	–	–	–	–	†	IIA
toluene	$C_6H_5CH_3$	−95	111	3.18	6	1.2	7	46	270	535	–	T1	IIA
toluidine§§	$CH_3C_6H_4NH_2$	−16	200	3.7	85	–	–	–	–	480	–	T1	IIA
triethylamine	$(C_2H_5)_3N$	−115	89	3.5	0	1.2	8	50	340	405	–	T2	IIA
α, α, α-trifluorotoluene	$C_6H_5CF_3$	–	102	5.0	12	–	–	–	–	–	–	†	IIA
trimethylamine	$(CH_3)_3N$	−117	3	2.04	–	2.0	11.6	49	285	(190)	–	(T4)	IIA
trimethylbenzene	$C_6H_3(CH_3)_3$	−45	165	4.15	–	–	–	–	–	470	–	T1	IIA
1,3,5,-trioxane	$OCH_2OCH_2OCH_2$	62	115	3.11	(45)	3.6	29	135	1110	410		T2	IIB
turpentine	Mixture	–	149	–	35	0.8	–	–	–	254	–	T3	IIA
vinyl acetate	$CH_3COOCH{=}CH_2$	–	–	–	−7	–	–	–	–	–	–	†	IIA
xylene (see clause **37**)	$C_6H_4(CH_3)_2$	−25	144	3.66	30	1.0	6.7	44	335	464	–	T1	IIA

*Sublimation temperature.
†T class data not available. Seek expert advice.
‡Applicable to both *trans* and *cis* forms.
§Data relate only to *m*-cresol; *o*-cresol is less hazardous.
‖Data relate to ortho form. *N,N*-dimethylaniline is slightly more hazardous (lower flash point).
¶In an enclosed vessel.
**Data relate to the form *di*-isobutyl carbinol but data for nonan-1-ol are close.
††Data relate to hexan-1-ol. Where data are available for other isomers they are similar.
‡‡Data relate to octan-1-ol. Data for other isomers give higher flash point.
§§Data relate to both ortho and para forms.
Classes in brackets have been derived using non standard means.

Note: The presence of impurities can affect the various properties.

Because several assumptions have been made and the point of change from one equation to the other (Equation 4.1 to Equation 4.3) the results of the two equations will be seen to vary but only by less than 5 per cent at the point of changeover and this will result in a small variation in the actual hazardous area defined. The changeover from Equation 4.1 to Equation 4.3 is quite rapid at $2 \times 10^5\,\mathrm{N/m^2}$ and, because of the small variation produced at critical pressure, utilizing either equation at the pressure related to the critical pressure ratio produces an acceptable result for mass of gas released in view of the type of exercise in which we are involved. It is, however, recommended that Equation 4.3 is used up to and including pressures of $2 \times 10^5\,\mathrm{N/m^2}$.

Calculation of the extents of hazardous areas is dependent upon the velocity of air at the point of leakage and the quantity of air which is available as, if sufficient air is not available, the leak will steadily increase the amount of flammable gas or vapour in air at any point and progressively increase the extent of the hazardous area throughout the period of leakage until equilibrium is reached. Therefore, the calculative methods described in this chapter (with the exception of those given in 4.4) are generally only valid in areas which are very well ventilated and where a large amount of unconfined air is available. This tends to limit the application of the equations given for calculating the extent of hazardous areas to outdoor areas or other areas with similar levels of ventilation.

If the release velocity of the flammable gas is high compared to the typical wind or ventilation velocity in the circumstances described above, the release will provide all the necessary energy for the necessary mixing to achieve the necessary dilution but, if the release velocity is low, then mixing will be due to the local wind conditions. In Europe these are normally considered to be of the order of 0.5 – 2 m/s. Because of the nature of release the effective cross-sectional area of the gas jet is normally less than the orifice cross-sectional area and the release velocity is higher than might at first be thought. This effect is, of course, taken care of in the derivation of Equations 4.1 and 4.3. A further problem is that the gas or vapour expands as soon as it leaves the leak orifice and it can be assumed that at, and above, an upstream pressure equal to the critical pressure the release velocity can be demonstrated to be at least at sonic velocity (e.g., the velocity of sound in the gas or vapour in question in the prevailing conditions). The gas or vapour will expand almost instantly on release and will leave the release orifice at around the speed of sound in the gas or vapour which velocity is given by the following equation:

$$v_s = [\delta RT/M]^{0.5} \qquad \mathrm{m/s}$$

where δR = ratio of specific heats

$$v_s = 108[T/M]^{0.5} \qquad \mathrm{m/s}\ \text{(Equation 4.5)}$$

The distance which the jet of gas or vapour will travel before mixing with air causes the resultant mixture to fall below the lower explosive limit

(LEL) in circumstances where the jet is at sonic velocity and is given by the following equation:

$$X = [2 \times 10^4\ d/EM] \times [\sigma_V/\sigma_a]^{0.5} \qquad m$$

where E = lower explosive limit (LEL) — %
σ_V = gas or vapour density at ambient pressure and temperature — kg/m^3
σ_a = density of air at ambient pressure and temperature — kg/m^3
d = diameter of release orifice corrected for pressure drop to ambient at release — m

Assuming, as previously discussed, sonic velocity, then the corrected orifice diameter is given by:

$$d = [4G/\pi\ \sigma_V\ v_s]^{0.5} \qquad m$$

Substituting for v_s in Equation 4.5 and using $1.2\,kg/m^3$ as the density of air at ambient pressure and temperature the distance to the LEL can be expressed as:

$$X = 2.1 \times 10^3 [G/E^2 M^{1.5} T^{0.5}]^{0.5} \qquad m\ (\text{Equation } 4.6)$$

The above equation remains valid as long as the jet velocity on release is sufficiently high in relation to the typical wind speed specified earlier (0.5 – 2 m/s). Where this is not so the flow of gas or vapour will cease to be the dominant factor and its dispersal will become more and more reliant on the atmospheric conditions local to the release. In the ultimate circumstance where the release has virtually no velocity (i.e., no energy of its own) it becomes more difficult to calculate dispersal and the derivation of the extent of the hazardous area becomes based on the following empirical formula which was produced by experimentation.

$$X = 10.8 [GT/ME]^{0.55} \qquad m\ (\text{Equation } 4.7)$$

This equation can only be used where the upstream pressure is such that the release velocity is not considerably higher than the wind velocity (say more than 20 times) and will not be valid unless that pressure is significantly less than the critical pressure, or the extent of hazardous area produced will be excessively large. The changeover will not be at a specific point but will be progressive. It is difficult to determine this progression as it will vary from gas to gas but Fig. 4.1 provides a graphical progression which will give an acceptable usable solution. This gives a smoothed changeover between Equations 4.6 and 4.7. This figure can be simply used by calculation of the mass release of gas or vapour at the critical pressure, and utilizing the result of this to calculate the extent of the hazardous area using Equation 4.7. This result is then multiplied by a factor produced from Fig. 4.1 for the actual pressure and the gas or vapour in question. It is considered best, although not essential, to utilize Equation 4.3 for calculation of mass

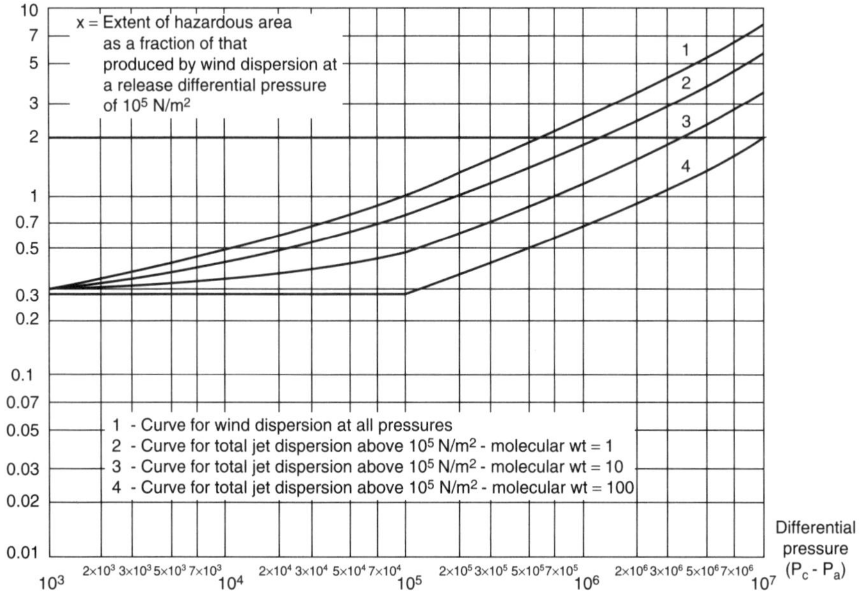

Fig. 4.1

release as, because of the assumptions made in derivation of the equations, it gives the slightly higher value for mass of gas/vapour released. Curve 1 gives the ratio of the extent of a hazardous area for a release at any pressure up to 107 N/m² to that at the critical pressure where dispersion is by the wind and curves 2, 3 and 4 give the ratio of the extent of a hazardous area for a release at any pressure up to 10^7 N/m² where dispersion is by the energy of the jet of gas/vapour alone to that at the critical pressure, where dispersion is by wind action. Curves 2, 3 and 4 are for gases and vapours with molecular weights of 1, 10 and 100 respectively, as the molecular weight has an effect on the extent of the hazardous area produced (not necessary in the case of the wind dispersion curve as the variation of molecular weight is already taken into account in this case). Curves 2, 3 and 4 are also based upon Equations 4.1 and 4.6 above the critical pressure, but below this pressure they are an estimate of the mixed effect of partial internal energy dispersion and partial wind dispersion. They will, therefore, give an estimated result below the critical pressure but this will generally be an overestimate, particularly for gases and vapours with high molecular weights. (It should be remembered that critical pressure is 2×10^5 N/m² which means that the effective pressure across the release orifice is half of that.) The calculated extent is in the direction of the jet and so it can be said that if the jet direction is known the hazardous area can be defined as in Fig. 4.2. This is only true where the wind does not play a part (above the critical pressure with no obstructions) and where the jet direction can be defined with confidence. Because of the unknown factors likely to come into

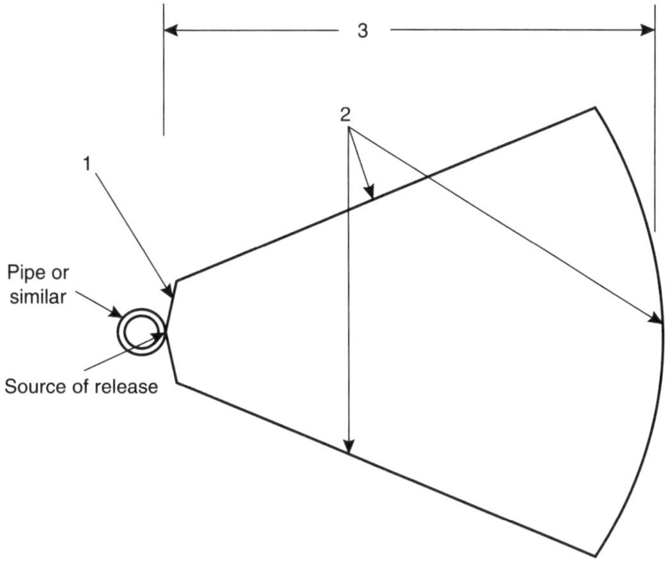

Fig. 4.2 Geometry of gas release formed hazardous area. (1) Rapid gas vapour expansion on release of pressure. (2) Envelope within which explosive atmosphere exists during turbulent mixing with air. (3) Extent of hazardous area (normally added to pipe or similar radius to give sphere radius due to varying orientation of leak)

play it is, however, felt that unless a high degree of confidence exists, the hazardous area should always be a sphere of radius equal to the distance to the lower explosive limit centred on the leak.

Where the release is at a pressure above the critical pressure, and an obstruction is present at a distance less that the distance to the lower explosive limit determined from Equation 4.6, then a composite solution is necessary. As the relationship between distance from release and concentration is linear (see Equation 4.6), Equation 4.8 can be used to determine the percentage of flammable gas/vapour in the mixture at the point of obstruction. (This of course is only necessary at pressures above the critical pressure.) The relationship is as follows:

$$B = 100 - L[(100 - LEL)/X] \qquad \% \text{ (Equation 4.8)}$$

where B = % gas/vapour in air — %
L = Distance to obstruction — m
X = Distance to LEL — m

As the volume ratio is now known a new effective molecular weight can be calculated as follows:

$$M(\text{Mixture}) = [M(\text{Gas}) \times \%(\text{Gas})/100] + [M(\text{Air}) \times \%(\text{Air})/100] \qquad \text{(Equation 4.9)}$$

(For this calculation the molecular weight of air can be taken as 29)

A figure for G of the mixture can now be calculated using the original released mass of gas plus the mass of air which is included in the mixture at the point of obstruction.

$$\text{V (gas)} = 0.082\text{GT/M (gas)}$$

$$\text{V (Mixture)} = \text{V (Gas)} \times [100/\%\,\text{Gas in Mixture}] \quad \text{m}^3 \text{ (Equation 4.10)}$$

$$\text{G (Mixture)} = \text{V (Mixture)} \times 12.19\,\text{M (Mixture)/T} \quad \text{kg (Equation 4.11)}$$

It is now necessary to calculate a new lower explosive limit (LEL) and this can be done simply by the following calculation:

$$\text{LEL (Mixture)} = \text{LEL (Gas} \times [100/\%\,\text{Gas in Mixture)} \quad \% \text{ (Equation 4.12)}$$

These new figures can then be inserted in Equation 4.7 and a distance to the edge of the hazardous area calculated. This distance, added to the distance between the point of release and the obstruction, will then define the extent of the hazardous area in the direction of the obstruction.

A further problem occurs when the release is close to the ground as the dispersion is affected. There are no mathematical procedures for determining the effects of this but the following are typical of the procedures adopted.

First, whatever the release pressure (e.g., above or below that defined by the critical pressure ratio), provided that the lower limit of explosive atmosphere is less than 3 m from the ground then Equation 4.7 should be used in all cases for extent of the hazardous area and the horizontal limits should be projected to the ground. (Chapter 3 deals with the results of this in more detail.)

Second, where the lower extremity of the explosive atmosphere is within 1.5 m of the ground the drift release equation (Equation 4.7) should be used and, again, the extremities of the explosive atmosphere projected to ground level but in this case the ground footprint should be multiplied by 1.5. (Chapter 3 deals with the results of this in more detail.)

Third, where the lower extremity of the explosive atmosphere touches the ground the extent of the hazardous area should be that produced when the result of the drift equation (Equation 4.7) is multiplied by 1.5 to take account of the distorting effect of the ground upon dispersion of gas in all directions. (Chapter 3 deals with the results of this in more detail.)

The above gives a calculative approach which will effectively deal with all normal circumstances where gas or vapour is released, provided that gas or vapour does not have a density dramatically different from air. In the case of sonic releases which are not impeded, and therefore utilize Equations 4.1 and 4.6 density will not have a significant effect for any normal circumstance (including hydrogen) as the energy in the released gas by virtue of its velocity will overcome any significant effect of density differences, but where releases become subsonic (typically where Equations 4.3 and 4.7 are relevant) differences of density will become increasingly relevant. It is difficult to determine the exact effect of these, but as a rule of thumb the vertical extents of explosive atmosphere should be doubled wherever the density is more than 1.5 times the density of air, or less than 0.7 times the density of air. This will mean, for instance, doubling the upward extent for such gases as hydrogen in such circumstances and doubling the downward direction for such gases as pentane – indeed this latter will apply for most of the hydrocarbon gases

4.1.1 Examples of gas and vapour release

Example 1

A pipe flange gasket fails producing an orifice of $4 \times 10^{-5}\,m^2$. The contained gas is ethylene (M = 28) and the pressure inside the pipe is $4 \times 10^5\,N/m^2$. Ambient temperature is 22 °C. The contained gas is at ambient temperature. Assuming the jet direction cannot be defined with confidence, what will be the hazardous area surrounding the pipejoint? The lower explosive limit of ethylene in air at 22 °C temperature and atmospheric pressure is 2.7 per cent.

The release pressure is in excess of critical pressure and thus:

$$G = 0.006aP\,(M/T)^{0.5} \qquad \text{kg/s (Equation 4.1)}$$

$$G = 0.006 \times 4 \times 10^{-5} \times 3 \times 105\,(28/295)^{0.5} \qquad \text{kg/s}$$

$$\underline{G = 0.03\ \text{kg/s}}$$

Dispersal is by jet energy and so distance to LEL is:

$$X = 2.1 \times 10^3 (G/E^2 \times M^{1.5} \times T^{0.5})^{0.55} \qquad \text{m (Equation 4.6)}$$

$$X = 2.1 \times 10^3 (0.03/2.7^2 \times 28^{1.5} \times 295^{0.5})^{0.55} \qquad \text{m}$$

$$\underline{X = 2.7\ \text{m}}$$

The hazardous area will be a sphere extending 2.7 m from the source of release in all directions.

Example 2

An obstruction is present at a horizontal distance of 1 m from the leak location described in example 1. What will the extent of the hazardous are be? The mass release remains at 0.03 kg/s as in the first example and it is necessary to calculate the amount of gas in the mixture at the obstruction as follows:

$$B = 100 - (100 - \text{LEL})\,L/X \qquad \text{\%(Equation 4.8)}$$

$$B = 100 - (100 - 2.7)1/27 \qquad \%$$

$$\underline{B = 64\,\%}$$

The volume release rate of gas at the point of leakage will be:

$$V = 0.082GT/M \quad m^3/s \text{ (Equation 4.4)}$$

$$V = 0.082 \times 0.03 \times 295/28 \quad m^3/s$$

$$\underline{V = 0.026\,m^3/s}$$

The volume of the gas/air mixture at the point of obstruction will be:

$$V_m = V \times (100/\%\,\text{gas in mixture}) \quad m^3/s \text{ (Equation 4.10)}$$

$$V_m = 0.026 \times 100/57.7 \quad m^3/s$$

$$\underline{V_m = 0.04\,m^3/s}$$

The molecular weight of the mixture at the point of obstruction needs now to be calculated and is given by the following:

$$M_m = [M_{gas} \times (\%\,\text{gas}/100)] + [M_{air} \times (\%\,\text{air}/100)] \quad \text{(Equation 4.9)}$$

$$M_m = [28 \times (64/100)] + [27 \times (36/100)]$$

$$\underline{M_m = 27.6}$$

Rearranging Equation 4.4 to give Equation 4.10, the mass of mixture at the point of obstruction is as follows:

$$G_m = 0.04 \times 12.19 \times 27.6/295 \quad kg/s$$

$$\underline{G_m = 0.04\,kg/s}$$

In addition, the new LEL will need to be calculated as follows:

$$LEL_m = LEL \times (100/\%\,\text{gas in mixture}) \quad \% \text{ (Equation 4.12)}$$

$$LEL_m = 2.7 \times (100 \div 57.7) \quad \%$$

$$\underline{LEL = 4.68\,\%}$$

The foregoing figures can now be inserted into Equation 4.7 to give the extent of the hazardous area beyond the obstruction as follows:

$$X_m = 10.8\,(0.046 \times 295/27.6 \times 4.21)^{0.55} \quad m$$

$$\underline{X_m = 3.3\text{ m}}$$

The hazardous area in the direction of the obstruction will, therefore, extend to 4.3 m from the source of leakage and vertically upwards and downwards from the obstruction for 3.3 m if this is larger than the vertical extent derived from the basic release ignoring the effect of the obstruction (see Equation 4.7). No adjustment for relative density is necessary but any effects due to ground proximity need to be taken into account.

4.2 Release of liquid below its atmospheric boiling point

The release of a liquid below its atmospheric boiling point from an orifice will take the form of a jet or, where the upstream pressure is sufficiently high, a mist. The classic formula for release of a liquid from an orifice or nozzle is as follows:

$$G = Ca[2\sigma_1(P - 10^5]^{0.5} \qquad \text{kg/s}^4$$

where G = Mass release — kg/s
a = Orifice area — m^2
p = Upstream pressure — N/m^2
C = Discharge coefficient — –
σ_1 = Liquid density at atmospheric conditions — kg/m^3

As before, C has a maximum value of around 0.8 and therefore the equation becomes:

$$G - 1.13\ a\ [\sigma_1(P - 10^5]^{0.5} \qquad \text{kg/s (Equation 4.13)}$$

If no mist is formed then no significant hazardous area will surround the leak (unless liquid is further contained around the point of leakage) and a liquid jet will exit the orifice, forming a pool of liquid where it reaches the floor or ground. The time taken for this jet to reach the ground can be calculated using Newton's Laws of Motion:

Using $v = u + at$, where v is the final velocity, u is the initial velocity, and a is the acceleration due to gravity, the following is the case for a jet released at an angle above horizontal:

$$v\ \sin\Phi - gt_1 = 0$$

where Φ = Angle of release above horizontal
g = Gravity acceleration ($9.81\,m/s^2$)
t_1 = Time to apex of jet (final velocity = 0 at apex)

Alternatively:

$$t_1 = v\sin\Phi/g \qquad \text{Secs}$$

Using the relationship $v^2 = u^2 + 2gS$, where S is the vertical distance above the release point which the apex reaches,

$$(v\sin\Phi)^2 - 2 \times g \times S = 0$$

$$S = (v\sin\Phi)^2/2\,g \qquad \text{m}$$

If the initial release is at height h then the total height becomes $[h + (v\sin\Phi)^2/2\,g]$ and the time for the jet to reach the ground or floor can be calculated using the relationship;

$$S = ut + 0.5gt^2$$

where u = 0

Thus:

$$[h + (v \sin \Phi)^2/2g] = 0.5 \times g \times t^2$$

$$t^2 = 2h/g = (v \sin \Phi)^2/g^2 \qquad \text{s}$$

$$t^2 = [2h/g = (v \sin \Phi)^2/g^2]^{0.5} \qquad \text{s}$$

Adding this to t_1 and rationalizing this, gives a total time t as follows:

$$t = [(2gh + v^2 \sin^2 \Phi)^{0.5} + v \sin \Phi]/g \qquad \text{s}$$

As the horizontal element of velocity is $v \cos \Phi$ where Φ is the angle of release above horizontal, the distance travelled by the liquid jet neglecting the friction of the air through which it moves will be;

$$= v \cos \Phi(2gh + v^2 \sin^2 \Phi)^{0.5} + v \sin \Phi]/g \qquad \text{m (Equation 4.14)}$$

where the jet is horizontal, $\sin \Phi = 0$ and $\cos \Phi = 1$ which simplifies the equation to:

$$X = (2v^2h/g)^{0.5} \qquad \text{m (Equation 4.15)}$$

It is recommended that this simplified equation is used wherever the jet release direction is not specified, as the equations are idealized and it is unlikely that the release will in fact be ideal. Therefore all that is produced is an estimate and, because of the turbulence in a jet which is not an ideal orifice, the horizontal figure will in most cases give a distance which is larger than that which will practically occur. Where this is not so, however, then Equation 4.14 should be differentiated for a maximum and the angle giving the maximum introduced into Equation 4.14 to obtain the necessary distance.

Where the jet is directed at an angle below the horizontal, the equation changes to the following:

$$X = v \cos \Phi[(v \sin \Phi - 2gh)^{0.5} - v \sin \Phi]/g \qquad \text{m (Equation 4.16)}$$

From Equation 4.13:

$$\text{Velocity} = 1.13[(P - 10^5)/\sigma_1]^{0.5} \qquad \text{m/s (Equation 4.17)}$$

The distance travelled by the jet before it reaches the ground can now be calculated but it is difficult to define the angle which gives the maximum range for a leak which is not directionally defined (the normal case), and also it may not be possible on occasion to confirm that the jet will not be ideal. To overcome this the differentiation approach described earlier will be necessary. At the point where the jet lands a pool will form and, if not physically contained, will increase in size until the evaporation rate from its surface is equal to the release rate from the leak orifice.

The evaporation rate from a pool is given by the following equation:

$$G = A\ kg\ \blacktriangle p\ M \qquad \text{kg/s (Equation 4.18)}$$

where G = vapourization rate kg/s
A = pool area m^2
$\blacktriangle p$ = partial pressure of vapour over liquid as a fraction of atmospheric pressure
kg = overall mass transfer coefficient

This equation can be converted into a volume vaporization rate by using Equation 4.4 and results in the following volume vaporization rate:

$$Q = 8.2A\ kg\ \blacktriangle pT/10^2 \qquad m^3/s \text{ (Equation 4.19)}$$

where T = ambient temperature k

The partial pressure of vapour above a liquid is also known as its vapour pressure and below boiling point is a fraction of atmospheric pressure, which also indicates the ratio of vapour to air. Where this is not known an estimation can often be made using the figures in Table 4.2.

Table 4.2 Vapour (partial) pressure of liquids at various ambient temperatures

Liquid boiling point(°C)	Vapour (partial) pressure as a fraction of atmospheric pressure				
	T_a = 32 °C	T_a = 40 °C	T_a = 60 °C	T_a = 80 °C	T_a = 100 °C
35 °C	0.96	1	1	1	1
40 °C	0.76	1	1	1	1
50 °C	0.54	0.72	1	1	1
60 °C	0.38	0.56	1	1	1
70 °C	0.26	0.42	0.72	1	1
80 °C	0.18	0.3	0.56	1	1
90 °C	0.13	0.2	0.42	0.72	1
100 °C	0.092	0.14	0.3	0.56	1
110 °C	0.062	0.1	0.2	0.42	0.72
120 °C	0.042	0.072	0.14	0.3	0.56
130 °C	0.028	0.058	0.1	0.2	0.42
140 °C	0.018	0.027	0.072	0.14	0.3
150 °C	0.01	0.018	0.058	0.1	0.2

Note 1 The values in the table are approximate only.
Note 2 T_a is ambient temperature.
Note 3 Figures are typical for hydrocarbons. Other materials are likely to be lower in general.

These figures are derived from a monograph by Lippincott and Lyman[6]. If the partial pressure is known, however, it should be used, as the simplification executed will give answers which are higher than the actual figure in accordance with the estimation procedure used throughout this book.

The mass transfer coefficient kg can be found from the following formula:

$$kg = 3.6\ 10^{-2}\ Gm/ß^{0.67}\ R^{0.2}\ M \qquad \text{(Equation 4.20)}$$

where ß = schmidt number (kinematic viscosity of material divided by diffusivity of vapour in air)
R = Reynolds number
G_m = mass flow of air — kg-mole/s

The classic formula for Reynolds number is:

$$R = v\ d\ \sigma/\tau$$

where v = air velocity — m/s
d = characteristic dimension — m
σ = density of air at ambient temperature and pressure — kg/m^2
τ = absolute viscosity of air — Ns/m^2

Using the kinematic viscosity this equation simplifies to:

$$R = v\ d/\tilde{n}$$

where ñ = kinematic viscosity — m^2/s

Taking the wind velocity as 2 m/s and the kinematic viscosity of air as 1.5 $\times 10^{-5}$ this simplifies to:

$$R = 1.33\ d\ 10^5 \qquad \text{(Equation 4.21)}$$

As *R* is the only parameter subject to significant change with pool size then:

$$Kg = 2 \times 10^{-3}/R^{0.2}$$

We can now calculate the mass of vapour released from the pool using Equation 4.18 as follows:

$$G = 2 \times 10^{-3}\ A\ \blacktriangle p\ M/R^{0.2} \qquad kg/s$$

(Figure 4.3 gives values of $R_{0.2}$ for various pool sizes.)

This must equal the release rate of liquid from Equation 4.13 and thus the following relationship must be true if the pool size is not restricted physically:

$$1.13\ a\ [\sigma_1(P - 10^5)]^{0.5} = 2 \times 10^{-3} A\ \blacktriangle p\ M/R^{0.2} \qquad kg/s$$

where A = pool area — m^2
a = leak orifice area — m^2

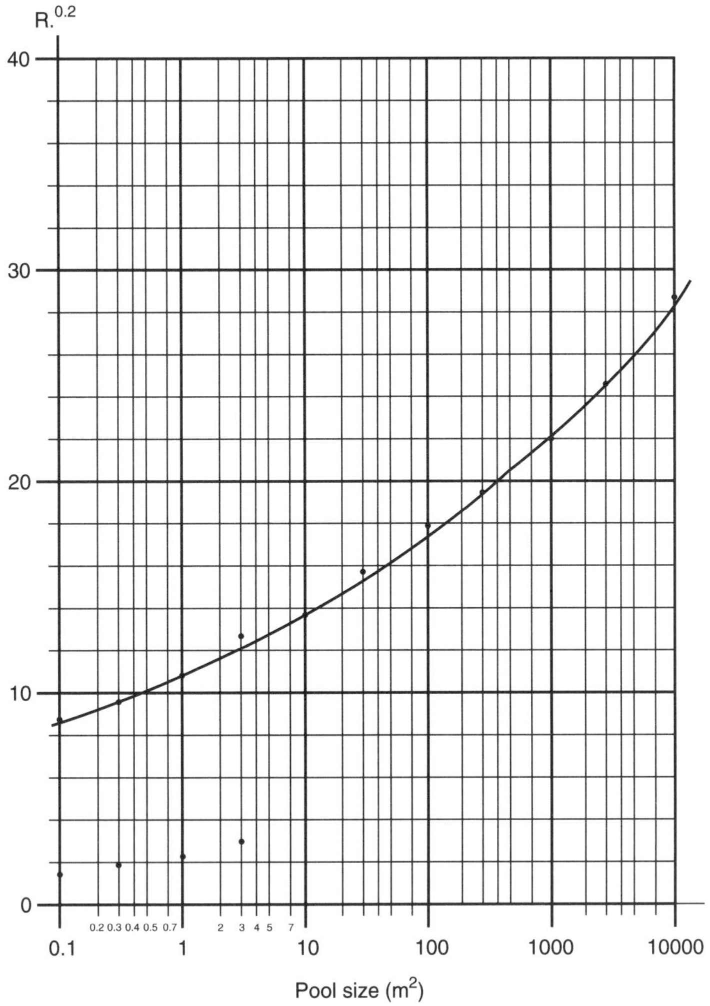

Fig. 4.3 (Reynolds Number $R^{0.2}$ against pool area)

This gives a pool area as follows:

$$A = 5.65 \times 10^2 \text{ a } [\sigma_1(P - 10^5)]^{0.5} R^{0.2} \blacktriangle p \text{ M} \qquad m^2 \text{ (Equation 4.23)}$$

The equation for extent of the hazardous area is again empirical and is:

$$X = [625 \text{ Q/LEL(mixture)} \times \text{source length}]^{1.14} \qquad \text{m (Equation 4.24)}$$

From Equation 4.19 the volume release of gas is as follows:

$$Q_g = 1.64 \times 10^{-4} A \blacktriangle p \text{ T}/R^{0.2} \qquad m^3/s$$

Thus the total volume of mixture leaving the pool edge is given by Q_m (volume of air plus gas mixture):

$$m = Q_a + Q_g \qquad m^3/s \text{ (Equation 4.25)}$$

where Q_a = volume of air leaving pool m^3

The percentage gas in the mixture leaving the pool then is:

$$Q_g \times 100/(Q_a + Q_g) \qquad \%$$

Using Equation 4.12:

$$LEL_m = LEL_g(Q_g + Q_a)/Q_g \qquad \%$$

The source length is half the perimeter of the pool and this equals $\pi d/2$. Expressed as area, this is 1.77 $A^{0.5}$. The volume of air flowing over the pool is assumed as given above (Qa). Substituting in Equation 4.24 gives the following hazardous area beyond the pool edge:

$$X = \{[625(Q_a + Q_g)Q_g]/[LEL(Q_a + Q_g) \times 1.77A^{0.5}]\}^{1.14} \qquad m$$

$$X = [353 \times Q_g/LEL \times A^{0.5}]1.14 \qquad m$$

Substituting the Equation for Q_g this becomes:

$$X = [353 \times 1.64 \times 10^{-4} \times A^{0.5} \times \blacktriangle p \times T/LEL_g \times R^{0.2}]^{1.14} \qquad m$$

$$X = [5.8\ A^{0.5}\ \blacktriangle p\ T/10^2\ LEL_g\ R^{0.2}]^{1.14} \qquad m$$

where LEL_g = lower explosive limit of vapour %
A = pool area m
$\blacktriangle p$ = partial pressure as a fraction of atmosphere
T = temperature K
R = reynolds number for airflow (Equation 4.26)

The above equation gives the horizontal extent of hazardous area from the edge of the pool which should also be used for the vertical extent. There remains the problem of mist and this is very difficult to quantify. Mists have been shown to be formed at pressures as low as $3 \times 10^5\ N/m^2$ and thus it cannot be assumed that no mist will be formed from any leak of liquid above the critical pressure ($2 \times 10^5\ N/m^2$). Thus the only method is to assume the worst case unless precautions are taken to avoid mist production. This means that the entire leak should be assumed to evaporate and Equation 4.4 should be used to determine the vapour equivalent this would have. Equations 4.6 and 4.7 can then be used to determine the extent of the hazardous area which will occur around the point of leakage. This will generally produce a result which is much more onerous than what will actually occur but, unless clear evidence as to the extent of formation of a flammable mist and its ignition limits is available in a particular case, it is hard to see how any alternative action can be taken.

4.2.1 Example of liquid release below its atmospheric boiling point

Example 3

Acetone is transported in a pipe with normal flanged joints at 22 °C and is at a guage pressure of $10^5\,N/m^2$. A failure in one of the flanged joints occurs and presents an orifice of $4 \times 10^{-5}\,m^2$. The pipe is some 3 m off the ground.

Relevant parameters of acetone are:

Liquid density	=	$791\,kg/m^3$
Vapour density	=	$2.58\,kg/m^3$
Boiling point	=	56 °C
Partial pressure at 22 °C	=	$2.2 \times 10^4\,N/m^2$ (0.22 Atm.)
Molecular weight	=	58
Lower explosive limit	=	2.1% in air

It is first necessary to calculate the rate of liquid release from the leak and to do this Equation 4.13 is used giving:

$$G = 1.13 \times 4 \times 10^{-5}(791 \times 10^5)^{0.5} \qquad kg/s$$

$$G = 0.4 \qquad kg/s$$

In calculating the extents of hazardous areas created by such a leak two assumptions must be made and the first of these is that the liquid reaches the ground without evaporation. To determine the distance from the leak where the liquid reaches the ground Equation 4.15 is used, with velocity being determined from Equation 4.17 assuming the leak to be horizontal.

$$\text{Velocity of jet} = 1.13(10^5/791)^{0.5} = 12.7 \qquad m/s$$

$$\text{Distance travelled} = (2 \times 12.7^2 \times 3/9.81)^{0.5} \qquad m$$

$$\underline{\text{Distance} = 9.93\,m \text{ (say } 10\,m)}$$

A pool will therefore form with its centre at a horizontal distance of 9.85 m from the point at which a vertical line from the leak orifice strikes the ground. This can be in any compass direction unless the direction of the jet of liquid can be established with confidence. This pool will, unless contained, expand until the vaporization from its surface equals the leakage rate from the orifice. The area of the pool can be calculated from the Equation 4.23 as follows, initially using a median value of 16 for $R^{0.2}$:

$$A = \{5.65 \times 10^2 \times 4 \times 10^{-5}[791 \times 10^5]^{0.5} \times 15\}/0.22 \times 58 \qquad m^2$$

At this size of pool from Fig. 4.3 $R^{0.2}$ is around 19 and so the calculation for pool area should be repeated using this figure and the result is:

$$A = 299 \qquad m^2$$

$$\underline{\text{The pool diameter is thus (d)} = 22\,m}$$

It is now necessary to know how far beyond the edge of (and above) the pool the explosive atmosphere will extend and for this Equation 4.26 is used giving:

$$X = \{[5.8 \times 10^{-2} \times 17.3 \times 0.22 \times 295]/[2.1 \times 19]\}^{1.14}$$

$$X = 1.75 \text{ (say 2)} \qquad \text{m}$$

Thus there will be a hazardous area 2 m high to a distance in all directions of 12 m from the point at which a vertical line from the leak touches the ground. It is now necessary to consider the second assumption which is that the entire release forms a mist but in this case, as the driving pressure is so low, it can be ignored. Thus the following solution holds for this circumstance: There will be no significant hazardous area created around the pipe where the leak occurs but from a point on the ground vertically below the leak a 2 m high hazardous area will exist for a radius of 22 m (10 + 10 + 2).

Example 4

With the same liquid transmission system and leak orifice as that described in example 3, isoprene is transmitted at a gauge pressure of 2×10^5 N/m^2. Temperature is 22 °C as before.

Relevant parameters for isoprene are:

Liquid density	=	680 kg/m^3
Vapour density	=	3 kg/m^3
Boiling point	=	34 °C
Partial pressure	=	7.1×10^4 N/m^2 (0.71 Atm.)
Molecular weight	=	68
Lower explosive limit	=	1 % in air.

The initial approach to this problem is exactly the same as that for Example 3 in that the first action is to determine the mass rate of liquid release using Equation 4.13:

$$G = 1.13 \times 4 \times 10^{-5} \times [680 \times 2 \times 10^5]^{0.5} \qquad \text{kg/s}$$

$$G = 0.53 \qquad \text{kg/s}$$

It is now necessary to determine the distance travelled by the liquid jet before it strikes the ground using Equation 4.15:

$$\text{Velocity of Jet} = 1.13(10^5/680)^{0.5} = 13.7 \qquad \text{m/s}$$

$$\text{Distance} = (2 \times 13.7^2 \times 3/9.81)^{0.5} \qquad \text{m}$$

$$\underline{\text{Distance} = 10.7 \text{ (say 11)}} \qquad \text{m}$$

The pool will now form with its centre at a horizontal distance of 11 m from a point on the ground vertically below the leak orifice. It is now possible using Equation 4.23 (assuming $Re^{0.2} = 15$) to determine the pool area and diameter as follows:

$$A = 5.65 \times 10^2 \times 4 \times 10^{-5} \times [680 \times 2 \times 10^2]^{0.5} \times 15/0.71 \times 68 \qquad m^2$$

$$A = 81.2 \text{ (say 82)} \qquad m^2$$

The figure for $R^{0.2}$ at this size of pool is around 17 and thus the equation should be solved using this figure which will give:-

$$A = 93 \qquad m^2$$

From the normal circular relationship the diameter can be calculated:

$$\underline{d = 11} \qquad m$$

For this part of the exercise it remains only to calculate the extent of the hazardous area from the edge of, and above, the pool using Equation 4.26:

$$X = [5.8 \times 10^{-2} \times 9.6 \times 0.71 \times 295/1 \times 17]^{1.14}$$

$$X = 9 \qquad m$$

Thus there will be, due to the pool and liquid jet, a hazardous area 9 m high for a circle of radius 26 m from a point on the ground vertically below the leak orifice.

We now have to consider, in this case because of the pressure, the possibility of a mist comprising all of the released liquid being formed at the point of leakage. To decide if this release is diluted by wind action or by its own energy it is necessary to determine the velocity of the liquid release as this will give an indication of the effect which the wind will have on dispersion. The velocity of release can, as already indicated, be determined by using equation 4.13 but dividing by σ_1 to convert to volume, and by the orifice area to give velocity. Thus:

$$\text{Velocity} = 13.7 \qquad m/s$$

This is a fairly low velocity and it has to be assumed that the wind will play a large part in dispersion. The hazardous area around the leak orifice has to be assumed to be that which would be produced by total vaporization of the release diluted by wind action. (Equation 4.7). Thus:

$$X = 10.8[0.53 \times 295/68 \times 1]^{0.55} \qquad m$$

$$X = 17 \qquad m$$

As the hazardous area touches the ground then this figure needs to be multiplied by 1.5 as previously stated. Thus:

$$X = 26 \qquad m$$

The hazardous area produced by this example will therefore be a horizontal radius of 26 m to a height of 10 m with a partial sphere above it described by a radius of 26 m from the source of release. This is a very onerous result but, in the absence of knowledge of the release orifice geometry, a necessary one.

4.3 Release of liquid above its atmospheric boiling point

This is the final one of the three 'outdoor' scenarios and addresses a situation where the flammable material would be a vapour in normal ambient circumstances but is maintained as a liquid by the containment pressure. In these circumstances some of the liquid will evaporate on release and the energy necessary to cause this evaporation will so lower the temperature of the remainder that further evaporation will only occur as it gains heat from its environment. It is assumed that this gain will be insignificant during its 'jet' life but rapid as soon as it comes into contact with the ground, due to the short duration of its travel between the point of release and the ground. Once on the ground, however, it is presumed that the assumption of additional energy is so rapid that instant evaporation will take place. The first necessity therefore is to calculate the amount of liquid which will flash off as vapour at the point of release. This is not normally necessary for calculation of the hazardous area at the point of release.

There is a problem in that mist may be formed by the nature of the release and that the hazardous area created by the release will be multiplied by 1.5 to allow for this, unless this would vaporize the whole of the release when this will be assumed to be the case. The fraction of the flammable material reaching the ground is based upon the heat capacity of the material which can be used in the vaporization process before the temperature lowers to boiling point, the latent heat of vaporization of the liquid which identifies the heat required to vaporize it, and the difference between the boiling point of the liquid and its actual temperature, which also identifies the amount of heat available. Thus:

$$\text{Fraction of liquid vaporizing} = [(T_l - T_b)/\delta]C_l \qquad \text{(Equation 4.27)}$$

where T_l =	release temperature of liquid	K
T_b =	boiling point of liquid	K
δ =	latent heat of vaporization	kj/kg
C_l =	liquid heat capacity	kj/kg/K

The release of the liquid is also more complicated as it is possible for vaporization to take place in the leak path if it is long, thus reducing the amount of the release. This can be said to occur where the length of the leak path is greater than 10 × the effective diameter of the leak path (given by the relationship, Diameter = $[4 \times \text{area}/\pi]^{0.5}$ for a non-circular orifice). At and above this figure the release equation is modified as the amount of liquid/vapour released will total significantly less than would be derived from Equation 4.13 which is used where vaporization does not occur in the leak path. In these circumstances the basic equation remains as Equation 4.13 but atmospheric pressure is replaced by P_c where P_c is 0.55 × the saturated vapour pressure of the contained liquid at operating temperature of the process. This may not, of course, be the same as the actual containment pressure, which may be higher if additional external means of pressurization are used but such is not normally the case – the maintenance of the material as liquid being secured by its own vapour pressure acting upon the containment. In addition, the density of the released mixture of combined liquid and vapour is the composite of the two elements of the mixture. Thus:

$$G = 0.8A[2\sigma m(P_1 - P_c)]^{0.5} \qquad \text{kg/s (Equation 4.28)}$$

where A = cross-sectional area of leak — m^2
σ_m = density of released mixture — kg/m^3
P_1 = containment pressure — kg/m^2
P_c = 0.55 × vapour pressure — kg/m^2

In order to calculate σ m it is necessary to investigate the conditions relative to a pressure of P_c and to do this it is necessary to have the vapour pressure curve for the material in question. From this a value can be obtained for the temperature at which a vapour pressure of P_c would be exerted (T_c). This allows the calculation of the fraction of the release which emerges as vapour as follows:

$$M_g = (T_1 - T_c)C_l/L \qquad \text{(Equation 4.29)}$$

where M_g = fraction of mass release which is vapour
T_1 = process temperature — K
T_c = temperature giving P_c — K
C_l = heat capacity of liquid — kj/kg °C
δ = latent heat of vaporization — kj/kg

This allows the density of the mixture to be calculated as follows:

$$\sigma_m = 1/[(M_g/\sigma_v) + \{(1 - M_g)/\sigma_l\}] \qquad kg/m^3 \text{ (Equation 4.30)}$$

where σ_m = density of released mixture — kg/m^3
σ_v = density of vapour at T_1 — kg/m^3
σ_l = density of liquid at T_1 — kg/m^3

The results of these equations allow the velocity of release to be calculated, together with the amount of liquid in the jet. This jet can then be treated using Equations 4.14, 4.15 or 4.16 as appropriate. The amount of liquid reaching the ground is then assumed to evaporate instantly and the extent of the hazardous area due to this calculated using Equation 4.7, corrected for a low-level point source.

4.3.1 Example of liquid release above its atmospheric boiling point

Example 5

Liquid propylene is contained in a vessel at a temperature of 15 °C and a pressure equal to its own vapour pressure at that temperature. It leaks down a drain line of 0.019 m bore ($2.8 \times 10^{-4}\,m^2$ area) and 0.3 m length.

Basic information is as follows:-

Storage pressure (vapour pressure)	=	$8.94 \times 10^5\,N/m^2$
Process temperature	=	288 K
Material boiling point	=	225 K
Temperature to give P_c	=	267 K
Latent heat of vaporization	=	469 kj/kg
Heat capacity of liquid at 288 K	=	2.26 kj/kg/K
Liquid density	=	$520\,kg/m^3$
Vapour density	=	$9.43\,kg/m^3$
Molecular weight	=	42
Lower explosive limit	=	2% in air

Due to the relationship between the drain length and its bore vaporization will take place within the leak path and thus the fluid leaking will be a mixture of vapour and liquid. In such cases it is necessary to calculate a density for the mixture and the first step is to calculate the amount vaporizing in the leak path. From Equation 4.29 the fraction vaporizing in the leak path as a percentage of leakage is given by:

$$M_g = (288 - 267)2.26/469$$

$$M_g = 0.1$$

Using this fraction the density of the mixture can now be calculated using Equation 4.30 as follows:

$$\sigma_m = 1/[(0.1/9.43) + (0.9/520)] \qquad kg/m^3$$

$$\sigma_m = 81.3 \qquad kg/m^3$$

The fraction of release flashing-off as vapour inside the release orifice and outside at the point of release is given by Equation 4.27 and this gives the following:

$$= (288 - 225)2.26/469 \qquad kg/s$$

We can now calculate the mass release using this density figure in Equation 4.28 as follows:

$$G = 0.8 \times 2.8 \times 10^{-4}[2 \times 81.3(8.94 \times 10^5 - 4.92 \times 10^5)]^{0.5} \qquad kg/s$$

$$\underline{G = 1.81} \qquad kg/s$$

Of this there will be some which appears at the outside of the orifice as vapour and some which will flash-off in the immediate locality of the orifice and this amount is given by Equation 4.27 as follows:

$$G_v = 1.81(288 - 225)2.26/469 \qquad \text{kg/s}$$

$$G_v = 0.55 \qquad \text{kg/s}$$

This gives the liquid which is assumed to reach the ground as:

$$G_l = 1.81 - 0.55 = 1.26 \qquad \text{kg/s}$$

That vaporizing at the orifice will behave as a vapour and will be jet dispersed in accordance with Equation 4.6 as follows:-

$$X = 2.1 \times 10^3(0.56/2^2 \times 42^{1.5} \times 288^{0.5})^{0.5} \qquad \text{m}$$

$$X = 11.5 \text{ (say 12)} \qquad \text{m}$$

Due to the nature of the release it is necessary to assume that some mist will occur and an allowance will be made for this by increasing the distance by 50%. Thus:

$$X = 18 \qquad \text{m}$$

The mass of liquid reaching the ground will be assumed to vaporize immediately and thus no pool will form. The vapour released will be wind dispersed and Equation 4.7 is appropriate. In this case no mist will be assumed.

$$X = 10.8(1.29 \times 288/42 \times 2)^{0.55} \qquad \text{m}$$

$$X = 24.5 \qquad \text{m}$$

The distance travelled by the jet before it reaches the ground is calculated as before. There will be a hazardous area extending 24.5 m plus the distance travelled by the jet before it reaches the ground in a horizontal plane, and there will be a hazardous area around the source of release extending in all above horizontal directions for 18 m which will be projected vertically down to the ground hazardous area.

4.4 Summary of use of equations

The foregoing equations are used as follows:

4.4.1 Gas and vapour releases

First determine the mass release of gas or vapour using Equation 4.1 if the release pressure is greater than $2 \times 10^5\,\text{N/m}^2$, and Equation 4.3 otherwise. Then convert this to a volume using Equation 4.4 If the release pressure is greater than $2 \times 1 - 0^5\,\text{N/m}^2$ calculate the extent of hazardous area using Equation 4.6. If the release pressure is less than $2 \times 10^5\,\text{N/nm}^2$ calculate the extent of hazardous area using Equation 4.7. In all cases multiply the result obtained by 1.5 if the release is within 1.5 m of the ground. If the release is at a pressure greater than $2 \times 10^5\,N/m^2$, but there is an obstruction within the distance calculated using Equation 4.6 then calculate the amount of gas in the mixture using Equation 4.8. Then calculate the molecular weight of the mixture using Equation 4.9 after which the total volume of the gas/air mixture at the obstruction can be calculated using Equation 4.10.

The Lower explosive limits of the mixture when further mixed with air can now be calculated using Equation 4.12, after which the wind dispersal distance can be calculated using Equation 4.7 taking account of the ground proximity. This should be added to the distance between the release and the obstruction to give the extent of the hazardous area from the release point in the direction of the obstruction.

4.4.2 Liquid releases below boiling point

The mass of liquid released is calculated using Equation 4.13. The distance travelled by the jet of liquid is then calculated using Equation 4.15 if the release is above horizontal, or 4.16 if it is below horizontal. If the release trajectory is not known use Equation 4.15. In both cases it is necessary to calculate the release velocity using Equation 4.17. Using Equation 4.19 calculate the vaporization rate and then Equation 4.23 will permit calculation of the pool area. Finally, using Equation 4.26, the extent of the hazardous area above and beyond the pool edge can be calculated.

The hazardous area can then be normally defined as the horizontal distance from the leak to the pool centre, plus the pool radius, plus the extent beyond the pool and the vertical distance just the extent beyond the pool. This takes no account of mists and if these are present they should be assumed as vapour and treated using the procedure in section 4.4.1

4.4.3 Liquid releases above boiling point

It is first necessary to calculate the amount of liquid vaporizing in the leak path using Equation 4.29 and, from this, the amount of vapour in the emerging mixture using Equation 4.27 and mixture density of the gas/liquid mixture emerging from the release using Equation 4.30, after which the mass of mixture released can be calculated using Equation 4.28.

The mass of vapour immediately outside the leak due to that released and that flashing-off immediately can be calculated using Equation 4.27 again, but at atmospheric pressure, and the extent of the hazardous area thus formed can be calculated using Equation 4.6 taking account of ground proximity. This figure is multiplied by a further factor of 1.5 because of the likelihood of mist formation.

The remaining liquid is assumed to reach the ground and the point at which it does is calculated as for liquids below their boiling points, using Equations 4.15 or 4.16 as appropriate.

Vaporization is expected immediately contact is made with the ground and the extent of the hazardous area is calculated as for gas/vapour using Equation 4.7 with the result multiplied by 1.5 because of ground proximity.

The hazardous areas are thus around the leak due to vaporization at the leak, and at ground level with an extent from the leak of the distance travelled by the jet plus the radius of the area created by vaporization at ground level. The height of this will be the radius created by ground level vaporization.

4.5 Releases in areas which are not well ventilated

All of the foregoing calculations depend upon wind reaching all parts at around 2 m/s. In poorly ventilated areas, such as indoors, this wind does not exist in the same form and is replaced by artificial ventilation in most circumstances. In addition, the enclosed volume inside the containment which limits the natural ventilation is not unlimited. Thus all of the foregoing calculations must be considered suspect unless the ventilation in all nooks and crannies of the enclosure can be considered as equivalent to natural ventilation. In BS/EN 60079-10[3] which will replace BS 5345[1] there is an attempt to define more globally the extents of and persistence of explosive atmospheres in a more general set of circumstances and the following equations are based upon that.

In general, therefore, the only way to deal with indoor areas is to install ventilation taking account of the leaks present. The minimum flow of air to dilute a given release of flammable material to below its lower explosive limit is as follows:

$$Q_a = 0.12 \times G_f \times T_a^2/T_o \times M \times LEL \qquad m^3/s \text{ (Equation 4.31)}$$

This simplifies to:

$$Q_a = 0.03 \times G_f \times T_a^2/M \times LEL \qquad m^3/s$$

where
Q_a = theoretical minimum air flowrate required — m^3/s
G_f = maximum mass release rate of flammable material — kg/s
T_a = ambient temperature — K
M = molecular weight of flammable material
LEL = lower explosive limit — % v/v

If Q_a can be related to the number of air changes around the source of release (i.e., the airflow velocity) then a further calculation can be carried out to determine the size of the explosive atmosphere around the gas cloud as follows:

$$V_m = Q_a/C \qquad m^3$$

Because of the degree of uncertainty in this two safety factors need to be added, one for the uncertainty in LEL and another for the uncertainty in ideal airflow. This gives:

$$V_m = Q_a f/C\,k \qquad m^3/s \text{ (Equation 4.32)}$$

where V_m = volume of explosive atmosphere — m^3
Q_a = airflow at leak source — m^3/s
f = Effectiveness of ventilation
(1 = ideal airflow)
(2–4 = intermediate grades of airflow)
(5 = most obstructed airflow)
C = number of air changes per second based on airflow around source of release
k = safety factor applied to LEL
(0.25 for continuous and primary grades of release)
(0.5 for secondary grades of release)

In the case of an enclosed (defined) area, C can be calculated as follows:

$$C = Q_a/V_o \qquad m^3 \text{ (Equation 4.33)}$$

$$V_o = \text{volume of enclosed space}$$

The above equation relates to defined (enclosed) spaces only. For the open-air situation a further equation is derived from Equation 4.32 and is:

$$V_o = Q_a/C\,k \qquad m^3$$

If one takes a volume of air in an unrestricted area (outdoors) of around 1000 m^3 (assumed to be circular as that is the worst case) then it will be swept with air in around 6 seconds (C = 1/6 = 0.16). Thus:

$$V_m = Q_a/0.16\,k \qquad m^3 \text{ (Equation 4.34)}$$

Due to the nature of airflow in outdoor conditions this latter equation is likely to give a pessimistic (overlarge) volume of explosive atmosphere.

The equations in this series also include the following equation which is intended to allow the calculation of dispersion time after the release has stopped:

$$t = (f/C)L_n \text{ (LEL kUL)} \qquad s\ \%\ v/v \text{ (Equation 4.35)}$$

where LEL = lower explosive limit — % v/v
UL = maximum concentration

To assist in the use of this equation where ventilation is poor (indoors where no extra ventilation is added) Table 4.1 may be used. This is derived from a table produced from the guide book of the Building Services Institute[7] which was used to calculate the heating necessary for any building to take account of losses due to natural ventilation occurring.

4.5.1 Example of gas release using BS/EN 10079-10[3] formulae

Example 6

The ethylene release discussed in Example 1 occurs indoors in a building which is well ventilated (i.e., having a factor f of 1). From Example 1 we know that the mass release rate is 0.55 kg/s.

Using equation 4.31 airflow required at leak:

$$Q_a = 0.03 \times 0.475 \times 2952/28 \times 2.7 \qquad \text{m}^3/\text{s}$$

$$Q_a = 16.4 \qquad \text{m}^3/\text{s}$$

This value can now be used in Equation 4.34 to give the maximum volume of flammable atmosphere present in the enclosed space if it is ventilated at the same rate as an open space ventilated by the wind, as follows:

$$Q_m = 16.4/0.16 \times 0.5 \qquad \text{m}^3$$

$$Q_m = 205 \qquad \text{m}^3$$

This volume will give a larger overall hazardous area than would actually exist outdoors (estimated at between 20 m and 45 m in the direction of ventilation flow from the leakage source) as the volume is not a sphere. Thus this equation is not applicable to the outdoor situation but only to enclosed finite spaces where the ventilation conditions are similar.

If we now apply Equation 4.35 to this situation we obtain the persistence time after release ends as follows:

$$t = (1/0.16)L_n(0.5 \times 2.7/100) \qquad \text{s}$$

$$t = 27 \qquad \text{s}$$

Again, this is a very high figure for an outside location but more realistic for an indoor situation where overall volume is more limited.

4.6 Conclusion

This chapter contains a relatively comprehensive set of calculations which may be used for determination of extents of hazardous areas. Those concerned with outdoor areas for vapours and for liquids have been extensively used for several years and basically agree with the subjective judgements found in several codes and thus have some pedigree. The formulae in Section 4.4, however, are newer. Until they have been in use for a considerable time and evidence ammassed, they should be used with extreme care. It is suggested that initially, they are used as yardstick calculations only (i.e., to determine if the persistence time in a particular circumstance would cause a secondary source of release to produce a Zone 1 indoors where it occurs). It is stressed that there is no intent to suggest that they are not accurate, but merely that work needs to be done to increase experience in their use by practicing engineers to further our understanding of the parameters within which they can be used. This set of formulae also will be more difficult to use in cases of liquid release, particularly where that liquid is below its boiling point.

Finally, Table 4.1 is included (Fig. 4.5 from BS 5345 Part 2[1]) and gives some of the information necessary to use the calculative methods used in this chapter. This table also includes two columns titled respectively 'Group' and 'Temperature Class'. These will be described in more detail in Chapter 7 as they refer to apparatus performance. They are listed here to identify the relationship of the explosive atmospheres occurring to the type of apparatus which should be used.

References

1 BS 5345 — Selection, Installation and Maintenance of Electrical Apparatus for use in Potentially Explosive Atmospheres (other than mining applications or explosives processing or manufacture). Part 2 (1983). Classification of hazardous areas.

2 RoSPA/ICI — Engineering Codes and Regulations, Electrical Installations in Flammable Atmospheres (1973). Group C (Electrical), Volume 1.5.

3 BS/EN 60079-10 — Electrical Apparatus for Explosive Atmospheres/ Classification of hazardous areas (1996).

4 — Chemical Engineers Hardbook (Editions 1-6). Latest edition. Edition 6 (1984) R.H. Perry and O. Green.

5 BSI 79/27013 — BSI Committee GEL/114/5 Draft Document produced in preparation of BS 5345.

6 — Lipincott, S.B. and Lyman, M.L. (1946). Vapour Pressure/Temperature Monographs. *Industrial Engineering and Chemistry* (38) **3**.

7 — Chartered Institution of Building Services (1970). Natural Infiltration into Buildings (guide book).

— 5 —

Area classification practice for gases, vapours and mists in areas which are not freely ventilated

In Chapter 3 the effects of releases of flammable materials in freely ventilated areas was considered in much detail. It will be remembered that in such areas there was, theoretically, an unlimited amount of diluting air and much turbulence was produced by normal winds and breezes. While this is useful in the majority of oil-refining installations and other process plants, there are cases where it is necessary to enclose the sources of possible release for operational or other safety reasons. Paint Spraying, for instance, needs a carefully controlled environment and where such things as cyanide are processed it is often necessary to enclose that process as leakage could have catastrophic effects if this were not done. Once a source of release of flammable material is enclosed, however, it is denied the large quantity of diluting air and the natural turbulent conditions present in an outside area, and its dilution and dispersion becomes a more significant problem. Not only is it extremely difficult to introduce sufficient diluting air into an enclosed space to accurately mimic the external situation in all parts of that enclosed space, but it can cause adverse personnel reaction. Typically, in external situations air movement in excess of 1 m/s occurs for much of the time, but in normal indoor conditions an air movement of more than 0.2 m/s in the general space is likely to cause discomfort to those normally working indoors. The problem is, therefore, a complex one to approach.

While places where ventilation is limited tend to be equated with buildings, many places which are not buildings are included in this consideration. Often, such places as tanker loading bays are covered to protect operations from the environment. Where this is done the enclosure is usually just a roof and without walls and in these circumstances, although the ground-level air movement is similar to that which would be expected in a freely ventilated situation, there will be areas near the roof where ventilation is restricted. There are four scenarios in which natural ventilation must be considered as restricted. In such circumstances the important objective is to ensure that such ventilation as exists is used to best effect, and this means that sources of release need to be identified and ventilation arrangements need to take account of their location so that ventilation is best at points where releases can occur.

5.1 Typical areas of restricted ventilation

The following are typical of the areas where ventilation can be expected to be restricted. (restriction will, of course, also appear in other areas).

5.1.1 Open areas surrounded by walls

Where walls are present, containing otherwise open areas, then such walls can restrict ventilation. BS 5345, Part 2[1] suggests that to have an open area, a building should have no walls below a significant height (say 3 m) to be assumed to be freely ventilated but a more relaxed approach is used in a Netherlands Directorate General of Labour Guide[2] which presumes that, provided 50 per cent of a building's walls are open construction, the building is considered as a freely ventilated area if the 50 per cent is evenly distributed over at least three walls and openings are at least 2.5 m high. While differing in approach, both of these statements confirm the fact that walls have an obstructing effect on airflow which must be taken into account.

5.1.2 Covered areas (dutch-barn type)

In areas, such as tanker loading bays, drum storage areas, and the like, it is often necessary to provide a cover to prevent rain penetration. These covers take the form of either flat roofs (e.g., as those on garage forecourts) or hipped roofs (e.g., as those in dutch-barn type construction), the latter often having apex vents. Both of these types of cover have a possibly deleterious effect on airflow, even though there are no walls in such cases. The degree of effect depends upon the flammable gas or vapour being handled and the height of the cover, even though the open wall requirements specified above are met.

5.1.3 Above-ground rooms

Above-ground rooms constitute a room which has four walls and a roof with no effective deliberate ventilation. In such cases there will be air movement by natural ventilation via cracks in the structure or around doors and windows, etc. Table 4.2 shows the level of ventilation which may be expected in such cases and this will be seen as airflow equivalent to the volume of the room in around one hour in most cases. This will not mean an air change in the building in one hour as the internal air currents will not be uniform and pockets of the room will require more time to be purged of air. To completely change the air in the room it is expected that several hours will need to elapse and, therefore, the retention time of any flammable gas or vapour will be long. This retention time may be sufficiently long to disrupt the source of release/classification of area relationship, certainly in pockets in the room. While this ventilation may be improved by the inclusion of openings in room walls, this is not necessarily as good an option as is at first thought. Most such openings are fitted with louvres which are necessary to maintain the integrity of the room in such circumstances. Louvres and similar devices such as meshes have a severely deleterious effect on ventilation. Experiments have shown, for example that strategically placed openings in walls of buildings produce significant airflows (up to 0.3 m/s) up to 10 m from the walls, but the inclusion of louvres has a significant negative effect in that when a louvre is present in an opening which would otherwise produce the airflow described above, no significant airflow is detectable more than 3 m from the walls[1].

5.1.4 Below-ground rooms

Below-ground rooms produce the most adverse situation possible because only the entry is above ground there is no possibility of effectively introducing openings, and crack ventilation is effectively absent. The time for the totality of the air in the room to change, while not being infinite, is very long (many hours). Any release in such rooms would be expected to persist for long enough to cause the room to be classified as Zone 0, even if the release was from a secondary source of release.

5.2 Effect of walls on hazardous areas

The effect of a wall close to an area which is classified as hazardous will be the same as that of ground proximity, although density of the flammable material will not have such a marked effect. Neglecting prevailing winds, which has to be the case in general, the presence of a wall will adversely affect mixing of gas and air, as will any other obstruction. The effects of the presence of a single wall will have the effect of changing the geometry of a hazardous area in the same way as ground proximity (see Figs. 3.4 and 3.5 for details). Where the wall is not of sufficient length or height to completely obstruct the gas/air mixture then the hazardous area will flow around and over it (See Figs. 5.1 and 5.2). The resultant wrap around hazardous area has been based on the entire leak exiting the edge of the wall.

This approach may be extended to cases where the source of release is contained in an area bounded by two walls or by three walls. Figures 5.3, 5.4 and 5.5 indicate how the hazardous area is affected. Identification of the hazardous area will basically be as in the case of one wall, but it should be noted that unless the walls are extremely long in the case of the two-wall scenario, the hazardous area will always extend at least to the end of both walls. In the three-wall scenario, the extention should be at least as far as the outboard end of both wing walls, with all of the enclosed area forming the hazardous area. Vertical extents should follow the single wall approach. In

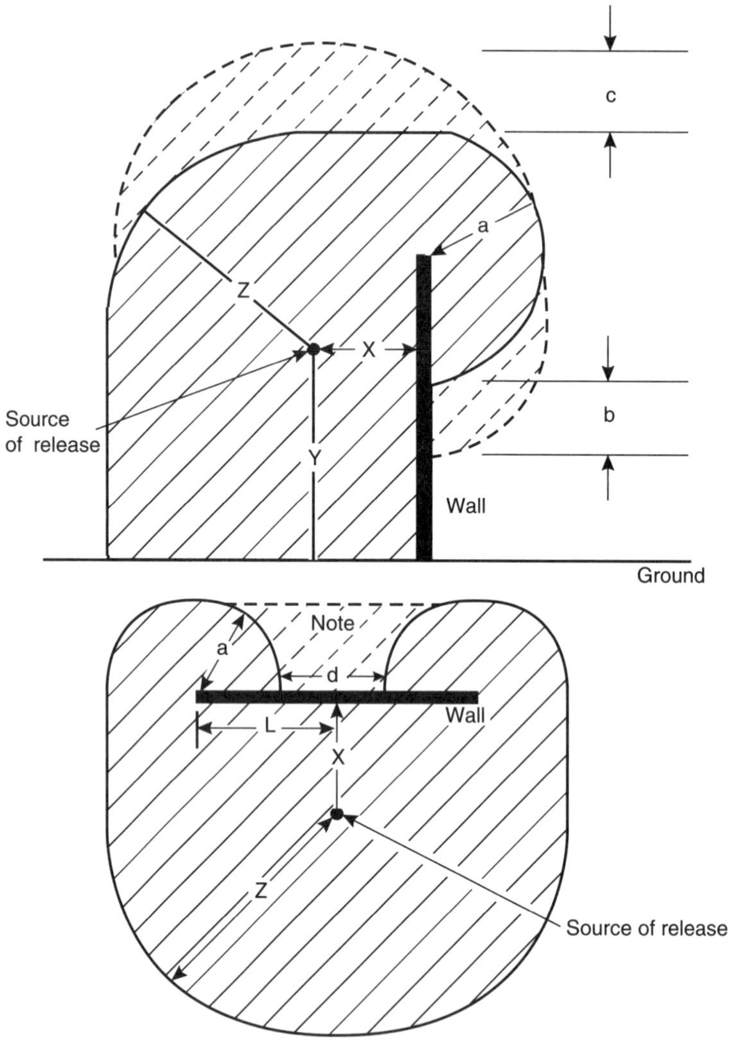

X = Distance wall/source of release (1.5–3 m)
Y = Distance source to ground (Z – Y = 1.5–3 m)
Z = Extent of hazardous area
a = Z – X (vertical) or Z – L (horizontal)
b = 0.5 Z (for densities greater than 1.3 only)
c = 0.5 Z (for densities less than 0.7 only)
d = wall length from edges of hazardous area
Note: Where *d* is less than *Z* it is prudent to continue the hazardous area across the rear face of the wall as shown

Fig. 5.1 Effect of single walls within 1.5–3 m of sources of hazard

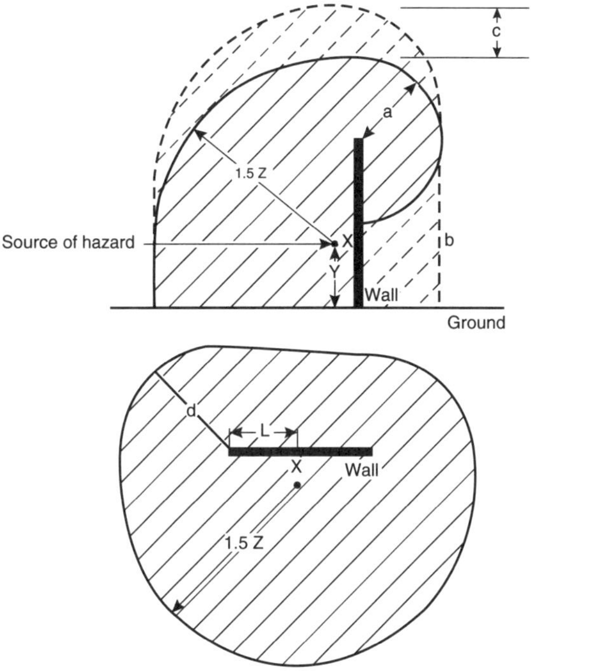

X = Distance wall/source of hazard (< 1.5 m)
Y = Distance source to ground (Z − Y =< 1.5 m)
Z = Extent of hazardous area (unmodified)
a = 1.5 *Z* − *X*
b = Distortion of hazardous area (densities greater than 1.3 only)
c = 0.75 Z (Densities less than 0.7 only)

Fig. 5.2 Effect of single walls within 1.5 m of source of hazard

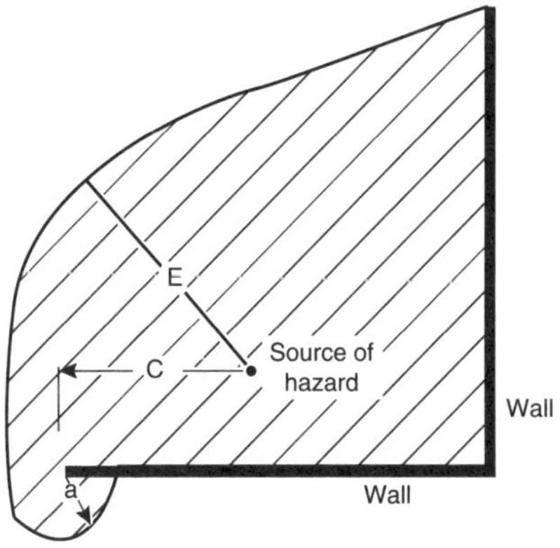

E = Extent of hazard taking account of wall proximity,
C = Distance source of hazard/wall end
a = E − C

Fig. 5.3 Typical two-wall effect (a)

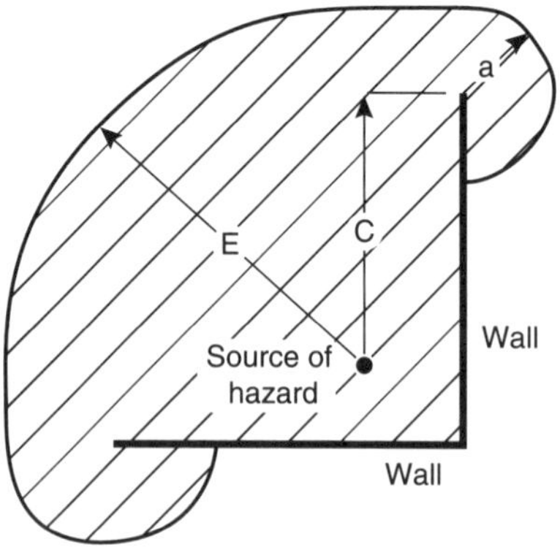

E = Extent of hazardous area with adjustments for wall proximity,
C = Distance source of hazard/wall end
a = E − C

Fig. 5.4 Typical two-wall effect (b)

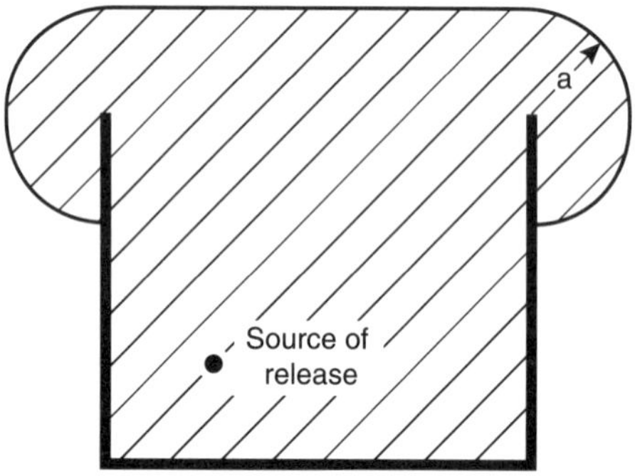

a = Taken from Table 3.2 on the basis of maximum release with a minimum of 0.5 m

Fig. 5.5 Typical three-wall effect

all cases this approach will be valid for both primary and secondary sources of release and, in general, the retention of explosive atmosphere will not be sufficient to increase the severity of classification (i.e., Zone 1 from a secondary source of release).

5.3 Roofs without walls or associated with one, two or three walls

5.3.1 Roofs without walls

There are two scenarios which must be considered here. The first is the flat roof, which is so typical of petrol station canopies and the second, the hipped roof (dutch-barn construction) which is more common in industrial loading and unloading areas. This latter may be with vents or without vents, although, in most cases, vents are present particularly in cases where the flammable gas or vapour is lighter than air.

Where no walls are present the effect of a flat roof is dependent upon the proximity of the roof to the edge of the hazardous area which would be created if the release were in free air (see Fig. 5.6). If the roof is more than 5 m beyond the extent of hazardous area predicted by Fig. 3.4 and 3.5 (in Chapter 3) the roof is unlikely to have any effect but in other cases the hazardous area is expected to reach the roof. Where a hipped (dutch-barn) type roof is present without walls and if the top of the hazardous area defined in the absence of the roof is within 5 m of the roof, the entire area contained by the roof will become a hazardous area of the same severity,

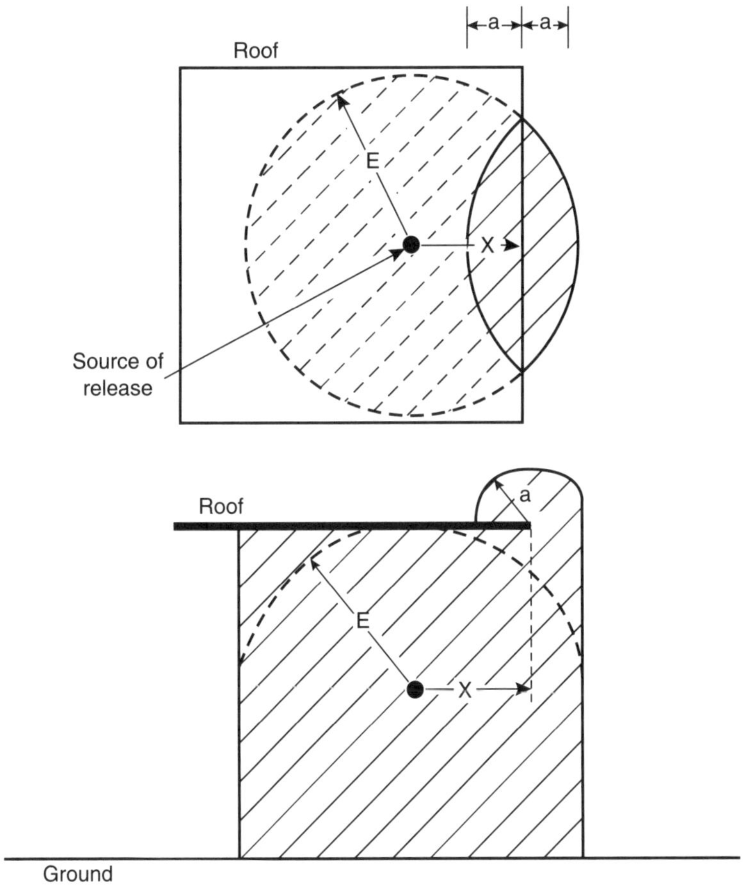

E = Extent of hazardous area neglecting effect of roof,
X = Distance source of release/wall,
a = E − X

Fig. 5.6 Effect of flat roof within 5 m of free ventilation limit of explosive atmosphere

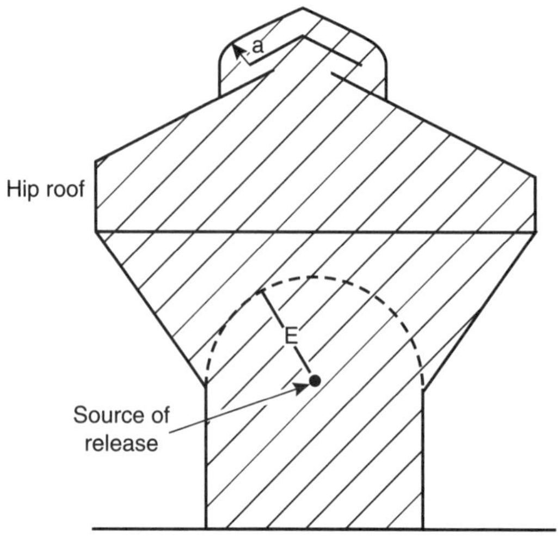

E = Extent of hazardous area neglecting roof,
a = 1 m

Fig. 5.7 Effect of hip roof within 5 m of E

provided that in cases where the flammable material is not heavier than air, vents must be provided in the apex of the roof. Figure 5.7 shows this situation and suggests a notional 1 m of hazardous area around the vents. This latter is difficult to predict but, at 1 m, is felt to be sufficiently large for most normal situations.

5.3.2 Roofs associated with one wall

Where a wall is present in addition to the roof, the situation is further complicated and the hazardous areas described in Fig. 5.1 and 5.2 become modified to give the situation shown in Fig. 5.8. The main thing to notice here is the extension of the hazardous area over the roof for a small distance, given by the difference between the extent of the hazardous area produced when the wall is present and the length of the wall. The length is used in preference to the height as the overlap will only occur if the wall length is less than the horizontal extent of the hazardous area, which is already distorted by being extended up to the roof level. The situation is similar in respect of the situation with a hipped roof, but here the effects shown in Fig. 5.7 must also be taken into account.

5.3.2 Roofs associated with two walls

Where two walls are present, then the entire area covered by the hazardous area shown in Figs. 5.3 and 5.4 will form part of the hazardous area up to

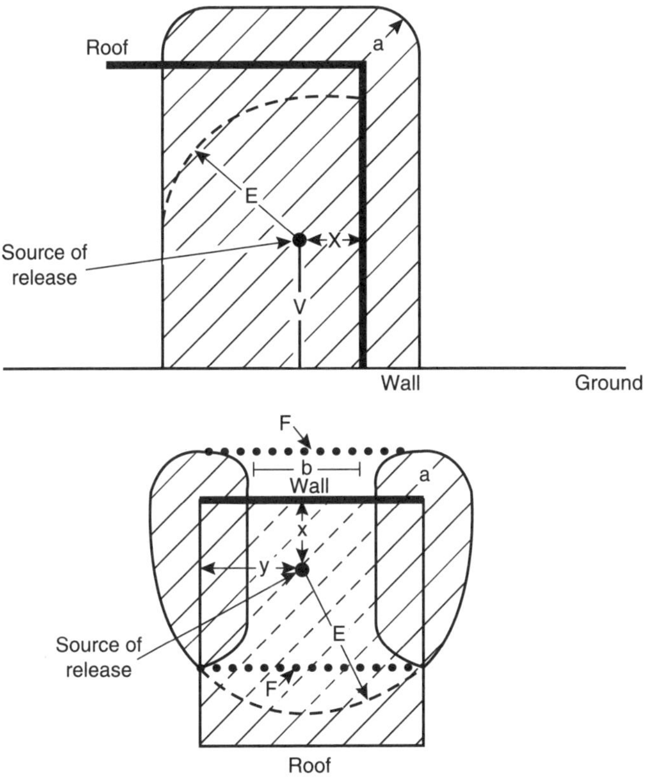

E = Extent of hazardous area taking account of wall proximity but in absence of roof
V = Height of source of release
X = Distance source/wall
a = $E - Y$ (with a minimum of 0.5 m over roof)
b = $2y - 2a$
Note: Where *b* is less than *E* hazardous area extends behind and over roof to *F*

Fig. 5.8 Effects of roof over single wall

the roof and down to the ground (see Fig. 5.9). As for one wall, the extents of hazardous area above the roof line will be determined using Fig. 5.3 and 5.4.

5.3.4 Roofs associated with three walls

Where three walls exist, the situation is entirely different and the area should be treated as a room as described later in this chapter, giving a hazardous area as described in Fig. 5.10, which is based on Table 3.2 in the same way as would be the case for an opening, such as a door in a room.

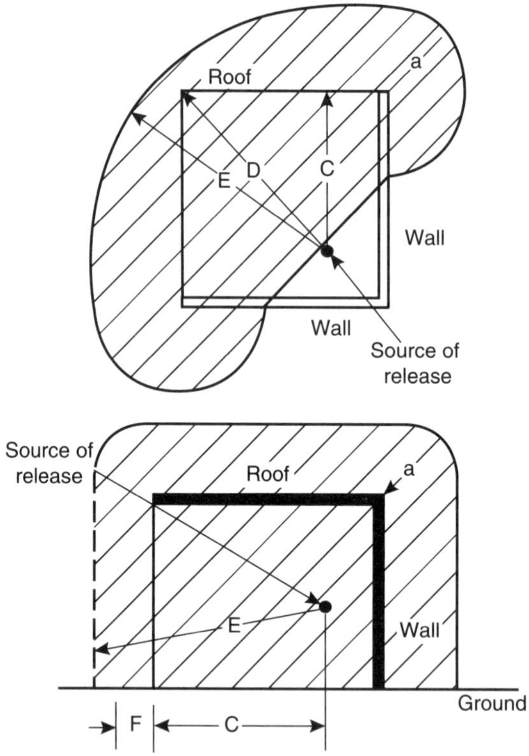

E = Extent of hazardous area taking account of walls if roof is not present
C = Distance from source to end wall
D = Distance from source to furthest corner of roof
F = E − D
a = E − C

Fig. 5.9 Effect of roof over two walls

5.4 Rooms above ground

As previously stated, an above-ground room with no attempts made to give ventilation will have a very long retention of any release of flammable material. A method of calculating this is given in Chapter 4 based upon a proposed new British Standard[3]. It is difficult, however, to be sure that all pockets of a room will be swept clear within this specified time by crack ventilation, and retention must be assumed to be capable of removing the source of hazard/classification relationship. It is not considered possible to countenance a room with no specifically included ventilation requirements being used for any purpose which means that it will contain sources of release more onerous than secondary grade sources of release. In such circumstances the interior area classification will, because of the paucity of ventilation, give an internal classification of Zone 1, which will clearly introduce significant difficulty in the use of the room.

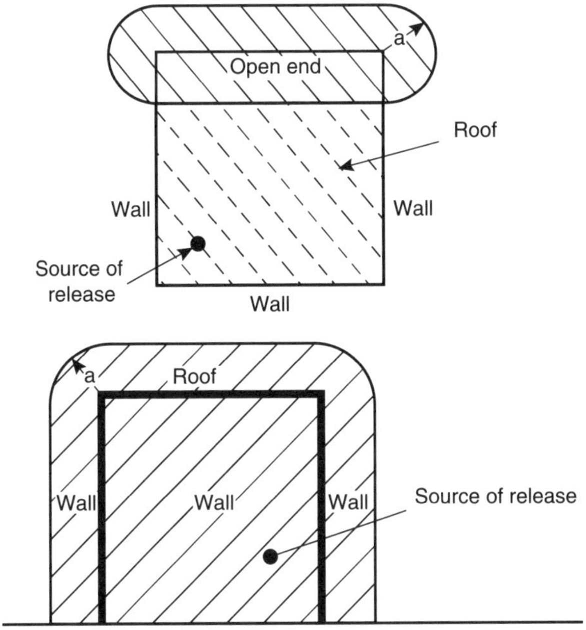

a = Taken from Table 3.2 on the basis of maximum release (minimum figure 0.5 m)

Fig. 5.10 Effect of roof on three-wall system

Any door which enters the room will be considered as a source of release equivalent to the quantity of vapour released within the room and Table 3.2 should be used to determine the extent of the hazardous area outside the room, around the door or other opening. Where liquids above their flashpoints but below their boiling points are contained within the room, drainage should be provided to ensure that a significant pool cannot form, and the external hazardous area should be based on Table 3.8 with a minimum of 0.5 m in cases where no mist is assumed. This latter is a safety factor to take account of unknowns. Where the room contains a liquid contained above its boiling point then the area outside the room (which is a hazardous area) should be based on Table 3.10. These areas outside the room will, be Zone 2 in the case of secondary grade sources of release (the only sources of release considered as acceptable in these circumstances) even though the retention problem is likely to lead to the classification of the room as Zone 1.

5.4.1 The application of additional general ventilation

Where a room contains sources of release then it is almost certain that additional ventilation will be necessary. A room may be provided with additional ventilation in one of three ways.

Openings (normally louvered) may be fitted to create more airflow in the building

Where openings are provided they do increase ventilation, but in no way as significantly as artificial ventilation unless they satisfy the criteria set out earlier in this chapter. Such openings are not in many cases practicable unless louvred, however, as they remove much of the protection from the environment which is often the reason why a room is necessary. The effect of such additional ventilation is to reduce the retention of explosive atmosphere in the building to a level where the source of hazard/classification relationship (i.e., secondary grade source of release gives Zone 2) is maintained. Because of the limited effect which they have, however, they do not allow parts of the building to be delineated as particular risks (e.g., parts Zone 1 and parts Zone 2) and the entire building will adopt the classification produced by the most onerous source of release contained within it. They must also be strategically placed to take maximum account of the internal situation. In buildings where internal activities produce temperature gradients of in excess of 3 °C between the interior of the building and the outside air, then significant chimney effects can occur and movement of explosive atmospheres within a building will be affected to some extent by their density relative to air. The results of these considerations generally result in louvered openings being placed at both the top and the bottom of the building.

In addition, care must be taken to ensure that the effect of any air entering through louvered openings is general, rather than limited, to specific areas as the airflow is not sufficient to ensure that releases do not contaminate all of the building. The layout of equipment within the building is also important as it could produce blindspots. In most cases considerations such as this tend to create a scenario where louvres are necessary all around the building, as shown in Fig. 5.11, at both high and low level which is not always ideal. The result will still usually lead to the entire interior of the building being classified as Zone 1 if a primary grade source of release is present which, because of toxic and asphyxiant considerations, may often mean that access to such buildings is severely restricted.

To sum up, buildings which merely have openings to allow enhanced natural ventilation without meeting the criteria described in Section 5.1.1 normally require ventilation openings as shown in Fig. 5.11 and, in the main, will only be suitable for secondary grade sources of release. Even in such cases, layout inside the building is of critical importance.

Where buildings ventilated naturally by openings not complying with the criteria for unrestricted ventilation, provided the ventilation openings have been provided with sufficient thought to internal airflow, secondary grade sources of release within the building will produce a Zone 2 classification and external Zones 2 at the openings, based upon the maximum single secondary grade release and using Table 3.2 as a basis, with a minimum of 0.5 m.

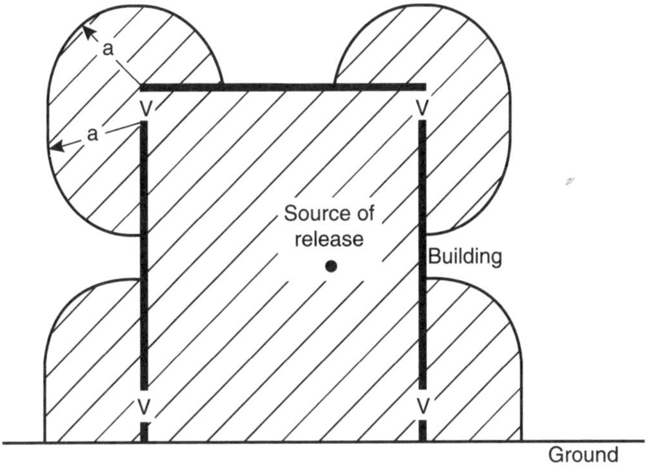

V = Vents (louvres or otherwise)
a = Extent of hazardous area (Table 3.2) with a minimum of 0.5 m

Hazardous area		Source of release
Not acceptable	–	Continuous grade
Zone 1	–	Primary grade
Zone 2	–	Secondary grade

Fig. 5.11 Hazardous area is a room with openings (with or without louvres)

Where a building (as described above) contains primary grade sources of release, unless local forced ventilation is fitted in a way which removes the release separately, the entire interior of the building will be Zone 1, and a Zone 1 will exist at all ventilation openings based upon the maximum number of primary grade sources of release which are considered as releasing at the same time, based upon Tables 3.1 and 3.2, with a minimum of 0.5 m (not normally acceptable for personnel entry).

It is not considered as acceptable to have any continuous grade sources of release releasing into such a building without additional precautions.

Buildings provided with forced ventilation

General forced ventilation is the most common way in which the building may be scoured with air. The objective is normally to ensure that the building is swept with air while at the same time, ensuring that the forced ventilation provided does not create hazardous areas around the building. To do this it is necessary to first determine the maximum release of flammable material from any one secondary grade source of release (it is not considered as necessary to consider more than one secondary grade source of release releasing at any given time) and, if greater, the maximum release from any possible combination of primary grade sources of release considered possible from the application of Table 3.1 (if it is decided that it is acceptable in any given circumstance to have a building which is all Zone 1).

If it is not considered as acceptable for the entire building to be Zone 1, then each primary grade source of release must have local ventilation applied to remove the material released before it can access the generality of the building. In no circumstances is it considered possible to allow any continuous grade source of release to freely release into the building where only general ventilation is present.

Having determined the maximum quantity of flammable material released into the building, it is then necessary to ensure that the amount of air supplied by the ventilation system is sufficient to ensure that, if a release occurs when the ventilation is on, the mixture of air and flammable material exhausted from the room is below the lower explosive limit and it is wise to apply a safety factor here. Chapter 4 provides equations which will allow this to be done. When the ventilation has been properly designed it can be accepted that, provided that early repair of the ventilation system is executed so that it is not off for a long time (say repair is to be completed well within a shift), then a secondary grade release will not occur while the ventilation is off and there is little likelihood of the building filling with explosive atmosphere and then exhausting when the ventilation is switched on, creating an explosive atmosphere outside the building. Unfortunately, this does not hold for primary grade sources of release and these must be expected to release at times when the ventilation has failed but, as failure of the ventilation is abnormal, such releases can be considered as secondary grade giving rise to Zone 2 within the building and not Zone 1. There remains, however, the problem that when the ventilation is repaired and switched on, an explosive atmosphere will be exhausted from the building. This, together with the fact that if input forced ventilation is used there will be some leakage of explosive atmosphere from within the building at all openings, demands that any ventilation system used is extract ventilation so that the pressure in the building will be very slightly lower than outside, resulting in release of explosive atmosphere to the outside only at the ventilation exhaust. Figs. 5.12 and 5.13 show how this situation exists in practice.

Where only secondary grade sources of release exist with general extract ventilation, the inside of the building will be Zone 2 and no external hazardous area will exist. Even in these circumstances, however, it is advisable to have an indirectly operated fan with the drive motor outside the ducting and clear of the ducting end, as if the ventilation fails for a long time the fan will be necessary to remove a possible explosive atmosphere from within the building. Although this is so unlikely as not to be within the area classification considerations it is clearly not acceptable to use a source of ignition to try to clear an explosive atmosphere, however unlikely that atmosphere may be.

Where primary grade sources of release exist without local ventilation, as described earlier, the inside of the building will be Zone 1 and a Zone 2

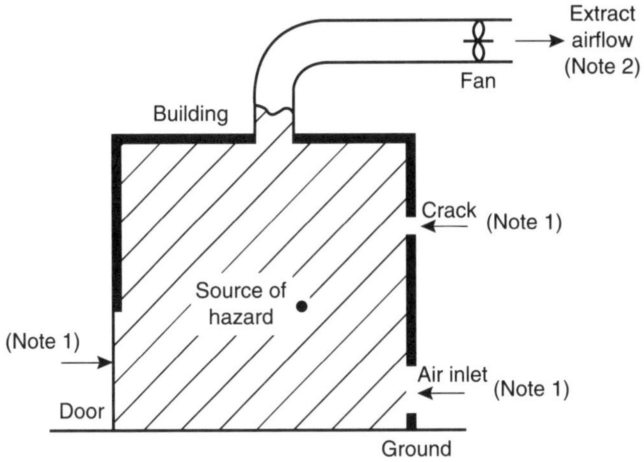

Fig. 5.12 Secondary grade source of release with forced ventilation. *Notes*: (1) Extract ventilation ensures that airflow at all apertures will be into building. (2) Extract airflow sufficient to dilute maximum secondary grade source of release to required fraction of LEL

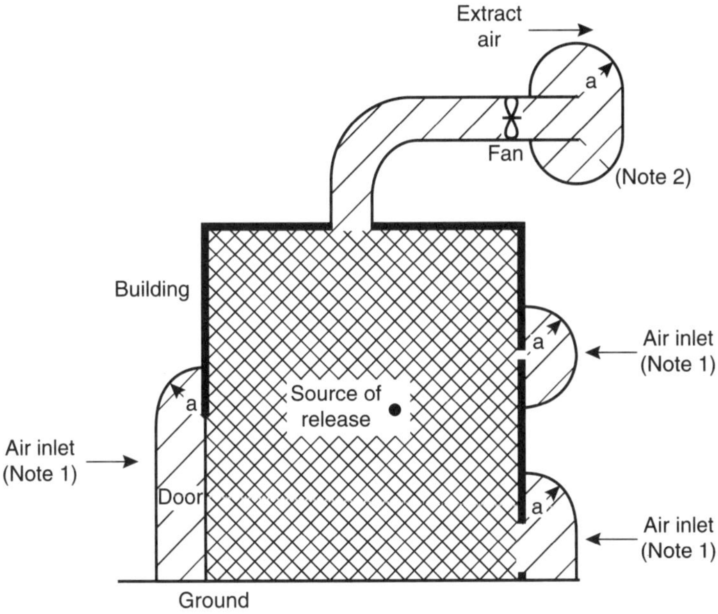

a = Table 3.2 but 0.5 m minimum

Fig. 5.13 Primary grade source of release with extract ventilation. *Notes*: (1) Ventilation ensures airflow is into the building in normal operation restricting Zone 1 to inside building. (2) In abnormal circumstances explosive atmosphere may leak from extract vent in addition to building openings (based upon Table 3.2 taking account of the maximum release of the source of hazard, but with a minimum of 0.5 m) will exist where the ventilation exhausts into the outside air. In this case, the fan motor will need to be considered as previously to allow for repair delays. This will have already been considered as the fan motor will be in a Zone 2 if in-line.

As previously, the use of extract ventilation will mean that all leaks of air will be into the building and so no external Zone 1 will occur. Any air inlets, however, will be surrounded by Zone 2 based upon the maximum leakage rate and should be sized in accordance with Table 3.2, with a minimum of 0.5 m.

Continuous grade sources of release are not considered as acceptable in normal circumstances within this type of building.

5.4.2 The application of additional local ventilation

Section 5.3.1 describes the situation which arises when general ventilation only is provided for. It is possible to additionally arrange for local ventilation at a single point of release or location to limit the extent of hazardous areas produced by specific sources of release in areas which are not generally freely ventilated; be they unventilated or provided with general natural or forced ventilation. There are two basic ways of doing this.

Provision of specific ventilation for individual sources of release

Where a particular source of release is provided with individual ventilation then, provided that such ventilation is properly conceived, the size of the hazardous area around that source may be described, even though the area in which it is sited is not generally freely ventilated (e.g., is in a building). The ventilation provided here must be local to the source of release and must be sized to ensure that the airflow in the area of the release is greater than the release velocity. It must also ensure that the quantity of ventilation air provided is sufficient to dilute the maximum release of the source in question to some fraction of the lower explosive limit of the flammable material released, so as to ensure that the gas vapour/air mixture exhausted from the area is below the lower explosive limit. Chapter 4 provides a method of defining the quantity of air necessary, but determination of the velocity of airflow depends upon detailed knowledge of the geometry around the release and the release velocity. This approach is generally only effective for extract point source ventilation as in other cases the effect of the ventilation would be to push the released gas/vapour into the effectively enclosed area. Also, the nature of secondary grade sources of release, in that they are often large and at high velocity, means that the approach is only effective in limiting Zones 0 and 1 caused by continuous and primary grade sources of release. In such cases, however, it has significant value in that it can be used to maintain a general Zone 2 classification in such places as buildings containing continuous and primary

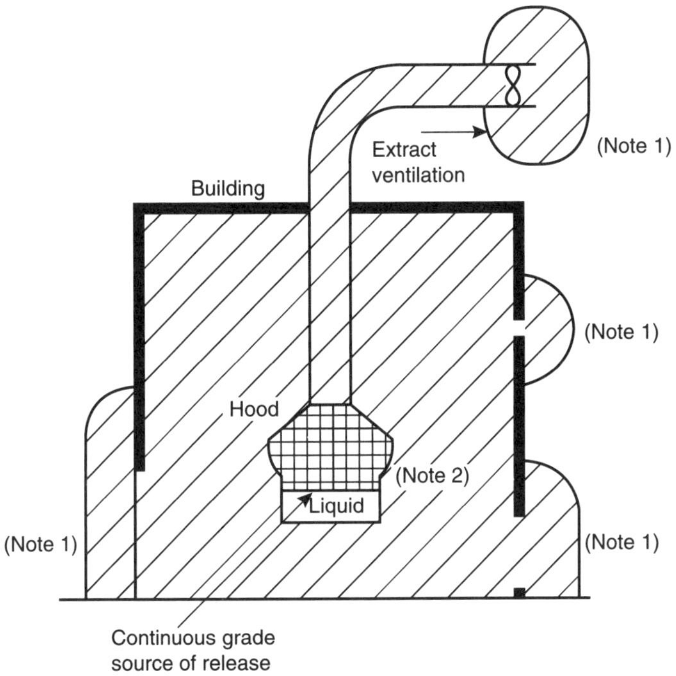

Fig. 5.14 Effects of point source ventilation. *Notes*: (1) Interior of building and exterior around openings are Zone 2 to take account of ventilation failure. (2) Immediate area around continuous (or primary) grade source of release is Zone 0 (Zone 1). (3) Where source is a point source and ventilation velocity local to it is 2 m/s Zone 0 (Zone 1) is restricted Table 3.2 with a minimum of 0.5 m

grade sources of release. The effects of this ventilation may also be considered when deciding on the additional level of general ventilation necessary for such a location. These situations are described in Fig. 5.14.

Where a continuous grade source of release is present in an area which is not freely ventilated, local extract ventilation (e.g., for an oil/water separator in a building) may be provided locally to the source of release to remove any gas or vapour which is normally released. Unless the source of release has additional modes of release it is, in such cases, reduced, as far as the area in question is concerned, to a secondary grade source of release on the basis that it will release into the area only when the local ventilation fails. This does suppose that the ventilation is quickly repaired if it does fail and here repair within the hour will be necessary. If the source can behave in other modes then these must be separately considered. Where the source of release can be described as a point source then, provided that the airflow around the source as a result of the ventilation is at least 0.5 m/s, the Zone 0 will be less than 0.5 m.

Where a primary grade source of release is protected by local ventilation, the situation is similar to that existing for a continuous grade source of release except that, because the release is not continuous, the time taken to repair the ventilation may be longer and a period of within one shift (i.e., eight hours) is considered appropriate.

Where a secondary grade source of release is protected by local ventilation, only the area local to the source of release is considered as Zone 2, as far as that release is concerned. Failure of the ventilation coincident with the actual release of flammable material is considered as not happening within the scope of area classification, provided the ventilation is repaired expeditiously (again, within one shift – eight hours – is appropriate). The Zone 2 limited to the immediate locale of the source of release if it is the only source of release in the area. It should be stressed, once again, that because of the velocity of release and quantity of material released from most secondary grade sources of release this type of limitation by point source ventilation is not easy or, in some cases, possible.

Use of dividers in buildings together with selective ventilation

Hazardous Areas within an area, such as a building, which is not freely ventilated may also be achieved by the use of dividing walls or curtains, with ventilation arranged so that airflow is normally into the space enclosed by the walls or curtains. This technique is often used where manual loading activities are involved and releases in normal operation cannot be excluded. It is not considered that such an approach is acceptable for continuous grade sources of release as the entire part of the area enclosed by the walls or curtains will adopt the classification appropriate to the source of release which would be Zone 0 in this case. The approach, could of course be used where a continuous grade source of release has additional local ventilation as described earlier in this chapter.

Where a primary grade source of release, inside an area which is not freely ventilated, is further enclosed in walls or curtains in such a way that the ventilation in the enclosed place causes a general inflow of air through all apertures, the classification of the area within the walls or curtains will normally be Zone 1 (if the ventilation within the enclosed area is sufficient – see Chapter 4). However, the effect of the source of release on the area outside the curtains will be that of a secondary grade source of release, giving only Zone 2 in those areas. This, of course, presumes that ventilation failure is corrected within one shift, as before.

Where a secondary grade source of release, inside an area which is not freely ventilated, is further enclosed in walls or curtains achieving the above objectives, the source of release need not be taken into account in determination of the zonal classification of the remainder of the area, provided that the ventilation is expeditiously repaired after breakdown (say within one shift – eight hours)

The walls or curtains used for the above purposes should be of gas-tight construction, apart from openings intended to be present, such as doorways, as the amount of air necessary if this were not so would be prohibitive. It is worth noting, however, that vertical overlapping strip curtaining has been used with success in this activity.

5.4.3 High integrity ventilation

All of the above is based upon the fact that forced ventilation can fail and that failure is an abnormal effect and, therefore, it is only considered where continuous or primary grade sources of release are involved. The types of failure involved are normally mechanical or electrical failure of the ventilation itself. This problem may be overcome by duplicating the ventilation system so that a failure particular to one will merely bring the standby system into operation. Provided the separation between the two ventilation systems is sufficient (e.g., different mechanical parts and different electrical supplies) then failure of both systems can be neglected as it would require two abnormal events (which need not be considered for area classification purposes). In such cases it is possible to define limits of Zones within the building as the ventilation can be relied upon and tests can be carried out to show the extent of hazardous areas produced by particular releases in cases where no experience exists.

In such situations there remains the possibility of total electrical failure which is not likely to coincide with a release where secondary grade sources of release are involved, and in cases where continuous grade and primary grade sources of release are involved all electrical equipment will be de-energized by the failure. In such circumstances, provided that residual hot surfaces in equipment are addressed, then a pre-purge of the area before energizing the electrical equipment will ensure that the situation is acceptable. This can be achieved by introducing a delay between restoration of the airflow and energization. The time for this delay will depend upon the geometry of the building but if the building is properly designed to minimize the risk of unventilated pockets, which should be the case, the time should not need to exceed that required for an airflow equivalent to five times the volume of the building to pass through it.

In such circumstances the extent of any hazardous area can be calculated on the basis of the Equations in Chapter 4. The extents of the hazardous areas produced should be based upon the volume of explosive atmosphere expected.

Example

A volume of vapour of mass 2.5×10^{-3} is released by a source of release inside a building which has high integrity ventilation. The material released is at 295 K, has a molecular weight of 50, and a lower explosive limit of 2 per cent.

In an open air situation near the ground the extent of the hazardous area would be given by Equation 4.7 multiplied by 1.5 in accordance with Fig. 3.3.
This gives:

$$X = 1.5 \times 10.8[GT/ME]^{0.55} \qquad \text{m}$$

$$X = 16.2[2.5 \times 10 - 03 \times 295/50 \times 2]^{0.55} \qquad \text{m}$$

$$X = 1.1 \text{ (in an open air situation)} \qquad \text{m}$$

If we assume the minimum amount of air is used in the ventilation system of the indoor area then Equation 4.31 can be used and the following is the case:

$$Q_a = 0.03 \times 2.5 \times 10^{-3} \times 2952/50 \times 2 \qquad \text{m}^3/\text{s}$$

$$Q_a = 0.065 \qquad \text{m}^3/\text{s}$$

If the room is $100\,\text{m}^3$ in volume then the number of air changes per second is 6.5×10^{-4}. At this low flow there will be badly ventilated parts and so a low airflow efficiency is expected and factor f (see Chapter 4) will be 5 and, if the source of release is a primary grade source of release, then k will be 0.25. If we now use Equation 4.32 from we have the volume of explosive atmosphere:

$$Q = 0.065 \times 5/6.5 \times 10^{-4} \times 0.25 \qquad \text{m}^3$$

$$Q = 2000\,\text{m}^3$$

This would give a linear extent of hazardous area in the best case of:

$$X = 7.8\,\text{m}$$

Therefore, the extent of the hazardous area is around 8 m if the volume was a sphere but as it will not be due to the directional nature of ventilation it will be considerably larger.

In addition the volume of the room would need to be much greater than the explosive atmosphere or it would result in the entire room being a hazardous area.

5.5 Rooms below ground

Rooms below ground should be treated as rooms above ground but, as natural ventilation via openings is not possible, only the forced ventilation solutions are possible. Provision of mechanisms to remove the gas vapour/air contents of the room become much more important as there is no other mechanism for changing the air in the room. Unless it is forcibly changed before energization of electrical equipment the risk of explosion is much greater as the persistence of an explosive atmosphere in an underground room with no forced ventilation is theoretically infinite.

5.6 Rooms without any internal release but which abut external hazardous areas

While no opening should exist in the part of a room which is adjacent to an external hazardous area, such an ideal situation is not always possible. Installations, such as cable ducts in walls, can be effectively sealed but it is often necessary to have a door in a wall, the other side of which is a hazardous area. In such circumstances the ideal solution would be to produce a situation where the explosive atmosphere does not access the room, as it is usually required to install electrical equipment which may be a source of ignition. This is not always possible, however, and as a result there are a variety of situations where partial or total invasion of the room by the external hazardous area occurs. The principal situation is where a room has a door or window which opens on to a hazardous area.

Where a room has an opening which abuts a hazardous area then, even if the opening is a door which is not used normally, the interior of the room must be assumed to be contaminated with the explosive atmosphere from the outside. As the ventilation inside the building is not normally free ventilation, the entire room must normally be assumed to adopt the external classification at least.

Where a room has a normal door or other opening which abuts a Zone 1 or 2 the entire room should be assumed to be itself a Zone 1 or 2 (i.e., the external classification) at best. If ventilation within the room is unusually poor then the interior would be Zone 1, even if the external classification is Zone 2, but this more severe situation would not be likely in the case of normal above-ground rooms. It is not considered acceptable for any room openings to abut Zone 0 as such zones are normally expected to be contained.

There are several ways to mitigate the effects described above in the Zone 1 and Zone 2 situations. If, for example, a door is present in a room and is only used in emergencies, then an essentially gas-tight door could be fitted and be made either self closing or to alarm if it is left open. Such doors are assumed not to transmit the hazardous area to the inside of the room. An airlock comprising of two self-closing doors is assumed to have a similar effect, as is a single self-closing gas-tight door coupled with fresh air inlet ventilation into a room which keeps its pressure slightly positive. The argument in this latter case is that even if the door is used regularly there will only be a problem if the ventilation fails and the time for which the door would be open in these circumstances would be unlikely to create a scenario where any significant amount of gas entered the room, bearing in mind that personnel would be aware that the ventilation had failed.

The ideal solution is to design the process or installation so that all walls, etc., which abut hazardous areas are effectively sealed and this should be possible in the majority of circumstances.

5.7 Particular circumstances

Quite often, rooms are employed for particular circumstances where flammable materials are used. Typical of these are the paint-spray booth (and similar rooms where personnel work) and the paint-drying oven.

5.7.1 The paint spray booth

In a paint-spray booth an operative actually releases a flammable material (the solvent in the paint) as both a vapour and a mist in their work. The booth will obviously become a hazardous area and, as spraying is going on for most of the time, would normally be a Zone 0. The gun is not in the same place all the time and moves during the spraying process which means that no part of the booth will contain an explosive atmosphere for more time than is appropriate to Zone 1 classification. There is also a risk to the operative and both of these problems give rise to a very careful design whereby airflow is carefully controlled to ensure that solvents are swept to the back of the booth and not spread around. This is done by keeping the ventilation velocity relatively high and ventilating by extract via a grid (or similar) at the rear of the booth to even-out airflow. Also, the spraying activity is normally interlocked with the ventilation to ensure that spraying cannot take place unless the ventilation is on. This is normally achieved by creating curtain flow across the aperture of the booth and to arrange activities so that the spraying activity is normally directed to the back of the booth. This coupled with the velocity of airflow which should be more than 0.5 m/s creates a scenario where any Zone 1 is within the booth and for a small distance in front of it. In these circumstances, even with the airflow, it is prudent to classify an area to the front of the booth as Zone 1 for a small distance in front of the booth (say 1 m) and to take account of misdirection of spray, to define a Zone 2 for 3 m in front of the booth.

Figure 5.15 shows a typical classification for a booth of this type. It should, however, be remembered that other precautions will need to be taken for reasons of toxicity or situations where other sources of release occur (e.g., vehicle petrol tanks). HSE Note PM 25[4] should be consulted in this regard).

5.7.2 The paint drying oven

Painted equipment is often dried in an oven giving a situation where solvents in the paint are evaporated in an enclosed space. What is worse

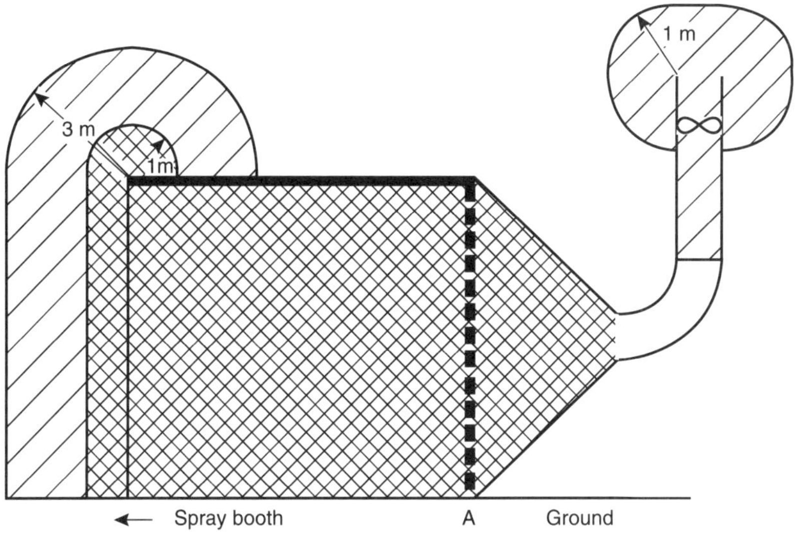

Fig. 5.15 The paint-spray booth

is that the airflow through the oven is recirculated as it is heated to a significant degree and the cost of fresh-air ventilation would be abortive. This situation leads to enhancement of the problem in that the level of flammable material in the drying air grows until an equilibrium is reached because some of it is fed back into the oven and added to that which is evaporating. This effect is mitigated by the fact that much of the solvent produced is evaporated within the spray booth or in transit between the booth and the oven and the interior of the oven may normally be classified as Zone 1. As it is an enclosed space additional precautions are necessary and HSE Note PM 25[4] should be consulted.

The exhaust of the oven should be classified as Zone 2 to take account of the fact that the ventilation may have to extract an explosive atmosphere from the oven on start-up, but such classification will be nominal as the solvents in question will have relatively high boiling points. Therefore, on start-up there will be at ambient temperature which will be very much lower. A distance of 3 m around the exit is suggested.

The oven should also be arranged so that in normal ventilation circumstances air is drawn in through any aperture, such as those used for entry of samples, and then a nominal hazardous area of (say) 3 m should be defined around these apertures to take account of abnormal circumstances.

References

1 BS 5345 Selection, Installation and Maintenance of Electrical

	Apparatus in Potentially Explosive Atmospheres (other than mining applications or explosive processing or manufacture). Part 2 (1983). Classification of hazardous areas
2 Directorate of Labour (Netherlands)(1980)	Guide to the Classification of hazardous areas in Zones in Relation to the Gas Explosion Hazard and to the Installation and Selection of Electrical Apparatus. First Edition.
3 BS/EN 60079–10 (1996)	Electrical Apparatus for Explosive Atmospheres. Classification of hazardous areas.
4 HSE Guidance Note PM 25	Vehicle Finishing Units: Fire and Explosion Hazards.

— 6 —

Area classification practice for dusts

In previous chapters the area classification of explosive atmospheres constituted of gases, vapours and mists and air have been discussed together with the legislation which addresses the total problem of explosive atmospheres. Among this legislation are requirements for the handling of combustible dusts (the term combustible is synonymous with the term flammable which is applied to gases, vapours and mists). As discussed in Chapter 1, Regulation 31(1) and 31(2) of the Factories Acts[1] requires certain actions where Combustible Dusts may be present or released.

First, it requires that processing plant which may produce dust clouds or release dust be enclosed as far as possible to prevent the general development of a dust cloud. This is already done in the case of such things as cyclones where the dust is contained by the cyclone during processing, but it also requires further action to restrict the travel of any release (in other words it requires positive attempts to be made to contain and define the limits of travel of released dust).

Second, it requires that, where dust can be released, accumulation of dust in these enclosed areas be limited by housekeeping which removes layers of dust and the like to prevent accumulation over time. It must be remembered that on release dust does not, like gas or vapour, disperse over time but settles as a layer and, to prevent such layers accumulating, dust which settles should be regularly removed either automatically or manually. Sources of ignition should be excluded where dust clouds or layers can occur in such density or thickness to constitute a hazard.

Third, it requires exclusion or effective enclosure of any source of ignition in an area where, even after taking all of the actions described above, dust clouds or layers may occur and sources of ignition cannot be excluded.

The differences between the performance of gases and dusts cannot be overstressed. In the case of gases, vapours and mists great reliance is placed on providing the most effective means of dispersion possible, while in the case of dusts, housekeeping and containment come to the fore. The one thing that both have in common is the requirement placed upon industry to minimize the risks of release of either, and to approach the protection of the results of release only when the release cannot reasonably be prevented.

The areas where dust is present, to an extent where ignition could occur, have historically been been classified only where dust could be released from process as Zone Z and Zone Y. The definitions of these two Zones are given in Chapter 2 and clearly address only problems of release in that

Zone Z (by definition) appears similar to Zone 1 for gases and Zone Y to Zone 2. This is further reinforced by the fact that BS 6467, Part 2[2] excludes the interior of vessels from its scope. This exclusion was clearly based upon the understanding that the inclusion of electrical apparatus inside vessels and silos, etc., was generally only acceptable in special circumstances. There has now been a change of view in this regard as IEC 1241–3[3] recognizes three Zones of risk in respect of dusts. These definitions are much more synonymous with those for gases and vapours, giving the relationship shown in Table 6.1. In this chapter the new three-Zone approach will be used as the document referred to is a draft British Standard, is based upon a draft IEC (International Electrotechnical Commission) Standard and will become a British Standard in the near future. In addition, this three-Zone technique has been used in one large company since 1973 with considerable success and, because of its relationship with the gas and vapour classification, the approach appears more logical.

Table 6.1 Approximate relationship between Zones

BS 5345, Part 2 (1983) Zone	BS 6467, Part 2 (1988) Zone	IEC 1241–3 (1994) (Draft) Zone
0		20
1	Z	21
2	Y	22

IEC 1241–3[3] also envisages dust releases outside buildings, which is an unusual situation as the effect of the environment is such that areas where dust is handled, stored or processed are normally indoors, or at least protected. The use of materials producing combustible dusts outdoors should be treated with caution. While in some cases (e.g., the outlets of extract ventilation systems where, in abnormal cases, the possibility of dust release cannot be ruled out) the presence of a loading facility (particularly a manual one) where dust is subject to normal exterior air currents provided by wind is difficult to justify as the distribution of any dust release becomes much more difficult to determine. Some external situations may be acceptable but the control which can be exercised within buildings in the case of dust releases is so advantageous it is hard to ignore. Even if outside operations are considered, partial enclosure to give some degree of confidence as to the performance of dust layers and clouds should be addressed.

6.1 Properties of dusts

Two properties of dusts are important to area classification and these are the ignition temperature required for a dust cloud and the ignition temperature required for a dust layer. It should be noted that ignition energy is not mentioned. This is not because dusts do not have an ignition energy (see Table 6.2) but because the methods of protection of electrical apparatus in areas made hazardous by dusts rely on adequate exclusion of dust from the electrical parts within the apparatus. Therefore, ignition energy is not a necessary piece of information in general.

Information on both of these values for a variety of dusts is given in Table 6.2. It should be noted that the layer ignition figures are based upon a layer thickness of 5 mm, as thicker layers are not normally acceptable because they could clearly be in contravention of Section 31 of the Factories Acts[1] and it is required that housekeeping normally maintains layers at smaller thicknesses. If, in a particular case, this is not possible then the figures in Table 6.2 are not appropriate and tests must be carried out to determine the ignition temperature at the relevant thickness. In addition, particle size and distribution in dusts, together with moisture content varies and with it both ignition energy and temperature. Table 6.2 is based upon particular particle size make-up of dusts, which is in some cases identified. Once again, if the dust in a particular case, while being included in Table 6.2, has a significantly different constitution then the figures in Table 6.2 may not be accurate and it may be necessary to determine its particular ignition temperature. The figures in Table 6.2, however, are a good yardstick as they are based on relatively fine dusts and may be used with a fair degree of confidence in most practical situations.

Having stated that ignition energy is not a necessary item of information for dust releases it should not be overlooked that many plants contain both flammable gases/vapours and combustible dusts and protection is necessary against the ignition of both. Also, some dusts may decompose to give off flammable vapours. Where flammable gases/vapours do occur ignition of these may well ignite the dust cloud or layer and protection against both risks must be provided. (It is worthy of note that, although the manufacture of explosives is specifically excluded by the majority of the Standards and Codes to which this book refers, both flammable vapours and combustible dusts are present in the early stages of explosives production and the approaches in this book may need to be implemented to prevent the ignition of such vapours and dusts which could otherwise act as triggers for detonation of the explosives.)

6.1.1 The ignition of dust clouds

When dust is mixed with air to the degree necessary to form an explosive atmosphere, the mixture is very dense and clearly visible. Dust clouds of any size which exhibit this possibility will be rare because of the environmental problems which they may create. The ratio of dust to air is a variable quantity depending upon particle size, etc., and no specific ideal mixture is given, unlike the situation in respect of gases and vapours. It is also not possible to ensure an even concentration of dust throughout the cloud.

Table 6.2 Properties of Combustible dusts (part from BS 6467, Part 2 (1988))

Dust	Particle size distribution					Median	Ignition temperature		Cloud	Min
	<500 µm	<125 µm	<71 µm	<32 µm	<20 µm		of cloud	of layer	Ign. energy	Explosive conc.
	Percentage by mass									
						µm	°C	°C	mj	g/l
Natural Products										
Wood, Flour			55	23		65	490	340	80	–
Cork			83	19	7	42	470	300		–
Cellulose			75	31		45	520	410	80	–
Grain, mixed dust from filter			63	48	40	37	510	300		0.06
Cocoa/Sugar, mixture of milkshake, most of oil removed	53	20				500	580	460		–
Milk powder, skimmed, spray dried			35	18	11	90	540	340		–
Soya meal			85	63	50	20	620	280	100	–
Starch, Cornstarch			99	85	65	15	460	435	–	0.15
Tea, black, from dust separator		64	48	26	16	76	510	300	–	–
Sugar, Milk			98	64	32	27	490	460	48	0.045
Caramel, dried		93	46	16		75	490	455	–	–
Cocoa Powder							500	200	120	–
Organic products										
Activated charcoal			86	56		29	660	400	–	–
Lignite			76	50	29	32	380	225	30	–
Bituminous coal medium-volatile			99	84	60	17	550	260	–	–
Phenolic resin			98	93	80	11	530	No glowing to 450 °C	–	0.015
Synthetic rubber		66	46	18	9	80	450	240	–	–
Polyacrylonitrile			99	66	38	25	540	No glowing to 450 °C	–	–

Polyethylene, low pressure				95	86	10	420	Melts	–	0.02
Polymethacrylate, from filter			90	70	48	21	550	Melts	–	–
Polyvinyl acetate, copolymerized			66	22	8	52	570	Melts	–	–
Polyvinyl chloride, from cyclone		41	35			98	700	No glowing to 450 °C	–	–
Poly Acrilonitrile						540	400		20	–
Methyl cellulose			45	12		75	420	320	–	–
Paraformaldehyde			89	65	41	23	460	No glowing to 450 °C	–	–
Calcium stearate			99	90	75	12	560	No glowing to 570 °C	–	–
Detergent raw material, based on olefin sulphonate		60	28			105	390	No glowing to 590 °C	–	–
Dye, phthalocyanine, blue			98	86		10	770	355	–	–
Metals										
Aluminium, from extraction system			65	47	37	36	590	No glowing to 450 °C	–	0.03
Bronze powder (gold bronze)				97	60	18	390	260	–	–
Sponge iron			88	74	65	12	470	390	–	–
Zinc dust, from separator					99	10	570	440	200	–
Lead							460	240	200	–
Inorganic products										
Molybdenum disulphide			92	75	53	19	520	320	–	–
Sulphur			96	70	51	20	280	–	–	–
Soot, from filter (lampblack)						10	810	570	–	–
Sintering powder, from filter	46		66	37	20	44	520	380	–	–
Immersion polishing medium						600	580	340	–	–
Toner					98	10	470	No glowing to 450 °C	– –	– –

The ignition energy of a dust cloud can be determined by dispersing dust suspended in a cloud, in air which is inside a tube and then introducing an ignition source. Some figures for this are given in Table 6.2. While this has been done for a variety of dusts, and figures exist, the information is only of value in respect of the use of electrical equipment which creates arcs or sparks to which the dust cloud has access. This situation is unusual as the normal approach is to exclude the dust from the interior of the equipment where such arcs or sparks could occur. Historically, there has been no internationally recognized test method and the available information is from a series of tests which were, nonetheless, carried out by those expert in the field.

At the time when the dust cloud ignition temperatures listed in Table 6.2 were produced there was no officially recognized international method for determination of dust-layer ignition temperature. One of the common historic methods for determination of a dust-cloud ignition temperature was, however, to determine the minimum temperature at which a cloud of the dust in air will ignite in a series of tests in a Godbert–Greenwald furnace or similar apparatus. A series of tests is required because of the difficulty of achieving the worst case, and a uniform cloud. If one addresses the figures given in Table 6.2 it will be noted that, with the exception of sulphur, for all of the materials included the temperature is around 400 °C or above.

An International Standard (IEC 1241 – 2[4]) now exists, produced by the International Electrotechnical Commission (IEC) for the standard test methods for these ignitions.

6.1.2 The ignition of dust layers

The ignition of dust layers is a complex phenomenon, depending upon the particle size of the layer and the environment in which ignition is to be achieved (e.g., whether it has been pre-heated, etc.). Again, there was no standard test for this when the figures given in Table 6.2 were produced and, in general, the ignition temperature was achieved by heating a 5 mm layer of dust on a hotplate and determining the temperature at which ignition occurs. This is difficult as dusts tend to smoulder when ignited and while some will continue to burn, and to progress along the layer away from the source of ignition, some will not and will extinguish as soon as the source of ignition is removed. Notwithstanding this difference, the ignition temperature is considered to be the temperature at which smouldering begins, even if it extinguishes on removal of the heat source. It should be noted that the layer ignition temperature is, in most cases, lower than the cloud ignition temperature. An International Standard now exists for the method of measuring this parameter – IEC 1241–2[4].

6.1.3 Production of flammable gases and vapours by dusts

Some dusts, particularly when heated, give off gases and vapours. This action is caused by the dust beginning to decompose and it is possible that the gases and vapours given off may be flammable. Initially, to determine the situation, the dust in question is heated in a tube with a flame applied above it. If any flammable gases or vapours are emitted during the decomposition of the dust then an ignition will occur. If an ignition is obtained then the released gases and vapours need to be identified and, if the dust can reach the temperature necessary to release them in the practical handling and process situation, then precautions to prevent their ignition have to be taken.

6.1.4 Other important dust properties

While the objective of the construction of electrical equipment for use in dust situations is to exclude the dust from the interior, insofar as is necessary to prevent an ignition, this may not mean total exclusion. The dust may, however, be conducting and, in such cases, must be totally excluded from the apparatus to prevent malfunction.

6.2 Area classification for dust releases

The method of classifying a hazardous area where dust presence is the problem is little different from that of classification in the case of gases or vapours. It is first necessary to identify the possibility of the presence of a dust cloud or layer from process information or likely release possibilities. These will then be graded as sources of release in the same way as for gases and vapours, after which the type and extents of hazardous areas may be identified.

6.2.1 Sources of dust release

Sources of Release of dusts are graded exactly as in the case of gas or vapour release and are classified as follows:

Continuous grade source of release

A continuous Grade Source of Release is one which releases a dust cloud for a large part of the time and, is in definition, synonymous with its gas or vapour counterpart. Typical of such areas are those inside process equipment such as hoppers, silos, etc.

Primary grade source of release

Primary Grade Sources of Release in the case of dusts are those areas where uncontrolled layers or clouds of dust are not normally present but may occur during the normal operation of the plant. Again, these are synonymous in derivation with their gas and vapour counterparts and are not expected to be present for more than 10 per cent of the time. Typical of such releases are the interior of some process vessels and loading points, and access doors to dust processing vessels or transport systems.

Secondary grade sources of release

Secondary Grade Sources of Release are those which are not normally expected to release except in abnormal operation, such as the failure of extract filters and similar situations.

6.2.2 Definition of Zones

Hazardous zones are related to the grade of release in much the same way as in the gas or vapour situation, except that the presence of dust layers can give rise to a more severe classification than would otherwise be the case (see Table 6.3) as, instead of dispersing, the dust settles on the ground. In many ways an indoor situation, where air movement is small, can be advantageous insofar as longevity of dust clouds is concerned. While this appears to be an advantage it is mitigated by the fact that the layer of dust so formed can be disturbed and create a cloud and is, itself, ignition capable.

Zone 20

A continuous grade source of release will give a Zone 20 from the cloud it creates, be it indoors or outdoors and only the extent will vary dependent

Table 6.3 Grade of release/Zone relationship (including effect of layers)

Grade of source	Dust clouds	Dust layers		
		Uncontrolled thickness	Controlled thickness disturbed	
			often	rarely
continuous	20	20	21	22
primary	21	20	21	22
secondary	22	20	21	22

(From BS/94/213454 DC[4])

upon its dispersion and settling of the dust to form a layer. The layers of dust formed also create the following hazardous areas.

An uncontrolled dust layer (i.e., one not contained in depth by housekeeping) will produce a Zone 20. Such layers are normally limited to the inside of vessels, etc., and because they are so thick (in excess of 5 mm) may have properties which are different to those of controlled layers. Such layers would not be acceptable outside containment such as process vessels in view of Section 31 of the Factories Acts[1].

A controlled dust layer (i.e., one which is contained in depth to less than 5 mm by housekeeping or other means) formed by a continuous grade source of release will only give a Zone 21 if disturbed often, and only a Zone 22 if rarely disturbed. The problems are principally the clouds produced by the layers when disturbed as the electrical equipment is designed to operate in this depth of dust layer.

Where the layer of dust can be controlled to less than 0.5 mm thickness with confidence it is unlikely that there will be enough dust to create an explosive atmosphere and, therefore no hazardous area is presumed to exist as a result of its presence, as when disturbed it is not capable of the production of an ignitable dust cloud.

Zone 21

A primary grade source of release will give rise to a Zone 21 if it produces a cloud. The extent of that Zone 21 will depend upon the dispersion of the dust cloud or the settling of the dust to form a layer. As before, the layer will be considered to produce the following Zones.

Where an uncontrolled dust layer (one not controlled to less than 5 mm by housekeeping, etc.) is formed the result is a Zone 20 in the area covered by the layer.

Where a controlled dust layer whose thickness is controlled to less than 5 mm is formed, but is regularly disturbed, then the result is a Zone 21 in the area around the layer. Where the layer is not regularly disturbed then the hazardous area reduces to Zone 22.

Where a dust layer is controlled to less than 0.5 mm no hazardous area is presumed to exist for reasons already described.

Zone 22

Where the source of release is of secondary grade then any cloud produced will give a Zone 22. As before, in the case of layers produced by this cloud the following is the case.

Where an uncontrolled dust layer is formed then, once again, a Zone 20 will exist in the region of the layer.

Where the dust layer is controlled by housekeeping or other means to less than 5 mm, a Zone 21 will exist where it is disturbed regularly, and a Zone 22 will be formed where it is only disturbed rarely.

Where the thickness of any dust layer produced can be controlled to less than 0.5 mm, then no hazardous area is assumed to exist.

When considering the possibility of dust layer-formation it has to be recognized that it is not necessary to have a dust cloud capable of forming an explosive atmosphere in order to have the possibility of a dust layer capable of forming such an atmosphere or being ignited. As already mentioned, a dust cloud has to be very dense to become an explosive atmosphere (50–100 g of dust per m^3 of air on average). Very much lower concentrations are well capable of depositing layers exceeding 5 mm, and hazardous areas due to dust layers may exist even when no dust cloud risk is identified. In addition, in all cases it will be necessary to institute actions to ensure that the dust layers produced in any area do not exceed 5 mm as only in exceptional circumstances will the situation be such that such limitation will be naturally achieved. The limitation of dust layers to less than 0.5 mm is even more unlikely and can only be expected to occur in outdoor areas where ventilation is very good, giving confidence of wind dispersion of any dust produced.

6.2.3 Extents of hazardous areas

Where dusts are processed it is likely that there will be a cloud within the processing equipment and, because it will not be possible to determine where in most cases, the entire interior of the equipment will be assumed to be contaminated with the dust cloud. An exception to this would be, for instance, where product particles were being separated from dust received with them by a cyclone (see Fig. 6.1). In such cases, the product stream after separation would probably not be a hazardous area.

Where dust clouds are formed due to failure of containment or loading or offloading activities, the extent will be small outside any sort of process containment as the density of the cloud would make it impossible for people to work because the cloud will be opaque and it will be difficult to breathe in such a cloud. The process equipment will have been designed to ensure this is not so. In addition, the density of the cloud will rapidly reduce as the mixture of dust and air leaves the point of release due to the addition of air by turbulence, and the settling of the dust which is, heavier than air. This leads to the conclusion that dust clouds caused by release of dusts from process equipment will extend no more than 1–1.5 m from the source of release. once again, because the dust is heavier than air, the hazardous area will have to be assumed to exist below the source of release down to the ground, unless the process design prevents this (for example by drawing into the process any dust released). The projection down to the ground will also only be valid if there is no excessive air movement which could distort it and so loading and unloading points should be protected from excessive air movement, such as wind. Typical examples of loading arrangements and the hazardous areas which they produce are given in Fig. 6.2 and 6.3. (See also Table 6.3.)

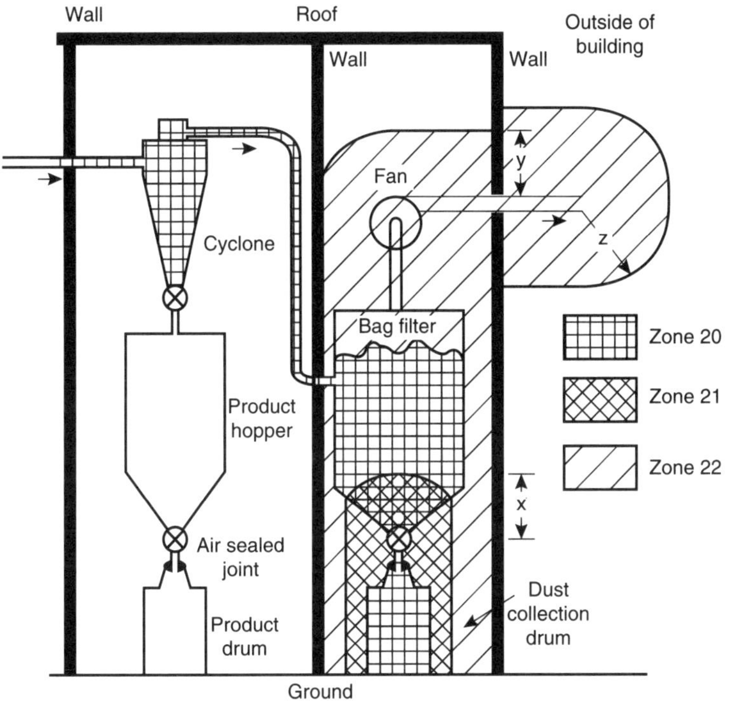

Fig. 6.1 Cyclone and bag filter. x = 1.5 m, y = 1.5 m, z = 2 m

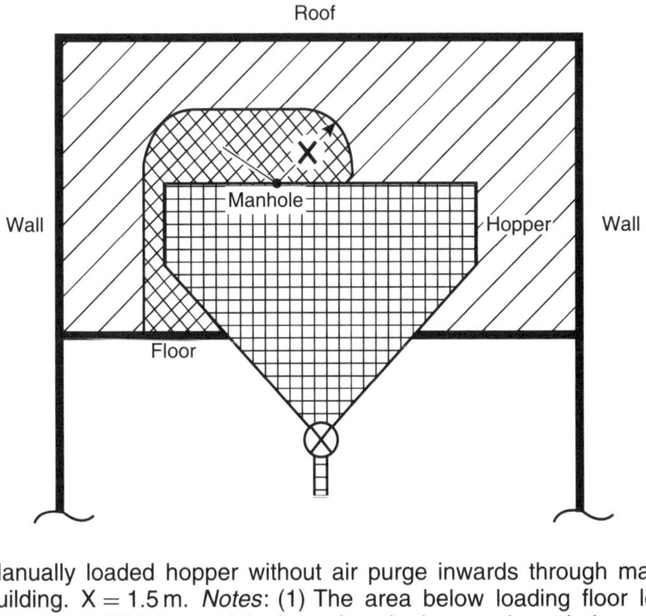

Fig. 6.2 Manually loaded hopper without air purge inwards through manhole in a building. X = 1.5 m. *Notes*: (1) The area below loading floor level is not addressed. (2) Where air is drawn into the hopper through the manhole, the dust cloud producing the Zone 21 will not exist provided airflow at manhole mouth is at least 1 m/s inwards. (3) If housekeeping is sufficient to prevent any layers forming the Zone 2 may be limited to 2–2.5 m around the hopper

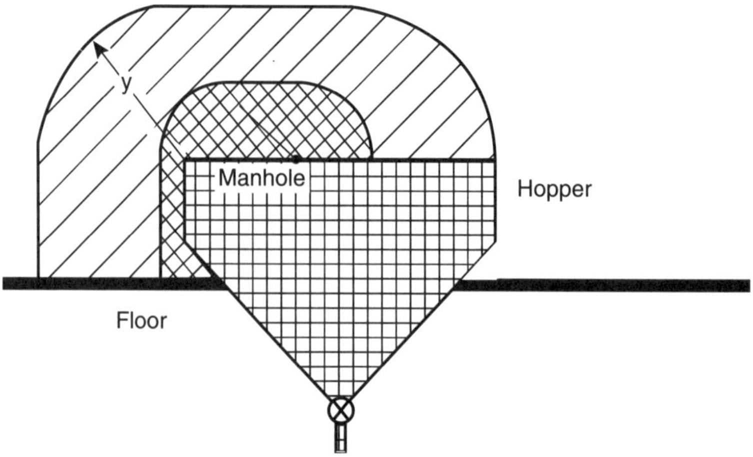

Fig. 6.3 Manually loaded hopper without air purge inwards through manhole outside a building. X = 1.5 m, y = 2.5 m. *Notes*: (1) The area below the loading floor is not addressed. (2) Where air is drawn into the hopper through the manhole, the dust cloud producing the Zone 21 will not exist provided the airflow at the manhole mouth exceeds 1 m/s

Layers of dust are formed wherever dust is released, even if that release is not sufficient to produce an explosive dust cloud. The extent and thickness of such layers is, to a degree, dependent upon the level of housekeeping in the area of release, particularly if this is indoors. While the level of housekeeping will always need to be sufficient to ensure that extensive, thick dust layers will not form from releases which occur in normal operation (from primary grade sources of release), only a very high level of such housekeeping can be assumed to have a significant limiting effect upon the extent of hazardous areas from dust-layer formation from secondary grade sources of release. These are usually from rare failures of process equipment containment and are less predictable and usually larger (for example, from the rupture of a bag being brought to the discharge point). For this reason it is not unusual to find the entire area of a building containing dust processing equipment classified as Zone 22. In addition, it is quite normal to classify the entire height of such a building as Zone 22, even though the dust layer will only be at floor level. Dust layers can form on beams, stanchions and similar items which produce ledges at higher levels and these must be taken into account, which is why a height limit is often not used.

Where dust is stored rather than processed the situation may be different depending upon the method of containment. Where drums and similar containers are used, the likelihood of leakage is small, and coupled with good housekeeping it is not difficult to ensure that dangerous layers of dust do not occur. Where the material is stored in such things as paper sacks this ceases to be true and it is likely that the storage area should be classified as Zone 22.

6.3 Practical situations

6.3.1 Cyclones and bag filters

Figure 6.1 shows a cyclone which is separating the product of a process which is formed of granules from dust of the same material produced by the process. The cyclone and bag filter are in separate small rooms with the bag filter air exhausting to the outside of the building. The hazardous area situation is as follows.

Zone 20

Both the interior of the cyclone and the bag filter on the powder side of the filter will be Zone 20, because dust is always present in both. As the process works by extracting air, the system is at a pressure slightly lower than that of the atmosphere and leakage from the pipework and the two vessels may be ignored.

Zone 21

As the system works at slightly lower than atmospheric pressure there is no leakage of dust from the system in normal operation. The dust from the filter is, however, discharged into a bag and release is possible in normal operation around the discharge duct. The discharge nozzle is a primary grade source of release and a Zone 21 will exist for a distance of 1 m above and around it and down to floor level.

Zone 22

The release of dust from the discharge duct can produce layers of dust, but in normal operation it is expected that housekeeping will limit the extent of these layers to within the Zone 21. It must occasionally be expected, however, that due to misalignment of the dust receptacle, failure of the receptacle/duct sealing arrangements (usually an air-operated expanding seal) significantly more dust will be released. While this will not greatly affect the extent of the dust cloud for reasons already mentioned, it will increase the amount of dust-forming layers and probably the housekeeping will not be sufficient to limit the extent of the layers in this case. Therefore, a Zone 22 will exist for a larger distance because of these circumstances and, as it will be difficult to define its extent, it will be assumed to cover the entire building. If there were no ledges, etc., in the building it may be possible to assume the Zone 22 is limited in height to 3 m or so.

6.3.2 Loading hoppers within buildings

It is quite common to use hoppers as a means of loading powders into process and quite often these hoppers will be on upper floors with effective sealing arrangements to prevent spilled dust from accessing the process floors. In these circumstances the following is the Zonal classification of the loading area. (See Fig. 6.2.)

Zone 20

The hopper is normally filled, or partially filled, with feedstock which is loaded into it by discharging containers, such as sacks of raw material. There will normally be thick layers of feedstock and possibly small clouds of the material within the confines of the hopper. For this reason the interior of the hopper will be considered as Zone 20.

Zone 21

The area around the manhole will be contaminated with dust clouds during loading of sacks if extreme care is not exercised and, as it is so likely that this situation will occur, the clouds produced by emptying of sacks, etc., into the hopper will be considered as a primary grade source of release giving a Zone 21 around the charging manhole, extending to 1 m above and around the manhole and down to the top of the manhole or the floor as appropriate.

The Zone 21 can effectively be removed by extracting room air into the hopper so that any dust released is effectively sucked into the hopper. In this case, there will be no Zone 21 around the manhole. The minimum airflow considered necessary to achieve this will produce a velocity of 1 m/s at the manhole mouth.

Zone 22

Dust will settle from the cloud but will normally be taken care of by housekeeping. This, however, will not always be so and occasionally there will be spillage from the bags in the room. These situations will constitute secondary grade sources of release, which will give rise to Zone 22 in the room. As before, unless the room is large the Zone 22 will be assumed to extend for the whole area of the room and its height, unless there can be guaranteed to be no ledges at high level in which case a height restriction of 3 m may be appropriate.

If the housekeeping is of such a standard that spillages are removed at the time which they occur and the hopper is arranged so that air is extracted from the room into it, then the Zone 22 can be limited to around 2 m surrounding the hopper manhole, as dust will only be released from the loading procedure abnormally when the air extract system fails.

6.3.3 Loading hoppers outside buildings

Where hoppers are in well-ventilated areas (outdoors) the Zones 20 and 21 are as described in Section 6.3.2. The Zone 22 however is different. (See Fig. 6.3.)

Zone 22

The outdoor situation is one in which there is assumed to be significant air movement and this will limit the deposition of dust so that the Zone 22 will have a finite size. Because of the air movement, spillage will be blown away rapidly and housekeeping will cover the unusual situation where it is not. The size of the Zone 22 in these circumstances is unlikely to exceed 3 m in dimension.

Care should be taken, however, to identify any places where obstructions, such as walls, could cause build-up of wind-borne dust to allow layers of dangerous thickness.

References

1 The Factories Act 1961.

2 BS 6467 Electrical Apparatus With Protection by Enclosure for Use in the Presence of Combustible Dust. Part 2 (1988). Guide to Selection, Installation and Maintenance.

3 IEC 1241–3 Electrical Apparatus for Use in the Presence of Combustible Dust. Part 3. Classification of Areas Where Combustible Dusts are or may be Present. (Draft 1994) (BS 94/213454 DC)

4 IEC 1241–2 Electrical Apparatus for Use in the Presence of Combustible Dust. Part 2, Test Methods: Section 1 (1994). Method for the Determination of the Minimum Ignition Temperature of Dust; Section 2 (1993). Method for the Determination of the Ignition Temperature of Dust in Layers; Section 3 (1993). Method for Determination of Minimum Ignition Energy for Dust/Air Mixtures.

— 7 —

Design philosophy for electrical apparatus for explosive atmospheres

General approach and applicable standards

The preceding three chapters discuss the various facets of the classification of areas made hazardous by the possible presence of explosive atmospheres of air mixed with gas, vapour, mist or dust. From these, it is possible to identify the areas where the hazard exists, together with the severity of the hazard. It now becomes necessary to address the construction of electrical equipment which should be installed in such areas to minimize the risk of fire or explosion. In doing this, it has to be recognized that however well protected electrical equipment may be, there will always be residual risk if it is placed in areas where explosive atmospheres may occur. To this end, the first golden rule is: *Only that electrical apparatus which is really necessary should be placed in or communicate with explosive atmospheres.*

The necessity of placing electrical equipment in explosive atmospheres has to be determined not only on safety grounds but also on operational and economic grounds. However, the yardstick which should always be applied is that of real benefit and unless such benefit can be recognized the equipment should not be installed.

7.1 History

The construction of electrical equipment specifically for use in areas where explosion risks might occur due to clouds of gas, vapour, mist or dust was a problem first addressed in the early part of the twentieth century and initially was aimed at the coal-mining industry. This initial addressing of the problem concentrated upon the problems associated with methane (firedamp) and the problems of coal dust.

7.1.1 Gas, vapour and mist risks

The types of protection envisaged for coal mining were those associated with protection against gas clouds and the levels of overall protection envisaged were those which were suitable for underground areas where men normally worked. They also presumed the equipment to be switched off if any gas was detected. Although it was relatively rare for significant outbursts of firedamp to occur (i.e., those which would engulf the men and the equipment before the latter could be switched off) the difficulty of escape from a mine was significant and a relatively high level of protection was adopted. This level later became the norm for Zone 1 above ground. Therefore the oldest types of protection currently used for electrical equipment in surface industry are those appropriate to Zone 1.

Surface industry did not, in the early days, consider the installation of electrical equipment in Zone 0, a situation contemporarily familiar to those dealing with dust hazards, and it was only with the rapid development of instrumentation that any such demand became significant. It must be remembered that Zone 0 generally occurs inside such things as process vessels and so, until the demand for automatic process monitoring increased with the development of sophisticated instruments at a much later date, there was no demand for protection suitable for Zone 0. Even now it is generally only necessary to site instrument sensors in Zone 0 and only the type of protection suitable for such devices has been developed for Zone 0. The Zone 2 scenario did not exist underground and was very much a surface industry phenomenon. Initially, it was presumed that good quality industrial equipment, which did not spark or get hot in normal operation, was suitable for Zone 2 and little work was done on Standards for Zone 2 equipment until relatively recently; industry being content with a Guide to Selection of Electrical Equipment for Zone 2[1].

The approach to Zone 2 has become less and less acceptable over the years and although it is still possible to utilize it there are now construction Standards for Zone 2 equipment and EU Directives[2] are making the old 'Selected Industrial Apparatus' approach less and less acceptable.

The above explains why, in respect of gas and vapour risks, the Standards for Zone 1 equipment are much more developed than those for Zone 0 or Zone 2 equipment at present, although much is being done to correct this.

7.1.2 Dust risks

A similar situation exists in respect of equipment for dusts as, historically it has not been considered as acceptable to put equipment inside dust-processing vessels, etc. and the Standards for such equipment did not recognize the interior Zone[3]. There is now a three-Zone system for dusts and it is expected that the equipment Standards in this area also will develop in the future. (It is worthy of note that one Code used a three-Zone system in the early 1970's[4] and this gives some idea of the inertia in developing ideas in the explosive atmospheres field.)

Fortunately, there is now an international three-Zone system for dusts, which is similar to that used for many years for gases, vapours and mists, with similar definitions and it is hoped that some parallelism will now develop in addressing the problems of explosive atmospheres.

7.2 Protection of electrical apparatus for gas, vapour and mist risks

As previously noted, released gas, vapour or mist clouds disperse relatively quickly after release and do not form layers on equipment as dust does. If equipment is protected against condensation, particularly in the case of hot vapours or mists, access of these to the inside of the equipment is not necessarily a problem, provided that the electrical components and circuits within the enclosure do not spark incendively or become excessively hot. If they do spark incendively or become excessively hot then their entry does, of course, have to be prevented unless the results of the resultant ignition can be effectively dealt with. There are thus four basic approaches which can be adopted to prevent uncontrolled ignitions of gas, vapour or mist and air clouds.

1. The gas, vapour or mist/air cloud can be excluded by mechanical barriers or other equivalent means.
2. The components of the electrical circuits can be prevented from sparking or becoming sufficiently hot to ignite the gas, vapour or mist/air cloud.
3. The gas,vapour or mist/air cloud can be permitted to enter the equipment enclosure and ignited, but the ensuing propagation of the explosion outside the enclosure can be prevented by some form of quenching.
4. The electrical components within the enclosure can be permitted to spark, but the energy fed to the enclosure will be limited to a level which is not capable of igniting the gas, vapour or mist/air cloud.

The above are the four main approaches to the limitation of explosion risk to an acceptable level. Clearly, they will, in many cases, have significant effect upon the design of the equipment and it should never be forgotten that there will be certain basic requirements for the equipment in a particular location, even if the explosion risk is not taken into account (e.g., equipment sited out of doors will normally need to be weather proof). The operational reliability of the equipment relies upon these basic requirements, which protect it from its general environment and the explosion protection techniques applied to the equipment are normally based upon its operational reliability. This means that, in general, the explosion protection features of equipment will be additional to, and not instead of, the basic operational requirements, such as protection from the environment.

Using the four criteria described above, specific types of protection have been developed over the years and are mostly referred to in detailed construction Standards.

7.2.1 Exclusion of the explosive atmosphere (criterion a)

Three methods of satisfying this requirement in the construction of explosion protected apparatus have been developed and are in general current use. These are immersion of the electrical circuits in oil, encapsulation of the electrical circuits, and pressurization of the enclosure containing the electrical circuits with non-flammable gas.

Oil immersion (symbol 'o')

In this protection concept (type of protection) the electrical components are immersed in oil within their enclosure, thus preventing access of the explosive atmosphere. It is dealt with in detail in Chapter 9. There are limitations on the type of oil which may be used and requirements to ensure the security of the oil within the enclosure, so that the electrical circuits remain immersed. The technique is considered as suitable for Zone 2 only, at present, within the UK but is used in more hazardous areas in other countries. This is likely to change in the not-too-distant future (see Chapter 9) and will be the protection concept permitted in Zone 1.

Encapsulation (symbol 'm')

This protection concept is dealt with in detail in Chapter 9. Again, the explosive atmosphere and electrical circuits are separated from one another, this time by encapsulating (potting) material. The types of material used are defined and the encapsulated block is arranged so that surfaces presented to the outside are hard enough to give protection. The technique is considered as suitable for both Zone 1 and 2.

Pressurization (symbol 'p')

This protection concept is dealt with in detail in Chapter 11. In this technique the explosive atmosphere is kept out of the equipment enclosure by pressure of air or inert gas. Air is normally used as there are asphyxiation problems with inert gas. Because the protection is by a gas (air) it is almost always necessary to provide ancillary equipment to ensure that the air pressure is maintained in spite of small leakages, which are almost certain to occur. Because of this the technique almost always requires a pressure-control system, together with a purge system to ensure that on start-up any internal explosive atmosphere is removed, and this gives added complication which must be set against its added flexibility because of the ease of depressurizing for repair. The technique is considered as suitable for both Zone 1 and 2 or only Zone 2, depending upon the pressure-control systems used.

7.2.2 Prevention of sparking (criterion b)

There is only one formal protection concept which is suitable for both Zone 1 and 2 in this area.

Increased safety (symbol 'e')

This protection concept is dealt with in detail in Chapter 12. The technique accepts that there is ignition-capable energy within the equipment but relies upon the quality of construction to ensure that the energy is not released in a way which could cause ignition. This is achieved by the quality of construction of the equipment. The technique is considered as suitable for both Zone 1 and 2.

7.2.3 Containment of explosions (criterion c)

There are two protection concepts which use this technique.

Flameproof equipment (symbol 'd')

This is the oldest protection technique. The explosive atmosphere is permitted to enter the equipment enclosure and to be ignited by the components within. The equipment is, however, provided with a very special strong enclosure which will withstand the internal explosion without sustaining damage and, in addition, will prevent the flames associated with the internal explosion from exiting the enclosure in a way which would permit them to ignite any surrounding explosive atmosphere. The technique is considered as suitable for both Zone 1 and 2.

Powder filling (symbol 'q')

Here the equipment enclosure is filled with quartz, sand or some similar inert small-grained filling. The technique is an extension of an old technique involving the use of stone chambers to prevent the passage of flame up-ducting. These chambers served to quench the flame, or so it was thought. The filling does not prevent the explosive atmosphere from accessing the equipment and coming into the proximity of a source of ignition. The fine-grained filling, however, serves to quench any ignition, thus preventing an explosion. The technique is considered as suitable for Zone 2 only in the UK, but is used in more hazardous areas in other countries and is expected to be acceptable for use in Zone 1 in the UK in the not-too-distant future (see Chapter 9).

7.2.4 Energy limitation (criterion d)

There is only one protection concept in this area but it is the protection concept offering the highest level of security.

Intrinsic safety (symbol 'i')

In this technique the electrical energy fed to the equipment is below that which will cause ignition if released in a spark or as a hot surface, and all energy storage in the equipment is closely controlled to ensure that stored energy is limited. As with pressurization, this equipment relies to a large extent upon other equipment, which feeds it with electricity and the technique is somewhat complex. It is also limited in its application to instrumentation because of the energy limitations imposed, but within this limitation it is very flexible.

There are two grades of intrinsic safety, the higher grade 'ia' being suitable for Zone 0, Zone 1 and Zone 2, but the lower grade 'ib' being limited to Zone 1 and Zone 2.

7.2.5 Special situations

While the methods of equipment protection given in Sections 7.2.1 to 7.2.4 cover most situations normally encountered, there is an additional type of protection for use where the types already described are not appropriate because of advances in technology or special circumstances.

Special protection (symbol 's')

Special protection is not a fixed type of protection, as in the above but is used to describe equipment which is suitable for use in explosive atmospheres on the basis that its individual type of protection is equivalent to one of the more classic types, although different. Its typical use is to permit advances in technology where such advances do not easily fit into standard types of protection. It has been typically used for encapsulated equipment 'm' prior to the publication of the construction Standard for that type of protection, and for sintered flame arresters prior to those being included in type of protection 'd' (flameproof enclosure). It has also been used where techniques contrary to existing standards such as bi-pin tubes in type 'e' (increased safety) fluorescent fittings are used on the basis of equivalent safety. It can also be used where equipment which has two independent types of protection, each of which is complete in itself (e.g., an increased safety 'e' terminal chamber in a flameproof enclosure), is used provided that the two protection concepts are each independent of the other. This latter approach must, however, be treated with caution.

Type 's' equipment is usable as specified in each particular case, and is only usable in Zone 0 and 1 where this is specifically stated.

7.3 Situation in respect of Zone 2 apparatus

While the techniques described in Sections 7.2.1 to 7.2.5 are all suitable for, at least, Zone 1 and 2 (with the exception of the current situation in respect of protection concepts 'o' and 'q') they offer a standard of protection which is higher than is necessary for Zone 2. For this reason a further type of protection has been developed.

Type of protection 'n' (historically in the UK, type of protection 'N')

This type of protection includes industrial equipment which does not get hot or spark, which was historically selected by users, and adds simplified forms of protection for sparking equipment or that which gets hot, based upon the Zone 1 types of protection. By producing detailed requirements, it removes the doubt which used to exist when only selection by somewhat general criteria was the order of the day, which led to excessive use of Zone 1 equipment in Zone 2, needlessly increasing operational expense.

7.4 Protection of electrical apparatus for dust risks

Unlike the situation in respect of gases, vapours and mists, the problems in relation to dusts are the settling properties which dusts have, and their conductivity. If dust enters an equipment enclosure in significant quantities, it will settle on the electrical components and by insulating them could cause excessive heating and, if it is conductive, partial short circuits and similar faults. The objective with dusts, therefore, is always to prevent significant amounts penetrating the enclosure. This leads to a very much simpler situation than that which exists with gases, vapours and mists, as there is effectively only one form of protection, which is to ensure the dust remains on the outside of the enclosure.

While some equipment constructed for gas/vapour/mist risks is also suitable for dusts, this does not necessarily follow, and it should not be assumed that because equipment is suitable for the one type of medium it is automatically suitable for the other. It is very important to remember this as dust risks and gas/vapour/mist risks often coincide and, in such cases, the electrical equipment must be protected for use in both types of risk, and the elements of this protection may be separate in each case.

7.5 Apparatus construction Standards

The harmonization of Standards is of paramount importance for members of the EU as these Standards will be acceptable throughout the EU and, by an agreement between the EU and the European Free Trade Association (EFTA), in EFTA countries also. To this end, those Standards which are harmonized may be called up in EU Directives as Standards with which compliance demonstrates fulfilment of the Directive, provided this is verified by a recognized (notified) certification body. Therefore, the Standards for equipment protection for gas, vapour and mist risks (with the exception of those methods restricted to Zone 2 use only) have been historically referred to in 76/117/EEC[2] and compliance with them allows the use of the Distinctive Community Mark (see Chapter 1). With the introduction of the newer Directive 94/9/EC[5], the EEC policy was changed to include essential technical requirements within the Directive. These are included in a relatively general form and it is intended to identify the harmonized standards (EN's) as a method of satisfying the essential requirements, by their approval by publication in the *European Journal*[7]. Unfortunately, it has been realized that the second editions of these current Standards do not necessarily satisfy the essential requirements and the Standards writing body, the Centre Europeen de Normalization Electrique (CENELEC), has been remitted to produce third editions which do in general, in 1997. This means that the new Directive[5] cannot be practically introduced until some time in 1997, and in the meantime the older Directive[2] will remain the only vehicle by which the Distinctive Community Mark can be awarded. Unfortunately, this Directive still refers to the first editions of the harmonized Standards and the second editions, now current, will not permit the use of the mark. Urgent action is being taken to introduce the second editions of the harmonized Standards into 76/117/EEC[2] but until that time certification in accordance with that Directive will be in line with the first editions.

While this seems to be a problem, it is not really, since the second editions do not vary widely from the first, and most equipment manufacturers are ensuring that their equipment will comply with both until the new Directive[5] comes into force . When this Directive[5] is enacted the third editions of the harmonized Standards will exist, and any equipment certified after that will comply to the new provisions.

7.5.1 Zone 0 and/or Zone 1 compatible apparatus for gases, vapours and mists

As already stated, there is a long world-wide history of utilizing only third-party certified equipment in Zone 0 and 1 and in some countries this is required by law. At the moment this is not the case in the UK, but the new Explosive Atmosphere Directive[5] from the EU will effectively ensure this by requiring that all equipment marketed in the EU complies with it (the Directive itself requiring third-party type certification as a minimum). While this will cause some restriction in the UK the impact will not be great, as industry in the UK has historically used only third-party certified equipment by choice. Therefore, subject to the resolution of the difficulties already identified in this chapter, the situation will not change greatly. What this historic situation has led to is a very high degree of detailed construction Standards which have become more and more international due to the international level of operation of the industry which needs the equipment. The current situation is that the Standards for electrical equipment intended generally for Zone 0 or Zone 1 (or both) are fully harmonized European Standards, and within the next 10 years will become fully harmonized International Standards. There are, however, historic national and European Standards which address this area and equipment is still available complying with these Standards. There is no suggestion that, in general, such equipment is not still safely usable in many circumstances, and the titles of those Standards are referred to in Chapters 8 to 15. Many of those standards are, however, obsolete or withdrawn and they should not be used for construction of new equipment. Where equipment complying with both current and historic Standards is available, the equipment to the current standards is always preferable.

The relatively large number of methods by which electrical equipment may be protected has meant that a large number of Standards exist, and it has been recognized that many of the requirements of these standards are common. The standardization structure is therefore to have a general Standard and a series of additional Standards which refer to the general Standard for many of their requirements, but contain additional requirements particular to the method used to protect the equipment. These are all European Standards and are structured as follows.

BS/EN 50014 (1993) – General requirements (see Chapter 8)

This is the general or common Standard and contains any requirements which apply to more than one of the specific methods of protection. Its requirements apply to all of the protection concepts (with the current exception of 'n'), unless they are specifically excluded and should be read in conjunction with all of the following individual protection concept Standards. It is currently at its second edition stage which should supersede the first edition, but equipment certified in accordance with this and one of the subsidiary protection concept Standards cannot, as already described, bear the Distinctive Community Mark referred to in Chapter 1, unless it also satisfies the first edition of the Standard. Therefore, it will not have free access to EU Member States (and EFTA States).

This, as already identified, is because Directive 76/117/EEC[2] currently refers to the first edition and the mark is controlled by the Directive, not the Standard. Again, as already identified, work is in hand to modify 76/117/EEC[2] and it is expected to allow the use of the second editions of this, and its subsidiary Standards, for equipment relating to the Directive in late 1996. A further complication which is preventing the activating of the new Directive[5] is the fact that there appear to be discrepancies between the second editions of these Standards and the essential requirements given in the new Directive. (As already stated, all new approach Directives carry the essential safety requirements within them, unlike their older counterparts which referred to Standards). This means that third editions of These standards will need to be produced and the production is expected to be complete in late 1997. When published, equipment complying with the third editions of these Standards will be deemed to comply with the Directive and will consequently be able to carry the 'Distinctive Community Mark' in accordance with the Directive's provisions. The need for continuing with the older Directive, 76/117/EEC[2], will then cease to exist for new equipment, although the older equipment will continue to be acceptable until the beginning of the twenty-first century (see Chapter 1).

This Standard, as already indicated, is supplemented by a series of specific Standards.

BS/EN 50015 (1994) – Oil immersion 'o' (see Chapter 9)

This is the second edition of this particular Standard. It suffers from the same problems in use as BS/EN 50014, second edition, and the resolution of those problems is being dealt with in the same way.

BS/EN 50016 (1996) – Pressurized apparatus 'p' (see Chapter 11)

This is the second edition of this particular Standard. It suffers from the same problems in use as BS/EN 50014, second edition, and the resolution of those problems is being dealt with in the same way.

BS/EN 50017 (1994) – Powder filling 'q' (see Chapter 9)

This is the second edition of this particular Standard. It suffers from the same problems in use as BS/EN 50014, second edition, and the resolution of those problems is being dealt with in the same way.

BS/EN 50018 (1995) – Flameproof enclosures 'd' (see Chapter 10)

This is the second edition of this particular Standard. It suffers from the same problems in use as BS/EN 50014, second edition, and the resolution of those problems is being dealt with in the same way.

BS/EN 50019 (1994) – Increased safety 'e' (see Chapter 12)

This is the second edition of this particular Standard. It suffers from the same problems in use as BS/EN 50014, second edition, and the resolution of those problems is being dealt with in the same way.

BS/EN 50020 (1995) – Intrinsic safety 'i' (see Chapter 13)

This is the second edition of this particular Standard. It suffers from the same problems in use as BS/EN 50014, second edition, and resolution of those problems are being dealt with in the same way.

EN 50028 (1987) – Encapsulation 'm' (see Chapter 9)

This is the first edition of this particular Standard. It is dual numbered and is also known as BS 5501, Part 8 (1987). It is not being rewritten at this time as it is felt to remain current and will not be amended until a third edition is published to comply with the essential requirements of 94/9/EC[5]. This produces a further complication as it refers to the first edition of EN 50014 and should be used with that edition. This is not, however, a major problem as those parts of EN 50014 which apply can be derived from either edition of EN 50014 without problems (see Chapter 9).

EN 50039 (1980) – Intrinsically safe electrical systems 'i' (see Chapter 13)

This is the first edition of this particular Standard and is dual numbered as BS 5501, Part 9 (1982). Fortunately it does not directly relate to EN 50014 but is stated to be a supplement to EN 50020 (1977) (BS 5501 part 7 (1977)), the first edition of that Standard. There is no practical problem here and this Standard can equally be used with the second edition of EN 50020 which is current (BS/EN 50020) (see Chapter 13).

7.5.2 The marketing situation in respect of European Standards

The value of the European Standards referred to in Section 7.5.1 lies in the fact that equipment which complies with them in their appropriate issue may bear the Distinctive Community Mark and has free access to both the EU and EFTA (European Free Trade Association) States. The problem lies in the difficulty in harmonizing the political (EU) documentation with the standards which are written by a separate technical body (CENELEC). For the time being, equipment must comply with the first editions of these standards to bear the Distinctive Community Mark but will also need to comply with the second editions of the Standards because of the imminent modification of the older Directive[2]. It is likely, for the time being, that equipment will need, to provide maximum flexibility for the manufacturer, to comply with both the first and the second editions.

In addition, because two of the above Standards are still current in their first editions, the situation appears even more complicated. These two Standards, however, make limited reference to EN 50014 and the change of edition of that Standard will make little practical difference. Also, the 'n' Standard is relatively contemporary and will include much of current thinking.

In addition to the above Standards, a certification Standard was issued for type of protection 's' by one of the UK third-party certification bodies. This may sound odd as, if an item of equipment is special it infers that it is non-standard. These was, however, a good reason for this issue and the Standard is used by both UK third-party certification bodies for the issue of national certificates, as opposed to the European certificates issued for equipment complying with European Standards.

SFA 3009 (1972) – BASEEFA Standard for type of protection 's' (see Chapter 9)

This Standard included many of the techniques developed, but not included, in formal Standards at the time (e.g., sinters, encapsulation, etc).

It has now been largely taken over by the second editions of the European Standards, but equipment certified to its requirements is still available and used in the UK.

7.5.3 Zone 2 compatible apparatus for gases, vapours and mists

In the case of Zone 2 apparatus there is no long history of third-party certification as in the more hazardous zones, and industry has historically selected its own using a British Standard Guide[1] for assistance. Within the UK, however, industry has always been slightly uneasy at this and has sought third-party certification for Zone 2 equipment also. Historically, there was no avenue for this and as no detailed certification requirements existed it was difficult to arrange one. This unhappy situation led to HM Factory Inspectorate issuing 'Letters of no Objection' for some items of equipment, which effectively said that the Factory Inspectorate had no knowledge or evidence to suggest the equipment was unsuitable. This difficult state of affairs led to the production in the UK of a Standard for Type 'N' equipment[6] to permit formal certification. The reason for the upper case 'N' was that there was an international symbol for this equipment 'n' and it was hoped that the use of the upper case letter would avoid confusion with the international concept, for which there was no Standard. There still remains only a National Standard for Type 'N' equipment and, unlike the situation in Section 7.4.1 where certification is valid across Europe, type 'N' certificates issued within the UK are valid only in the UK. The Standard in question is:

BS 6941 (1988) – Electrical apparatus for explosive atmospheres with type of protection 'N' (see Chapter 14)

This Standard covers all of the requirements for all of the methods used for protection of electrical equipment which is intended for Zone 2. It is based upon an international document published by the International Electrotechnical Commission – IEC 79/15 (1987), but because of the fact that the UK did not agree with some of the contents of IEC 79/15 there are significant differences.

IEC 79–15 (1987) – Electrical equipment for explosive gas atmospheres Part 15: electrical apparatus with type of protection 'n' (see Chapter 14)

This international document was the subject of considerable controversy as several countries objected to some parts of it. The principal objection of the UK was to the restricted breathing concept being used for sparking contacts and this concept does not appear in BS 6941. Because of these objections it was only possible to issue IEC 79–15 as an IEC Report not a Standard. This means that it is only a guidance document despite having the appearance of a Standard.

7.5.4 Electrical apparatus for dust risks

The British Standard for dusts based upon the International Standard is not yet published and the current British Standards[3] are limited to Zone 21 and 22 (Zone Z and Y). There are currently, therefore, no Standards for the construction of electrical equipment for Zone 20.

For Zone 21 and 22, equipment construction Standards exist. These mainly cover the degree of enclosure of the equipment, together with additional construction requirements covering such things as strength, etc. In one case, the relevant Standard covers the additional requirements necessary to make equipment constructed for gas/vapour and mist risks suitable for use in the explosive atmospheres of combustible dusts. The relevant Standards follow:

BS 6467 (1985) – Electrical apparatus with protection by enclosure for use in the presence of combustible dusts, Part 1: specification for apparatus (see Chapter 15)

It will be noted that the Standard particularly draws attention to the fact that protection is by enclosure. In addition, the Standard differentiates between equipment suitable for Zone 21 and Zone 22, and that suitable only for Zone 22.

BS 7353 (1992) – Guide to the use of electrical apparatus complying with BS 5501 or BS 6941 in the presence of combustible dust (see Chapter 15)

This Standard essentially specifies in what circumstances equipment complying with European Standards (ENs) is suitable for use in explosive atmospheres of combustible dust and air and what extra constructional features are necessary. It refers to these European Standards as BS 5501, as their first editions were given the numbers that follow:

BS 5501, Part 1 (1977) – EN 50014, first edition
BS 5501, Part 2 (1997) – EN 50015, first edition
BS 5501, Part 3 (1977) – EN 50016, first edition
BS 5501, Part 4 (1977) – EN 50017, first edition
BS 5501, Part 5 (1977) – EN 50018, first edition
BS 5501, Part 6 (1977) – EN 50019, first edition
BS 5501, Part 7 (1977) – EN 50020, first edition
BS 5501, Part 8 (1988) – EN 50028, first edition
BS 5501, Part 9 (1982) – EN 50039, first edition

While, as before, these European Standards are now, or soon will be, replaced by their second editions (which are numbered BS/EN50 and upwards with the exception of BS 5501, Parts 8 and 9) the differences so produced are not likely to be significant and it is likely that in most cases the second editions will, when used with this standard, produce satisfactory results.

IEC 1241–1 – Electrical apparatus for use in the presence of combustible dust, Part 1: electrical apparatus protected by enclosure (see Chapter 6)

This is the IEC document which is relevant to dust hazards and is a much newer document.

The requirements of this Standard are not dissimilar to BS 6467, Part 1 and at some time in the future it is expected that the two Standards will be harmonized. Until that time, however, it is expected that equipment to either the IEC Standard or BS 6467, Part 1 will be acceptable in the UK.

A further Part of IEC 1241 is also envisaged and will address at least some of the matters addressed by BS 7535. Work is in hand on sections to cover intrinsic safety 'i' and pressurization 'p' in dust risks. When they are published, unless the UK votes against them, they are expected to be acceptable in the UK as alternatives to BS 7535.

References

1 BS 4137 (1967) Guide to the Selection of Electrical Equipment for use in Division 2 Areas.

2 76/117/EEC Council Directive of 18 December 1975 (on the approximation of the laws of Member States concerning electrical equipment for use in Potentially Explosive Atmospheres)

3 BS 6467 Electrical Apparatus with Protection by Enclosure for Use in the Presence of Combustible Dusts. Part 2 (1985) Guide to Selection, Installation and Maintenance.

4 RoSPA/ICI Engineering Codes and Regulations, Electrical Installations in Flammable Atmospheres (1973). Group C (Electrical), Volume 1.5.

5 94/9/EC Directive of the European Parliament and Council of 23 March 1994 (on the approximation of the laws of Member States concerning equipment and protective systems intended for use in Potentially Explosive Atmospheres)

6 BS 4683 Electrical Apparatus for Explosive Atmospheres Part 3 (1972). Type of Protection N.

7 Official Journal of the European Communities.

— 8 —

General requirements for explosion protected apparatus (gas, vapour and mist risks)

Apparatus to European Standards

Before embarking upon a detailed examination of the general requirements[1] Standard it is necessary to understand the wording used in this and other Standards. First, the Standard does not have the imperative of legislation and cannot dictate what must or must not be done to comply with the law in any country.

The words which are important in this and other Standards are, first *shall*, the use of which indicates that a requirement is a necessity as far as the Standard is concerned. If this is not complied with compliance with the Standard cannot be claimed.

Second, the use of *should*, which indicates a strong recommendation but allows some flexibility in application of the Standard. In other words, it may be that, occasionally, an alternative approach producing the same effective result will be acceptable. The stress here is on the word *occasional* as the relaxation is not intended to allow a coach and horses to be driven through the Standard. It should be noted that the word *should* is only occasionally used in any event.

The word *must* is seldom used in Standards but where it does appear it means that a law exists at the time the Standard was written, and an imperative is appropriate. The Standard is not in this case making law but drawing attention to the existence of law.

Chapter 7 identifies the European Standards which exist for the differing types of explosion protected equipment. It draws attention to the fact that, unlike the preceding National Standards in the UK where all of the requirements were contained within the particular protection concept Standard, the European Standards contain only those requirements specific to the particular protection concept, with the more general requirements (i.e., those which applied to several of the protection concepts) being contained in a general requirements[1] Standard to which the protection concept Standards refer. The requirements of this Standard are then considered to apply to all of the particular protection concept Standards, unless a particular Standard specifically excludes one or more of these general requirements. This approach is considered to minimize the duplication of effort by the Standards writing committees and give a more rational approach. In practice, this approach has been shown to have significant drawbacks, in that any change to the general requirements Standard automatically impinges upon the particular protection concept Standards which are written by different European committees, comprising different sets of people to those involved in the writing of the general requirements Standard. To overcome this, particular protection concept Standards specify a particular issue of the general requirements Standard, but this means that, as the particular protection concept Standards are written in different time frames, it is necessary to have more than one issue of the general requirements Standard valid at any one time. Unless one is very careful, confusion can result. While the situation is less than perfect, it is unlikely to change and whenever a particular protection concept is addressed, it is necessary to ensure that it is addressed with the appropriate issue of the general requirements Standard.

The latest issue of the general requirements Standard is BS/EN 50014 (second edition) (1993)[1] which applies to all of the protection concepts with the exception of Ex m (BS 5501, Part 8 (1988) – EN 50028 (1987) at present. Its predecessor which applies to Ex m was BS 5501, Part 1 (1977) – EN 50014 (1977), first edition. A further complication is the fact that both of these Standards have been the subject of amendments issued after the publication of the Standards (seven in the case of BS 5501 part 1 (1977) and one in the case of BS/EN 50014 (1993)[1]. In general terms, amendments are considered to be part of the standard and thus will apply to all of the protection concept Standards from the date of amendment issue, unless these latter Standards are themselves amended to exclude the amendment to the general requirements Standard. To simplify the situation, therefore, the second edition of the Standard (BS/EN 50014 (1993)[1], including amendment 1) will form the basis of the content of this chapter and differences between it and the first edition (BS 5501, part 1 (1977), including amendments 1 to 7) will be highlighted to cover the situation until Directive 76/117/EEC is amended, as previously discussed.

8.1 BS/EN 50014 (1993) (including amendment 1 (1994))

It is better to deal with the amendment to this Standard first to avoid any confusion. It may appear that the necessity to amend a Standard so soon after its publication is worrying, but the amendment was issued only to the English text of the Standard which omitted the limitation of validity of the Standard to the second editions of the protection concept standards only. (All European Standards are written in three languages, English, French and German and in this case the English language text omitted a paragraph present in the French and German texts). It is worthy of note here that EN Standards may appear in other languages but those are national translations and in any dispute as to the meaning of the Standards the English, French and German texts must be referred to for clarification.

BS/EN 50014 (1993)[1] deals with those matters common to more than one of the protection concepts. Some of its content may not be appropriate to a particular protection concept Standard and, in this case, that Standard will, in its scope where exclusion is total, or in its detailed text where exclusion is only partial, define those parts of BS/EN 50014 (1993)[1] which do not apply. The basic matters dealt with in BS/EN 50014 (1993)[1] and its predecessor, BS 5501, part 1 (1977) are as follows:

1. Definitions of terms used in BS/EN 50014 (1993)[1] and its subsidiary protection concept Standards.
2. The method by which apparatus is divided into groups and temperature classes for utilization purposes.
3. Requirements for enclosures.
4. Requirements for fasteners used for enclosure securing, interlocking devices used to prevent protection being bypassed, bushings used for connections, and cements which may be used in enclosure construction.
5. Requirements for connection of conductors to the apparatus and for entry of cables to the apparatus.
6. Requirements which additionally apply to particular types of apparatus such as rotating machines, luminaires, fuses, etc.
7. Requirements for ex-components, which are components which form part of an apparatus but may be used in several types of apparatus, and be examined for compliance with the appropriate parts of the standard separately to avoid repeat evaluation.
8. Requirements for marking of complying apparatus to ensure that appropriate information is given to the purchaser.

It is worthy of note that BS/EN 50014 (1993)[1] draws attention to the fact that apparatus constructors need also to ensure that basic electrical safety requirements are met, and are assumed to guarantee this by application of the marking required by the Standard. (BS 5501, part 1 (1977) required a specific form of declaration for this purpose.)

8.1.1 Definitions

There are some 25 definitions in the Standard, some dealing with terms such as apparatus and some dealing with the meaning of some of the symbols used in the Standard and its supplementary protection concept Standards. In common with earlier chapters they will be detailed at the end of this book. While in the main, these definitions cover all of the group of Standards, they are not complete but need to be added to by additional definitions in the protection concept Standards (showing the problems associated with limiting the meaning of terms by definition).

8.1.2 Division of apparatus into sub-groups and surface temperature classes

As earlier indicated, electrical apparatus is divided into groups and classes according to its performance with regard to ignition capability. Initially, the apparatus is divided into Group I, which is intended for use in gassy mines (principally but not exclusively coal mines), and Group II which covers apparatus for use in other industries (which in effect means surface industry). This book is concerned with Group II Apparatus and the requirements for Group I will not be further explored.

Apparatus sub-grouping

As already stated, apparatus is divided into Group I and Group II. Group II apparatus may be further divided into sub-groups to identify particular factors appropriate to its use. At the moment, only one sub-grouping system is in common use and that is related to the energy which may be released in a spark within an explosive atmosphere, or with the ability of flame to transmit through small gaps and ignite any explosive atmosphere downstream of the gap.

Intrinsic safety and similar protection concepts do not seek to prevent the release of electrical energy, but only to limit its value to that which cannot cause ignition. Apparatus and systems which are said to be intrinsically safe will be sub-grouped as follows:-

Sub-group IIA: Apparatus and systems which will not ignite the most easily ignitable mixture of propane/air when tested in accordance with Clause 10.4 of BS/EN 50020 (1993). This test corresponds approximately to an equivalent released energy of 160 microjoules from an inductive circuit where energy release is very efficient. Gases, vapours and mists in mixture with air are associated with this sub-group where the minimum current required to cause their ignition (MIC) is more than 0.8 of that needed to ignite the most easily ignitable mixture of laboratory methane and air (laboratory methane is more than 95 per cent pure) in a spark test apparatus (see Annex B of BS/EN 50020 (1993)[1] using the calibration circuit specified in that Annex).

Sub-group IIB: Apparatus and systems which will not ignite the most easily ignitable mixture of ethylene/air when tested in accordance with Clause 10.4 of BS/EN 50020 (1993). This test corresponds approximately to a released energy of 80 microjoules from an inductive circuit where energy release is very efficient. Gases, vapours and mists in mixture with air are associated with this sub-group when their MIC is between 0.45 and 0.8 of that needed to ignite the most easily ignitable mixture of laboratory methane and air when tested in a spark test apparatus (see Annex B of BS/EN 50020 (1993)[1] using the calibration circuit specified in that Annex).

Sub-group IIC: Apparatus or systems which will not ignite the most easily ignitable mixture of hydrogen/air when tested in accordance with

Clause 10.4 of BS/EN 50020 (1993). This test corresponds approximately to a released energy of 40 microjoules from an inductive circuit where energy release is very efficient. Gases, vapours and mists in mixture with air are associated with this sub-group when their MIC is less than 0.45 of that necessary to ignite the most easily ignitable mixture of laboratory methane and air when tested in a spark test apparatus (see Annex B of BS/EN 50020 (1993) using the calibration circuit specified in that Annex).

In the case of sub-group IIC, the statement may sound a little odd as the apparatus or system is tested with hydrogen/air which has an MIC of around 0.45, and more sensitive gas/air mixtures may be ignited by the apparatus. The fact is that hydrogen/air is the most sensitive gas known and more sensitive gas mixtures can only be produced by additional oxygen in the mixture. Such mixtures are outside the scope of this Standard and need to be treated specially.

Flameproof enclosure and similar concepts do not limit the release of electrical energy within the apparatus but seek to prevent the progress of the flame to any explosive atmosphere outside their enclosure. To do this they have any apertures closely controlled to ensure that any internal conflagration is sufficiently cooled or otherwise treated such that no external ignition will take place. Flameproof apparatus for a specific group (the groups being IIA, IIB and IIC as before) is tested in specific gas/air mixtures to ensure that the transmission cannot take place. These test mixtures are arranged to give a safety factor in use and the situation is more complex than is the case for intrinsic safety. Gases, vapours and mists are, in this case, associated with the groups on the basis of tests in a special test apparatus. This has 25 mm long flanged joints of adjustable aperture, as described in IEC 79 – 1A (1975), titled 'Electrical Apparatus for Explosive Gas Atmospheres, Part 1: Construction and Test of Flameproof Enclosures of Electrical Apparatus. First Supplement 'Appendix D' Method of Test for Ascertainment of Maximum Experimental Safe Gap' (see Fig. 8.1).The apertures are adjusted until flame propagation from inside the test apparatus to the surrounding explosive atmosphere does not take place. This aperture is termed the maximum experimental safe gap (MESG). The mixtures, both inside the test apparatus and outside, are mixtures of the same gas and air but that inside is the stoichiometric mixture (the mixture where all the fuel gas and oxygen are consumed) and outside is the most easily ignited mixture, which may be slightly different. The reason for this is that the internal mixture produced gives the worst conditions for flame transmission and the outer mixture the worst condition for ignition if transmission occurs.

Sub-group IIA: Apparatus will not ignite an external explosive atmosphere when filled with and surrounded with a mixture of 55 per cent hydrogen in air (equivalent to an MESG of 0.65 mm) at atmospheric pressure. Gases, vapours and mists in mixture with air will be associated with sub-group IIA when their MESG is measured by the method described in IEC 79-1A (see Fig. 8.1) at above 0.9 mm. A safety factor is produced by using a more sensitive test mixture for the apparatus.

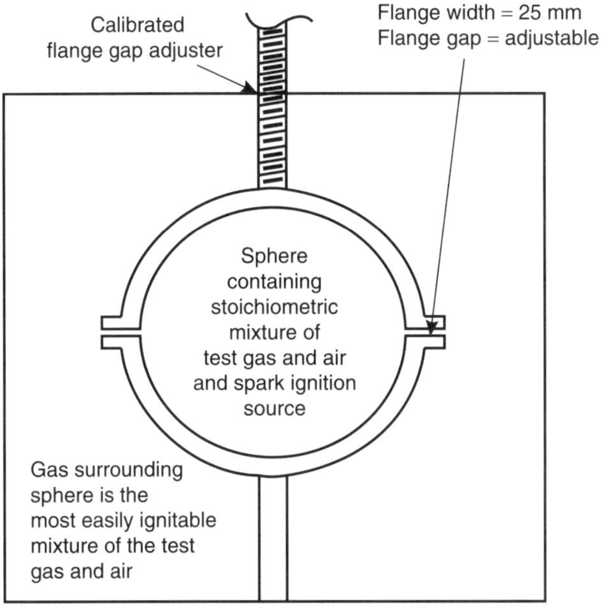

Fig. 8.1 Method of determination of maximum experimental safe gap. (For full details see IEC 79-1A (1975), Appendix D)

Sub-group IIB: Apparatus will not ignite a surrounding explosive atmosphere when filled with, and surrounded by a mixture of 37 per cent hydrogen in air (equivalent to an MESG of 0.35 mm) at atmospheric pressure. Gases, vapours and mists in mixture with air will be associated with sub-group IIB when their MESG is measured by the method described in IEC 79-1A (see Fig. 8.1) **ia** between 0.5 mm and 0.9 mm. A safety factor is produced by using a more sensitive test gas for the apparatus.

Sub-group IIC: Apparatus testing is very different here as achieving a safety factor on the test gas is more difficult. The safety factor is achieved by increasing the gaps specified by the manufacturer and then testing with the most sensitive mixtures of both hydrogen and acetylene with air. (These are 28 per cent hydrogen in air and 7.5 per cent acetylene in air). Gases, vapours and mists in mixture with air will be associated with sub-group IIC when their MESG is measured in accordance with the method described in IEC 79-1A (see Fig. 8.1) at less than 0.5 mm. In this case, the safety factor normally achieved by enlargement of gaps is rather more sensitive than test mixtures.

Once again, as in the case of intrinsic safety the IIC statement is based upon the fact that hydrogen and acetylene are the two most sensitive gases known and more sensitive mixtures can only be achieved by adding further oxygen, which is outside the scope of this Standard and requires special treatment.

Fortunately there is a relationship between MIC and MESG and to allocate a gas, vapour or mist to a particular sub-group it is only necessary to carry

out either an MIC or an MESG test and not both. This ceases to be true, however, at the upper limits and where both need to be carried out. In such cases the following will be true: where MIC is between 0.8–0.9 mm, MESG will determine the sub-group; where MIC is between 0.45–0.5 mm, MESG will determine the sub-group; where MESG is between 0.5–0.55 mm, the MIC will determine the sub-group.
These criteria are necessary to ensure that the most sensitive parameter is used to determine the sub-group.

To assist in sub-grouping gases, vapours and mists which have not been tested, it is often possible to identify them as one of a range of materials of similar structure, in which case it is highly likely that their sub-group will be the same as other gases, vapours and mists within similar materials which have a lower molecular weight. In all cases, however, care must be taken with materials not already allocated to a sub-group to ensure that no special feature of the material may make allocation unacceptable. Ethyl nitrate, for instance, will produce an explosion pressure in excess of any allocated material. There is no guarantee that flameproof apparatus will withstand an internal explosion of this material and special precautions are necessary.

The system for sub-grouping now used was preceded by different systems intended to achieve the same objective in the UK and other countries. The approximate relationship between the current system and these historic systems is given in Table 8.1.

Surface temperature classification

Any unprotected surface to which an explosive atmosphere has access may cause ignition. This means that while for such protection concepts as flameproof enclosure or pressurization, only the external enclosure temperature is important. When intrinsic safety and increased safety are considered, the temperature of internal components becomes important as the explosive atmosphere has access to them and there is no method of preventing flame transmission. For all apparatus surfaces where any ignition caused would produce uncontrolled burning, be they inside or merely on the outer enclosure of the apparatus, it is necessary to identify the attained temperature in the worst case of operation, which includes supply variation (which in the case of mains-fed apparatus is normally plus or minus 10 per cent.)

This is done by temperature classifying apparatus into six temperature classes on the basis of the maximum temperature it reaches in the extreme of its designed operating conditions (with a safety factor) and associating gases, vapours and mists with those classes on the basis of their ignition temperatures, and giving apparatus a temperature classification . Because of the greater difficulty in causing thermal ignition due to the effects of air movement, etc., the safety factor in this case is smaller than that normally used for grouping. The temperature classes are as follows.

Table 8.1 Current european grouping system showing relationship to historic German and UK systems and current USA system

Test gases	European grouping	Historic UK groups and classes		German class	US groups and classes
		FLP GRP	IS CLS		
Propane	IIA	II	2c	1	Class 1[2] Group D
Ethylene	IIB	III	2d	2	Class 1[2] Group C
Hydrogen	IIC	IV	2e	3a	Class 1[2] Group B
Acetylene	IIC	IV[1]	2f	3c	Class 1[2] Group A
Carbon disulphide	IIC	IV[1]	2f	3b	Not specifically allocated
All gases				3n	

Notes:
1 Although Group IV was allocated for these gases the Standard appropriate at the time (BS 229) excluded construction requirements for these gases and thus no equipment exists.
2 Class I in the USA National Electrical Code was for gases, vapours and mists only. Dusts were Class II, and fibres and flyings Class III.

T1

For T1 the maximum apparatus temperature must not exceed 440 °C. (As temperature classification is normally done at 40 °C ambient temperature, this usually means an elevation due to self heating of 400 °C.) Gases, vapours and mists associated with this temperature class will have ignition temperatures in excess of 450 °C.

T2

For T2 the maximum apparatus temperature must not exceed 290 °C. (As temperature classification is normally done at 40 °C ambient temperature, this usually means an elevation due to self heating of 250 °C.) Gases, vapours and mists associated with this temperature class will have ignition temperatures of between 300 °C and 450 °C.

T3

For T3 the maximum apparatus temperature must not exceed 195 °C. (As temperature classification is normally done at a 40 °C ambient temperature, this usually means an elevation due to self heating of 155 °C.) Gases, vapours and mists associated with this temperature class will have ignition temperatures of between 200 °C and 300 °C

T4

For T4 the maximum apparatus temperature must not exceed 130 °C. (As temperature classification is normally done at a 40 °C ambient temperature, this usually means an elevation due to self heating of 90 °C.) Gases, vapours and mists associated with this temperature class will have ignition temperatures of between 135 °C and 200 °C.

T5

For T5 the maximum apparatus temperature must not exceed 95 °C. (As temperature classification is normally done at a 40 °C ambient temperature, this usually means an elevation due to self heating of 55 °C.) Gases, vapours and mists associated with this temperature class will have ignition temperatures of between 100 °C and 135 °C.

T6

For T6 the maximum apparatus temperature must not exceed 80 °C. (As temperature classification is normally done at a 40 °C ambient temperature, this usually means an elevation due to self heating of 40 °C.) Gases, vapours and mists associated with this temperature class will have ignition temperatures of between 85 °C and 100 °C.

As indicated, the self elevation of the apparatus permitted in all cases depends upon the ambient temperature at which temperature classification is carried out. If an item of apparatus is temperature classified as T3 at an ambient temperature of 100 °C its permitted self heating will be reduced to 95 °C, as the overall maximum temperature must remain the same.

It is also recognized that small components can exceed the ignition temperature of a particular gas, vapour or mist without causing ignition, and this has been demonstrated as the case. In general, this difference depends upon factors such as the convection performance of the particular gas, vapour or mist and the configuration of the hot surface. For this reason, there is no general relaxation (except in the case of intrinsic safety, see Chapter 13) and each type of small component must be treated individually. To do this it is necessary to determine the temperature at which the surface in question actually ignites a gas representative of the most sensitive in the temperature class, and then ensure that the surface does not exceed the following temperatures in service:

T1 – ignition temperature minus 50 °C
T2 – ignition temperature minus 50 °C
T3 – ignition temperature minus 50 °C
T4 – ignition temperature minus 25 °C
T5 – ignition temperature minus 25 °C
T6 – ignition temperature minus 25 °C

A system of temperature classification similar in concept to this existed in Germany and the relationship between this and the current system is shown in Table 8.2. In the United States of America there was initially a system whereby apparatus classification (their equivalent of grouping) determined the maximum apparatus temperature (see Table 8.1) but in recent years they have adopted a variation on the European temperature classification system (see Table 8.2).

Table 8.2 European temperature classification system and its relationship with German and US systems

Temperature	European system (Note 1)	Historic German system (Note 2)	US systems	
			Current (Note 3)	Historic (Notes 3 and 4)
450 °C	T1	G1	T1 (842 °F)	Groups A, B, C and D
300 °C	T2	G2	T2 (572 °F)	Groups A, B, C and D
			T2A (536 °F)	Groups A, B, C and D
			T2B (500 °F)	Group C
			T2C (446 °F)	Group C
			T2D (419 °F)	Group C
200 °C	T3	G3	T3 (392 °F)	Group C
			T3A (356 °F)	Group C
			T3B (329 °F)	–
			T3C (320 °F)	–
135 °C	T4	G4	T4 (275 °F)	–
			T4A (248 °F)	–
100 °C	T5	G5	T5 (212 °F)	–
85 °C	T6		T6 (185 °F)	–

Notes:
1 The UK did not have a temperature classification system prior to the introduction of the European system.
2 The historic German system did not have the equivalent of T6.
3 The USA works on the Fahrenheit scale but the basic T classes are equivalent.
4 The original US temperature classification was associated with its grouping system whereby the following was the case: Groups A and B were associated with a maximum temperature of 536 °F Group C was associated with a maximum temperature of 356 °F.

8.1.3 Requirements for enclosures

In all protection concepts, the enclosure of the apparatus is, to some degree, important to the continued security afforded to the apparatus. It is clearly important that the integrity of the enclosure is maintained and it has to be understood that there are often components within the enclosure which either retain ignition capable electrical charge, or ignition capable temperature after isolation of the apparatus for some identifiable time. For these reasons enclosures are subjected to significant impact and drop tests to ensure that they have sufficient strength for their purpose. They are tested with the contents inside them and the strength of fixings within are also tested at the same time. All apparatus is subjected to impact tests at a basic level of 7 joules or, if the apparatus is intended to be installed where impact risks are small, 4 joules. In general, this means the 7 joule approach is used to give maximum flexibility of use, although in such cases as indoor risks in pharmaceutical plants, the reduced level can be of assistance. Guards on parts of the apparatus can also mitigate the impact test requirement and Table 8.3 shows the possible reductions of impact severity. In addition, portable apparatus will be subjected to a drop test from a height of 1 m to verify its reliability in service. The tests are normally carried out at normal laboratory temperature as the effects of changes in ambient temperature (normally −20 °C to +40 °C) are not considered significant. If, however, this is not true because of unusual ambient temperature variations or particular features of enclosure material (plastic enclosures are dealt with later in this section) it may be necessary to carry out impact and, if appropriate, drop tests at the limits of ambient temperature envisaged.

Glass is recognized as a weakness, when used for such things as viewports in enclosures, and is subjected to a thermal shock test by spraying water at a relatively low temperature onto it when it is elevated to its maximum service temperature.

Several of the protection concepts identify a required enclosure integrity against the ingress of solid or liquid foreign bodies, or both. This is identified as an 'IP' number, such as IP54. The first numeral identifies the protection against solid foreign bodies, such as tools or dust, and the second numeral identifies the protection afforded against liquid ingress. IP specification is derived by testing enclosures in accordance with BS/EN 60529 1991[2] and Table 8.4 identifies the numerals used in IP rating. Typical IP ratings are:

IP20: This is considered as sufficient protection to prevent insertion of fingers, etc., and is assumed to prevent electric shock.

IP54: This is considered as weather proof for outdoor mounting. All outdoor-mounted apparatus be it for hazardous-area mounting or not should meet at least this criterion.

IP65: This is considered to be dust tight. Once again it must be stressed that the enclosure integrity is often identified by the general situation and not by the minimum permitted by the protection concept. For example, outdoor apparatus is almost always IP54 to ensure operational reliability,

Table 8.3 Test Requirements for resistance to impact

	Mechanical details	Impact energy in Joules	
	Risk of mechanical danger	High	Low
1	Guards, protective covers, fanhoods, cable entries	7	4
2	Plastics enclosures	7	4
3	Light metal or cast metal enclosures	7	4
4	Enclosures of other materials than 3 with wall thickness of less than 1 mm	7	4
5	Light transmitting parts without guard	4	2
6	Light transmitting parts with guard (tested without guard)	2	1

(*from BS/EN 50014*[1])

Note: Impact test is normally with a 1 kg mass with a hardened steel 25 cm ball at its impact point. The height for dropping purposes is one tenth of the required impact energy in metres.

and apparatus for use in the presence of conducting dusts is likewise almost always required to be IP65.

As far as residual charge or temperature after isolation is concerned, the only way to overcome this problem if it cannot be avoided by design is to identify the time taken for decay, and label the apparatus with a warning indicating a delay which should be observed before opening. For residual charge, figures are given as follows:

Group IIA – The residual charge must not exceed 0.2 mJ when the enclosure is opened;

Group IIB – The residual charge must not exceed 0.06 mJ when the enclosure is opened;

Group IIC – The residual charge must not exceed 0.02 mJ when the enclosure is opened.

These figures allow the calculation of the necessary time to be included on the warning label.

Where the charge cannot be dissipated in a sensible time, or the temperature likewise is retained for a very long time, an alternative approach is to

Table 8.4 Degrees of protection of enclosures

Number	First numeral Protection against solids afforded	Second numeral Against liquids
0	No protection of persons against contact with live or moving parts. No protection of equipment against ingress of solid foreign bodies.	No protection
1	Protection against accidental or inadvertent contact with live or moving parts inside the enclosure by a large surface of the human body, for example, a hand, but not protection against deliberate access to such parts. Protection against ingress of large solid foreign bodies.	Protection against drops of condensed water. Drops of condensed water falling on the enclosure shall have no harmful effect.
2	Protection against contact with live or moving parts inside the enclosure by fingers. Protection against ingress of medium size solid foreign bodies.	Protection against drops of liquid. Drops of falling liquid shall have no harmful effect when the enclosure is tilted at any angle up to 15° from the vertical.
3	Protection against contact with live or moving parts inside the enclosure by tools wires or such objects of thickness greater than 2.5 mm. Protection against ingress of small solid foreign bodies.	Protection against rain. Water falling in rain at an angle of up to 60° with respect to the vertical shall have no harmful effect.
4	Protection against contact with live or moving parts inside the enclosure by tools wires or such objects of thickness greater than 1 mm. Protection against ingress of small solid foreign bodies.	Protection against splashing. Liquid splashing from any direction shall have no harmful effect.
5	Complete protection against contact with live or moving parts inside the enclosure. Protection against harmful	Protection against water jets. Water projected by a nozzle from any direction under stated conditions shall have no harmful effect.

Table 8.4 *(continued)*

Number	First numeral Protection against solids afforded	Second numeral Against liquids
	deposits of dust. The ingress of dust is not totally prevented, but dust cannot enter in an amount sufficient to interfere with satisfactory operation of the equipment enclosed.	
6	Complete protection against contact with live or moving parts inside the enclosure. Protection against ingress of dust.	Protection against conditions on ships' decks (deck watertight equipment). Water from heavy seas shall not enter the enclosure under prescribed conditions.
7	No prescription.	Protection against immersion in water. It shall not be possible for water to enter the enclosure under stated conditions of pressure and time.
8	No prescription.	Protection against indefinite immersion in water under specified pressure. It shall not be possible for water to enter the enclosure.

from BS/EN 60529[2]

warn that the enclosure should not be opened unless the area of installation can be specified as gas-free at the time of opening.

Aluminium alloys and plastics can present significant additional problems when used as enclosure material, both from the strength point of view, and in respect of their ability to become ignition sources. To this end, both are additionally addressed in detail in BS/EN 50014 (1993).

Specific requirements for non-metallic (plastic) enclosures

In order to ensure that the performance of the enclosure is repeatable, the plastic(s) of which the enclosure is made needs to be clearly identified by its complete composition, including fillers etc., and its manufacturer's name. In addition, its surface treatment (e.g., varnish) needs to be specified. To assist in this it is always better to use a plastics formulation which is in-line with

International Standards Organization (ISO)[3] Standard as, in cases where a manufacturer ceases production of a particular plastic, the search for a substitute will be easier.

The Temperature Index (TI) (taken from the 20 000 hour point on the thermal endurance graph for the plastic) needs to demonstrate that at 20 °C above the maximum temperature achieved by any part of the enclosure at maximum operating temperature for the apparatus, the plastic has lost less than 50 per cent of its flexing strength to demonstrate that the plastic is of sufficient strength for the purpose. (While demonstration of this for the purposes of BS/EN 50014 (1993) is by the manufacturer of the apparatus specifying the particular value, the older Standard BS 5501, part 1 (1977) required that the entire graph be produced to confirm this situation.) IEC 216–1[4], IEC 216–2[5] and ISO 178[6] or ISO R527[7] will need to be consulted for the methods of producing this figure.

In addition to being chosen to comply with this figure, enclosures made of plastics need to be tested for their resistance to heat, cold and, where the enclosure or parts thereof are not protected from normal incident light which is the general situation, their resistance to light. Likewise the impact tests and, if appropriate, drop tests normally carried out at laboratory temperature, will need to be carried out at the maximum and minimum service temperatures, with safety factors of around 10 °C for plastics enclosures.

Most plastics also have the propensity to hold charge when subjected to friction, such as being rubbed with a dry cloth, and this static charge is often capable of igniting an explosive atmosphere. It is necessary, therefore, to ensure that such the material cannot support such charge or, if its generation is possible, precautions are taken to ensure that it is not generated.

In general terms, electrostatic charges only become a problem where an enclosure, which is capable of sustaining such a charge is rubbed with a dry cloth or similar. BS/EN 50014 (1993)[1] identifies these conditions as the only conditions needing to be addressed by limiting the requirements for prevention of, or dealing with, electrostatic charge to plastics surfaces of portable and transportable (non-fixed) apparatus, and apparatus which is likely to be rubbed or cleaned on site. In the latter case, only apparatus in clean rooms or such places as pharmaceutical plants, where cleanliness is of great importance, is likely to be affected. On typical chemical plants or oil refineries, for example, it is more likely that equipment will be hosed down rather than cleaned with dry cloths.

There are two methods of dealing with plastics enclosures to prevent the build up of ignition-capable electrostatic charge. First, selection of material so that it has a surface resistance of less than 1 G ohm when measured between two 100 mm conducting lines, 10 mm apart, which are painted on the plastics enclosure surface or the surface of a flat plate of the same plastic, or by design of the enclosure such that development of charge is unlikely.

Second, by limitation of the surface of the enclosure projected in any direction (any single surface) to the following maximum sizes. For apparatus given Group IIA or IIB, limitation to 100 cm^2 is necessary unless the plastic surface is surrounded with a conductive frame which is earthed (see Fig. 8.2), when the area of the particular surface can be increased to 400 cm^2, and for apparatus given Group IIC, limitation to 20 cm^2 is necessary unless the plastic surface is surrounded with a conducting frame which is earthed (see Fig. 8.2), when the area of the particular surface can be increased to 100 cm^2.

The Standard also permits the use of a warning label indicating how charge is to be avoided if the above measures are not possible. Historically, the words 'not possible' have been taken in the UK to mean 'have not been taken' because of the difficulty in defining what is and is not possible. In practice, therefore, the two most common solutions for fixed apparatus have been to either load the plastics material with some conducting medium, such as carbon (although this can give problems with insulation within the apparatus) or to utilize the warning label. Portable apparatus has tended to rely on an overall cover of non-plastics material, such as leather or, again, loading the plastic with conducting material. BS 5501 part 1 (1977). (The first edition of this Standard did not limit the requirements to non-fixed apparatus and apparatus likely to be cleaned but the introduction of this limitation is unlikely to have significant effect upon design as manufacturers tend to design their apparatus for the widest possible market.

The final problem with plastic enclosures is the problem which can be associated with using fastening screws (for example, to hold the lid, in place). Plastic being somewhat softer than metal in most cases, it is more subject to thread stripping and where threads for fixing screws, which hold covers in place and other parts likely to be opened in service for adjustment etc., are tapped directly into the plastic, the Standard requires the thread form to be compatible with the plastics material. No further guidance is given but fine or shallow threads should be avoided as these are more likely to strip, particularly if plastic screws are used. Many manufacturers solve this problem by casting into the plastic metal thread bosses and this is probably the best way to solve the problem.

Specific requirements for light metal (aluminium and similar) enclosures

While such enclosures offer a similar advantage to plastic enclosures in weight and ease of casting, they mainly exhibit greater strength. They do, however, have similar drawbacks in respect of threads for fastening screws and such threads should be treated in the same way as those for plastics enclosures. There is also a problem associated with so-called thermite sparking, where magnesium content of alloy enclosures is high. This means that where the enclosure comes forcibly into contact with oxidized iron or steel (rust), the resultant spark is enhanced by the presence of the magnesium and the spark is much more powerful and is ignition capable in most cases. To avoid this situation, alloys with more than 6 per cent magnesium are not permitted by the standard.

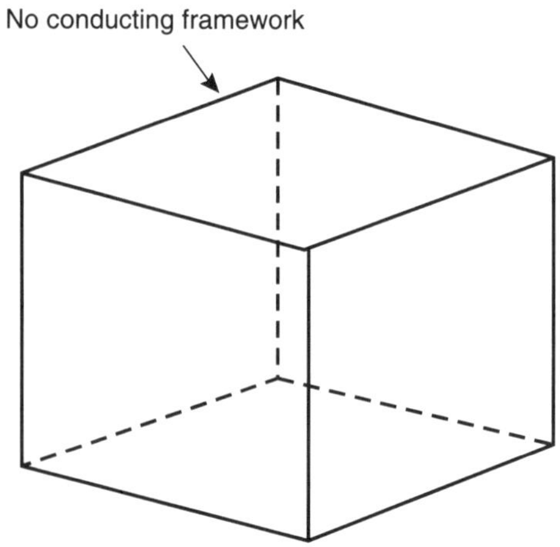

Maximum area of each of six external surfaces
IIA and IIB = 100 cm^2
IIC = 20 cm^2

Maximum volume
IIA and IIB = 1000 cm^3
IIC = 90 cm^3

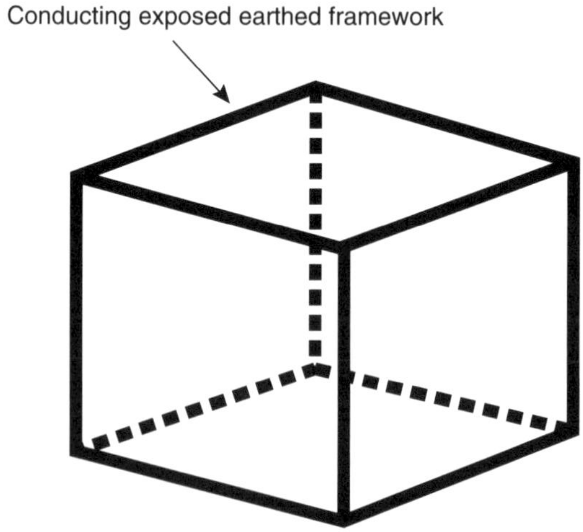

Maximum area of each of six external surfaces
IIA and IIB = 400 cm^2
IIC = 100 cm^2

Maximum volume
IIA and IIB = 8000 cm^3
IIC = 1000 cm^3

Fig. 8.2 Insulating plastics enclosures

8.1.4 Fasteners, interlocking devices, bushings and cements

Once again the Standard identifies those facets of fasteners, interlocking devices, bushings and cements; the performance of which are important to the protection concept and these apply to all the subsequent individual protection concept Standards, unless the particular protection concept Standard specifically excludes them.

Fasteners (including special fasteners)

The only general statement made about fasteners which fix parts necessary to maintain the protection concept (apart from the obvious one that the fastener in material and construction must be compatible with the enclosure it fastens) is that such fasteners must be releasable only with the aid of a tool. The term 'tool' is not defined but in a subsequent Clause dealing with interlocking devices, screwdrivers and pliers are specifically defined as not being acceptable as a method of defeating an interlock. Some certification bodies have used this wording or wording of similar import in BS 5501 part 1 (1977) as justifying the non-use of screwdrivers and pliers for fasteners in general, and it is wise to utilize such things as hexagon and socket-headed bolts and screws in this regard, unless prior knowledge of the attitude of the chosen certification body is obtained in advance of completion of the particular apparatus design.

Some of the protection concept standards call up 'special fasteners' which are intended to give a greater degree of security than the norm. To ensure this, the screws, nuts and threads used are carefully defined, as are the holes, (either clearance or tapped through) which the screws or studs pass. The basic requirements for threads are as: all threads shall be coarse pitch metric in accordance with ISO 262 (1973)[8]; tolerance of fit of threads shall be 6g/6H in accordance with ISO 965 (1980)[9].

The heads of screws or the nuts, where studs and nuts are used to secure a cover or similar part essential for the protection concept, are required to be one of the following:

1. Screws with hexagon heads to ISO 4014 (1988)[10] or ISO 4017 (1988)[11]. (Note: only the head must comply with the named Standard.)
2. Hexagon nuts to ISO 4032 (1986)[12].
3. Cap screws with hexagon socket heads to ISO 4762 (1989)[13]. (Note: only the head must comply with the named Standard.)
4. Hexagon socket set screws to ISO 4026 (1977)[14], ISO 4027 (1977)[15], ISO 4028 (1977)[16] or ISO 4029 (1977)[17] provided that the set screw does not protrude from the threaded hole in which it is fitted when it is tight.

In the case of screws with heads, the Standard also requires that the land under the head from the edge of the clearance hole, or the threaded hole in the case of a reduced shank fastener, is no more than that which would occur with a standard screw when the hole was a clearance hole with the maximum tolerance permitted by medium fit H13 as defined in ISO 286–2 (1988)[18].

BS 5501 part 1 (1977) included a requirement for shrouds on special fasteners (see Fig. 8.3 and 8.4) to make it difficult to gain purchase on them by such things as adjustable wrenches, etc. This requirement has been dropped in the case of BS/EN 50014 (1993)[1], except for mining applications which are not dealt with here.

The objective of all of the above in the case of fasteners is to create a situation where fasteners do not become loose or cannot easily be inadvertently loosened. The difference between normal fasteners and special fasteners is the degree of security which is considered necessary by the particular protection concept standard. It is worthy of note that in more than one case the protection concept Standard requires even a higher level of security as will be seen when the individual protection concepts are discussed.

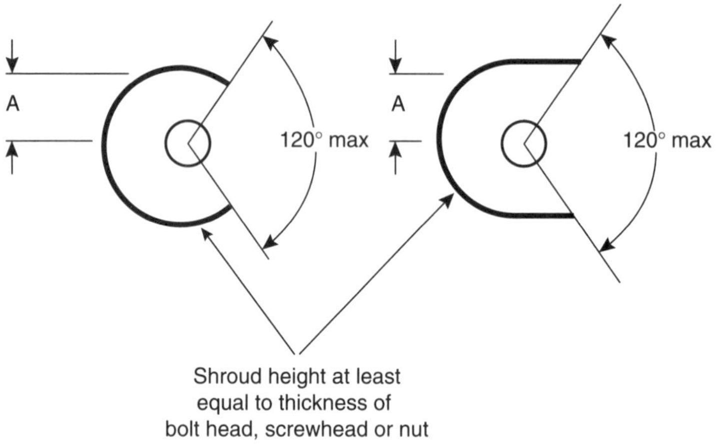

Thread size	A in mm (normal)
M5	9.0
M6	9.5
M8	12.0
M10	14.0
M12	17.0
M14	19.0
M16	21.0
M20	24.0
M24	30.0

Fig. 8.3 Typical shrouds for fasteners

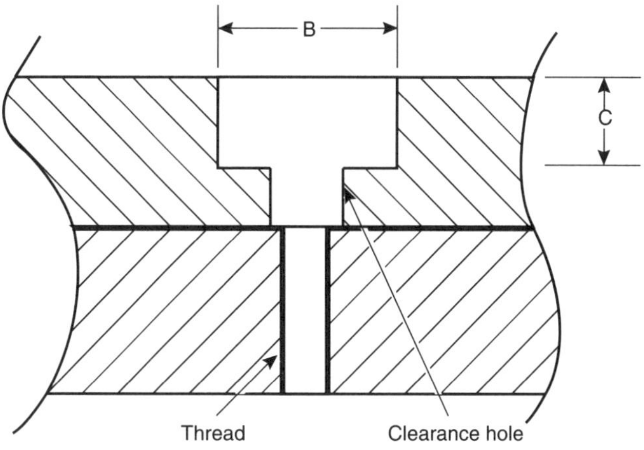

Thread size	Clearance hole size (mm)	*B* (mm)
M5	5.5	18
M6	6.6	19
M8	9.0	24
M10	11.0	28
M12	14.0	34
M14	16.0	38
M16	18.0	42
M20	22.0	48
M24	26.0	60

C = at least height of bolthead, screwhead or nut

Fig. 8.4 Typical recesses for shrouding purposes

Interlocking devices

Interlocking devices, may in some cases, be used instead of high security fasteners in such a way that the interlock isolates the electrical equipment and removes any residual sources of ignition (e.g., stored energy) before the apparatus enclosure can be opened. There is no formal specification for such devices in BS/EN 50014 (1993)[1] except indications to give some idea as to the difficulty which should be encountered by those seeking to circumvent them. The Standard requires that they are to be incapable of being defeated by screwdrivers or pliers. In addition, as no specification for them is given, they may be either mechanical or electrical.

The requirements are very much more relaxed then those in BS 5501, Part 1 (1977) (the first edition of this Standard) as the requirements there were that the interlock could only be defeated by a tool specifically designed for the purpose and, by inference, it should not be susceptible to being defeated by any tool in the normal range of tools used by personnel.

Bushings

Insulated bushings are sometimes used for communication between different parts of an enclosure or through a barrier within the enclosure. In these cases, normal industrial practice is used. Sometimes however, the bushing is used as a terminal (connection facility) and it is possible that if a screw connection is made, or if the connection is by a post and nut terminal, a turning moment will be applied to the terminal. The Standard requires that the terminal be secure against this when a specified maximum torque test is applied (see Table 8.5). If the bushing cannot be made secure by tightening then a set screw may be used to prevent turning. Where this set screw is within the enclosure (i.e., not accessible from outside the enclosure) it need not comply with the special fastener requirements.

Table 8.5 Test Torque to be applied to bushings used for connection facilities

Diameter of the stem of the bushing (metric thread size)	Torque Newton metres
M4	2.0
M5	3.2
M6	5.0
M8	10.0
M10	16.0
M12	25.0
M16	50.0
M20	85.0
M24	130.0

(*from BS/EN 50014*[1])

Note: Torque values for sizes other than those specified above may be determined from a graph plotted using these values. In addition, the graph may be extrapolated to allow torque values to be determined for bushings larger than those specified.

Cements

Cements are often used for such things as the construction of fabricated enclosures, or securing of such things as bushings. There are no specific requirements for these except that they must remain stable up to 20 °C above their maximum service temperature. This represents a significant relaxation with regard to BS 5501, part 1 (1977) which also required chemical stability and proven resistance to solvents or protection from their effects.

The current Standard merely requires that the cements be satisfactory in the set of conditions agreed by the manufacturer and user, removing the involvement of the certification body.

8.1.5 Connection facilities and cable entries

There are two elements to be considered here. First, the terminals and their terminal box (if one is used) are addressed to ensure that effective connection can be made, and second, the method by which the cable enters the enclosure is addressed. Obviously, neither the connection facilities, connection box, nor the conductor or cable entry mechanisms should adversely affect the protection concept but there are also more general requirements.

Connection facilities and terminal compartments

The basic requirements in BS/EN 50014 (1993)[1] for connection facilities are fairly straightforward, merely requiring that they allow proper connection of conductors and do this without reducing such things as clearances within the apparatus. While much of the wording used refers to terminal compartments, it is clear that a terminal compartment is not specifically required and the terminals may be in the main enclosure. In this latter case, however, it must be stressed that the arrangement needs to adequately protect the electrical equipment within the enclosure from damage during connection.

Connection facilities for earthing (bonding conductors) are more specific, requiring that the connection facilities can handle conductors of at least specific maximum sizes (see Table 8.6) and, where the apparatus enclosure is metal, that connection facilities satisfying these requirements appear both inside and outside the enclosure with the outside facility being capable of terminating a 4 mm^2 conductor as a minimum, if earthing is required. Strangely, corrosion and connection of light metal (aluminium) conductors is identified as a problem with earth connections but not for other connections. Clearly other connections should be examined for this problem and, if present, steps should be taken to minimize it.

Table 8.6 Minimum cross-sectional area of protective conductor

Cross-sectional area of phase conductors of the installation (mm^2)	Minimum cross-sectional area of corresponding protective conductor (mm^2)
up to 16	16
16 to 35	16
over 35	0.5 × phase conductor

Conductor entry (cable or conduit entries)

In the UK it is normal to use cables and cable entry devices are the norm. These may form part of the enclosure (typical German practice) or be separate from the enclosure and form a range of standard devices (typical UK practice). The requirements in both cases are effectively the same.

There should always be sealing between the cable sheath and the gland body (i.e., that part of the gland which is directly fixed to the enclosure) and this may be either by a sealing ring around the cable sheath or by compound filling, in which case the sheath is cut back and the compound seals to both the sheath and conductor insulation (see Fig. 8.5 and 8.6). The Standard also requires that sealing compounds be treated as cements and elsatomeric (rather than metal) sealing rings pass an ageing type test. There are also clamping requirements which are intended to ensure the cable is clamped by the sheath or armouring in such a way as to prevent stress on the conductors and lead in requirements to prevent sheath damage if the cable is moved (see Fig. 8.7). BS/EN 50014 (1993)[1] contains a whole range of type tests to ensure that cable entries are basically suitable and this results in a series of standard glands from which the manufacturer or user chooses for his apparatus.

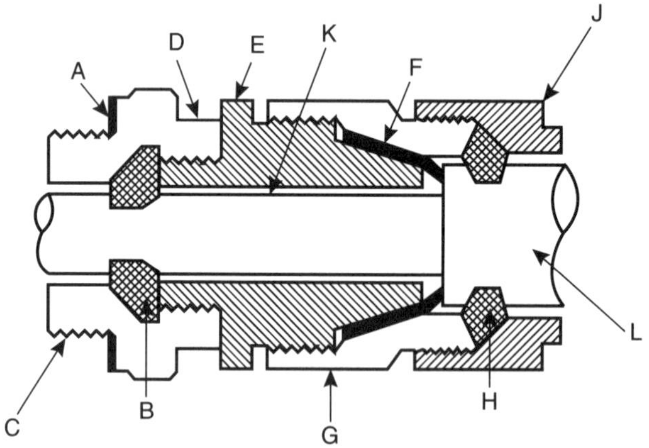

A = Sealing washer between enclosure and gland
B = Sealing ring on cable inner sheath of armoured cable (is also weatherseal for non armoured cable where items F, G, H, J and L are not present)
C = Thread for fixing gland to enclosure
D = Gland body (entry element)
E = Cable seal compression element
F = Cable armouring
G = Armour clamp
H = Weather sealing ring
J = Weather seal compression element
K = Cable inner sheath (or outer sheath for non-armoured cables)
L = Outer sheath of armoured cables

Fig. 8.5 Typical compression gland for armoured cable

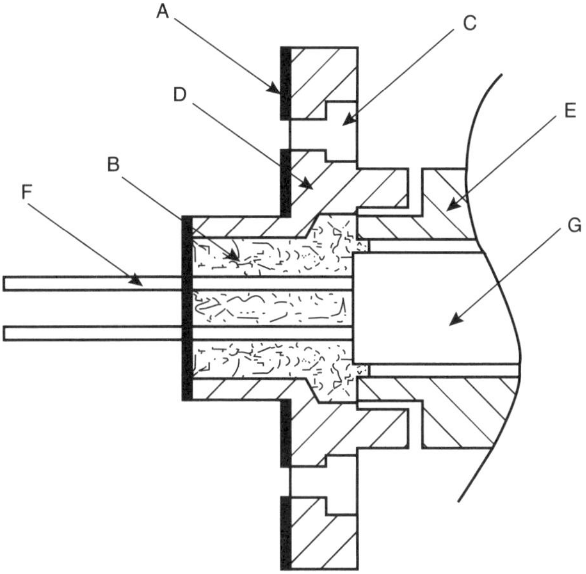

A = Sealing washer between enclosure and gland
B = Filling compound
C = Gland fixing holes
D = Gland body
E = Compound retaining element
F = Insulated cable cores
G = Cable inner/outer sheath
Note: Armoured cables will additionally have an armour clamp and outer weather seal

Fig. 8.6 Detail of compound sealed gland

Conduit entries are not usual in the UK but may be used. The normally acceptable conduit is solid drawn to ensure protection from the environment, and screwed entry into the apparatus. As the conduit forms part of the earthing or bonding network, inadvertently if not deliberately, its joints and entries should be protected against environmental damage, and the prevention of passage of explosive atmosphere down its inside sealing, by such things as stopping boxes, is required.

The manufacturer of apparatus normally provides entry holes for cable or conduit, and often more than one to permit flexibility. It is essential that these are closed when not used to protect the enclosure integrity, and plugs for such holes need to be secure. They should only be removable with the aid of a tool with the problems which that creates (see Section 8.5.1).

8.1.6 Additional requirements for particular types of apparatus

Certain types of apparatus are considered to have specific problems and there are thus additional requirements for these.

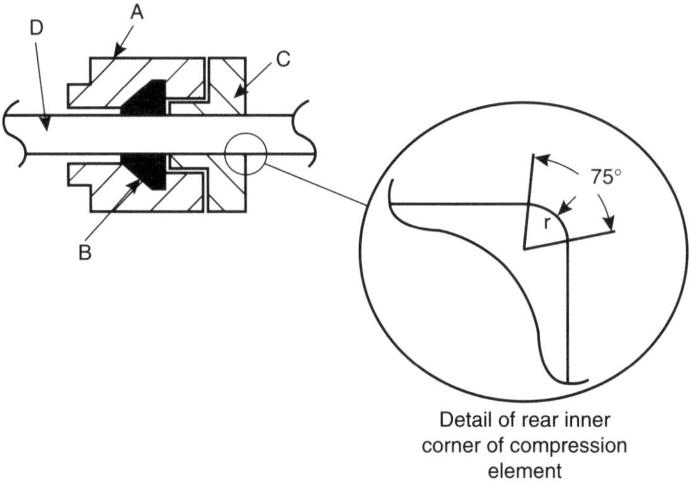

A = Gland body
B = Sealing ring
C = Cable seal compression element
D = Cable outer sheath
r = 0.25 × maximum cable diameter or 3 mm whichever is smaller

Fig. 8.7 Entry protection for flexible (non-armoured) cables

Rotating machines

Rotating machines often have external fans for cooling purposes. While these fans do not form part of the basic protection of the machine, not permitting access to the interior of the machine enclosure, they do form rotating parts and can generate friction heating or sparking due to the fan catching on its guard. For this reason BS/EN 50014 (1993)[1] contains requirements for such fans and hoods to prevent them from becoming sources of ignition, or to prevent the loading of the machine beyond its design rating and the ratings considered in its protection concept. These requirements include limitations on materials used, mounting restrictions, and enclosure requirements, most of which are drawn from the basic requirements of the Standard (e.g., limitations on plastics and on magnesium content of light metals).

The ventilation openings of fans are required to be IP20 on the air inlet side, and IP10 on the outlet side, the latter reduction only being permitted when the geometry of the outlet is such that foreign bodies above 12.5 mm in size cannot access the moving parts, either by falling into them (e.g., if the outlet is vertical) or by vibration causing their access to be possible. The IP rating in this case is produced by compliance with a special Standard, BS 4999, part 105 (1988)[19]. In addition, running clearances are required to be a minimum of 1/100 of the maximum fan diameter with a maximum figure of 5 mm. This maximum figure may be reduced to 1 mm for fans of high machining accuracy and long-term stability.

Switchgear

Switchgear is a potential source of ignition if failure occurs or if it is operated inadvertently. For these reasons, the Standard contains limitations on the types of switchgear (i.e., no oil-filled switchgear is permitted because of the possibility of discharge of burning oil if the gear fails). In addition, it requires locking capability to prevent inadvertent operation and, in the case of disconnectors, all poles (including the earth) are required to be disconnected to prevent sparking due to circulating earth currents during such activities as maintenance.

Warning labels are also required for such things as off-load isolators to prevent their operation on-load, which could cause an ignition, and for doors and covers giving access to automatic switchgear, unless those doors or covers are interlocked. Where some parts need to remain energized within cabinets containing switchgear after an interlock has operated, those parts must remain protected by a recognized protection concept or be protected to IP20 (BS/EN 60529[2]).

Fuses

Enclosures containing fuses are required to be either interlocked, to prevent opening while the fuses are energized, or are required to be fitted with a warning label to identify the danger of removing fuses live in a hazardous area.

Plugs and sockets

In general, plugs and sockets should not be used in a hazardous area but where they are, the ideal situation is one where they are interlocked to ensure that they are de-energized before separation. BS/EN 50014 (1993)[1] recognizes this as not always possible and allows as the alternative a label with a warning against energized separation. If de-energization is not possible, a warning not to separate in a hazardous area is permitted, although this is felt to be of little value for fixed equipment. It does, however, clearly identify the acceptance of energized separation at times when the absence of explosive atmosphere can be guaranteed.

In addition, it is recognized that a socket can be designed so that during removal of the plug, the arc is in an enclosure which has protection by one of the recognized protection concepts and, after separation, the energized conductors in the socket remain so protected. Typically Ex-d during separation and Ex-e after separation is complete is possible. It should be noted that this relaxation applies to the socket (fixed part of the arrangement) only and not the plug.

Luminaires (lighting fittings)

BS/EN 50014 (1993)[1] does not permit naked bulbs or tubes in lighting fittings but requires them to be covered by a light transmitting cover. In addition, it requires isolation before opening to relamp, for example, unless the cover operates an interlock isolating the supplies to the luminaire. Where this latter route is chosen, the isolating switch is required to have its own recognized protection concept as it remains live when the rest of the luminaire is isolated, and the spark on isolation together with the contact separation after isolation needs to be secure. Its external terminals also need to remain protected against interference in this state and it must therefore be enclosed to IP20 (EN 60529 (1991)[2]) standard when the transparent cover is removed.

8.1.7 Ex components

As an Ex component is not a complete item of apparatus it only needs to satisfy the appropriate requirements of BS/EN 50014 (1993)[1]. These vary according to the type of component but the Standard identifies the following as *not* being applicable to any components: First, the requirements for surface temperature classification. (It must, however, have a maximum operating temperature defined); and Second, the definition of the delay time necessary to ensure that any residual charge or high temperature remaining after isolation is dissipated before opening.

The other clauses of the Standard apply as appropriate (i.e., the Clauses relating to an apparatus enclosure only apply if the component is an empty enclosure).

8.1.8 Marking requirements

The marking requirements of the Standard include identification of the manufacturer, the certification Code and other relevant information. While a certification mark is not a requirement, unless the apparatus is certified, there are several requirements for intervention of 'the test station' in the marking clause. This means that it is normal to have certification and such a mark will normally be present. Typical of the certification coding are the following.

EEx: The first 'E' shows compliance with this Standard and one of the subsequent protection concept Standards, and the subsequent 'Ex' identifies the equipment as explosion protected. Although the 'Ex' appears on all explosion protected apparatus the first 'E' only appears on that protected to BS/EN 50014 (1993), its predecessor and its subsidiary protection concept Standards.

d: The symbol for the protection concept follows the 'EEx', the one shown here being for flameproof enclosure. This symbol will vary depending on the protection concept used as follows:

o – oil immersion (Chapter 9)
p – pressurization (Chapter 11)
q – powder filling (Chapter 9)
d – flameproof enclosure (Chapter 10)
e – increased safety (Chapter 12)
ia – intrinsic safety (Chapter 13)
ib – intrinsic safety (Chapter 13)
m – encapsulation (Chapter 9)

In some cases the apparatus may use two or more types of protection. In such cases, both protection concept markings will appear with the main protection concept coming first. (e.g., a luminaire which is type 'e' with an isolating switch which is type 'd' will be marked 'de'

II: this shows the apparatus is Group II for surface industry. (Equipment for coal mining use is Group I.) Where surface industry apparatus is sub-grouped, typically because it is intrinsically safe or flameproof, and its performance is different with different gases from the spark ignition or flame transmission point of view, the symbols will be 'IIA', 'IIB' or 'IIC'. (If only Group II is present the apparatus is suitable for all Group II gases, vapours and mists. In some cases the apparatus may be intended for a specific gas or vapour only, and in these cases the group or sub-group marking is not used being replaced by the chemical formula of the gas or vapour in question (e.g., NH_3)

T: T1 to T6 is marked to show the temperature classification of the apparatus. Exceptionally, if the apparatus has a maximum surface temperature less than a particular class maximum, it may be marked, for example 35 °C (T1). If the maximum temperature reached by the equipment is greater than the T1 class limit (>450 °C), then no class limit is shown and the equipment is marked only with the actual maximum temperature reached (e.g. 600 °C). Where the apparatus is marked for use with one particular gas or vapour only, as above, no temperature classification marking will appear.

Ta: Where an ambient temperature range, other than −20 °C to +40 °C is used the symbol 'Ta' or 'Tamb' may appear, together with the actual ambient temperature range, for example, Ta(−30 °C to +55 °C)

X: The symbol 'X' appears when there are special conditions necessary for the safe use of the apparatus and these cannot be identified effectively on the apparatus label. This symbol does not appear with the certification code marking (e.g., EEx q II T4) but as after the certificate number or test house reference (e.g., BAS 92 3054X)

U: This identifies the fact that the equipment in question is an Ex component and cannot alone be used in an explosive atmosphere. Components are also not normally marked with a temperature class as this is determined by its ultimate use. In addition, it is not normal for an 'X' mark to appear on a component as this is concerned with safe use, and as the component cannot be used without further certification or testing it is not appropriate. Typical examples of apparatus marking are given in Fig. 8.8 and 8.9.

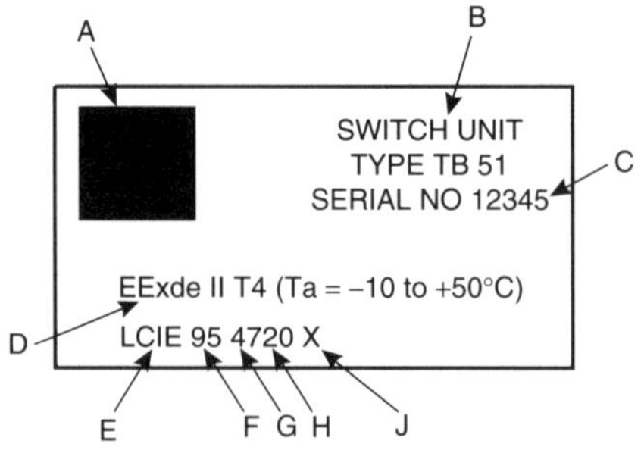

A = Manufacturers logo for identification
B = Apparatus description and type no.
C = Apparatus serial or batch no.
D = Certification Code: note dual protection (EExd) switch with EEx e connection facilities; Ta, ambient temperature range. Marked only because it is not the normal one used by the Standard.
E = Identification of the certification body (test house)
F = Year of issue of certificate
G = Identification of Principal Protection Concept
H = Number of certificate within that year
J = X indicating special conditions for safe use (certificate must be consulted for these)

Fig. 8.8 Example of apparatus marking

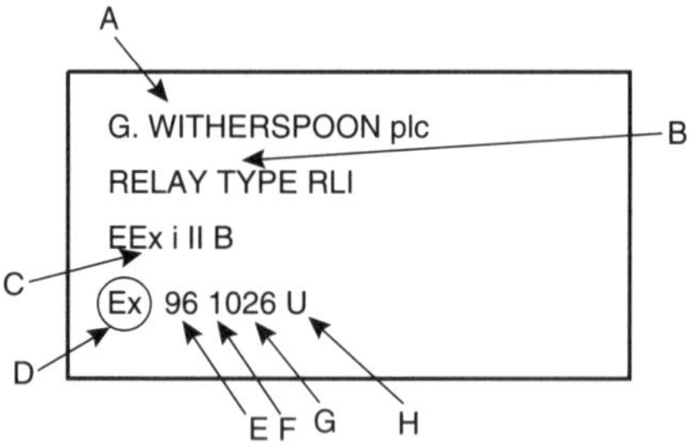

A = Manufacturers name
B = Manufacturers type no. (note serial no. not necessary)
C = Certification Code (note no temperature classification)
D = Certification body identification logo
E = Year of certificate issue
F = Identification of Principal Protection Concept
G = Number of certificate in year
H = U indicates a component

Fig. 8.9 Example of component labelling

Additional marking

In some cases, such as pressurization 'p' it is necessary to provide additional information, such as the purge rate and time necessary to ensure that the user is aware of the settings which must be applied to the control apparatus. Where possible, this should be marked on the apparatus but if it is not possible, then it must be referred to in the certification/approval documentation. The individual protection concept standard identifies how this information should be provided and how any user needs to be made aware of it. In some cases, specific unusual installation requirements must be met. These must be marked on the apparatus or, if this is not possible, the apparatus must be marked with an 'X' and these conditions referred to in the certification/approval documentation.

References

1 BS/EN 50014 (1993) Electrical Equipment for Potentially Explosive Atmospheres General Requirements.

2 BS/EN 60529 (1991) Specification for Degrees of Protection Provided by Enclosures (IP Code).

3 ISO The International Standards Organization (the non-electrical equivalent of CENELEC).

4 IEC 216–1 Guide for the determination of thermal endurance properties of electrical insulating materials. Part 1 (1987) General Guide-lines for Ageing and Evaluation of Test Results.

5 BS 5691 (1971) Guide for the Determination of Thermal Endurance Properties of Electrical Insulating Materials (IEC 216–2 (1974)).

6 BS 2782 (1975) Methods of Testing Plastics. (ISO 178 (1975)) Part 3. Mechanical Properties.

7 IEC R527 (1966) Plastics – Determination of Tensile Properties.

8 BS 3643 (1981) Metric Screw Threads. ISO 262 (1973) Part 1. Principles and Basic Data.

9 BS 3643 (1981) Metric Screw Threads. (ISO 965–1 (1980)) Part 1. Principles and Basic Data. General Purpose Metric Screw Threads – tolerances. ISO 965–2 (1980) Part 2. Limits of Sizes for General Purpose Bolt and Nut Threads, Medium Quality.

10 ISO 4014 (1988) Hexagon Head Bolts – Product Grades A and B.

11 ISO 4017 (1988) Hexagon Head Screws – Product Grades A and B.

12 ISO 4032 (1986) Hexagon Nuts, Style 1 – Product Grades A and B.

13 BS 4168 (1981) Hexagon Socket Screws and Wrench Keys – Metric Sizes. (ISO 4762 (1989)) Part 1. Specification for Hexagon Socket Head Cap Screws

14 BS 4168 (1981) Hexagon Socket Screws and Wrench Keys – Metric Sizes (ISO 4026 (1977)). Part 2. Specification for Hexagon Socket Set Screws with Flat Point.

15 BS 4168 (1981) Hexagon Socket Screws and Wrench Keys – metric Sizes. (ISO 4027 (1977)) Part 3. Specifications for Hexagon Socket Set Screws with Cone Point.

16 BS 4168 (1981) Hexagon Socket Screws and Wrench Keys – Metric Sizes (ISO 4028 (1977)) Part 4. Specification for Hexagon Socket Set Screws with Dog Point.

17 BS 4168 (1981) Hexagon Socket Screws and Wrench Keys – Metric Sizes. (ISO 4029 (1977)) Part 5. Specification for Hexagon Socket Set Screws with Cup Point.

18 BS 4500 (1990) ISO Limits and Fits. (ISO 286–2 (1988)) Part 1. General tolerances and Deviations. Section 1.2, 1990 Tables of Commonly Used Tolerances and Grades and Limit Deviations for Holes and Shafts.

19. BS 4999 (1988) General Requirements for Rotating Electrical Machines. Part 105 Classification of Degrees of Protection Provided by Enclosures for Rotating Machines.

— 9 —

Apparatus using protection concepts encapsulation 'm', oil immersion 'o', and powder filling 'q'

(BS/EN 50015 (1994))
(BS/EN 50017 (1994))
(BS 5501 part 8 (1998))

This is the first of eight chapters dealing with specific protection concepts (types of protection). It will deal with three types of protection which are not yet in common use in the UK, were not developed in the UK, but are included in the protection concepts covered by Directives 76/117/EEC[1] and 94/9/EC.[2] Although the use of protection concepts 'o' and 'q' is currently limited to Zone 2 in the UK, it is very likely that they will be permitted in Zone 1 when the Directive concerned with safety at work eventually becomes law. They are permitted in Zone 1 in the countries from which they originated.

9.1 Encapsulation – 'm' BS 5501 part 8 (1988)[3] (EN 50028 (1987))

The first matter which must be dealt with in this Standard is the fact that it still exists in its first edition and relates to the first edition of EN 50014 which is BS 5501, Part 1 (1977).[4] It does, however, exclude many parts of that Standard and there is little difference between those that remain and their equivalents in the second edition, BS/EN 50014 (1993).[5]

9.1.1 Exclusions from BS 5501, Part 1 (1977)

The parts which are excluded are:

1. Requirements for maximum surface temperature in respect of Ex-m components.
2. Time delays for opening of enclosures (obvious as it is not possible to open encapsulation without destroying it).

3. Definition of enclosure material for non-metallic enclosures (encapsulation is not, strictly speaking, a non-metallic enclosure although non-metallic in substance).
4. Encapsulation is not required to be given a temperature index as, although it is non-metallic, it is not a plastic as defined in BS 5501, Part 1 (1977). The encapsulant is, however, required to pass the thermal endurance tests prescribed by that Standard.
5. The requirements for threaded holes in plastics enclosures do not apply to encapsulation as there are no parts of the encapsulant which can readily be dismantled without destruction of the encapsulant.
6. Because no parts are intended for removal the requirements for interlocking are excluded, together with those for fasteners.
7. The requirements for cable and conduit entries are excluded as in this protection concept, the cable is sealed into the encapsulant.
8. The requirements for switchgear and fuses are also excluded as they mostly address the prevention of access and no access is possible when encapsulated.
9. The warning label for luminaires is also not necessary as they also cannot be opened if encapsulated.
10. A group of the tests is excluded as follows:

    (a) it is not necessary to impact test Ex 'm' components;
    (b) tests for degree of protection of enclosures are irrelevant;
    (c) tests in explosive mixtures are irrelevant as the explosive mixture does not have access to the electrical circuits;
    (d) tests for cable clamping are not necessary because the end of the cable is sealed in the encapsulant.

BS 5501, Part 8 (1988) also contains further definitions which supplement those in BS 5501, Part 1 (1977)[4] and BS/EN 50014 (1993)[5]. These will be included in the list of definitions at the end of this book.

9.1.2 Specification of the encapsulation

The compound used for encapsulation must be fully defined including its exact material with detail of fillers, other additives and any surface treatment given after encapsulation (e.g., varnishing). Its temperature range needs to be defined together with its maximum continuous operating temperature (which may be higher than the upper range limit as the temperature range is the range through which the material satisfies BS 5501, Part 8 (1988)[3]). It is helpful if an encapsulating material with an IEC reference number can be used.

The encapsulant is also tested to confirm its insulating properties and its resistance to water absorption, the latter test only being specified as necessary if the encapsulated apparatus is intended for use in a moist environment. In reality the water absorption, test will be necessary in all cases as manufacturers would find the limitations to dry environments very restrictive for general usage purposes.

Both tests require discs of encapsulant of 50 mm diameter and 3 mm thickness. For the electric strength test the disc has two 30 mm diameter electrodes placed centrally one on each side. The disc is then heated to a temperature equal to the maximum temperature of its specified operating range and 4000 V at nominally 50 Hz is applied between the electrodes. Any flashover or insulation breakdown within 5 minutes means that the encapsulation is not suitable for use in association with BS 5501, Part 8[3] (1988).

For the water absorption test, dry samples are weighed and then immersed in tap water at laboratory temperature (23 °C) for 24 hours. After drying and reweighing, the weight must not have increased by more than 1 per cent.

Encapsulation may be hard or soft but in the latter case it is likely that it would need to be in a mould which formed part of the apparatus.

9.1.3 Types of apparatus for encapsulation

Examination of the requirements of BS 5501, Part 8[3] (1988) leads immediately to the conclusion that the concept is intended for 'light current' electrical equipment and instrumentation only.

Although the Standard specifically only limits apparatus to that which operates below 11 kV, it also states that apparatus must be capable of operation within the terms of the Standard from a supply of 4000 A Prospective current capability. This prospective is typical of the requirements which were placed on mains-powered instrumentation in the protection concept in BS 5501, Part 7 (1977).[6] This requirement was reduced to 1500 A in BS/EN 50020 (1995)[7] (the second edition of the Intrinsic Safety Standard) because of the use of standard IEC fuses to BS/EN 60127, (1991) Parts 1, 2 and 3[8] of which are identified and deal with miniature fuses. Thus, the requirement is typical of one which is applied to instrumentation and low-power electrical apparatus.

It is highly unlikely that switchgear could satisfy the prospective current limits specified above, or the 4000 A specified in BS 5501, Part 8 (1988) and, in any event, it is not considered likely that switchgear which has to be destroyed to gain access would be economical.

Luminaires which have to be destroyed to change lamps or tubes would not be economical and only small low-voltage lamps in such things as annunciators are likely to be suitable for protection in accordance with this concept.

Although the Standard contains requirements for encapsulation of stator windings of rotating machines, the magnetostrictive forces involved do not lend the protection concept to rotating machines of significant size, and other more historically applied techniques are proving adequate.

Taking the view above then, the requirements of the concept become more understandable and realistic.

9.1.4 Encapsulated circuits and components

The Standard permits a wide range of electrical and electronic components to be encapsulated, provided that the operating temperature of such components does not exceed their rating at the maximum ambient temperature envisaged for operation (normally 40 °C). Even components such as relays and switches are permitted, provided that they are themselves enclosed before being encapsulated. In the case of these components, however, the maximum volume of their enclosure is limited to 100 cm^2 and, if they switch more than 6 A, their enclosure is required to be inorganic to prevent combustion of its material on arcing or sparking. The rating of the components used needs to be sufficient to ensure that they remain within it in case of a single fault elsewhere, or their failure in the worst possible way assumed to be a part of that fault. The types of fault which are considered include, but are not limited to, short or open circuit of any component, or faults in printed circuitry such as open circuit failures or shorts between tracks. The apparatus is not permitted anywhere to exceed its specified operating temperature range in normal operation or fault conditions, and this may be ensured by an internal thermal trip provided such a trip, is not self-resetting which, in effect, means that if it operated the apparatus would be at the end of its useful life.

Some components are considered as not subject to faults in the protection concept if operated at less than two third of their voltage and power ratings in normal operation, and less than their voltage and power ratings in a fault condition and these are: carbon or metal film type resistors; wire wound resistors with the wire in a single helical layer; plastic foil, paper and ceramic capacitors.

In addition, the following components are considered as not subject to fault when they satisfy the requirements applied to them in normal operation and do not exceed their ratings in a single fault situation.

First, optocouplers supplying isolation between separate circuits if the sum of the voltages of the separated circuits is less than 1000 V rms and the rated voltage of the optocoupler between these circuits is at least 1.5 times that voltage sum.

Second, transformer and other windings complying with BS 5501, Part 6 (1977)[9] (this will include its second edition BS/EN 50019 (1994)[10] the requirements of which are not dissimilar). In addition, windings which use wire of less than 0.25 mm diameter which are not permitted by BS 5501, Part 6 (1977)[9] or its successor BS/EN 50019 (1994)[10] are permitted, provided they otherwise comply with those standards and, in addition, are protected against inadmissible internal temperatures by embedded thermal cut-outs or similar devices.

Third, transformers complying with the requirements for infallible mains transformers in BS 5501, Part 7 (1977)[6] (and its successor BS/EN 50020

(1994)[7] which is not dissimilar), except those which have one winding wound over the other and are not separated by an earthed screen (type 2a transformers).

9.1.5 The encapsulation process

The standard recognizes two types of encapsulation which are, first, embedding, which is the situation where normally the encapsulant is poured over the electrical circuits in a mould which is later removed, leaving the encapsulant as the outer part of the apparatus. (A mould may not be necessary, the important fact being that the encapsulant is the outer part of the apparatus and is in contact with the environment.

Second, potting, which is a similar process except that the mould remains adhered to the encapsulant and forms the external surface of the apparatus protecting the encapsulant from the environment. Where the mould does not have a lid, it is acceptable to cover the encapsulant with another encapsulant which adheres to the main encapsulant but protects it from the environment.

The Standard defines the minimum thickness of encapsulant between conductors and the surface of the encapsulant as 3 mm but reduces this requirement to 1 mm where the encapsulated apparatus has no single surface greater than 2 cm^2 or is potted in a metallic mould or housing. Where the mould is an insulator there is no minimum limit, provided the mould is at least 1 mm thick. In addition, the thickness of encapsulant round a void, such as a relay box within the encapsulant, is required to be 3 mm unless the void is less than 1 cm^3 when the thickness is reducible to 1 mm.

Anything exiting the encapsulant is a possible route for entry of explosive atmosphere and must be effectively sealed. The Standard suggests that 5 mm of bare conductor within the encapsulant is acceptable to ensure effective sealing of connection cables which exit the encapsulant.

There are also minimum requirements for separation of bare live parts be they within the same circuit, in two separate circuits or one circuit and the frame (earth) of the apparatus and these are given in Table 9.1. Obviously they only apply, as do all other requirements, where failure will affect the protection concept.

9.1.6 Particular component problems

As in many of the other Standards, certain types of component are singled out as having particular problems insofar as the protection concept is concerned.

Fuses

To avoid problems with ingress of encapsulant into the fuse cartridge, fuses are required to be enclosed types to BS 4265 (1977) (1984)[11] or IEC 269.[12] It is recognized that during rupturing such fuses might exceed the temperature

Table 9.1 Separation between live parts through encapsulant

Minimum distances between bare live parts of the same circuit, different circuits and any circuit and earthed metallic parts	
Maximum voltage between live parts at maximum rated supply voltage taking account of faults and recognized overloads[1] (Volts rms)	Minimum permissible separation[2] (mm)
380	1.0
500	1.5
660	2.0
1000	2.5
1500	4.0
3000	7.0
6000	12.0
10 000	20.0

(*From BS 5501, Part 8*[3])

Notes:
1 The voltage in practice may exceed the values above by up to 10% without the necessity to move to the next highest figure.
2 Where the separation is between two live parts via an interposing isolated conducting part the separation required will be formed by the total of the separations of the two live parts and the interposing part.

limits applied to the apparatus, but provided this does not damage the encapsulant or cause the external encapsulant temperature to exceed the temperature classification, such a situation is acceptable.

Cells or batteries

Only primary and secondary cells, batteries or accumulators which do not release gas or electrolyte in the normal operating conditions specified by the manufacturer of the cell or battery may be encapsulated. It is, however, recognized that in abnormal circumstances such cells or batteries may release gas (but not electrolyte) and there must be a method of release of the gas which does not defeat the protection concept. This often takes the form of a plug of porous encapsulant or a capillary from the top of the cell or battery to the outside of the encapsulant. It is also necessary to consider any dimension variation due to such things as charging and this is usually accommodated by surrounding the cells or batteries in soft encapsulant before the overall encapsulation is applied. In such cases it is also necessary to carefully define the charging conditions necessary to achieve this objective if the charger is not a component part of the encapsulated apparatus.

9.1.7 Type testing

Encapsulated apparatus is subject to type tests to ensure that the protection concept is not breached within the specified operating conditions.

Temperature testing is carried out to ensure that internal heating does not cause the maximum temperature of the encapsulant, or the maximum operating temperature of the apparatus, to be exceeded.

The apparatus is also subjected to a temperature cycling test (see Fig. 9.1) to ensure that no deterioration takes place. These tests are carried out at the worst possible input voltage in the range of the apparatus. For mains supplies this is assumed to be plus or minus 10 per cent. There are also electric strength tests between separate circuits, discharge tests at above maximum ambient temperature for cells and batteries, and pull tests on cables which exit the encapsulant to ensure their integrity. These are all detailed in BS 5501, Part 8 (1988)[3].

9.2 Oil immersion–'o' (BS/EN 50015, (1994))[13]

This type of protection is again one where the explosive atmosphere is prevented from accessing the electrical circuits by their immersion in oil. Originally a wide range of apparatus was covered by the Standard including switchgear (see BS 5501, Part 2 (1977))[14] but the second edition, BS/EN 50015 (1994)[13], limits the protection concept to apparatus which is not capable of causing an ignition of an explosive atmosphere in normal operation (see Chapter 15) and would be usable in Zone 2 without oil immersion. Apparatus in accordance with BS 5501, Part 2 (1977)[14] will not be discussed as no apparatus other than that which would comply with BS/EN 50015 (1994)[13] has been used in the UK and it is not recommended that any is in the future. If any apparatus is constructed for oil immersion before Directive 76/117/EEC[1] it is recommended that it complies with the requirements in BS/EN 50015 (1994)[13] in respect of construction of the electrical apparatus itself.

9.2.1 Construction of the apparatus

The basic constructional requirements for the apparatus itself do not appear in this Standard. Instead, it refers to apparatus complying with IEC 79-15 (1987)[15] which covers apparatus with type of protection 'n'. This standard is not yet fully accepted in the UK and the constructional requirements should be those given in the UK equivalent which is BS 6941 (1988).[16] In reality, this makes little difference as the differences between the British Standard and the IEC Standard centre around the restrictive breathing concept which does not lend itself to oil immersion in any event. Chapter 15 of this book should be consulted for the basic apparatus construction requirements.

9.2.2 Containment of the oil

The oil is required to be contained within the apparatus by one of the following two methods. It may be within an apparatus sealed at the manufacturing stage, in which case the enclosure must be capable of withstanding the maximum internal pressure which occurs at maximum temperature with the apparatus in operation and the oil at maximum level. The Standard requires a pressure relief device installed at the time of manufacture which operates at 1.1 times that pressure, and is sealed to prevent interference. Sealing in this context does not necessarily mean fusion-type sealing and gasketted enclosures are acceptable for this purpose. While sealing of enclosures is not specifically identified in BS 5501, Part 2 (1977)[14] as a means of oil containment, the wording in that Standard is sufficiently vague to permit it. Sealed enclosures are subject to overpressure tests at 1.5 times the setting of the pressure relief device and leakage tests at reduced pressure to ensure their strength and sealing capabilities. These tests were not required by BS 5501, Part 2 (1977)[14].

Alternatively, it must be in an enclosure which has at least an IP rating of IP66 to BS/EN 60529 (1991)[17] (see also Chapter 8). In this case, there must be a device to permit breathing of vapours from the oil without any pressurization of the enclosure and the breathing device will have to have a desiccant to prevent the ingress of water or water vapour which will degrade the oil. The Standard requires the breathing device to achieve at least IP 23 to BS/EN 60529 (1991)[17]. While this is a fairly low level of ingress protection, care needs to be taken to ensure that any breathing device is suitable for intended locations of installation. If, for example, the apparatus is in normal outdoor process plant locations hosing of those locations must be expected and the breathing device will need some form of downward facing outlet to stop ingress of water which would overburden the desiccant. A typical arrangement is shown in Fig. 9.1.

Non-sealed apparatus is required to have a trip which isolates the electrical supply to the apparatus in conditions of fault (internal arcs or excessively high temperatures caused by significant overcurrent due to internal faults) where oil decomposition is likely. Because the circumstances giving rise to this problem are almost certain to produce either transient or continuous overcurrent, an overcurrent trip is the most likely method of achieving this, but it must also be noted that the trip must not be self resetting or capable of being reset remotely. Such a trip must only be capable of being reset locally and manually. Non-sealed enclosures need no leakage test but must be capable of withstanding a pressure test at $1.5 \times 10^5\,N/m^2$ absolute to ensure they have sufficient strength. This test was not required by BS 5501, Part 2 (1977)[14].

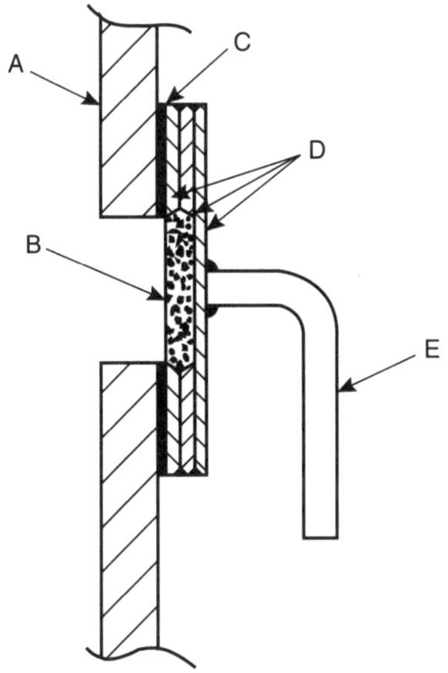

Fig. 9.1 Example of breathing device to exclude Water. A = Enclosure Wall, B = Desiccant, C = Gasket, D = Desiccant holder where all three parts are secured together by welding, soldering, cementing or have interposing gaskets to prevent moisture entry, E = Downward facing vent secured to desiccant holder by welding, soldering or screwing. *Note*: The desiccant Holder is fixed to the enclosure in a manner acceptable to BS/EN 50015 (1994)

All apparatus, both sealed and non-sealed, needs to have an indicator which identifies the maximum and minimum oil levels acceptable in all normal conditions. In the case of apparatus which is not sealed, this may take the form of a dipstick if it is secured to the apparatus in normal conditions (this means it forms part of the enclosure and satisfies the ingress protection requirements at times when not in use, to check oil levels). Alternatively, it may be a device, such as a sight tube or level windows in the enclosure, in which case the material must not be degraded by the oil in a way that will cause loss of strength or obscuration, and it must be arranged so that, unless it is protected from such things as impact so that damage can be ignored in normal service, its failure will not permit the oil level to fall below the minimum acceptable level. All fasteners which are germane to the protection concept need to be protected against accidental removal or loosening by personnel, or such things as vibration. While neither this Standard or its predecessor calls up special fasteners (see BS/EN 50014 (1993)[5]) suggestions are made in BS/EN 50015 (1994)[13] as to what is acceptable and the following are mentioned: shrouds around boltheads; cementing of threads; fitting of locking washers; and wiring of boltheads. The choice of any of these or equivalents is up to the manufacturer in particular cases, but appropriateness will need to be justified and, in the case of equivalents, equivalence.

9.2.3 Requirements for the protective fluid (oil)

The protective fluid is required to immerse any electrical circuits to a depth of at least 25 mm with the oil at its lowest level. Clearly, this 25 mm does not apply to separation between those circuits and the enclosure but faults to the enclosure need to be taken into consideration during design to ensure that the enclosure cannot be ruptured by electrical faults.

BS 5501, Part 2 (1977) limited the oil to that conforming to IEC 296 (1969).[18] This was quite restrictive and to overcome this BS/EN 50015 (1994),[13] while still permitting oils to the updated IEC Standard (IEC 296 (1982))[19] also permits other oils provided they satisfy the following:

their fire points must be above 300 °C (IEC 836 (1988), first method);[20]

their flash points shall exceed 200 °C (BS 6664, Part 5 (1990), closed cup);[22]

their maximum kinematic viscosity at 25 °C must not exceed 100 cSt (ISO 3014 (1976)).[21]

their electrical breakdown strength must be at least 27 kV (BS 5874 (1980)[22] or, in the case of silicone fluids, IEC 836 (1988));[20]

their volume resistivity must be at least $10^{14}\Omega$ at 25 °C (BS 5737 (1979));[23]

their pour point must be −30 °C or lower (BS 2000 Part 15 (1993));[24]

their acidity must not exceed 0.03 mg KOH/g (IEC 588–2 (1978)).[25]

Clearly these are fairly restrictive specifications but the reason for each of them is apparent and they represent a widening of choice, particularly as all that is required is to demonstrate that the specification of the oil used by its manufacturer meets these requirements, rather than have to prove it by test.

9.2.4 External connections

It is highly unlikely that the external connection facilities could practically be immersed in oil and so it must be assumed that they exit the oil. To achieve safety, therefore, they need to be protected by another protection concept (e.g., Increased Safety BS/EN 50019)[10] where the oil immersion is ineffective, which means from the point where they exit the oil-filled enclosure or, if the oil has a free surface within the terminal chamber, from a point 25 mm below the oil surface to and beyond the surface.

9.2.5 Type testing

Specific type testing of oil-immersed apparatus is limited to following testing of enclosures. Sealed Enclosures are subjected to both overpressure and underpressure tests. The overpressure test is intended to identify enclosure strength and consists of an overpressure of at least 1.5 times the pressure setting of the pressure relief device applied to the enclosure, filled with oil for 60 seconds. No significant enclosure damage or distortion is expected. The underpressure test is designed to test the sealing. This consists of filling the enclosure to its maximum level with oil and then reducing the level to the minimum. The reduced pressure must be maintained for at least 24 hours with no variation greater than 5 per cent. Unsealed enclosures are subjected only to the overpressure test which, in this case, is carried out at 1.5 times atmospheric pressure, all other test parameters being the same.

9.3 Powder filling – 'q' BS/EN 50017 (1994)[26]

At first glance, this protection concept is a further method of separating the electrical circuits from the explosive atmosphere by surrounding them with powder. This is not strictly true, however, as unlike such things as oil immersion the explosive atmosphere can penetrate the filling and, theoretically, may be ignited if ignition-capable parts are within the filling. What actually happens here is that the ignition cannot propagate outside the filling material because of the quenching effect produced. In this context the filling material has a somewhat different function and is more critical.

9.3.1 The filling material

The filling material is limited to quartz or solid glass particles with size limits which will permit it to pass through a metal sieve of 1 mm aperture but not one with an aperture of 0.5 mm (see ISO 565 (1990)[27]). The filling material is also required to have a leakage current of less than 1 μA when 1000 V dc is applied to an electrode system shown in Fig. 9.2, which is immersed in the filling material so that it is surrounded to a distance of at least 1 cm (see also Section 9.3.5).

9.3.2 The enclosure

In general terms the enclosures must be mechanically robust but no special tests other than those in BS/EN 50014 (1993)[5] are considered necessary. The method of enclosure must also be such that no filling escapes and BS/EN 50017 (1994)[26] specifies any enclosure aperture as not having any opening more than 0.1 mm less than the minimum filling dimension. IP54 to BS/EN 60529[17] is specified as the minimum ingress protection and, where the enclosure protection exceeds IP55, a breathing device giving IP54 is required. All enclosures are subjected to a type test of $1.5 \times 10^5\,N/m^2$ absolute, to ensure their adequate strength but where they do not contain breathing openings and do contain large electrolytic capacitors, for example, (capacitor volumes greater than one eighth of the filling material volume) this pressure test is increased to $15 \times 10^5\,N/m^2$ absolute. When filling the

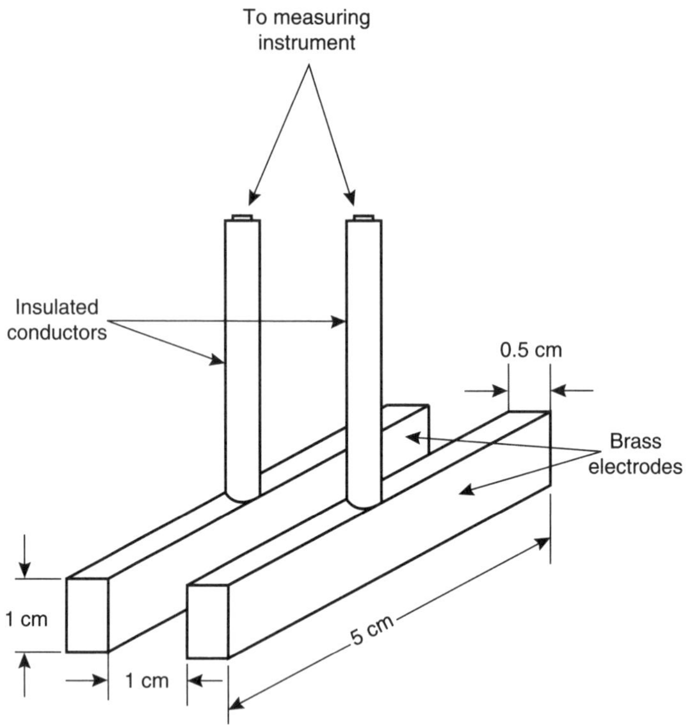

Fig. 9.2 Leakage Measuring Technique. *Notes*: (1) Electrodes should be surrounded by filling material with a depth of at least 1 cm in all directions. (2) Measuring Instrument should apply 1000 V dc. to electrodes

enclosure it is necessary to ensure total penetration of the filling material and this may require shaking during filling. The filled enclosure is then not intended to be opened in service and closure should be by welding, soldering or cementing to prevent this.

9.3.3 Electrical components and circuits

The electrical components and circuits inside the filling are required to be separated from the enclosure through the material by the distances shown in Tables 9.2 and 9.3 even when the voltages are derived with any possible overloads and fault conditions, such as component short circuits, open circuits and printed circuit board failures, applied to the electrical circuits. In considering these fault conditions, the following limitations can be applied:

transformers, coils and windings complying with BS/EN 50019[10] (1993) are not subject to fault;

transformers complying with 8.1 of BS/EN 50020 (1994),[7] other than type 2a transformers, are not considered as subject to fault;

Table 9.2 Separations between conducting parts and insulating parts and/or the enclosure through the filling material

Maximum voltage taking account of supply voltage variations, recognized overloads and faults[1] (Volts rms ac/dc)	Minimum separation[2] (mm)
0 to 275	5
276 to 420	6
421 to 550	8
551 to 750	10
751 to 1000	14
1001 to 3000	36
3001 to 6000	60
6001 to 10 000	100

(*from BS/EN 50017*)

Notes:
1 This is the voltage through the filling between electrically conducting parts and insulating parts and/or the inner surface of the enclosure.
2 This separation applies even when the electrically conducting part is isolated.

optocouplers and relays which are designed to separate circuits having at least 1.5 times the voltage differential which actually exists, are not subject to fault provided the voltage separated does not exceed 1000 V peak;

plastic foil, ceramic and paper capacitors are not considered as subject to short-circuit fault provided they do not operate at more than two thirds of their maximum rated voltage;

film type and wire wound (single layer) resistors will only fail to higher resistance.

In addition, separations in accordance with Table 9.3 are not considered as subject to short circuit failure.

Components such as relays are permitted within the filling material, provided they have their own enclosure which will withstand faults within them and their internal volume is less than 30 cm^3, however, if the internal volume is more than 3 cm^3 a 15 mm minimum is applied when Table 9.2 is used. This requirement accepts that the explosive atmosphere can enter the inner void so produced, but an ignition will not cause damage to the apparatus which will produce danger and its flame will likewise be quenched by the filling material.

As the protection concept recognizes faults, then some form of temperature limitation is often going to be necessary. This can be provided

Table 9.3 Separations of conducting parts within the filling

Peak Voltage[1] (Volts)	Creepage distance[2] (mm)	Minimum CTI value[3]	Creepage distance under coating[4] (mm)	Distance through filling material[5] (mm)
10	1.5	N/A[6]	0.6	1.5
30	2.0	100	0.7	1.5
60	3.0	100	1.0	1.5
90	4.0	100	1.3	2.0
190	8.0	175	2.6	3.0
375	10.0	175	3.3	3.0
550	15.0	175	5.0	3.0
750	18.0	175	6.0	5.0
1000	25.0	175	8.3	5.0
1300	36.0	175	12.0	10.0
1575	49.0	175	13.3	10.0

(*from BS/EN 50017*)

Notes:
1 This is the maximum peak voltage between any two live parts at maximum rated voltage with recognized overloads and faults. Where energized parts do not have a common reference the sum of the two voltages concerned will be used.
2 This is the minimum distance along an insulating surface within the filling.
3 Comparative Tracking Index (CTI) is a measure of the quality of insulation against breakdown by contamination (see BS 5901 (1980). Method of Test for Determining the Comparative and proof Tracking indices of Solid Insulating Materials Under Moist Conditions).
4 The conformal coating must be such as to totally cover the conducting parts, adhere to both the conducting parts and the insulation, and effectively exclude moisture.
5 The shortest direct distance through the filling material between two conducting parts.
6 CTI is not considered relevant below 10 V.
7 Where voltages between conducting parts are in excess of 1575 V failure is always considered.

by fuses to BS/EN 60127[8] or IEC 269[12] within the filling, or thermal trips provided the latter are not self resetting.

The Standard also discusses any insulating materials which may be present between the component parts of the apparatus and the enclosure wall in the area defined as filled by Table 9.2 and, with the exception of the insulation of the wiring which exits the filling, for example, to connect to the connection facilities and the filling itself, and requires it to not burn for more than 60 seconds after removal of the flame and resist more than 60 mm of the test piece length being destroyed when tested in accordance with BS 2782, Part 1 (1992).[28] This requirement will apply to support members in plastic and such things as bushings.

This set of requirements is very different to those in the first edition of the Standard BS 5501, Part 4 (1977).[29] In that Standard a very severe test to ensure that ignition could not be transmitted from within the enclosure was included, filling materials were required to be much smaller in size, and clearances between electrical conductors within the filling were much larger. The reason for this is that the requirements of BS/EN 50017 (1994)[26] limit the apparatus protected to that which operates at less than 1000 V, 16 A and 1000 VA which limitation is not in its predecessor. The approach has, therefore, been significantly changed. For this reason, it is not recommended that powder-filled apparatus to BS 5501, Part 4 (1977)[29] is used in the future.

9.3.4 External connections

Any connection facilities for external circuits cannot be such as to fall within the scope of powder filling, particularly as the filled enclosure is sealed permanently at the manufacturing stage. There will, therefore, be the need to protect terminals and similar facilities by another protection concept (e.g., BS/EN 50019 (1994)[10]).

9.3.5 Type testing

The specific testing of this type of apparatus is limited to; pressure testing of the enclosure; flammability testing of its materials; electric-strength testing of the filling material; and maximum temperature testing of the outside of the apparatus.

Pressure testing of the enclosure

The enclosure is subjected to 1.5 times atmospheric pressure for 1 minute without deformation exceeding 0.5 mm.

Flammability testing of enclosure material

The test is carried out with a bunsen burner in accordance with BS 2782[28] and should not result in an average destroyed length of more than 6 cms with burning, not exceeding 60 seconds after removal of the flame. If this test is not possible alternatives are included in BS/EN 50017[26].

Electric strength testing

Using the electrode arrangement in Fig. 9.2, 1000 v dc is applied. With the temperature at $25 \pm 2\,^{\circ}C$ and relative humidity at 45–55 per cent, leakage current should not exceed 10^{-6} A.

Temperature testing

The maximum surface temperature of the enclosure should be measured in full load conditions and including all recognized overloads. Where the apparatus is protected by fuses, the temperature will be measured at 1.7 times the fuse-rated current. For other protective devices the current should be the maximum which can continuously flow without operation.

References

1 76/117/EEC Council Directive of 18 December 1975 on the approximation of the laws of the Member States concerning electrical equipment for use in potentially explosive atmospheres.

2 94/9/EC Directive of the European Parliament and Council of 23 March 1994 on the approximation of the laws of Member States concerning equipment and protective systems for use in potentially explosive atmospheres.

3 BS 5501 Electrical Apparatus for Potentially Explosive Atmospheres. Part 8 (1988). Encapsulation 'm'.

4 BS 5501 Electrical Apparatus for Potentially Explosive Atmospheres. Part 1 (1977). General Requirements.

5 BS/EN 50014 Electrical Apparatus for Potentially Explosive Atmospheres. Part 1 (1993). General Requirements.

6 BS 5501 Electrical Apparatus for Potentially Explosive Atmospheres. Part 7 (1977). Intrinsic Safety 'i'.

7 BS/EN 50020 (1994) Electrical Apparatus for Potentially Explosive Atmospheres. Intrinsic Safety 'i'.

8 BS/EN 60127 (1991) Miniature Fuses.

Part 1 Definitions for miniature fuses general requirements for miniature fuse-links.

Part 2 Specification for cartridge fuse-links.

Part 3 Specification for sub-miniature fuse-links

9 BS 5501 Electrical Apparatus for Potentially Explosive Atmospheres. Part 6 (1977). Increased Safety 'e'.

10 BS/EN 50019 (1994) Electrical Equipment for Potentially Explosive Atmospheres. Increased Safety 'e'.

11 BS 4265 (1977) (1984) Specification for Cartridge Fuse links for Miniature Fuses.

12 IEC 269 Series of Standards for low voltage fuses

13 BS/EN 50015 (1994) Electrical Apparatus for Potentially Explosive Atmospheres. Oil Immersion 'o'.

14 BS 5501 Electrical Apparatus for Potentially Explosive Atmospheres. Part 2 (1977). Oil Immersion 'o'.

15 IEC 79-15 Electrical Apparatus for Explosive Gas Atmospheres. Part 15 (1987). Electrical Apparatus with Type of Protection 'n'.

16 BS 6941 (1988) Electrical Apparatus for Explosive Atmospheres with Type of Protection 'n'.

17 BS/EN 60529 (1991) Specification for Degrees of Protection provided by Enclosures (IP Code).

18 IEC 296 (1969) Specification for New Insulating Oils for Transformers and Switchgear.

19 IEC 296 (1982) Specification for Unused Mineral Insulating Oils for Transformers and Switchgear.

20 IEC 836 (1988) Specifications for Silicone Liquids for Electrical Purposes.

21 ISO 3104 (1976) Petroleum Products – Transparent and Opaque Liquids – Determination of Kinematic viscosity and Calculation of Dynamic Viscosity.

22 BS 6664 Flashpoint of Petroleum Related Products. Part 5 (1990). Method for Determination of flashpoint by Pensky-Martens closed tester.

23 BS 5737 (1979) Method for Measurement of Relative Permittivity, Dielectric Dissipation Factor and dc Resistivity of Insulating Oils.

24 BS 2000 Methods of Test for Petroleum and its Products. Part 15 (1993). Determination of Pour Point.

25 IEC 588-2 Askarels for Transformers and Capacitors. Part 2 (1978). Test Methods.

26 BS/EN 50017 (1994) Electrical Equipment for Potentially Explosive Atmospheres. Powder Filling 'q'.

27 ISO 565 (1990) Test Sieves – Metal Wire Cloth, Perforated Metal Plate and Electro/Formed Sheet – Nominal Size of Openings.

28 BS 2782 (1992) Methods of Testing Plastics. Method 140A – Determination of the Burning Behaviour of Horizontal and Vertical Specimens in contact with a Small-Flame Ignition Source.

29 BS 5501 Electrical Apparatus for Potentially Explosive Atmospheres. Part 4 (1977). Powder Filling 'q'.

BS 5784 Method for Determination of Electrical Strength of Insulating Oils (1980)

— 10 —

Apparatus using protection concept flameproof enclosure 'd' (BS/EN 50018 (1995))

Flameproof enclosure is probably the oldest of the protection concepts considered in the UK and Europe as suitable for Zone 1 and less hazardous areas dating back to before the Second World War. There is much controversy as to who 'invented' it with both Germany and the UK claiming that accolade. While the truth of the matter is not fully clear, history shows it to have developed in the mining industry and that development was done in both Germany and the UK. The prime movers appear to have been the Bergerwerkshaftlische Versuchstrekke in Germany (now known as BVS and one of the German-recognized certification bodies) and the Safety in Mines Research Establishment in the UK (now known as the Health & Safety Laboratory of the Health and Safety Executive [HSE]), which is associated with the Electrical Equipment Certification Service (EECS/BASEEFA). Dr Ing Carl Beyling produced a document describing the application of what was later to become known as 'druckfeste kapselung' (flameproof enclosure) to electric motors in 1908 and was awarded the medal of the UK. Institution of Mining Engineers in 1938 for his work on safety in mines. This gives a lie to any suggestion of rivalry and shows the level of cooperation existing between the UK and Germany during this period. It is also worth noting that the protection concept (type of protection) takes its defining letter 'd' from the German title, although this may have its historical roots in compromises reached in the International Standards-making process and historical issues of German Standards than initial ownership.

It is further worthy of note that flameproof enclosure (called explosion-proof enclosure in the USA) is one of only three protection concepts accepted for Class 1 Division 1 in the USA. This is the equivalent of Zone 0 and 1, as historically the USA did not differentiate between the two. Now, however, in the latest edition of Chapter 5 (Article 500) of the National Electrical Code the USA has begun to accept the European three-Zone system for gases and vapours and is now actively considering other protection concepts currently not acceptable in the USA but used in Europe.

The development of the 'flameproof enclosure' followed very quickly upon the development of usage of electricity in coal mines (industrial problems on the surface not being prime mover during the early years of development) and the recognition that rotating electrical machines (electric motors), which were all dc in the early part of the twentieth century, produced highly ignition-capable sparking in normal operation. While it would have been ideal if the explosive atmosphere could be excluded from the interior of electrical equipment, removing the explosion risk, it was rapidly recognized that such an approach was not generally feasible, particularly in the light of the unreliability of equipment at that time. This resulted in the regular opening of apparatus for maintenance, breaking any seal with the attendant difficulty of remaking it with confidence. (This is still, to a degree, the case as it is still considered that to make and break a seal of the desired quality in the field with confidence is generally not possible). In addition, such things as rotating machines and other actuating devices also have shafts and rods which penetrate the enclosure of apparatus making sealing to the required degree and with the required longevity even more difficult.

Having accepted that the explosive atmosphere could not be excluded and, in general, neither could the ignition source because of the normal sparking which goes on in commutators and switches, the thought patterns turned to a method of allowing the internal explosion of the explosive atmosphere and making arrangements for it not to damage the equipment nor cause ignition of the external explosive atmosphere. Obviously, to withstand an internal explosion without damage the enclosure had to be strong which led to heavy metal enclosures (usually cast). It was discovered that the flamefront caused by the explosion could be rendered harmless by passing it through a small gap, (if the gap size could be guaranteed to have a specific *maximum* dimension during the explosion) the apparatus so enclosed would not constitute an unacceptable risk, even if the explosive atmosphere did penetrate its enclosure and was ignited internally (see Fig. 10.1). Thus was the concept of Flameproof Enclosure born. It must be noted that there is generally no minimum gap specified as the only gap that matters is that achieved in maximum deviation conditions.

In the early days, all flameproof enclosures were of metal construction and a myth developed that they had to be to perform their function, as the objective was achieved only by cooling the flame as it exited the enclosure via the gap. This is now known not to be fully true and the effect is accepted as being one of cooling while exiting through the flange gap and, in addition, rapid entrainment on exit from the gap with cool gases surrounding the enclosure (see Fig. 10.1). This is demonstrated by H. Phillips in his paper to the 1971 IEE conference[1] in which he demonstrates a method of the calculation of the Minimum Experimental Safe Gap (MESG) utilizing these two characteristics. Work in Europe, and particularly in Germany, confirmed this in demonstrating that plastic enclosures which, by definition, have less heat capacity than those of metal performed in essentially the same way. As a result of this, plastic enclosures are now accepted alongside their metallic counterparts provided they satisfy the same criteria, particularly as plastics have now been developed which exhibit similar rigidity and strength as metal. This gives the technique much more commercial attractiveness and flexibility. The requirements of a Flameproof Enclosure are therefore as follows: it must contain an internal explosion of the worst case explosive

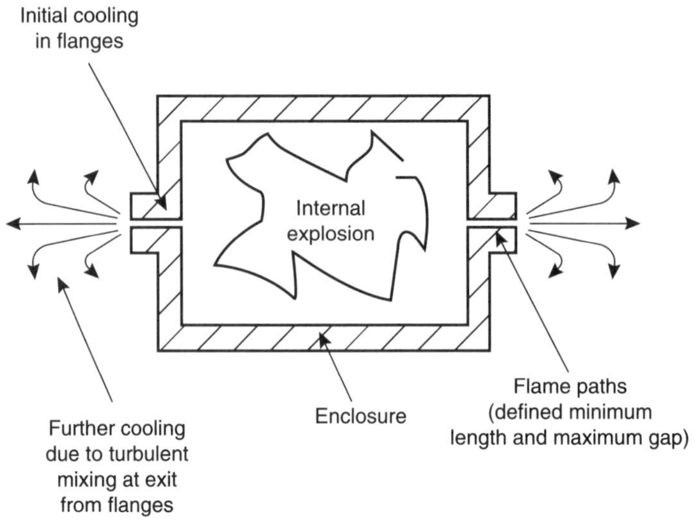

Fig. 10.1 Principle of operation of flameproof enclosure

atmosphere for which it is designed, without damage; the joints between its parts which access the external atmosphere must be of specified maximum dimensions and its strength must be such that those joints do not widen under conditions of internal explosion of the worst case explosive atmosphere for which it is designed, to a point where the flame is transmitted outside the enclosure and ignites the external atmosphere. In addition, its material of construction must not be damaged by the internal burning associated with an internal explosion of the worst case explosive atmosphere.

Obviously, the enclosure must not deteriorate in the environment in which it is installed, but this is not a specific explosive atmosphere requirement and is not included in the detail of the flameproof enclosure requirements, but is identified as something the user must consider when selecting equipment for a particular location.

10.1 Standards for flameproof apparatus

As befits its age, the protection concept has been addressed in several Standards applicable in the UK over the years, and it is probably worthwhile to address these because they identify the development of the technique.

The first Standard of significance was BS 229[2] which was first issued in 1926 with revisions in 1929, 1940, 1946 and 1957. This Standard did not require, in common with its contemporary Standards, that the parts of enclosures in direct contact with an external explosive atmosphere be temperature classified as it pre-dated the surface temperature classification system. Users were given no guidance on usage in respect of thermal ignition of an explosive atmosphere. In addition, it did not permit facilities for external connection to be within the main component enclosing parts of the enclosure, but insisted they be in a separate terminal box (see Section 10.2). It also limited enclosures to those made of metal, required far more severe glanding arrangements (the engaged thread of a gland within the enclosure wall was 18 mm, rather than the now permitted 8 mm (see Section 10.2) and, most importantly, it did not allow flameproof enclosures for use in what is now Group IIC gases, vapours and mists. Therefore, wherever hydrogen or acetylene was present, there was no Standard protection concept for electrical equipment which was, by its operation, ignition capable until pressurization came into use much later. BS 229[2] equipment is largely now historic and should not be selected for use, although some still exists in older installations.

BS 229[2] was effectively replaced in 1971 by BS 4683, Part 2[3] which included many of the ideas at that time being developed in Europe and internationally. This Standard was very close to the current European Standards in content. The Standard introduced the concept of non-metallic enclosures, already commonplace in Germany, to the UK, added requirements for Group IIC enclosures (although it still baulked at enclosures for acetylene mixtures) and reduced the gland thread engagement to 8 mm. This Standard was produced shortly before the European standstill agreement which prevented member states from issuing National Standards where CENELEC[4] was preparing a parallel Standard or it may never have appeared. It was, however, necessary as UK flameproof practice had fallen behind competition in Europe and urgent correction was necessary. This explains the short life of BS 4683, Part 2 which was superseded in the UK by BS 5501, Part 5[5] in 1977, this being the first edition of the European Standard, EN 50018. This European Standard was very similar in content to BS 4683, Part 2[3] as the UK was involved in its production in parallel to the European work, and a good degree of cross fertilization occurred. It is true that differences exist in relationship to testing methods and elsewhere but none of these would lead to a situation where concern would be expressed over the use of BS 4683, Part 2 apparatus, much of which still exists. In accordance with European agreements, however, it is withdrawn and all future equipment will be to the European Standard.

The European Standard, BS 5501, Part 5[5] has now been superseded by a second edition and, unlike the first edition, is not given a separate BS number but retains its European number and is titled BS/EN 50018[6]. This second edition was published in 1995 and was very significant in that it permitted breathing and draining devices, which did not comply with the dimensional constructional requirements of the standard and, did not have any measurable dimensions except the external size, in the protection concept for the first time. The significance of this is the introduction for the first time of compliance by test only, rather than by dimensional specification and test. As the second edition of EN 50018 is now current, this chapter will address that Standard. As already stated, however, most of the differences between this and its preceding first edition and, indeed, BS 4683, Part 2[3] are relatively small.

There is a further Standard in existence which is the International Standard, IEC 79–1[7]. This Standard is very similar to BS/EN 50018[6] but is voluntary only and in Europe it is necessary to comply with the European Standard, so the international document is not so important. An agreement between the European Standards body (CENELEC) and its international equivalent (IEC[8]) requires that the Standards of the two bodies are harmonized and IEC 79–1 and BS/EN 50018[6] may be expected to come together in the next few years.

10.2 Construction and testing requirements for flamepaths

The detailed requirements for the construction of flameproof enclosures are currently given in BS/EN 50018 (1995). As may be expected, much of the Standard is given over to description of the types of joint between, for example, enclosure and cover and enclosure strength as these are the two factors upon which the protection concept is based. It also contains additional requirements for cable entries, such as glands which also form entries into the enclosure, breathing and draining devices, which are the main change between this Standard and its predecessor, and additional requirements for such things as non-metallic enclosures and lamp caps where these form flameproof joints (e.g., in apparatus to BS/EN 50018[6]).

10.2.1 Joints between the interior of flameproof enclosures and the external atmosphere

There are effectively five types of joint used in flameproof enclosures. In addition, there are requirements for joints used for rotating shafts together with an additional type of joint. These are:

1. Flat flange joints.
2. Spigot joints.
3. Cylindrical joints, operating rod joints and partial cylindrical joints.
4. Threaded Joints.
5. Cemented Joints.

Flat flange joints

Flat flange joints are the oldest form of joint (together with cylindrical joints) and probably the easiest to construct. Figure 10.2 shows the basic flange-joint configurations. The joints are required to be of certain limiting quality. For example, the two faces of the flange are each required to be no rougher than 6.3 μm in accordance with ISO 468 (1982)[10]. This is not a particularly

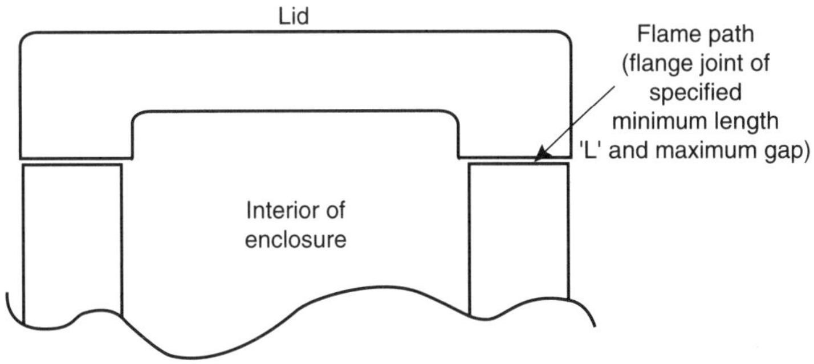

Fig. 10.2 Typical flanged joints

stringent specification but precludes such things as casting blowholes and deep scores in the surfaces, both of which could assist flame transmission out of the enclosure. The minimum length of joints is also specified, together with the matching maximum gap between flanges, and the current figures for these are given in Table 10.1 which relates to Fig. 10.2.

Table 10.1 Maximum permitted gaps for flanged joints of various widths

Joint width (L) (mm)	Permissible maximum gaps for given enclosure volumes and sub-groups (mm)											
	Volume ≤ 100 cm³			Volume ≤ 500 cm³			Volume ≤ 2000 cm³			Volume >2000 cm³		
	IIA	IIB	IIC	IIA	IIB	IIC	IIA	IIB	IIC	IIA	IIB	IIC
≥6.0	0.3	0.2	0.1	N/P	N/P	N/P	N/P	N/P	N/P	N/P	N/P	N/P
≥9.5	0.3	0.2	0.1	0.3	0.2	N/P	N/P	N/P	N/P	N/P	N/P	N/P
≥12.5	0.3	0.2	0.1	0.3	0.2	0.1	0.3	0.2	N/P	0.2	0.15	N/P
≥25.0	0.4	0.2	0.1	0.4	0.2	0.1	0.4	0.2	N/P	0.4	0.20	N/P
≥40.0	0.4	0.2	0.1	0.4	0.2	0.1	0.4	0.2	N/P	0.4	0.20	N/P

(from BS/EN 50018)
N/P = Flanged joints are not permitted for this volume of enclosure and this sub-group

Weather proofing of flat flanged joints

Historically it has been recognized that the introduction of such things as gaskets or 'o' rings for weather proofing between the joint surfaces could cause problems, as the gasket or 'o' ring could make it impossible to guarantee the maximum gap required, and this led to the virtual prohibition of such weather proofing techniques in flanged joints. This situation was

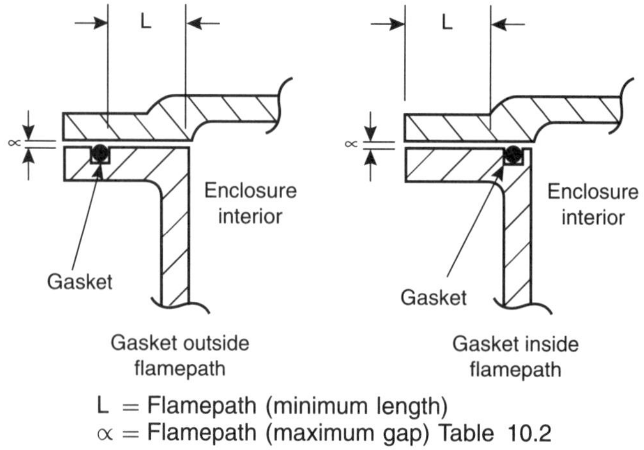

Fig. 10.3 Fitting of gaskets to flanged joints

relaxed to a degree in BS 5501, Part 5[5] (the first edition of the European Standard) by removal of any prohibitive statements and in BS/EN 50018[6] (the second edition of the European Standard) has been fully removed by the inclusion of guidance on the fitting of gaskets in a way which maintains the joint integrity. This guidance requires a groove to be inserted either inside the actual joint path or outside it and the fitting of an 'o' ring or similar style of gasket in that groove (see Fig. 10.3). This widens the flange and makes the enclosure more cumbersome but does overcome the problem of weather proofing the enclosure. It is recommended that the 'o' ring-type gasket is always fitted on the outside of the flange as, particularly in the case of metal joints, the flanges are subject to corrosion in the case of installation in outdoor and similar hostile environments, and such corrosion could damage the joint and permit flame transmission.

Facilities for fixings for parts of flat flanged enclosures

It is recognized that the parts of the enclosure forming the joint will require fixing, and if the fixings are outside the flanges the width of the flanges would be significantly increased. To this end, as a result of experimentation over the years, a situation where the holes for fixing may pass through the flange itself has been identified. This is based upon the conclusion that the bolt clearance hole is a passage to the outside environment or the interior of the enclosure and, in common with the other flamepaths, is usually most pronounced during an internal explosion, even after satisfying the dimensional requirements for joints. This enlargement is taken care of by a safety factor test.

The length of path (see Fig. 10.4 and 10.5) required between the unprotected bolt hole and the interior or exterior of the enclosure (depending upon the enclosure geometry) is defined in Table 10.2. It should be noted that the clearance holes for the fasteners and the threaded holes are required

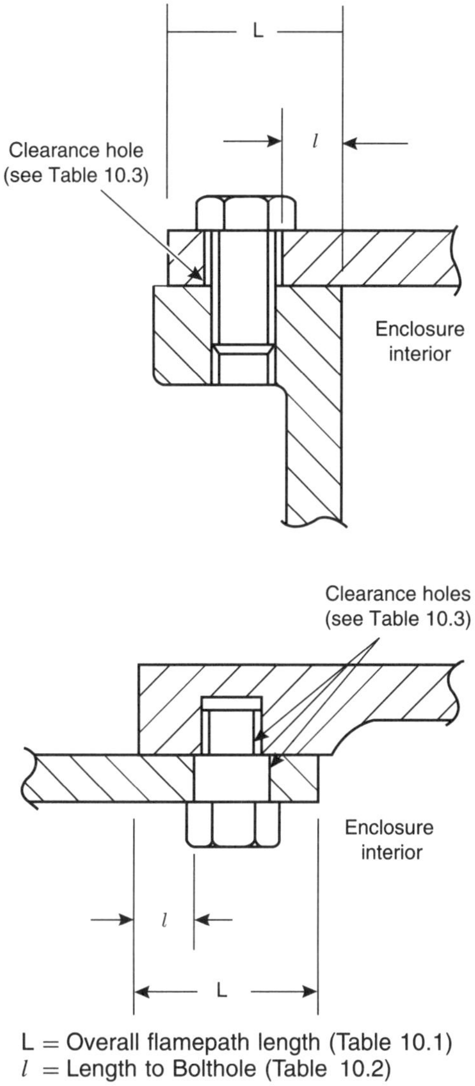

Fig. 10.4 Effects of boltholes through flanges

to satisfy certain criteria. The threads and bolt strengths will be dealt with later in this chapter but the clearance holes should satisfy the requirements of Table 10.3.

Where the fixing bolts enter the main body of the enclosure from outside there are certain requirements which apply to ensure they do not adversely affect the flameproof properties of the enclosure. The first is that if the thread penetrates the enclosure and therefore becomes a flamepath it must comply with the requirement for threaded joints. To avoid wear, it must also be secured to the enclosure by welding, rivetting or a method of similar security.

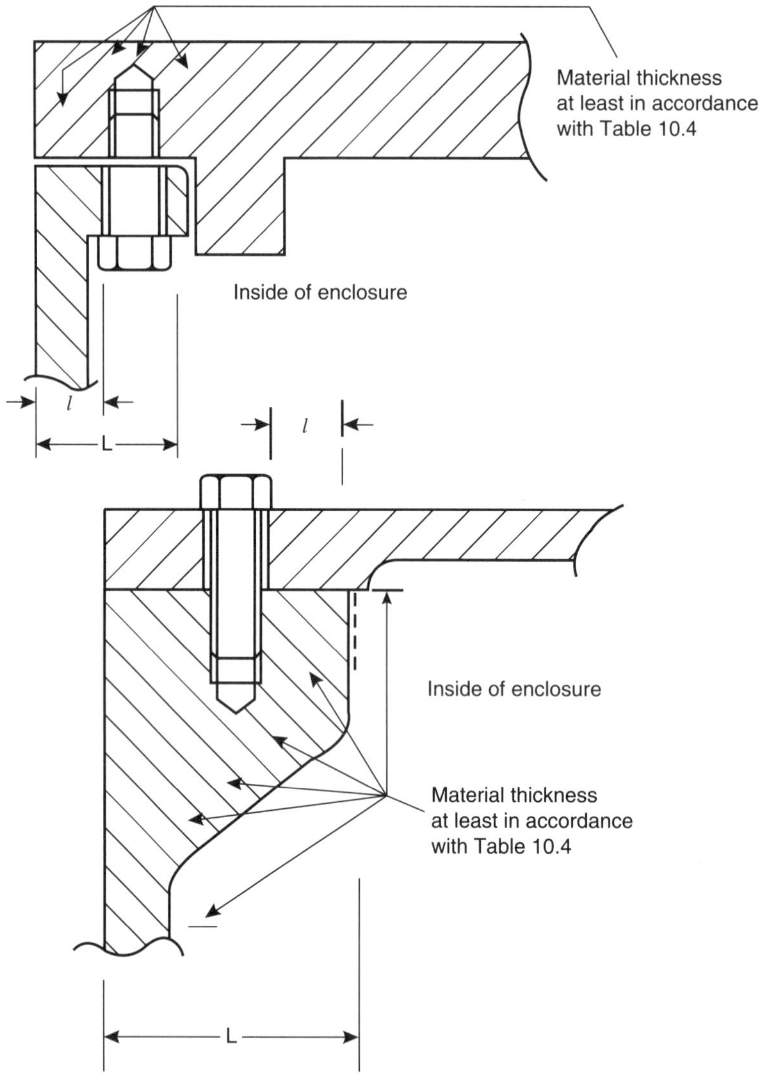

L = Overall flamepath length (Table 10.1)
l = Length to bolthole (Table 10.2)

Fig. 10.5 Threaded holes in enclosures walls

Where the threaded hole does not penetrate the enclosure wall the thickness of enclosure material between the threaded hole and the inside of the enclosure where the bolt head is outside the enclosure (see Fig. 10.5) or between the threaded hole, and the outside of the enclosure where the bolt head is inside the enclosure must have at least the thickness given in Table 10.4 to ensure that the enclosure and fixing have adequate strength.

Table 10.2 Geometry of joint where bolts pass through it

Joint width (L) (mm)	Length of flamepath between enclosure and exterior (l) (mm)
<12.5	6
≥12.5 < 25	8
≥25	9

See Fig. 10.4 to see geometry of reduced joint width where bolts pass through the flamepath.

Table 10.3 Bolt clearance holes which penetrate enclosure flange flamepath

Thread size (mm)	Diameter of clearance hole (nominal) (mm)
M 4	4.5
M 5	5.5
M 6	6.6
M 8	9.0
M 10	11.0
M 12	14.0
M 14	16.0
M 16	18.0
M 20	22.0
M 24	26.0

(*from BS/EN 50014*)
Note: For other sizes clearance holes should be in accordance with not worse than a medium tolerance fit of H13 in accordance with BS 4500 (1990).

Because of the severity of explosions where hydrogen is present there are severe limits on the size of enclosures with plane flanged joints for group IIC apparatus. Enclosures greater than 500 cm^3 volume with flanged joints are not permitted with any width of flange, and those over 100 cm^3 must have flanges which exceed 9.5 mm in width. Likewise, flanged joints are not permitted for acetylene atmospheres, even though acetylene is nominally in sub-group IIC because of the carbon formation associated with acetylene explosions, and the possibility that this formation will prevent proper seating of the joint when remade. There is also a real possibility of ejection

Table 10.4 Minimum thickness of wall between thread and interior of enclosure

Thread size (mm)	Minimum thickness of wall (T) (mm)
M 4	3.0
M 5	3.0
M 6	3.0
M 8	3.0
M 10	3.4
M 12	4.0
M 14	4.7
M 16	5.4
M 20	6.7
M 24	8.0

Note: For other diameters above 10 mm use one third of thread diameter for minimum thickness.

of incandescent carbon particles during an explosion and these may contain sufficient energy to cause ignition.

Similar, but less onerous, restrictions exist for sub-group IIB and IIA enclosures in that flanges of less than 9.5 mm are not permitted for IIB enclosures exceeding 100 cm^3 in volume, and flanges of less than 12.5 cm^3 are not permitted for those of more than 500 cm^3 although in this case, unlike the situation in sub-group IIC, larger enclosures are permitted and there is no limit on size provided the flange width is not less than 12.5 mm.

2 Spigot joints

Spigot joints are joints in which the critical gap forming the flamepath is contained, either totally within the cylindrical part of the joint ('a' in Fig. 10.6), or where it is partly contained within the cylindrical joint and partly within the plane part, which is similar to a flange (a combination of 'a' and 'b' in Fig. 10.6). Even joints where the flamepath is totally within the cylindrical part of the joint usually have a plane part to provide for the possibility of fixing bolts, even though this may not form part of the critical path (flamepath) through which the burning gases pass in case of an internal explosion. This is not, however, always true as alternative methods may be used to ensure that the joint is stable, for example, the fixing may be by an external clamp or by a thread on the cylindrical part outside, or inside the flamepath. The joint is more simple to manufacture if the flamepath is fully within the cylindrical part of the joint, but this may cause an enclosure to be significantly larger than if the first alternative is adopted.

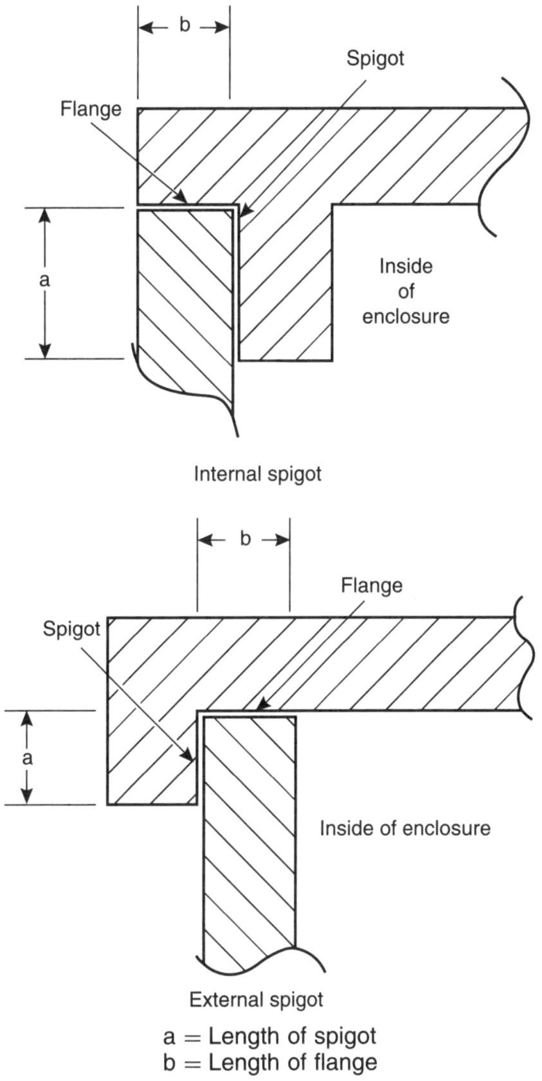

Fig. 10.6 Internal and external spigot joints

The overall advantage of spigot joints is the fact that, as this type of joint has a right angle either outside it or inside it, it is much less likely to emit ignition-capable particles and, as a result, there is no specific restriction in the use of such joints in acetylene atmospheres, unlike the situation in respect of their flat flanged counterparts.

Composite spigot joints (flamepath partly in the plane part of the joint and partly in the cylindrical part)

The limits of maximum gap size for various lengths of composite joints, where the flamepath is divided between the plane part and the cylindrical

Table 10.5 maximum permitted gaps for composite spigot joints of various widths

Joint width L^1 (mm)	Permissible maximum gaps for given enclosure volumes and sub-groups (mm)											
	Volume $\leq 100\,cm^3$			Volume $\leq 500\,cm^3$			Volume $\leq 2000\,cm^3$			Volume $>2000\,cm^3$		
	IIA	IIB	IIC	IIA	IIB	IIC	IIA	IIB	IIC	IIA	IIB	IIC
≥6.0	0.3	0.2	N/P	N/P	N/P	N/P	N/P	N/P	N/P	N/P	N/P	N/P
≥9.5	0.3	0.2	N/P	0.3	0.2	N/P	N/P	N/P	N/P	N/P	N/P	N/P
≥12.5	0.3	0.2	0.15	0.3	0.2	0.15	0.3	0.2	0.15	0.2	0.15	N/P
≥25.0	0.4	0.2	0.18	0.4	0.2	0.18	0.4	0.2	0.18	0.4	0.20	0.18
≥40.0	0.4	0.2	0.20	0.4	0.2	0.20	0.4	0.2	0.20	0.4	0.2	0.20

(*from BS/EN 50018*)
N/P = Spigot joints are not permitted for this enclosure volume and this sub-group.

part in various explosive atmospheres and for various sizes of enclosure, are given in Table 10.5. In addition, there are limits to the division of the flamepath between the plane part and the cylindrical part of the joint, in that the plane part of the joint must be at least 3 mm for joints in enclosures for use in sub-groups IIA and IIB, and 6 mm for those for use in sub-group IIC. In addition for joints in enclosures for use in sub-group IIC the cylindrical part of the joint must be at least half the total minimum required length of flamepath. No similar restriction exists for joints in enclosures for sub-group IIA or IIB.

In these circumstances it is likely that considerable machining difficulties would be encountered in forming the right angles in both the parts of the joint, and ensuring proper mating. For this reason the situation whereby the male right angle has a chamfer or radius on it has been carefully investigated. Such a situation is shown for both internal and external spigot joints in Fig. 10.7 and it has been shown that, provided the chamfer or radius does not have a linear dimension in either the plane of the plane part of the joint and in the cylindrical part of greater than 1 mm and, if a radius is convex rather than concave (resulting in less material removal), the aperture so produced will not cause any significant reduction in the security of joints made up of both plane and spigot portions of the joint. Therefore, provided the remaining parts and cylindrical parts ('a' and 'b' in Fig. 10.7) add up to at least the minimum required joint width specified in Table 10.5, and is divided between the two parts of the joint in accordance with the additional restrictions given in this chapter, the situation is acceptable. It has to be clearly understood, however, that the parts of the joint removed by the radius or chamfer do not form part of the length required ('f' in Fig. 10.7 does not form part of the joint length).

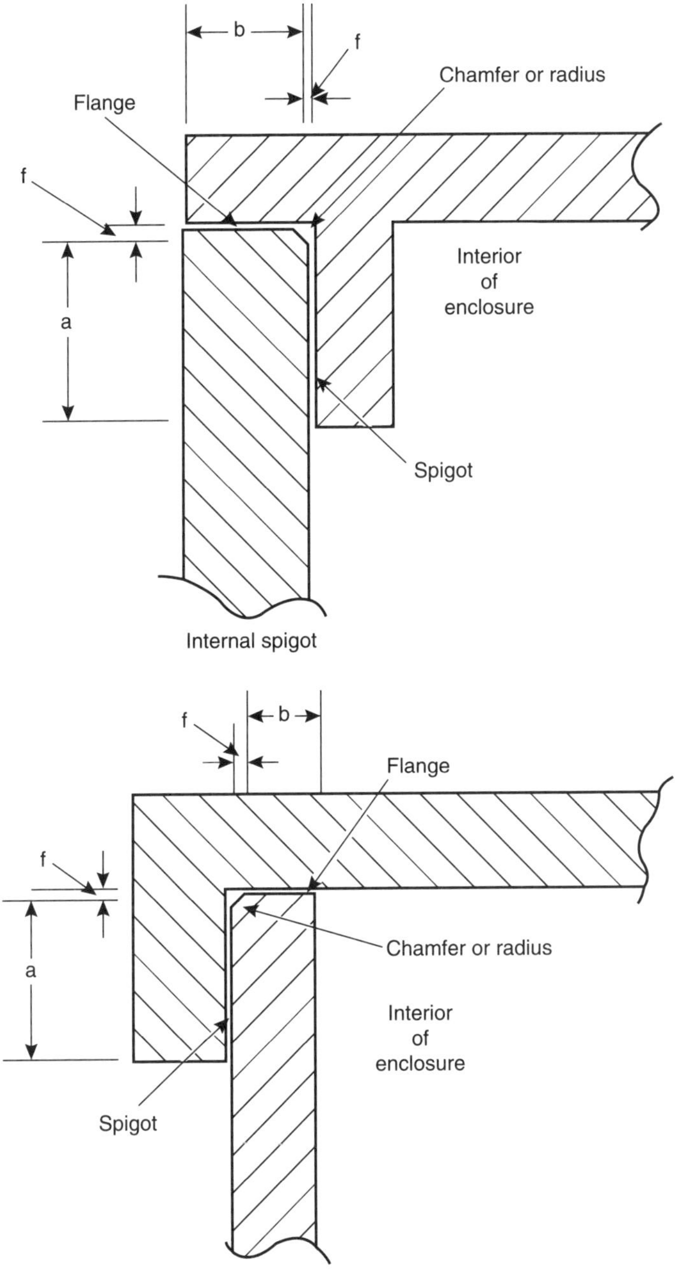

a = Actual length of cylindrical part to chamfer or radius
b = Actual length of plane part to chamfer or radius
f = Maximum encroachment of chamfer or radius into plane and cylindrical part (1 mm max) (e.g., in these examples width of wall = b+f

Fig. 10.7 Practical execution of spigot joint

As stated in the previous paragraph there are additional requirements for the division of the required length of joint between the plane part and the cylindrical part of joints which are as follows: first, the minimum width of the plane part of the joint must be at least 3 mm for sub-groups IIA and IIB and 6 mm for sub-group IIC; and second, the minimum length of the cylindrical part of the joint must be at least half of the minimum length specified in Table 10.5 for enclosures intended for sub-group IIC use. No restriction applies in this respect for enclosures intended for sub-group IIA or IIB use as the requirements for flanged joints and spigot joints are the same.

As previously stated, there is no specific restriction to the use of these joints in acetylene atmospheres and this has led to restrictions in the minimum length of flamepath permitted in sub-group IIC. The reason for this is the performance of composite (cylindrical part plus plane part) joints of shorter length in acetylene atmospheres and, to a degree, the performance of composite joints of short length in hydrogen atmospheres. Rather than create a very complex situation, therefore, the following restrictions apply:

> No composite joint with a length of less than 12.5 mm is permitted for enclosures for sub-group IIC.
>
> No composite joint with a length of less than 25 mm is permitted in enclosures with volumes greater than 2000 cm^3 for sub-group IIC.
>
> No composite joint with a length less than 9.5 mm is permitted in enclosures of greater than 100 cm^3 volume for sub-group IIA and IIB.
>
> No composite joint with a length of less than 12.5 mm is permitted in enclosures of greater than 500 cm^3 for sub-group IIA and IIB.

The above requirements are more severe than those applied to spigot joints where all of the flamepath is in the cylindrical part of the joint and which are dealt with in the following text.

Spigot joints with all of the flamepath in the cylindrical part of the joint

The requirements for flamepath length are the same as for a composite joint in the case of joints where the entire flamepath is in the cylindrical part of the joint ('a' in Fig. 10.6) and which are used in enclosures for sub-group IIA and IIB, but there are significant relaxations for joints in enclosures for sub-group IIC, as can be seen from Table 10.6 which defines the maximum gaps for this type of joint for various sizes of enclosure and the three sub-groups, IIA, IIB and IIC. The reduction of permissible gap for joints of enclosures intended for sub-group IIC use is 0.15 mm for joints where all of the flamepath is within the cylindrical part and the joint length is $\leq$ 25 mm. (This compares with 0.18 mm for composite joints).

The other differences are the permissibility of smaller joint lengths in cases where all of the joint is in the cylindrical part and the restrictions in joint length are much more in-line with those of flanged joints, although the spigot joint has the added advantage that it may be used in acetylene

Table 10.6 Maximum permitted gaps for simple spigot joints of various widths

Joint width (L) (mm)	Permissible maximum gaps for given enclosure volumes and sub-groups (mm)											
	Volume $\leq 100\,cm^3$			Volume $\leq 500\,cm^3$			Volume $\leq 2000\,cm^3$			Volume $>2000\,cm^3$		
	IIA	IIB	IIC	IIA	IIB	IIC	IIA	IIB	IIC	IIA	IIB	IIC
≥6.0	0.3	0.2	0.10	N/P	N/P	0.10	N/P	N/P	N/P	N/P	N/P	N/P
≥9.5	0.3	0.2	0.10	0.3	0.2	0.10	N/P	N/P	N/P	N/P	N/P	N/P
≥12.5	0.3	0.02	0.15	0.3	0.2	0.15	0.3	0.2	0.15	0.2	0.15	N/P
≥25.0	0.4	0.2	0.15	0.4	0.2	0.15	0.4	0.2	0.15	0.4	0.20	0.15
≥40.0	0.4	0.2	0.20	0.4	0.2	0.20	0.4	0.2	0.20	0.4	0.20	0.2

(from BS/EN 50018)
N/P = Spigot joints are not permitted for enclosures of this volume in this sub-group

atmospheres. These restrictions are: first, joints of less than 6 mm length are not permitted in enclosures of more than $100\,cm^3$ for sub-group IIC use. (Composite joints must have a length of 12.5 mm for such use.) and second, joints with lengths of less than 9.5 mm are not permitted in enclosures of greater volume than $500\,cm^3$ for use in IIC atmospheres. (Composite joints must have minimum lengths of 12.5 mm for such use.).

As can be seen, these restrictions are considerably less than those for composite joints and more in-line with those for flanged joints, except that in this case there is no overall restriction on enclosure size as there is in the case of flanged joints for their flanged counterparts gaskets, or 'o' rings may be fitted to make spigot joints weatherproof, provided these do not reduce the length of the flamepath achieved to less than that minimum specified in Table 10.5, and do not cause the spigot part or the flange part of any joint to cease to comply with the minimum lengths specified earlier in this chapter.

Gaskets for weatherproofing, etc., of both types of spigot joint

The use of 'o' ring-type gaskets, similar to those used in flat flanged joints, is shown in Fig. 10.8 for an 'o' ring in the plane part and the cylindrical part of the joint. In the latter case, both inside the flamepath and outside the flamepath. The 'o' ring must always be outside or inside the flamepath, not within it, and as can be seen from Fig. 10.8, the flamepath must be totally within the cylindrical part where the 'o' ring is outside the flamepath, but in the cylindrical part of the joint. Where the 'o' ring is in the plane part of the joint outside the flamepath, or in the cylindrical part inside the flamepath, composite joints are, of course, possible. The recess must fully

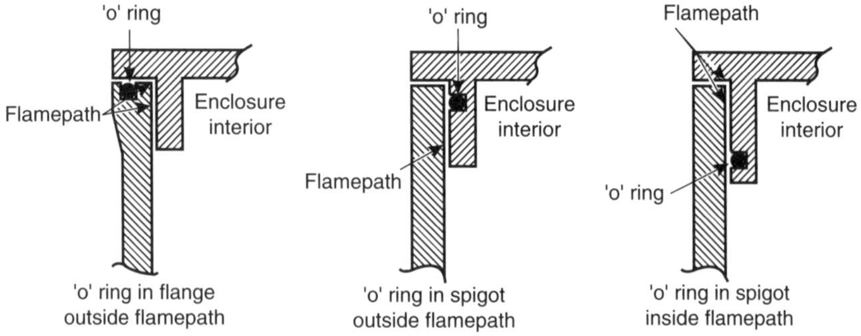

Fig. 10.8 Arrangement of 'o' ring type gasket

accommodate the 'o' ring to ensure that the joint is not distorted. This is particularly important in the case of the composite joint, where the 'o' ring is in the plane part of the joint. Again, for metallic enclosures the preferred solution for weatherproofing is to have the gasket outside the flamepath to avoid corrosion of the joint which could damage its flameproof properties.

Flat gaskets are, in this case, also permitted, either inside or outside the flamepath, and their position is shown in Fig. 10.9. In this case, the flamepath must be totally within the cylindrical part of the joint as the gaskets will prevent clear definition of the plane part of the joint. In addition, it will be necessary to ensure that the flamepath in the cylindrical part is always of adequate length, and the only effective way to ensure this is to ensure that the flamepath in the cylindrical part of the joint satisfies the requirements of Table 10.6 before compression of the gasket when the enclosure is fitted with a gasket of maximum dimension.

Fixings in the plane parts of composite spigot joints

The construction of the joints is, however, much more complex particularly where the plane part of the joint forms part of the flamepath (gap) and fixing

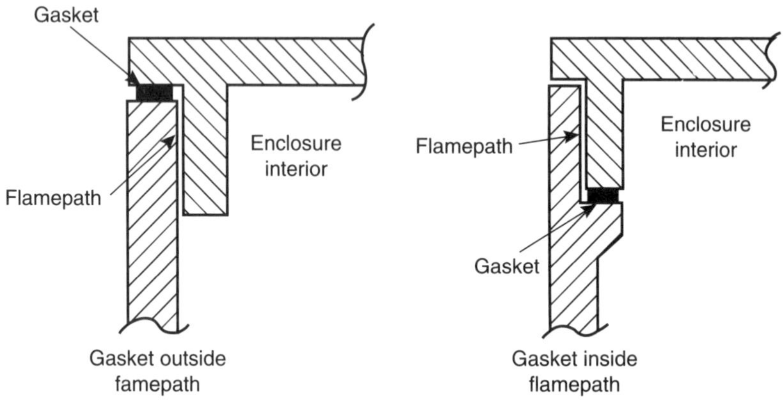

Fig. 10.9 Arrangement for flat compressible gaskets

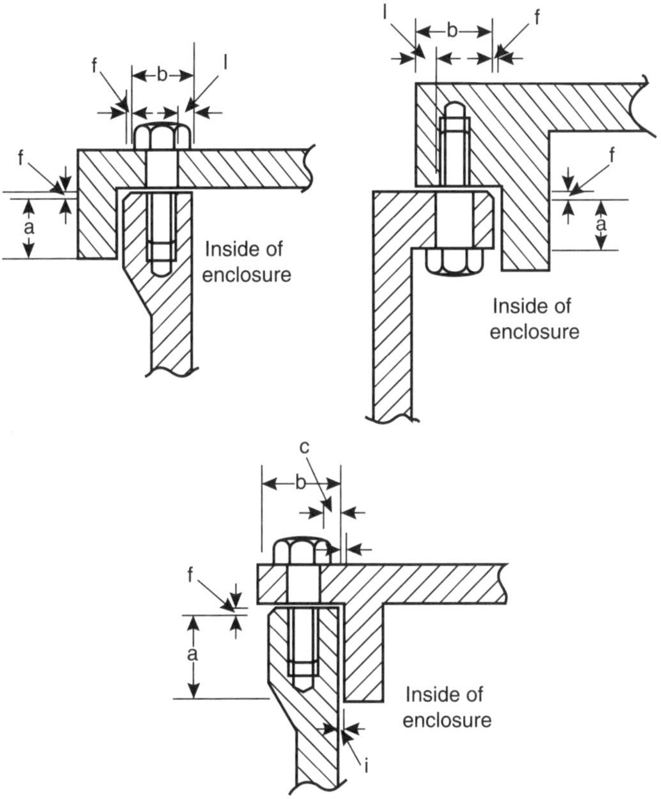

a = Length of cylindrical part of joint
b = Length of plane part of joint
f = Encroachment of chamfer or radius into plane or cylindrical planes
l = Length of flamepath up to bolt hole (a + c where l is composite of plane and cylindrical parts) (i = 0.2 mm max for sub-group IIA and IIB, 0.1 mm max for sub-group IIC)

Fig. 10.10 Effects of boltholes on joints

bolts pass through it. The passage of the bolt actually divides the flamepath in a similar way to that which occurs with flange joints with an external spigot joint with the bolt head either inside or outside the enclosure (see Fig. 10.10) or an internal spigot where the bolt head is inside the enclosure. In all of these cases it should be noted that the length of path between the bolt clearance hole and the outside of the enclosure, where the bolt head is inside the enclosure and the bolt clearance hole, and the interior of the enclosure where the bolt head is outside the enclosure, is formed totally in the plane part of the joint and thus the requirements of Table 10.2 apply to the minimum value of 'l'.

In the case of the internal spigot joint where the bolt head is external, however, the situation is very different. Here, the distance 'l' between the interior of the enclosure and the bolt clearance hole is composite, being made up of the part of the plane part of the joint and its cylindrical part of the joint. This is further exacerbated where there is a chamfer or radius on the male part of the joint to aid seating of the joint. In this case, as for the flamepath, the distance 'l' is made up of the length of the cylindrical part of the joint ('a' in Fig. 10.10) up to, but not including, the chamfer or radius and the distance between the edge of the chamfer or radius and the bolt clearance hole in the plane part of the joint ('c' in Fig. 10.10).

The integrity of spigot joints is based on two criteria. First, the Maximum Experimental Safe Gap (MESG) is larger than the gap permitted as maximum by the Standard, thus permitting the reduction to the bolt clearance hole specified in Table 10.2, and second, the volume created by the chamfer or radius in the male part of a spigot joint while adversely affecting the joint performance will not be added to the reduction of the distance 'l' as it does not form part of that path. Unfortunately, where the bolt head is outside the enclosure in cases where an internal spigot is used, this is not true as the reduced distance 'l' is composite, containing a plane part which is from the bolt clearance hole to the edge of the chamfer or radius, and a cylindrical part which is from the internal edge of the joint to the edge of the chamfer or radius. This gives the worst of both worlds in cases where a chamfer is present and a further restriction is necessary. This is achieved by restriction in the gap permitted in the cylindrical part of the joint to 0.2 mm for joints of enclosures intended for use in sub-group IIA and IIB and 0.1 mm for those intended for use in sub-group IIC. The total joint length 'L', the reduced length 'l' to the bolt clearance hole, and the gap permitted for the plane part of the joint remain unchanged, the latter being as specified in Table 10.5. If the chamfer or radius can be reduced to an encroachment of no more than 0.5 mm, then these figures may be increased to 0.2 mm for Group IIC joints of 25 mm or greater length, and 0.25 mm for such joints of not less than 40 mm length. In cases where no chamfer or radius exists, or where 'l' is achieved completely in the plane part of the joint, these figures for gaps in the cylindrical part of the joint do not apply and the required gaps are those in Table 10.5.

While this makes the application of spigot joints a little more complex than their flange counterparts, the inclusion of acetylene and the effective reduction in enclosure size which is possible makes this type of joint attractive particularly for instrument applications and the type of joint is becoming more and more popular.

The above information has all been based upon the spigot joint where of the part of the joint not in the plane part of the joint (which may form the entire flamepath) is cylindrical. There is no reason why this should not be conical, provided that the gap is uniform throughout the conical part of the joint and the conical part of the joint complies with the requirements of length and gap for a normal spigot joint. There are, however, restrictions in the case of sub-group IIC joints and in these cases the taper of the joint (the cone angle) is required not to exceed 5°. While being a special case of a spigot joint, these joints are normally referred to as conical joints.

3 Cylindrical joints, operating rod joints, and partial cylindrical joints

A basic cylindrical joint is no different to a spigot joint where all of the flamepath is in the cylindrical part of the joint and the limiting dimensions are contained in Table 10.6. These joints are, however, mainly used for operating rods and rotating shafts where eccentricity and wear can become problems. They have, therefore, special requirements applied to them in such circumstances. The requirements for shafts will be dealt with in a later section of this chapter but those for operating rods will be dealt with here. It must be stressed, however, that if the two parts of the cylindrical joint are firmly fixed, and the joint does not move or rotate as part of its normal operation, these requirements do not apply and the joint should be treated as a spigot joint with all of the flamepath in the cylindrical part of the joint.

In cases where the inner part of the joint is an operating rod, whereby eccentricity in assembly or due to movement must be taken into account, the joint gap required must be achieved even when the rod is at one side of the joint (which means that when it is central in the hole then the gap around it must be half of that normally required). In addition, the length of joint must comply with the required length of joint for static cylindrical joints given earlier in this chapter, but must also have a length at least equal to the diameter of the rod itself where this is less than 25 mm. Where the rod is in excess of 25 mm diameter, then the joint length requirements for static cylindrical joints alone apply.

If the inner part of the joint is an operating rod and the joint is subject to wear during the normal operating life of the enclosure because of the materials of construction and/or the frequency of operation, then the parts of the joint must be replaceable. This can be achieved by, for example, making the outer part of the joint of softer bushing material and making it replaceable. It is recommended that the approach is to take the view that wear is possible unless it can be clearly proved that it is not. In addition, the rod must not be removable from the outside of the enclosure nor must it be capable of moving totally inside the enclosure as either event would remove any flamepath and permit transmission of an explosion. It is likely that in most cases the rod will be secured to the necessary degree by the fixings necessary for its operation inside the enclosure, but if not then it needs to be secured against removal by internal fasteners (e.g., circlips or similar).

Partial cylindrical joints are permitted where such things as plates are used as covers on hollow cylinders, and an example is shown in Fig. 10.11. This type of joint should be treated exactly as for a flanged joint where gaps, joint lengths, gaskets, and introduction of fixing bolts are concerned but, in this case, a total prohibition of the type of joint for enclosures intended for sub-group IIC is applied so that, unlike the other types of joint, partial cylindrical joints may not be used in enclosures for sub-group IIC. This is probably because of the greater difficulty in achieving the coincidence of radius required between the two parts than is the case with achievement of the necessary flatness for flanged joints.

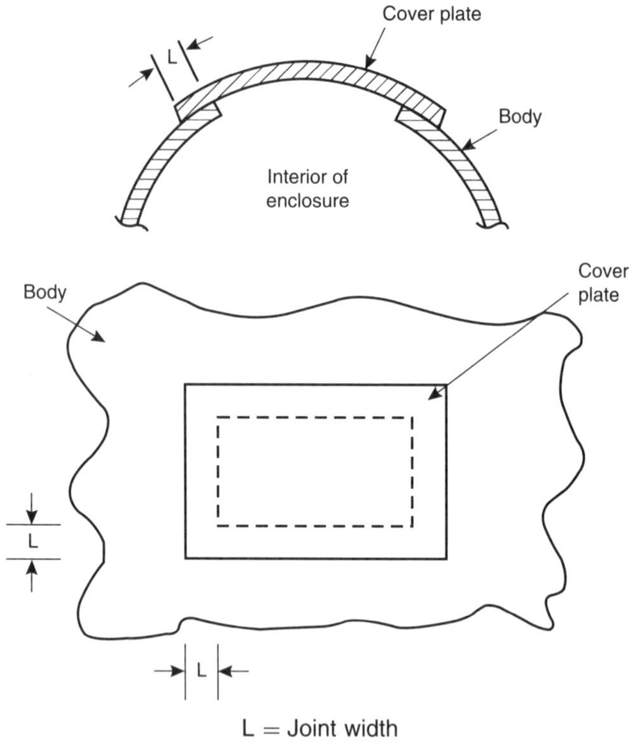

Fig. 10.11 Partial cylindrical joint

It is worthy of note that these joints were not specifically identified in BS 5501, Part 5 (the first edition of EN 50018). Their similarity to the flanged joint, however, means that they were probably so treated by at least some of the certification bodies involved and may exist in some apparatus – even that with a volume of less than 500 cm^3 intended for sub-group IIC use. The requirement in BS/EN 50018[6] (1995) (the second edition of EN 50018) represents an additional restriction on the use of such joints. As there has been no official notice that previous practice is unsafe, however, this does not require any retrospective remedial action but it would be wise to favour apparatus to BS/EN 50018[6] in the future.

A capillary can be considered as a cylindrical joint with the inside diameter equal to 0. Therefore, the maximum gaps specified in Table 10.6 will become the maximum internal diameter of the capillary.

4 Threaded joints

Joints between parts of flameproof enclosures may also be threaded. Where this is so the threads involved require either to be of specific named types with specific qualities of fit or to be specified, possibly to a lower level of quality, and be subject to additional requirements when testing for flame

Table 10.7 Thread requirements for cylindrical (parallel) threaded joints

Cylindrical (parallel) threaded joints	
Thread pitch	0.7 mm min to 2 mm max (see note)
Thread form and fit quality according to ISO 965/1 and ISO 965/3	Medium or fine tolerance
No. of threads engaged	Minimum 5
Depth of engagement in Enclosure wall:	
Enclosure Volume $\leq 100\,\text{cm}^3$	At least 5 mm
Enclosure Volume $>100\,\text{cm}^3$	At least 8 mm

(*from BS/EN 50018*)
Note: If this pitch is exceeded then requirements in addition to this table may be necessary (see text).

Table 10.8 Cylindrical (taper) threaded joints

Cylindrical (taper) threaded joints	
Pitch	At least 0.9 mm (see notes 1 and 2
Threads engaged	5 Nominal (see note 3)
Threads provided on each part	At least 6

(*from BS/EN 50018*)

Notes:
1 There is no maximum pitch in this case as the joint is tight fitting.
2 The cone angle on the taper shall be the same for both parts of the threaded joint.
3 It is accepted that at the limit of tolerance less than 5 threads may be engaged because the tightness of fit will allow the flameproof properties of the joint to be maintained even in such cases.

transmission is carried out. As a result, some specifications can be sacrificed provided that more onerous testing is carried out. The requirements for threaded joints are included in Table 10.7 for parallel threads and Table 10.8 for taper threads. In addition, the following requirements need to be complied with.

Where these threaded joints are used for lids, doors or the covers of flameproof enclosures, there is always the possibility that they could be loosened by inexperienced personnel and, to avoid this, such joints are required to be secured by fasteners of the same quality and operational requirements as bolts or screws of flanged and spigot joints. The typical way this is done with a cover is to fit a cap screw into the outer part outside the thread, so that when it is tightened it impinges on the inner part, again outside the thread, preventing loosening of the joint. The capscrew should be flush with the enclosure outside when tightened to prevent it being removed with pliers, etc.

Parallel threads

In respect of parallel threads the following limitations need to be taken into account. First, parallel threads with a pitch of less than 0.7 mm are not permitted because of their fineness which gives rise to shallowness, and the added possibility of stripping or partial stripping in use with resultant damage to their flameproof properties.

Second, where the threads pitch exceeds 2 mm the combination of coarse pitch and quality of fit may not be sufficient to achieve the necessary flameproof qualities and the apparatus could fail the tests in Table 10.7. In such cases it may be necessary to increase the number of threads engaged to more than five. No specific increase can be given as it will depend upon how much the pitch exceeds 2 mm, but as a starting point it is suggested that an additional thread be added for each 0.5 mm by which the thread pitch exceeds 2 mm. Alternatively, a test could be performed similar to that used for non-standard threads. These alternatives should be discussed with the appropriate certification body before being adopted in any given case.

Third, where threadforms and/or tolerances other than those permitted by Table 10.7 are used, the joints will be subjected to additional requirements which normally take the form of an increase in thread withdrawal for testing over that used for complying threads.

Taper threads

While taper threads should comply with the requirements of Table 10.8 it is recognized that, at their limit of tolerance, the number of threads engaged may be less than five.

Securing of threaded joints

Unlike flanged, spigot and cylindrical joints, it is not usually possible to secure this joint easily, as it needs to rotate in order to ensure it is fully made. It is, however, a screw similar to fastening devices and, provided that it needs a hexagon spanner or hexagon key for its removal, and should not have any protrusions which would make alternative opening possible, then it can be accepted as secured once it is fully screwed home. If there is doubt as to the quality of securing, then a socket-headed cap screw in the cylindrical assembly outside the joint threaded into the outside member of the joint, outside the thread forming the flamepath, will be adequate for securing purposes. This will elongate the cylinder only slightly. In the case of lids, doors and covers the additional screw is always considered necessary and it would be wise to utilize this approach in all cases to avoid problems due to differing views.

5 Cemented joints

Cemented joints are often used to insert such things as viewing ports into flameproof enclosures and it is often difficult to create a joint complying with joint requirements. In such circumstances, a joint may be made using cement and may be significantly shorter than its normal counterpart, needing only to comply with the length requirements of Table 10.9. Where the joint would comply with the requirements for flanged, spigot, cylindrical or threaded joints in the absence of the cement, including the securing needs of such joints, then no special requirements apply other than the leakage test to ensure the completeness of the cement seal, as neither the strength of the joint or its flameproof performance rely on the cement. (It is necessary to ensure that the cement seal allows no jets to cause abnormal flameproof performance and a sealing test is included in BS/EN 50018 (1995). In addition, the strength of the joint must not rely on the cement, and removal and replacement of the joint must be possible without damage to the cement. This can be achieved by making the cemented joint as a cartridge and its insertion into a further joint of more normal design the method of replacement. Where the joint forms part of the enclosure, however, and removal is not intended, then no additional action is necessary.

Table 10.9 Minimum lengths of cemented joints not complying with joint requirements in the absence of cement

Length of cemented joints Enclosure volume cm^3	Joint length mm
Less than 10	At least 3
Over 10 and up to 100	At least 6
Over 100	At least 10

(from BS/EN 50018)

Where the joint does not conform to the requirements of other joint types in the absence of the cement, but only to the length requirements of Table 10.9, an arrangement must be in place to ensure that the joint strength does not rely on the cement. Additionally, in these circumstances, the cement must not be damaged by the thermal resistance to heat and cold tests specified in BS/EN 50014 (1994)[12] (see also, Chapter 7).

10.2.2 Joints for rotary or longitudinal shafts and operating rods

Operating rods which pass through the walls of flameproof enclosures move in a longitudinal or rotary direction. In either case, cylindrical joints are appropriate as the use of flanged or spigot joints is not easily applicable. Although one could identify a situation where the use of a simple spigot joint (one where the flamepath is totally in the cylindrical part of the joint) may be possible, the securing of the joint would produce real problems. Where movement is only in the rotary direction it could be argued that a further specialist type of joint is also suitable. This is the labyrinth joint shown in Fig. 10.12. This joint is like a cylindrical joint except that the flamepath is via a set of interleaved cylindrical parts. If this specialist joint is used it would be wise to ensure that any certification body involved would accept it, as the way in which the Standard is written could be taken as excluding it depending upon how it is interpreted.

Where a cylindrical joint is used in this configuration, it must satisfy special requirements as one part of it moves and some wear must be assumed. While it needs to have a minimum joint length and maximum gap complying with Table 10.6, the length of the joint must also relate to the size of the operating rod which forms the moving part of the joint, and the joint length is, to a degree, determined by the circumference of the rod. It must, in addition to complying with Table 10.6, have a length at least equal to the diameter of the operating rod, up to a rod diameter of 25 mm.

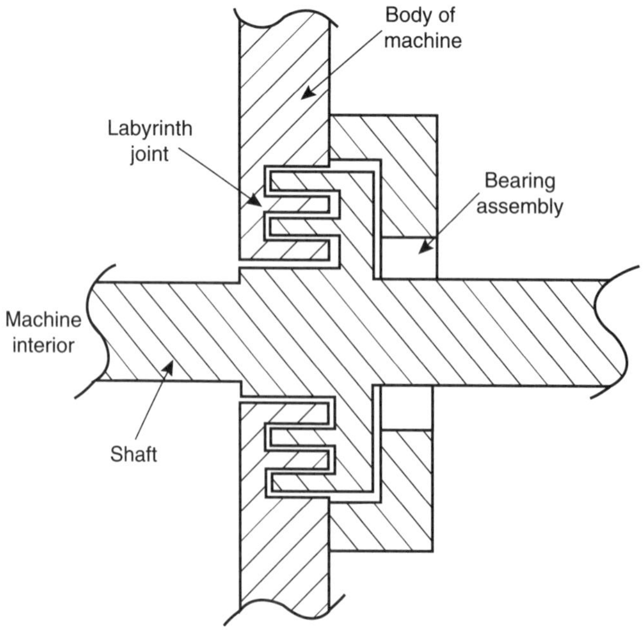

Fig. 10.12 Geometry of a labyrinth joint

Also, where the rod does not have a supporting bearing, other than the fixed part of the joint and significant wear of the joint in normal operation is expected, the fixed part of the joint should form a replaceable bushing so that the joint can be renewed with ease when necessary.

If the labyrinth-type joint (see Fig. 10.12) is considered to be appropriate a relaxation is permitted and these limits need not be complied with in the case of this joint, provided that it can be shown to be flameproof using the tests in BS/EN 50018, although it would be wise to ensure a joint minimum length and maximum gap in accordance with Table 10.6 with further allowance made for shaft diameter. This relaxation is possible because of the geometry of the joint, which is more likely to prevent flame transmission than its cylindrical counterpart.

To avoid joint wear in both types of joint, the rod may be fitted with a bearing which does not form part of the joint but keeps the rod away from the joint surface, effectively preventing wear. Two types of bearing are acceptable in principle, the sleeve bearing, where the outer part of the bearing is static, and the rolling element bearing, which introduces rolling elements between the rod and the enclosure. In both cases the minimum radial clearance between the moving part of the joint and the fixed part of the joint should not be less than 0.05 mm taking account of tolerances. In the case of the cylindrical joint the maximum radial clearance must not exceed that specified in Table 10.10 for sleeve bearings, and Table 10.11 for rolling element bearings for the length of joint in question but, as there is a relaxation in the case of the labyrinth joint, in cases where this type of joint is acceptable, no maximum limit of radial clearance is specified. The only requirement is the passing of the flame transmission tests. The use of a sleeve bearing for any joint associated with a rotating electrical machine is limited to sub-group IIA and IIB only.

Table 10.10 Maximum permissible gaps for cylindrical joints of operating rods and shafts of rotating machines with sleeve bearings

Joint width (L) (mm)	Permissible maximum gaps for given enclosure volumes											
	Volume ≤ 100 cm³			Volume 500 cm³			Volume ≤ 2000 cm³			Volume >2000 cm³		
	IIA	IIB	IIC	IIA	IIB	IIC	IIA	IIB	IIC	IIA	IIB	IIC
≥6.0	0.30	0.20	0.10	N/P	N/P	N/P	N/P	N/P	N/P	N/P	N/P	N/P
≥9.5	0.30	0.20	0.10	0.3	0.20	0.10	N/P	N/P	N/P	N/P	N/P	N/P
≥12.5	0.35	0.25	0.15	0.3	0.20	0.15	0.3	0.20	0.15	0.2	N/P	N/P
≥25.0	0.40	0.30	0.15	0.4	0.25	0.15	0.4	0.25	0.15	0.4	0.20	0.15
≥40.0	0.50	0.40	0.20	0.5	0.30	0.20	0.5	0.30	0.20	0.5	0.25	0.20

(BS/EN 50018)
N/P = Joints of this width and/or this sub-group are not permitted when sleeve bearings are used.
Note: Sleeve bearings are not permitted for subgroup IIC rotating electrical machines.

Table 10.11 Maximum permissible gaps for operating rods using rolling element bearings

Joint width (L) (mm)	Permissible maximum gaps for given enclosure volumes											
	Volume $\leq$100 cm^3			Volume $\leq$500 cm^3			Volume $\leq$2000 cm^3			Volume >2000 cm^3		
	IIA	IIB	IIC	IIA	IIB	IIC	IIA	IIB	IIC	IIA	IIB	IIC
$\geq$6.0	0.45	0.30	0.15	N/P	N/P	N/P	N/P	N/P	N/P	N/P	N/P	N/P
$\geq$9.5	0.45	0.35	0.15	0.40	0.25	0.15	N/P	N/P	N/P	N/P	N/P	N/P
$\geq$12.5	0.50	0.40	0.25	0.45	0.30	0.25	0.45	0.30	0.25	0.30	0.20	N/P
$\geq$25.0	0.60	0.45	0.25	0.60	0.40	0.25	0.60	0.40	0.25	0.60	0.30	0.25
$\geq$40.0	0.75	0.60	0.30	0.75	0.45	0.30	0.75	0.45	0.30	0.75	0.45	0.30

(*from BS/EN 50018*)
N/P = Not permitted for joints of this width and/or this sub-group.
Note: This table is not valid for shafts and rotating machines. For values of gaps for shafts and rotating machines see Table 10.12.

It is possible to use a combination of a cylindrical joint (or labyrinth joint where such a joint is acceptable) and a flanged joint to make a floating joint so that some latitude of lateral movement is permitted (see Fig. 10.13). In such cases, the length of the flange should be at least that required by Table 10.1 plus an amount equal to the maximum lateral movement expected in operation. Such joints should also be secured against rotation and are limited to enclosures intended for use in sub-group IIA and IIB.

10.2.3 Joints for shafts and rotating machines

A rotating shaft is a special case. Due to the rotation it is often unwise to have the flameproof joint forming the shaft support and a bearing is used. This approach is always necessary for rotating electrical machines.

With sleeve bearings, the same restrictions apply in the case of cylindrical joints and the joint dimensions must satisfy the requirements of Table 10.10. The joint length must be at least equal to the shaft diameter if that is below 25 mm. It is not, however, necessary to make the joint longer than 25 mm. The minimum radial clearance in the joint must be at least 0.05 mm (see '*k*' in Fig. 10.14) and the joints are usable only in enclosures intended for sub-group IIA and IIB. In the case of labyrinth joints (see Fig. 10.12) the same minimum radial clearance is necessary. Joint maximum gap requirements may, in this latter case, be waived as is the case for operating rods if the joint can be shown by test to be flameproof, but all other requirements are as for cylindrical joints.

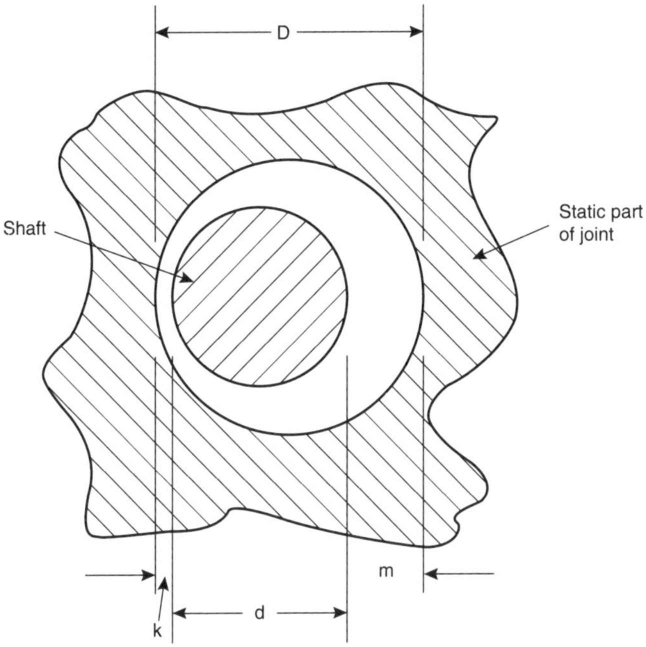

d = Shaft diameter
k = Minimum acceptable radial clearance
m = Maximum permissible gap for a cylindrical joint
D = d + m + k

Fig. 10.13 Geometry of a shaft joint

As, because of the speed of rotation, wear can be rapid it is also necessary in the case of sleeve bearings to ensure that one part of a cylindrical or labyrinth joint is non-sparking (e.g., leaded brass) to prevent sparking on bearing failure and, where the minimum radial clearance of the joint (0.05 mm) is smaller than the running stator rotor clearance of the machine, this joint part needs to be thicker than that running clearance to avoid joint sparking.

In the case of rolling element bearings, the same rules apply with the exception of the restriction to sub-group IIA and IIB, where machines with rolling element bearings are acceptable and the need to have one part of the joint non-sparking is also waived. The maximum radial joint gap is, however, reduced and must comply with Table 10.12.

In all cases the rotating shaft may be in a floating joint using both a flat flanged joint and a cylindrical joint (see Fig. 10.14). In no case is a rotating machine with such a joint permissible in sub-group IIC.

10.2.4 Bearing greasing arrangements

Where grease grooves are used in shafts to retain grease around the bearing, these should not interfere with the joint. Figure 10.15 shows an acceptable way of their use.

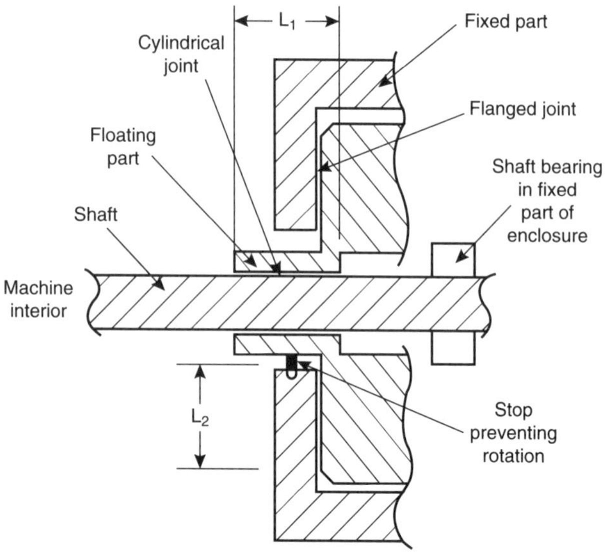

L_1 = Cylindrical joint
L_2 = Flange joint allowing cylindrical joint assembly to float

Fig. 10.14 Limiting dimensions for shaft joint of rotating machines

Table 10.12 Maximum permissible gaps for shafts and rotating electrical machines using rolling element bearings

Joint width (L) (mm)	Permissible maximum gaps for given enclosure volumes											
	Volume $\leq$100 cm^3			Volume $\leq$500 cm^3			Volume $\leq$2000 cm^3			Volume >2000 cm^3		
	IIA	IIB	IIC	IIA	IIB	IIC	IIA	IIB	IIC	IIA	IIB	IIC
$\geq$6.0	0.30	0.20	0.10	N/P	N/P	N/P	N/P	N/P	N/P	N/P	N/P	N/P
$\geq$9.5	0.30	0.23	0.10	0.27	0.17	0.10	N/P	N/P	N/P	N/P	N/P	N/P
$\geq$12.5	0.33	0.27	0.17	0.30	0.20	0.17	0.30	0.20	0.17	0.20	0.13	N/P
$\geq$25.0	0.40	0.30	0.17	0.40	0.27	0.17	0.40	0.27	0.17	0.40	0.20	0.17
$\geq$40.0	0.50	0.40	0.20	0.50	0.30	0.20	0.50	0.30	0.20	0.50	0.27	0.20

(from BS/EN 50018)
N/P = Not permitted for joints of this width and/or sub-group

10.2.5 Tests for flameproof joints

Testing of flamepaths for flame transmission is dynamic in that it involves filling the enclosure with a specified explosive atmosphere and surrounding it with the same atmosphere. The internal explosive atmosphere is then ignited and non-transmission has to be proved in a number of tests prescribed in BS/EN 50018.

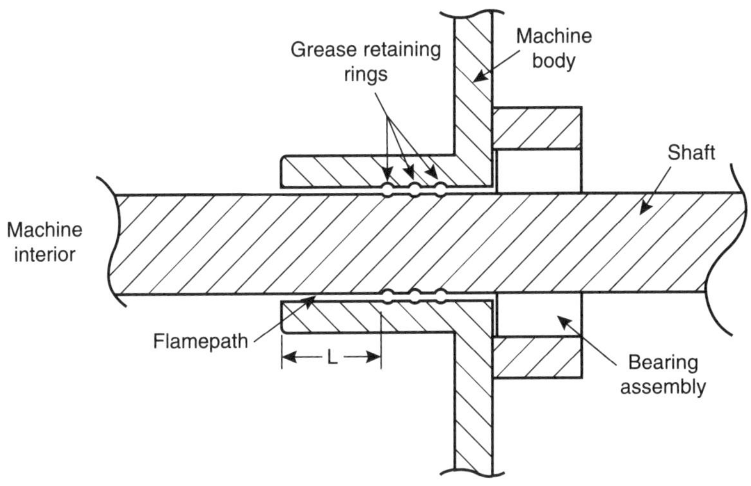

Fig. 10.15 Cylindrical joint with grease retaining rings

Table 10.13 Reduction in thread length for testing

Type of threaded joint	Reduction in engaged thread length by			
	Sub-group IIA and IIB		Sub-group IIC	
Test detail	A	B	C	D
Parallel thread to ISO 965 medium or better fit	None	1/3	1/3	None
Other parallel	1/3	1/2	1/2	1/3
Taper	None	1/3	1/3	None

(*from BS/EN 50018*)

A= Tests with enhanced mixtures
B= Tests with enhanced gaps
C= Tests with enhanced gaps
D= Tests at high Pressure

Note: Taper threaded joints are tested with minimum hand tightening using threads at extremes of tolerance. Length of engaged thread is achieved by machining off 1/3 engaged threads.

In this Standard the test is normally carried out with all flamepaths, excluding threaded and cemented joints, set at a figure which is at least 90 per cent of the maximum design figure, taking account of tolerances. Threaded flamepaths are dealt with as detailed in Table 10.13. The explosive atmosphere used to fill and surround the enclosure is then chosen to give a safety factor of <1.4 for enclosures for sub-group IIA and IIB (the actual safety factor in each case is defined in BS/EN 50018) and several tests are carried out with internal ignition points chosen to give the worst possible situation taking account of the contents of the enclosure. Alternatively, for sub-group IIA and IIB more onerous mixtures may be used with gaps which are at less than 0.9 times the maximum design gap (details again being given in the Standard), or by specified enlargement of the gap and the use of less onerous test explosive atmospheres.

The situation in respect of sub-group IIC is more complex in that the only way to increase test sensitivity would be to enrich the test explosive atmosphere with oxygen and, rather than do this, the tests are carried out with hydrogen or acetylene air mixtures with the flamepaths enlarged to greater than the maximum design gaps or with the test explosive atmosphere at greater than atmospheric pressure. The test requirements in BS/EN 50018 (the second edition of EN 50018) differ significantly from those in BS 5501, Part 5 and are considerably more onerous for sub-group IIA and IIB. It should not be assumed, therefore, that an enclosure which satisfied the requirements of the first edition will necessarily satisfy those of the second. This, again, is a good reason for recommending that equipment to BS/EN 50018 should be chosen in the future.

10.3 Construction of flameproof enclosures, entry facilities, fasteners and component parts

10.3.1 Enclosure construction

Flameproof enclosures may be constructed of metal or appropriate non-metallic material (usually plastic). Non-metallic enclosures are limited to volumes up to 3000 cm^3 if they are totally non-metallic, but where they are basically metallic with the non-metallic parts forming only parts of the enclosure this volume limit does not apply, provided that no non-metallic surface exceeds 500 cm^3. This 500 cm^2 restriction does not apply to light-transmitting parts of luminaires which exceptionally may have non-metallic parts up to 8000 cm^2 in surface area.

Where a metallic enclosure is constructed of cast iron, account needs to be taken of the fact that some grades of cast iron are very brittle, and to avoid their use the cast iron is required to comply with, at worst, quality 150 as described in ISO 185[14]. Brass and aluminium are also among the materials acceptable and construction may be by casting or fabrication with welding of similar types of securing parts of the enclosure together. Where enclosures are fabricated a routine pressure test, waived for enclosures type tested at four times the pressure developed in an internal explosion of the sub-group characteristic gas/air mixture (reference pressure), is always required to ensure the quality of fabrication as the level of confidence in repeatability of welding excellence is not as high as that for casting.

Non-metallic enclosures may be constructed by moulding or fabrication, with similar methods of securing one part of an enclosure to another but, as already stated, they have a volume limit of 3000 cm^3 unless the non-metallic parts form only part of an otherwise metallic enclosure. When this occurs an individual 500 cm^2 surface area limit is imposed on the non-metallic parts (excepting light transmitting parts of luminaires where the limit is increased to 8000 cm^2). After being tested to confirm their capabilities to withstand pressure in common with all flameproof enclosures, non-metallic enclosures having non-metallic or partially non-metallic joint surfaces are subjected to flame erosion tests. In these their flamepaths are subjected to the passage of burning gas by the carrying out of 50 tests, with plane gaps opened to their maximum values, using the explosive test mixture for explosion pressure testing, and to confirm that no significant erosion has taken place. Where the non-metallic parts are of plastics material, flammability tests are also carried out on the material.

In addition, non-metallic enclosures which have insulating properties can, unlike metal enclosures, be used to directly support conductors of differing voltages. In utilizing this advantage, however, care needs to be taken to ensure the insulation quality of the material, as unlike material chosen for insulation alone, it is chosen principally for its dimensional ability and strength. There are requirements for all apparatus in explosive atmospheres (see Chapter 8) to minimize the risk of static build up. One way of satisfying these is to load the plastic with a conducting material to limit its surface resistivity. Clearly, this will bring its insulating properties into question and it is therefore necessary to ensure that non-metallic enclosures used for such support satisfy the requirements of Table 10.14. The comparative tracking index (CTI) specified in that table is determined in accordance with BS 5901: 1980[15].

All enclosures, both metallic and non-metallic, are subjected to a hydraulic pressure test at 1.5 times the reference pressure. It is recognized that they may be subject to elastic movement during the explosion (they may temporarily enlarge due to their internal pressure) but no permanent distortion is acceptable and measurements on the enclosure after pressure testing are necessary to confirm this. Permanent distortion is not acceptable either in the enclosure parts themselves (e.g., bowed lids) or in the flamepaths. Elastic expansion of the flamepaths is, of course, taken account of during the flame transmission tests. The reference pressure is obtained by igniting a specific test mixture inside an enclosure with no gaps specially opened, and monitoring the rise and fall of pressure inside the enclosure during the explosion. Several tests are carried out and the worst case pressure taken as the reference pressure. Fig. 10.16 shows a typical pressure rise and decay curve obtained in such tests. There is a problem in cases where the interior of the enclosure is divided into separate parts (see Fig. 10.17) or a component within the enclosure has its own enclosure. An ignition within one enclosure can lead to pre-pressurization of the gas in the other as the shock fronts preceding the flame travel faster than the flame travelling at the speed of sound in the gas. The explosion pressure

Table 10.14 Creepage distance between bare live parts of flameproof apparatus supported by non-metallic enclosure

Maximum rms working voltage (U in volts)	Minimum creepage distance (mm)		
	Material Group I	Material Group II	Material Group IIIa
$0 < U \leq 15$	1.6	1.6	1.6
$15 < U \leq 30$	1.8	1.8	1.8
$30 < U \leq 60$	2.1	2.6	3.4
$60 < U \leq 110$	2.5	3.2	4.0
$110 < U \leq 175$	3.2	4.0	5.0
$175 < U \leq 275$	5.0	6.3	8.0
$275 < U \leq 420$	8.0	10.0	12.5
$420 < U \leq 550$	10.0	12.5	16.0
$550 < U \leq 750$	12.0	16.0	20.0
$750 < U \leq 1100$	20.0	25.0	32.0
$1100 < U \leq 2200$	32.0	36.0	40.0
$2200 < U \leq 3300$	40.0	45.0	50.0
$3300 < U \leq 4200$	50.0	56.0	63.0
$4200 < U \leq 500$	63.0	71.0	80.0
$5500 < U \leq 6600$	80.0	90.0	100.0
$6600 < U \leq 8300$	100.0	110.0	125.0
$8300 < U \leq 11000$	125.0	140.0	160.0

(*from BS/EN 50019*)
Material Group I = Comparative tracking index (CTI) over 600
Material Group II = Comparative tracking index at least 400 but less than 600
Material Group IIIa = Comparative tracking index at least 175 but below 400
Note: Comparative tracking index in accordance with BS 5901 (1980).

is a function of the initial pressure at the time of ignition and if this initial pressure is raised, the explosion pressure in the second part of the enclosure is significantly increased and, additionally, the pressure rise time in the second enclosure reduces. This phenomenon is called pressure piling. The evidence of such a phenomenon is the reduction of pressure rise time to less than 5 ms, or erratic maximum pressure values which can be identified by variation of more than a factor of 1.5 in the measured explosion pressures in separate tests. Enclosure and apparatus construction should, as far as possible, be arranged so as to prevent this. The use of enclosures where pressure piling does occur is not, however, precluded.

In small enclosures it is often very difficult to measure explosion pressure and to determine the pressure to be used in the pressure test. In these cases the values of pressure in Table 10.15 are used.

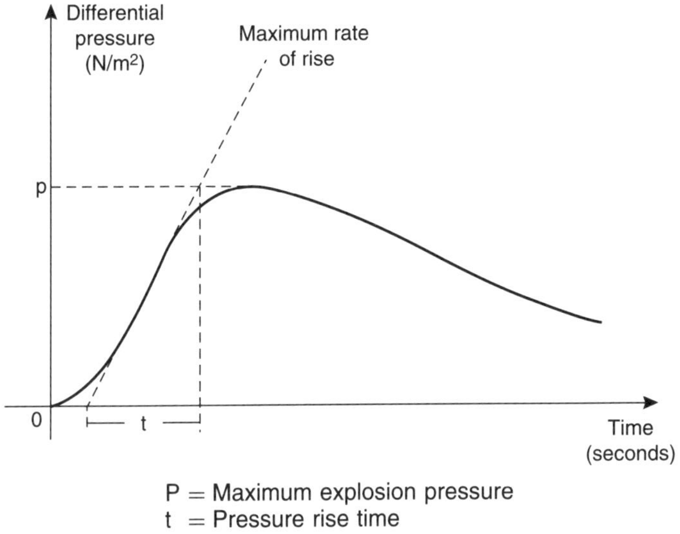

Fig. 10.16 Profile of pressure inside a flameproof enclosure resulting form an internal explosion

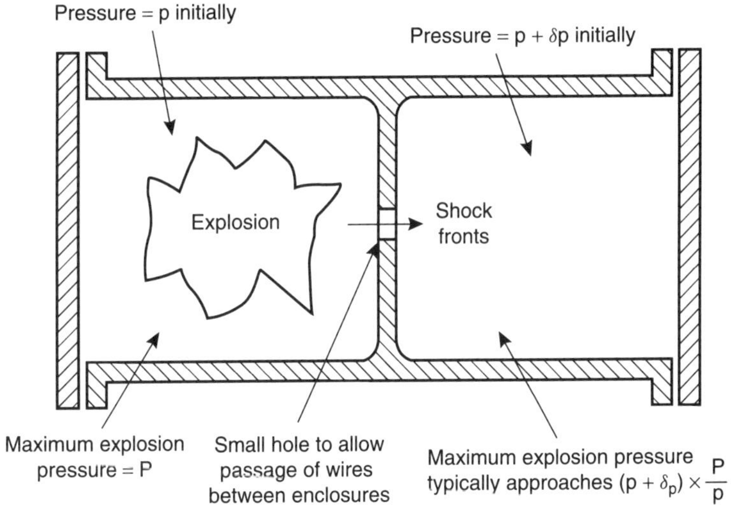

Fig. 10.17 Effects of pressure piling

A flameproof enclosure may be what is called direct entry or indirect entry (see Fig. 10.18 and 10.19). A direct entry enclosure has the connection facilities (e.g., terminals) for external connection in the same enclosure, as the enclosed apparatus and an indirect entry enclosure has a separate terminal box. This may be connected to the main enclosure by, for example, bushings and has the advantage that entry to the connection facilities does not access the main enclosure and, as the main enclosure may contain

Table 10.15 Test pressure for small enclosures where reference pressure cannot be measured

Enclosure volume (cm^3)	Test pressure (N/m^2)		
	Sub-group IIA	Sub-group IIB	Sub-group IIC
≤ 10	1×10^6	1×10^6	1×10^6
>10	1.5×10^6	1.5×10^6	2×10^6

(*from BS/EN 50018*)

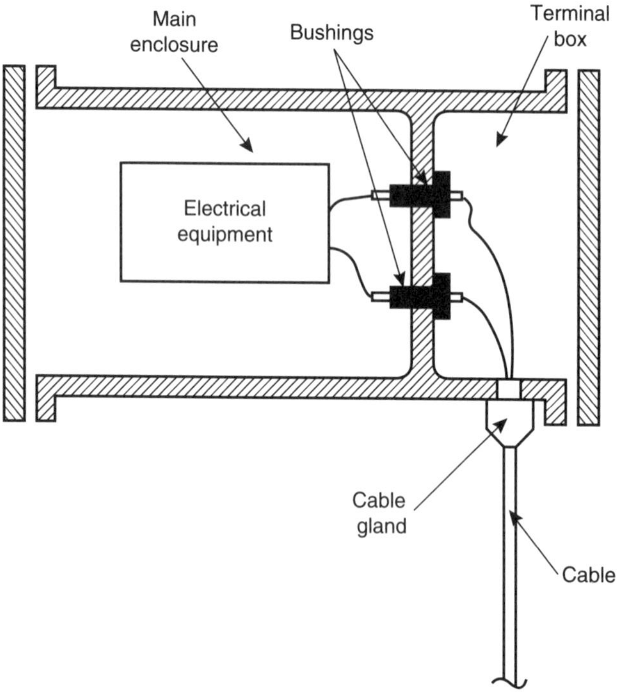

Fig. 10.18 Indirect entry flameproof enclosure. *Note*: The main enclosure and terminal box are entirely separate enclosures

normally sparking parts, it was felt to be an advantage. In BS 229 enclosures were not permitted to be direct entry and direct entry only became common with the advent of BS 4683, Part 2. As will be seen when installation is discussed, there are differences in permissible installation practices for the two types of enclosure.

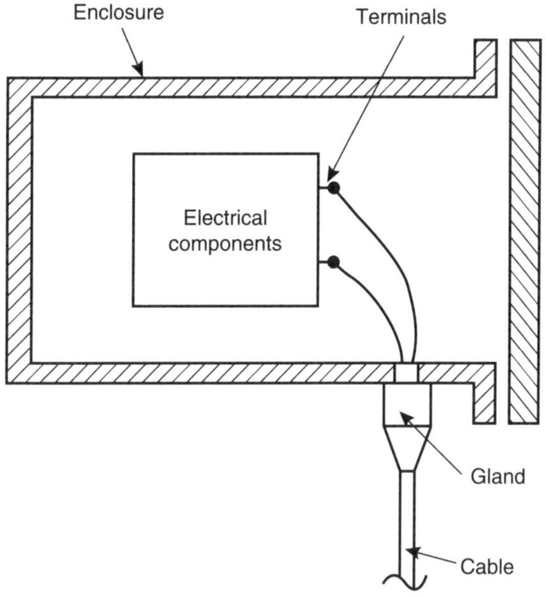

Fig. 10.19 Direct entry flameproof enclosure

10.3.2 Bushings

A bushing is a method of carrying a conductor through the wall of an enclosure or between two enclosures with a common wall. It is normally of insulating material containing one or more conductors. The conductors passing through the bushing are normally not insulated and adhesion of the bushing insulating material to the conductors gives the required seal against flame transmission. The normal construction used is either conductors cemented together and into a metal ring which forms a flamepath with the enclosure wall, or plastic moulded onto the conductors in which case the plastic itself forms the flamepath with the enclosure wall. The bushings are normally subjected to flame erosion tests and their material, if plastic, is subjected to flammability testing.

All bushings not unique to one flameproof enclosure are also subjected to pressure testing at $30 \times 10^6\,\mathrm{N/m^2}$ to ensure that no leaks occur along the conductors.

10.3.3 Arrangements for entry facilities

The usual method by which cables enter flameproof enclosures is via a cable gland or conduit. The most common method in the UK is a cable gland but the situation is quite the reverse in the USA – a fact which is quite important as flameproof enclosures in the USA are tested with a length of conduit attached, whereas in the UK this is not done. Therefore, the requirements for fitting stopper boxes (described later) are different in the UK to those used in the USA.

Glands enter the enclosure through its wall and the entry is normally a threaded hole which must satisfy the requirements for a threaded joint with the cable gland or conduit in place. This places significant requirements on the production of such holes and for this reason they are normally machined into the enclosure at the time of manufacture. This causes problems as entries may be required in different places for different applications. To overcome this the manufacturer machines in several holes, some of which are unlikely to be used in particular installations. To overcome this problem a series of closing devices have been develop for unused threaded openings. These devices must be secure and form, with the opening, a threaded flamepath. The acceptable methods of mounting are as follows: first, the closing device must be removable only from the inside of the enclosure. It must be fitted from the inside or secured from the inside after fitting (see Fig. 10.20); second, the closing device may be fitted from the outside but shall only have a narrow shoulder to minimize the possibility of its removal with a wrench, and its installation or removal must be with a hexagon head or socket of the same specification as those used for bolts and screws holding enclosures together (see Fig. 10.21); or third, the closing device must be fitted with a shearing head so that it is permanently installed when the head has been sheared off (see Fig. 10.22).

10.3.4 Fasteners

The fasteners used for flameproof enclosures are almost invariably screws, bolts, or nuts and bolts. These devices have to hold the enclosure together during an explosion but are not usually an integral part of it. These bolts or screws need to comply with the following : first, their threadform, tolerances and heads should comply with those for special fasteners to BS/EN 50014 which are discussed in Chapter 8; second, any screws bolts or nuts used

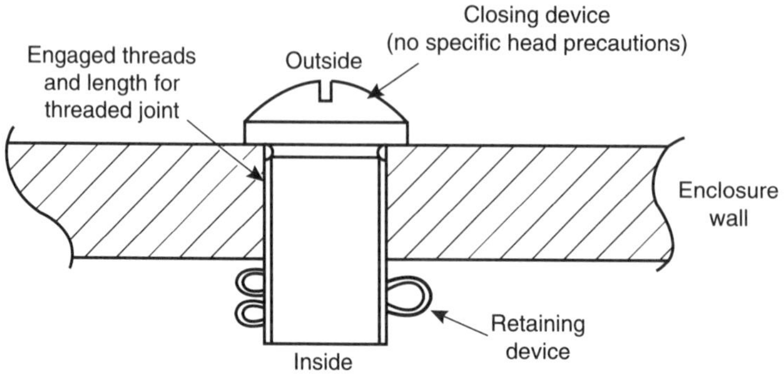

Fig. 10.20 Internally secured closing device

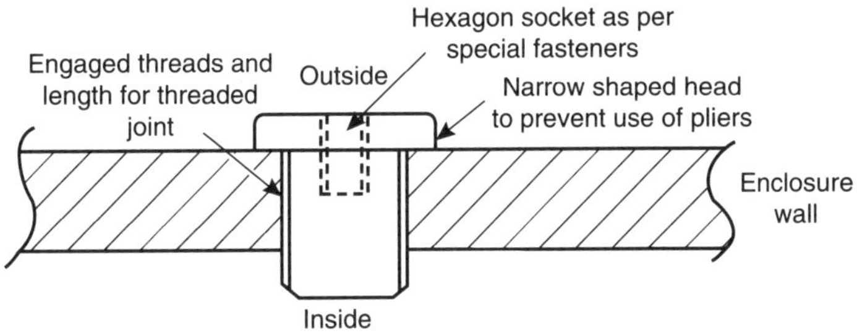

Fig. 10.21 Closing device with hexagon key type control

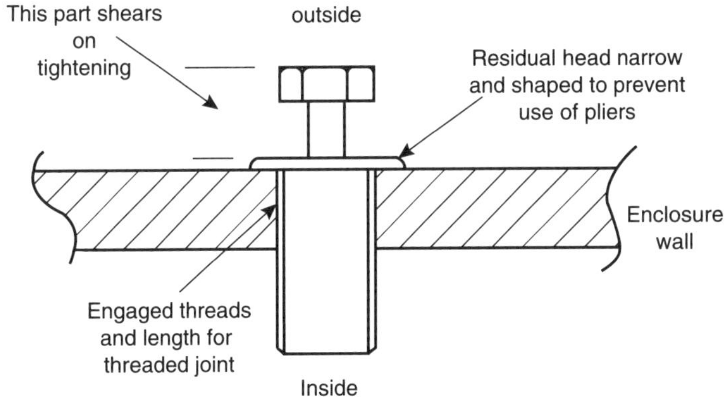

Fig. 10.22 Closing device with shearing head

as fasteners should have a lower limit yield stress of at last 240 N/mm^2 in accordance with ISO 6892 and, unless there is a real necessity to use fixings of a higher yield stress, it is recommended that these are always used. The use of any higher yield stress fixings is considered as special and will require the 'X' mark described in Chapter 8; and third, if any stud screw or bolt passes through the wall of the enclosure it must form a flameproof joint, as described in Section 10.2.1, and be non-detachable, being held to the enclosure by welding or a method which is equally effective (e.g., rivetting).

10.3.5 Component parts

In general there are no specific requirements for components within flameproof enclosures except those associated with such things as arcing parts.

Arcing or sparking parts

It is known that arcing parts placed near and in the plane of flange gaps can seriously affect the flameproof nature of an enclosure and, when this occurs, the information in this chapter may not be sufficient to ensure that an enclosure is flameproof. It is difficult to see how such parts could be placed in similar proximity to spigot and cylindrical parts, but in exceptional circumstances where such possible siting is identified the same problems arise.

Obstacles near flamepaths

Obstacles placed near flamepaths of flameproof enclosures are likewise known to affect the flamefront and allow transmission of flame where none would occur in their absence. This is important when constructing a flameproof enclosure where parts of the enclosure may have other items mounted on them (e.g., a flameproof telephone). Much work has been done on this problem, mainly to overcome installation problems, but the solutions identified are just as applicable for constructors. To avoid the possibility of an enclosure with outside fixtures, which otherwise satisfies the requirements for flameproof enclosures, failing flame transmission tests no obstructions should be placed in the exit area of a flamepath within 1 cm of the flamepath edge for sub-group IIA, within 3 cm of the flamepath edge for sub-group IIB, or within 4 cm of the flamepath edge for sub-group IIC.

Liquids

Flameproof enclosures may contain apparatus which either requires a liquid to operate (e.g., electrohydraulic devices) or operates on a liquid (e.g., a chromatograph). These situations are not prohibited but care needs to be taken to ensure that any liquid entering cannot decompose due to any situation occurring within the enclosure, even in abnormal conditions, and create a vapour belonging to a more onerous sub-group than that for which the enclosure is designed. In these circumstances the enclosure must be designed for the more onerous sub-group as the vapour produced may exit the enclosure at the flanges and form the external explosive atmosphere in addition to being present within the enclosure.

Any liquid or gas within the enclosure which may be pressurized must not pressurize the enclosure if released therein, or an effect similar to pressure piling may occur. If liquid or gas under pressure is permitted within an enclosure there must be a method of breathing or draining to ensure that the enclosure is not pressurized in the worst case of internal release. The method of breathing or draining needs to maintain the flameproof nature of the enclosure and is subject to specific construction requirements.

Breathing and draining devices

Breathing and draining devices are for draining liquids and gases from an enclosure without any significant pressure increase. They may not be used where a liquid core gas released within an enclosure increases the internal pressure by more than $1 \times 10^4\,\mathrm{N/m^2}$ and they may not be used to reduce internal pressure caused by an explosion, even though they themselves may withstand such an explosion. Therefore, an enclosure where the internal pressure is increased by liquid or gas release within it must withstand the internal pressure produced in the absence (blockage) of the device, and must not transmit the explosion to the outside atmosphere. This will require special construction requirements not included in those for flameproof enclosures. The internal pressure generated by an internal explosion must also be considered as that occurring with the device blocked.

Breathing and draining devices, due to their construction (which will be described later), are often manufactured in copper or brass. While this is generally acceptable it must be borne in mind that copper in the presence of acetylene may form copper acetylides, which are in effect solid explosives. For this reason devices containing copper or of alloys containing more than 60 per cent copper are not permitted in breathing or draining devices for enclosures for applications where acetylene may be present. This is necessary because, although users will identify enclosures containing copper as unsuitable and not use them, it may not be clear to that a copper-containing breathing or draining device is present in an otherwise copper-free enclosure.

There are two types of breathing or draining device, namely those with measurable flamepaths through their interstices, and those where these paths cannot be measured.

The requirements for breathing and draining devices, whose dimensions are all measurable and controllable to ensure that each measurement is repeatable within a specific tolerance or against a specific maximum value, are fairly straightforward. The measured gaps and interstices need not comply with the gap dimensions specified earlier in this chapter for flange, spigot and cylindrical gaps, provided the device does not transmit an internal explosion to the outside atmosphere when tested in the same manner as these gaps and, in addition, the device withstands an internal explosion within enclosure without damage when a pressure test is applied to the enclosure with the device blocked.

As with all divisions there are exceptions and in this case the crimped-ribbon breathing and draining device is one. These devices may have gaps within them which can be specified as to their maximum and minimum sizes and in this case they are breathing and draining devices with measurable gaps. In such cases they are tested for their ability to transmit an internal explosion to the outside atmosphere with the maximum gaps permitted. Their material of construction is, however, restricted in that no material used may contain magnesium, aluminium or titanium because these materials are active in that they can burn and, therefore, adversely affect the performance of the device in an unquantifiable manner. A preference for cupronickel or stainless steel is expressed but this is not mandatory, provided that the metal used is not subject to any reaction with the gases involved as this would adversely affect the performance of the device insofar as its flameproofness is concerned.

There are several types of breathing and draining device whose gaps and interstices cannot be measured and an alternative strategy is necessary to define these with regard to their ability to transmit an internal explosion to the outside atmosphere. The approach used is to define the overall dimensions of the devices. Their density in accordance with BS 5600 Part 3[16] is then determined, followed by their bubble pore size in accordance with the same British Standard. Although this Standard is concerned with sintered metal elements, the determination methods can be readily applied to other types of breathing and draining device. Determination and specification of these two parameters will adequately define the performance of the devices for the purposes of confidence in their flameproof properties, provided that they satisfy the flameproof requirements on explosion transmission type tests.

BS/EN 50018 places requirements on the methods used for determination of porosity or fluid permeability which determine the effectiveness of the device as a breathing or draining device, requiring them to be determined in accordance with BS 5600, Part 3. The reason for this is that the performance of the device as a breathing or draining device is pertinent to the pressure which can be developed within the enclosure prior to the initiation of an internal explosion. If the device does not perform effectively then the entry of fluids into the enclosure is not acceptable as it could lead to pre-pressurization.

Elements with non-measurable gaps are subject to four basic constructional requirements. First, crimped-ribbon elements shall, as for those with measurable elements, of metal and magnesium, aluminium, titanium, or alloys containing these materials are not acceptable. A preference for cupronickel or stainless steel is expressed but use of these metals is not mandatory, provided the metal or alloy chosen does not react with the fluids present in a way which would adversely affect the flameproof properties of the device. In particular, where acetylene is involved the upper limit of 60 per cent copper in any alloy used must be observed to avoid copper acetylides, which tend to behave as solid explosives.

Second, pressed wire elements are required to be metal and to satisfy the same requirements as crimped-ribbon elements, as far as their materials of construction are concerned. Their initial construction must also begin by the compression of the wire or wire braid into a die to form a homogeneous matrix which can then be treated as a solid material as far as further machining is concerned.

Third, sintered metal devices may be constructed of any metal but the same restrictions as for pressed wire elements apply to these. The preferred metals in this case are stainless steel or, where acetylene is not present, 90/10 copper – tin bronze.

Fourth, the construction of metal-foam elements is much more specific because of the method of production of as metal foam. The elements need to be produced by coating a reticulated polyurethane foam with nickel and then removing the polyurethane by thermal decomposition. The nickel must then be converted into nickel/chrome alloy by a process such as gaseous diffusion and subsequent compression of the metal foam produced. After compression the devices should contain at least 15 per cent chromium by weight.

Cable glands

Not current practice

Cable glands used in flameproof enclosure may be of two types; a normal compression gland with a sealing ring (see Fig. 10.23), or a gland using a sealing compound (see Fig. 10.24). The type chosen depends upon the type of cable used for a particular installation, in that a compression gland is only suitable where effective sealing of the cable interstices is possible by compression. In both cases the thread on the part of the gland which is screwed into the enclosure is required to satisfy the requirements for threaded joints and, in addition, required to be at least 8 mm long and comprise at least six full threads to ensure the five thread minimum specified for a threaded joint. If the gland has an undercut to ensure that its base is flush with the enclosure side, washer must be provided and be sufficiently non-compressible to ensure that the undercut does not enter the female thread and reduce the engaged thread length to less than five threads.

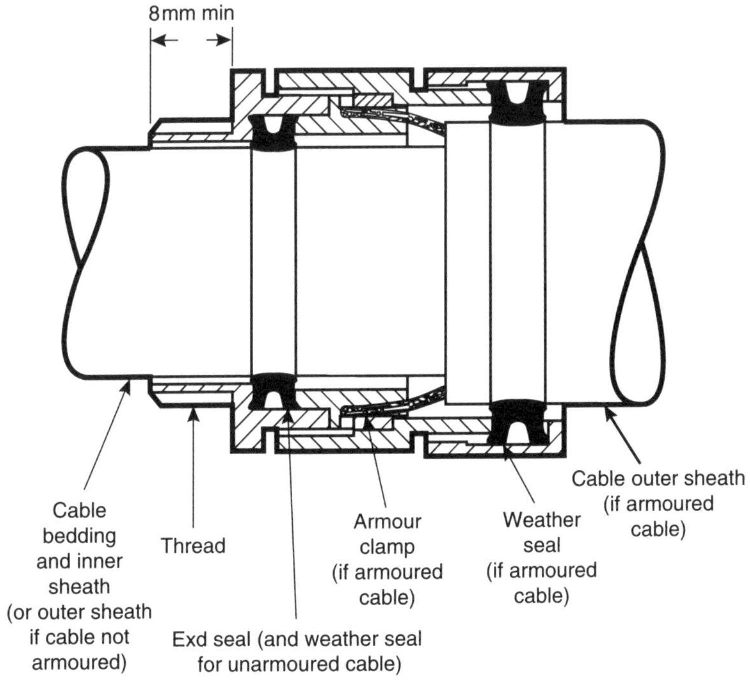

Fig. 10.23 Flameproof compression gland

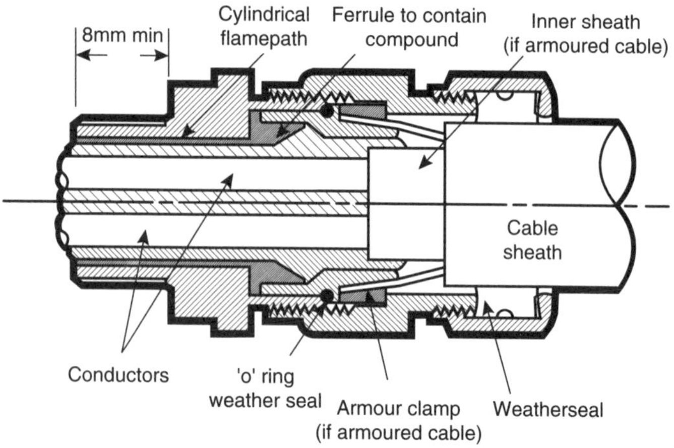

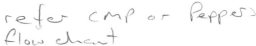

Fig. 10.24 Compound filled gland

refer CMP or Peppers flow chart

A compression gland for general use will be capable of accepting a range of sealing rings all with the same outside diameter but with differing internal diameters, matched to the size of cable for which they are designed. These sealing rings are required to have an uncompressed axial length of 20 mm for cables of less than 20 mm diameter (60 mm circumference for non-circular cables), rising to 25 mm for larger cables. If the gland is designed to accept only one sealing ring and is intended for one cable diameter only, the axial length may be reduced to 5 mm, provided the enclosure is not intended for use in sub-group IIC and does not have a volume greater than 2000 cm^3.

Cable glands with sealing rings are subjected to a hydraulic pressure test with the sealing ring sealed onto a mandrill and $30 \times 10^5\,N/m^2$ applied to one side of the seal. Liquid leakage is then identified by drips from the other side onto blotting paper.

A cable gland using a sealing compound is arranged so that only the cores, after removal of the overall sheath and bedding elements (the inner sheath in the case of armoured cables), pass through the compound. It is necessary to ensure that sufficient sealing compound is present, with the maximum number of cores of the maximum size for which the gland is intended passing through the sealing element. To do this the sealing element should be constructed to ensure that there is always at least 20 per cent of the cross section of the element filled with the sealing compound.

Cable glands using sealing compounds are subject to a similar hydraulic test of sealing which involves applying the pressure of $30 \times 10^5\,N/m^2$ to a liquid in contact with one end of the seal, and looking for drips of liquid onto blotting paper from the other end of the seal.

Stopping boxes

A stopping box is merely a device through which conductors pass (i.e., not the cable but only the conductors) which is subsequently filled with

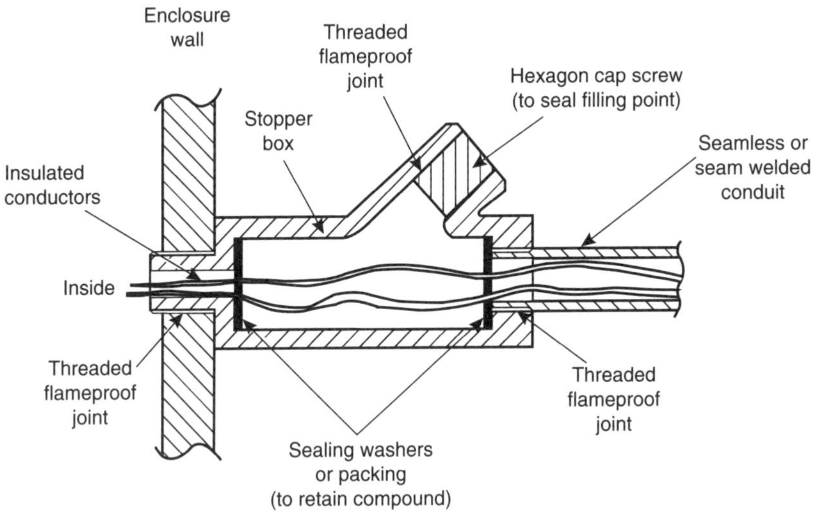

Fig. 10.25 Conduit stopping box

compound. The requirements for the box when assembled and filled with compound (and conductors) are the same as for cable glands using sealing compound. Figure 10.25 shows a typical stopping box.

10.3.6 Freestanding flameproof components

As with the other protection concepts, these are certain flameproof items which can be approved as components and used in other apparatus with a minimum of further investigation. This protection concept relies upon the enclosure almost exclusively for its operation, and the components within the enclosure are only subject to a minimum of requirements. It is possible to produce a flameproof enclosure with a specification of how it must be filled which is sufficiently flexible to permit a range of components therein with a minimum of further examination. This is dependent upon the enclosure itself having been subjected to the constructional and test requirements of the protection concept when empty. In addition certain elements, such as lampholders, are used in other types of protection but cannot satisfy the requirements of that particular type of protection. The flameproof protection concept can be used as a sub-protection in these cases.

Empty flameproof enclosures

A flameproof enclosure which has been examined and tested after construction with all entry holes, etc., in place is likely to remain flameproof after fitting of internal components, provided the following simple rules are applied:

1. No equipment installed in the enclosure should have its own enclosure. This will limit the possibility of pressure piling.
2. The installation of components in the enclosure must be such that any cross section of the equipment will demonstrate at least 20 per cent free space, made up of component-free spaces of 12.5 mm minimum dimension in any direction.
3. Rotating machinery and other items which rotate and cause significant turbulence inside the enclosure are prohibited as the turbulence created could affect the flameproof properties of the enclosure. This is not a total prohibition – positioning devices and small clock motors are not likely to cause significant turbulence and may be acceptable.
4. Where energy-storing devices, such as capacitors, are present in the enclosure they should not be readily accessible on taking the lid off the enclosure to avoid the creation of arcs and sparks by intervention inside the enclosure.
5. Rewirable fuses (non-cartridge fuses) should not be placed inside the enclosure because of the possibility of production of incandescent particles on their operation, which may be ejected from the enclosures via the flamepaths.
6. Oil-filled contactors should not be placed inside the enclosures because of the dangers associated with the operation of such contactors in case of an electrical fault, which may cause the release of hot or burning oil via the flamepaths. In addition, there may be the production of gas due to decomposition of the oil.

The above limitations presuppose that the enclosure is ultimately temperature classified on the basis of the power dissipated within it by the components installed. In all other respects (i.e., the closing of unused apertures and cable entries) the enclosure must be treated in the same way as any other flameproof enclosure.

Lampholders

It is recognized that lamp removal is a regular occurrence and that lamps can work loose in service. It is also clear that although a device to prevent lamps working loose and causing sparking can be provided, this device causes problems with the ease of lamp replacement and is, therefore, not acceptable in many circumstances. There is a need for a flameproof situation in the lamp connection mechanisms, so that any sparking which occurs when the lamp is either deliberately or accidentally disconnected is contained in what is effectively a flameproof enclosure.

With normal lamps the screwed lampcap will be E10, E14, E27 and E40. For the smaller sizes (E10 and E14) it has been shown that all that is

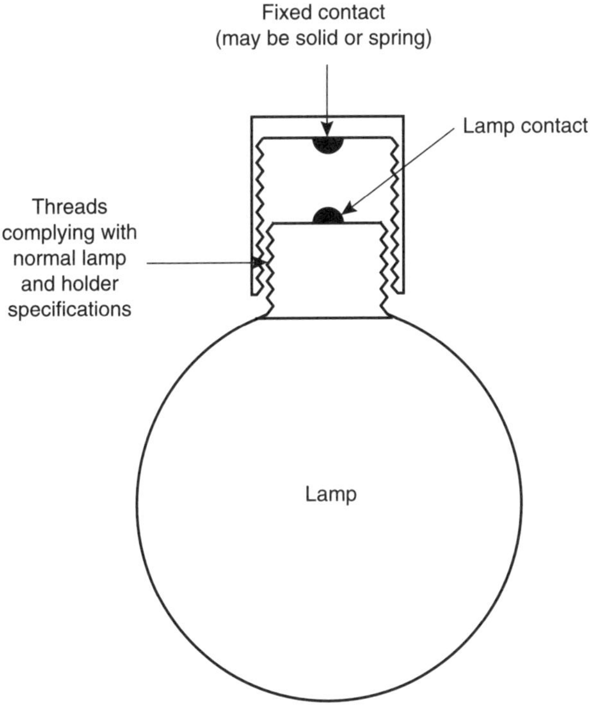

Fig. 10.26 Screw Lamps and lampcaps for E10 and E14 screw lamps. *Note*: Minimum two complete turns of thread engaged at time of separation of fixed and lamp contacts

necessary is for at least two complete threads of the lamp to be engaged at the moment of contact separation (see Fig. 10.26). For the larger threads (E27 and E40) it has been shown that the same requirement is acceptable for sub-group IIA but not for sub-group IIB or IIC. With these larger thread sizes it is also necessary to ensure that the contact is made by spring-loaded contact elements to lessen the risk of disconnection. For sub-group IIB and IIC, in addition to the above, the lamp and holder-engaged thread must also form a flameproof enclosure, with all of the requirements for flame transmission and strength which are applied to threaded joints (see Fig. 10.27).

For fluorescent tubes, the cold cathode TLX-type tube, with one pin at each end, is normally used (see Fig. 10.28). These are specified together with the requirements for holders in BS 5101[16] and compliance will satisfy the flameproof requirements for such lamp assemblies.

For other lamp/lampcap situations, the lamp and lampcap must form a cylindrical flameproof joint satisfying all of the requirements for such joints at the point of contact separation but, additionally, because of the nature of the joint, a minimum length of joint at the time of separation of 10 mm is required (see Fig. 10.28 and 10.29).

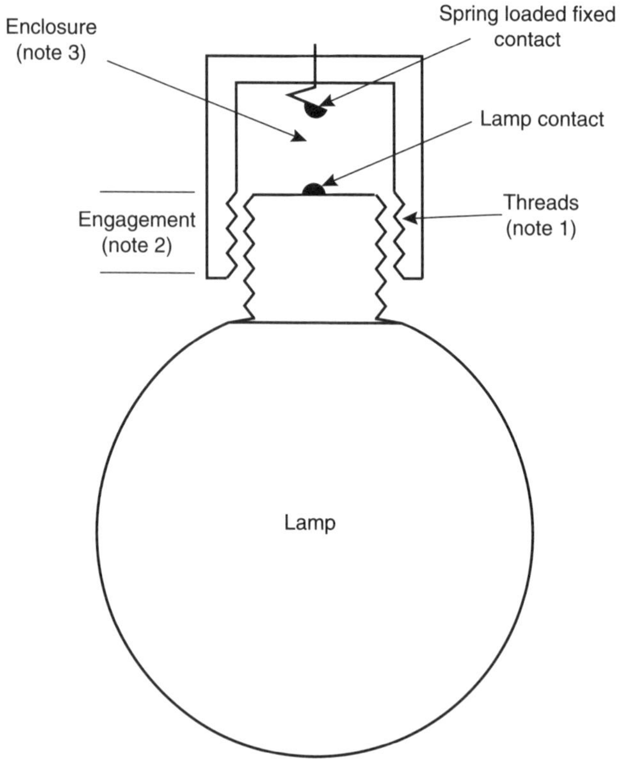

Fig. 10.27 Screw lamps and lampcaps E27 and E40. *Notes*: (1) Threads comply with normal lamp/lampholder requirements for group IIA but with threaded flameproof joint requirements for Group IIB and IIC. (2) At time of electrical separation 2 threads engaged for group IIA but must be a flameproof threaded joint for group IIB and IIC. (3) Must be a flameproof enclosure for groups IIB and IIC

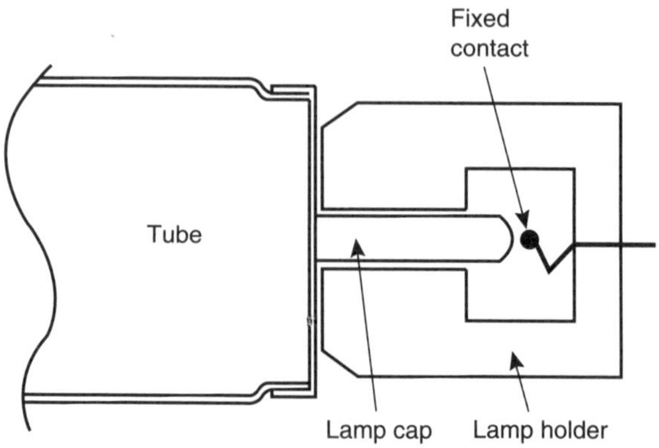

Fig. 10.28 Flameproof joint of single pin (TLX) fluorescent. *Note*: Lampcap and holder comply with data sheet Fab of IEC 61 to ensure no flame transmission

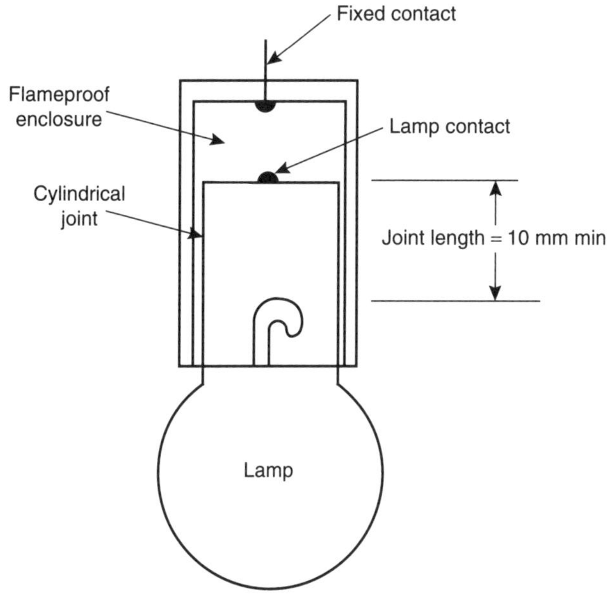

Fig. 10.29 Cylindrical (bayonet type) lamps. *Note*: The point must comply with the cylindrical joint requirements but must also have a length of at least 10 mm when the contacts separate

References

1 Phillips, H. (1971) (SMRE) Institution of Electrical Engineers conference, 'Electrical Safety in Hazardous Environments'. The Basic Theory of the Flameproof Enclosure.

2 BS 229 (1959) Flameproof Enclosure of Electrical Apparatus. (First published in 1926 and revised in 1929, 1940, 1946, 1957 and 1959).

3 BS 4683 Electrical Apparatus for Explosive Atmospheres. Part 2 (1971). The Construction and Testing of Flameproof Enclosures of Electrical Apparatus.

4 CENELEC Centre Européen de Normalization Electrique.

5 BS 5501 Electrical Apparatus for Potentially Explosive Atmospheres. Part 5 (1977). Flameproof Enclosure 'd'.

6 BS/EN 50018 (1995) Electrical Apparatus for Potentially Explosive Atmospheres. Flameproof Enclosure 'd'.

7 IEC 79-1A (1975) Electrical Apparatus for Explosive Atmospheres. Part 1. Construction and Test of

	Flameproof Enclosures of Electrical Apparatus. Appendix D, Method of Test for Ascertainment of Maximum Experimental Safe Gap.
8 IEC	International Electrotechnical Commission.
9 BS/EN 50019 (1994)	Electrical Apparatus for Potentially Explosive Atmospheres. Increased Safety 'e'.
10 ISO 468 (1982)	Surface Roughness, Parameters, Their Values and General Rules for Specifying Requirements.
11 BS 4500 (1990)	ISO Limits and Fits. Part 1. General Tolerances and Deviations. Section 1.2, Tables of Commonly Used Tolerances and Grades and Limits Deviations for Holes and Shafts.
12 BS/EN 50014 (1992)	Electrical Apparatus for Potentially Explosive Atmospheres. General Requirements.
13 ISO 6892 (1984)	Metallic Materials, Tensile Testing.
14 ISO 185 (1988)	Grey Cast Iron, Classification.
15 BS 5901:1980	Method of Test for Determining the Comparative and the Proof Tracking Indices for Solid Insulating Materials Under Moist Conditions.
16 BS 5600: (1979) (1988)	Powder Metallurgical Material and Products. Part 3. Methods of Testing Sintered Materials and Products, Excluding Hard Metals. Section 3.2, Determination of Density, Oil Content and Open Porosity. Section 3.5, Determination of Bubble Test Pore Size for Permeable Sintered Metal Materials. Section 3.6, Determination of Fluid Permeability.
17 BS 5101 (1975)	Specification for Lamp Caps and Holders Together with Gauges for the Control of Interchangeability and Safety. Part 1. Lamp Caps. Part 2. Lamp holders.

— 11 —

Apparatus with protection concept pressurization 'p' (BS/EN 50016 (1995))

Protection concept (type of protection) pressurization 'p' has been used for many years, although it has historically been considered as a code of practice (user) matter in the UK. Before the advent of a protection concept Standard, the technique has been considered as a method to be used on a fairly ad-hoc basis, when no other protection concept could effectively be used. This was not surprising as the protection concept relied heavily upon items outside the apparatus, such as ducting for the pressurization medium, the pressurization medium itself, and the electrical control devices which control the concept. Although the technique was referred to in BS/CP 1003, Part 2,[1] no National Standard was ever written for it and, it was considered that the matter was one not for certification as an apparatus protection concept but for installers and users as a practical installation matter.

The attitude in the UK (and elsewhere) began to change as the North Sea oil industry developed because much of the drilling equipment used could only be protected by pressurization, and the technique had been developed to a great degree in the USA as evidenced by its inclusion in the National Electrical Code.[2] Coincident with this, entrepreneurial activity in the UK led to a situation where the control equipment for pressurization became available 'off the shelf', rather than having to be developed individually for each use (which had largely been the case historically). These changes, together with similar changes in attitude in the other countries of Europe led to the first Standard being produced for apparatus with protection type 'p' and subsequently the protection concept became one of the Standard protection concepts, rather than an installation matter only.

11.1 Standards for pressurization 'p'

Such was the interest in the pressurization concept that when the first European Union Explosive Atmospheres Directive, 76/117/EEC[3] was published it referred to a CENELEC Standard, EN 50016 (1977)[4] which was published in the UK as BS 5501, Part 3: (1977)[5] in respect of pressurization, giving the protection concept legal status, rather than a 'user' approach.

BS 5501, Part 3[5] contained requirements only for apparatus which did not contain, or have brought to it, any flammable material. This effectively excluded its use with any analytical equipment and analyzer houses, which are normally prefabricated rooms containing analytical equipment into which personnel have access. It also excluded pressurized rooms which were also very important to industry as pressurization is the protection concept applied to such rooms in many circumstances.

This situation remained until the second edition of the European Standard was published in the UK as BS/EN 50016 (1996)[6] which introduced two new concepts. First, and most important, it introduced the concept of pressurized electrical equipment into which flammable materials were brought, and extended the technique to analytical equipment which continues to become more and more common as products become more sophisticated. Second it formalized static pressurization, which before its publication had not been considered by some to be included. This gave a clear and much-needed boost to the technique as static pressurization needs none of the ducts and gas supplies required by its counterparts in the mainstream of the technique, relying only on the quality of the seals it contained to hold the internal pressure. Analyzer houses and pressurized rooms are, however, still excluded from the standard and it is difficult to see how they could be included because of their very nature; in that they have regular human access and their content varies from time to time, both of which factors require a more dynamic approach as provided in codes of practice rather than Standards (see Installation section of this book). Figure 11.1 shows the current situation in regard to the interface between the apparatus parts of the protection concept and the user-controlled parts.

There are three principle approaches to pressurization contained in this Standard for application to individual items of apparatus. First, static pressurization, in which the apparatus is pressurized outside the hazardous area and relies on its seals alone for its continued safety.

Second, pressurization with leakage compensation, where the apparatus is sealed as far as possible and the pressurizing medium remains connected to allow entry of pressurizing gas to replace any lost by leakage caused by imperfect sealing.

Third, pressurization with continuous flow of protective gas, where a defined minimum flow of gas is arranged by design throughout the time for which the enclosure is pressurized.

The various uses of these three methods of pressurization are given in Table 11.1 and details of their implementation in the following text. All three pressurization systems are intended for use in Zone 1 and less hazardous areas, provided that the apparatus is de-energized if the pressurization fails, but may be restricted to Zone 2 where a lower level of security exists (e.g., alarm only on pressure failure).

Because they operate by exclusion of the surrounding atmosphere, pressurized enclosures are normally intended for all Group II gases, vapours and mists in this regard. Where, however, enclosures have been shown to only purge effectively with certain gases, or there is the possibility of internal release, there may be restrictions on the range of such gases, vapours and mists in which the enclosure may be used or which may

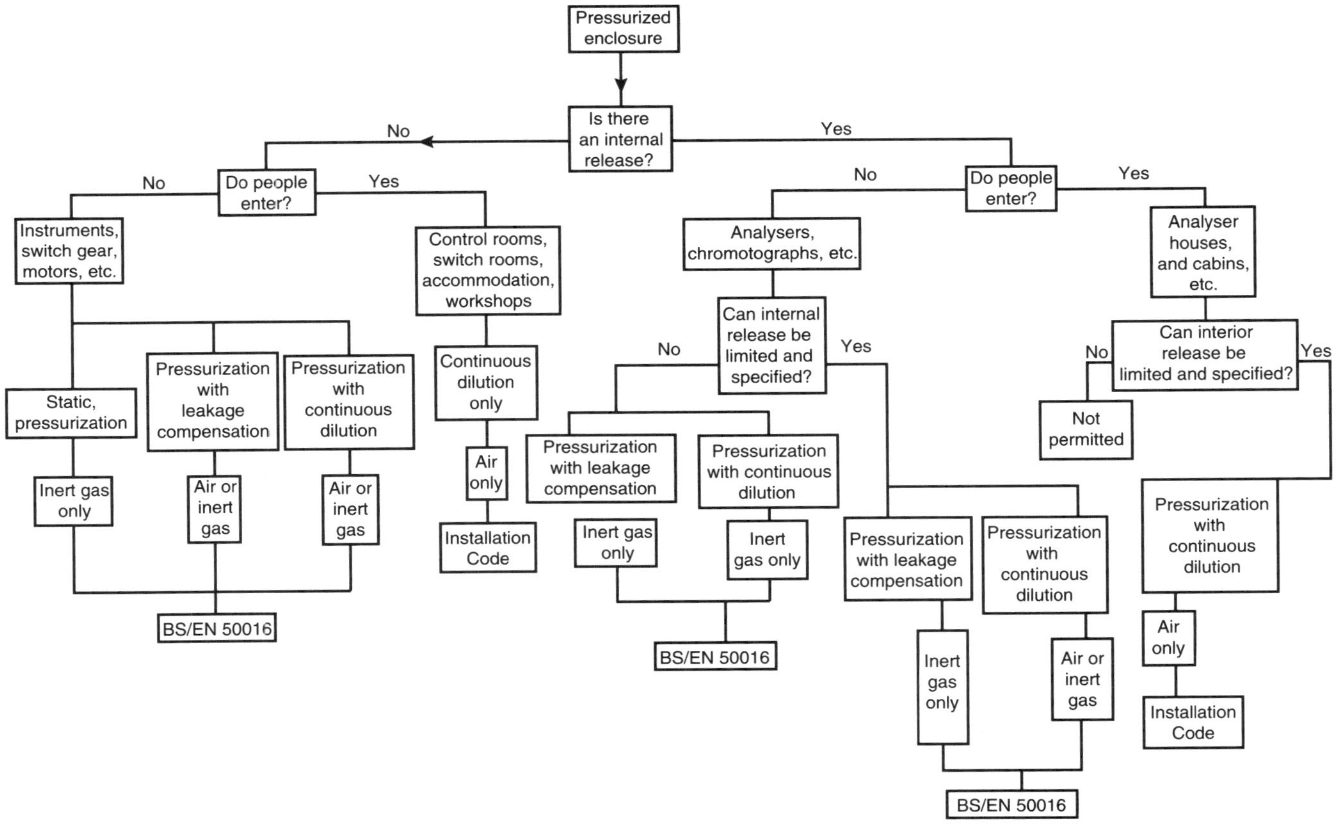

Fig. 11.1 Use of pressurization

Table 11.1 Type of pressurization vs release conditions

Release conditions	Type of pressurization					
	Static		Leakage Compensation		Continuous Dilution	
	Air	Inert[2]	Air	Inert[2]	Air	Inert[2]
No release of flammable material (note 1)	N[1]	Y	Y	Y	Y	Y
Deliberate release of flammable material	N[1]	N[3]	N[4]	N[4]	Y[6]	N[4]
Limited release of flammable material in fault condition	N[1]	N[3]	N[5]	Y[7]	Y[6]	Y[7]
Unlimited release of flammable material in fault conditions	N[1]	N[3]	N[5]	Y[7]	N[5]	Y[7]

1 Static pressurization with air is not permitted by BS/EN 50016.
2 Inert gas must contain less than 1% oxygen
3 Static pressurization cannot be used where there is any release of flammable material either deliberate or in fault conditions
4 Pressurization with leakage compensation cannot be used with either air or inert gas when the release is deliberate. Pressurization with dilution must use air in these circumstances
5 Pressurization with leakage compensation using air is not permitted where there is either a limited or an unlimited release in fault conditions. Pressurization with dilution using air is not permitted where the release is unlimited
6 When dilution with air is used the airflow must be sufficient to dilute the flammable gas concentration to less than 25% of its lower explosive limit in all but the dilution area of the enclosure, whether the release is a limited release in fault conditions or a specified normal release.
7 The protective gas in the enclosure must be such that the oxygen concentration is less than 2% by volume and the use of inert gas is not permitted when the flammable material has an upper explosive limit (UEL) of more than 80%

Note: In cases where the flammable material is contained in an infallible containment the enclosure may be treated as though it does not contain a flammable material.

be permitted inside the enclosure. This will not produce sub-grouping as described in Chapter 11, but may require limits to be defined for particular enclosures on the basis of, for example, gas density.

11.2 Methods of pressurization

The detail of the three methods of pressurization and their application are as follows:

11.2.1 Static pressurization

As already stated, static pressurization is a method of pressurization where the enclosure is filled with an inert gas at pressure, and then sealed to a degree which will allow operation for a length of time which will allow its operation and use, without the pressure falling sufficiently to cause danger. Typical of such uses are those which require the insertion of the apparatus into vessels, pipelines and similar locations where it would be impractical to utilize a pressurization system requiring continuous connection to a gas or air supply.

The pressurization medium for static pressurization must be an inert gas which contains less than 1 per cent oxygen, as pressurization with air is not considered to give the required level of security. This is because of its oxygen content which would support any combustion existing within the enclosure, allowing any burning occurring within the enclosure due to electrical fault, etc., to be perpetuated and allow damage to the apparatus even after isolation of the electrical supplies.

The enclosure should be pressurized with the inert gas outside the hazardous area and the technique used should be such as to ensure that all air is evacuated. This will normally require the pressurization method to include a purge, which is arranged to ensure adequate scavenging of the enclosure. This purge adequacy is determined by a type test in which the enclosure is purged and measurements taken at various places inside the enclosure to ensure that all air is removed by the purge. The time taken for this to happen is then the 'minimum purge time' and applying the purge in the same way, as for the test, for that time should always ensure that the air is removed from the enclosure. The criterion for a successful purge is when the oxygen concentration has fallen to less than 2 per cent. It is of course wise to specify a time slightly longer than the minimum to ensure some safety factor and a figure of 10 per cent additional time is suggested.

The enclosure is then pressurized, with the gas outlet sealed, to the pressure required. The leakage of gas from the enclosure should ensure that the time taken for the internal pressure to drop, from the design filling pressure, to $50\,N/m^2$ above external pressure is longer than the time for which operation demands that the apparatus be in use. The time needs to be longer if there are energy-storing devices or hot surfaces within the enclosure and needs to allow their charge or temperature to decay to a safe level (see BS/EN 50014 (1993))[7] after the electrical supplies have been switched off and before the lower limit of $50\,N/m^2$ is reached.

The apparatus requires two separate devices which indicate to a user that a pressure has been reached, such that within one hour, or 100 times the time taken for decay of charge or temperature (if this is longer), the pressure will have fallen to $50\,N/m^2$ at normal expected leakage rates. The 100 times figure is intended to allow a safety factor to ensure that with all possible variables at their worst, there is still a very high degree of certainty that the apparatus will have been switched off and removed from the hazardous area before the pressure falls sufficiently to allow an explosive atmosphere into the enclosure. Because of the nature of the static pressurization approach, these devices need to be fitted by the manufacturer of the apparatus. As, of necessity, these indicating devices will need to connect to circuits outside the pressurized enclosure, and normally remain energized after the removal of power to the apparatus, the circuits in which they are installed will need to be otherwise protected (for example, the devices may be in a flameproof enclosure within the apparatus, or the circuits in which they are installed may be intrinsically safe circuits).

The operation of these devices is as described above but the actions taken after operation are the responsibility of the user of the apparatus. Likewise, the control of the purging of the enclosure is a matter for the user, although it must comply with the specification provided by the manufacturer (see Section 11.5 of this chapter).

Finally, it must be recognized that the use of inert gas in the filling process could present an asphyxiation risk in confined places when filling the enclosure, and users of the technique need to be warned of this.

11.2.2 Pressurization with leakage compensation

This is the most economical method of pressurization, using a permanently connected supply of pressurizing gas to make up losses due to leakage, because the use of gas is determined only by the rate of leakage and loss of internal pressure. It, therefore, is more secure than static pressurization, and air is permitted as the pressurizing medium in some cases effecting further economy.

As for static pressurization, it is necessary to ensure that on pressurization failure the ingress of any external explosive atmosphere is sufficiently slow to permit any residual charge or hot surface to fall to a safe level before the gas can enter (see BS/EN 50014[7]). In this case, unlike the situation in static pressurization, deliberate opening of the enclosure must also take this problem into account. Normally some form of restriction in the exit duct, together with a warning notice, will be sufficient to ensure this in practice, but the restriction may have to be initiated by the identification of pressurization failure or the isolation of the electrical circuits within the enclosure.

No internal release of flammable material

Where the enclosure is intended to be purged and pressurized with an inert gas, the enclosure is tested as for static pressurization with that inert gas used as a purge medium to ascertain the time taken for the oxygen concentration inside the enclosure to fall to below 2 per cent. This then becomes the minimum purge time and, again, it is suggested that the time required be specified using a 10 per cent safety factor to cover variations in application. The disadvantage of purging and pressurization with inert gas is that there may be an asphyxiation risk, and this must be evaluated for each use.

Where the enclosure is intended to be purged and pressurized with air the situation is somewhat more complicated as the enclosure contains enough oxygen to support combustion after the purge is complete. This makes it much more important that no flammable gas exists in the enclosure after purging, and to this end account must be taken of the various densities of the gases involved (e.g., hydrogen has a density of only 0.07 relative to air, whereas some flammable hydrocarbons have densities in excess of 5 times that of air). The procedure for determination of purging time needs to be different, therefore, and two types of test are carried out; the first using an initial filling gas for the enclosure which is lighter than air (helium whose density is 0.14 that of air is normally used); and second using a gas which is heavier than air (possibilities here are carbon dioxide, which has a density of 1.6 times that of air, or argon which has a density of 1.4 times that of air).

The tests should determine the time taken for the concentration of the test gases (helium and carbon dioxide/argon) anywhere in the enclosure to fall in concentration to less than 1 per cent for helium or 0.25 per cent for carbon dioxide/argon, the enclosure having been filled with one of these gases to a minimum concentration of 70 per cent anywhere in the enclosure. The low levels of these gases that it is necessary to measure indicates that very sensitive oxygen monitors would be necessary if it is to be determined indirectly (i.e., by variation between the oxygen concentration of the purge gas and that of the gas samples taken from the enclosure, where for carbon dioxide a difference in oxygen concentration of 0.05 per cent is the limit situation) and direct measurement of the gas in question may be necessary. The longest of these two times is the one which should be specified as the purge time, and it is suggested that a 10 per cent safety factor is added to allow for variations.

In some circumstances, an enclosure may need to be specified as purged and pressurized by air or inert gas. In these cases the air purge test is sufficient if the inert gas has a density within ±10 per cent of air. In other circumstances the purge times will need to be determined with both air and the inert gas and the longest of these specified, or separate times specified, for each case (i.e., air purge and inert gas purge).

After purge the outlet of the enclosure is closed and the enclosure is permitted to rise to its design pressure which must be above $50\,N/m^2$ gauge, the purge gas remaining connected and replacing any gas lost by leakage thereby maintaining the pressure.

Unlike the situation in static pressurization there is no pressure decay unless a fault occurs and only one low pressure sensing device needs to be fitted. In this case, the device can be fitted by the manufacturer and be part of the enclosure package, but it may also be provided by the installer to the specification of the manufacturer. Unlike static pressurization, purging is in situ and if the gas supply fails the enclosure must go through its purge cycle again as soon as the gas supply is reinstated and before the apparatus is energized if the apparatus was switched off during the failure. In addition, because the installation will have ducts or pipes to carry the purge and compensation gas to the enclosure these also must be purged, and the purging time must be extended for this purpose. (Unfortunately, the volume of such ducts or pipes is only determined at installation and the user of the apparatus must decide on the total purge time necessary. The devices to ensure proper purging and purge control (i.e., timers, flow detectors etc.) may also be fitted by the installer to the manufacturer's specification and often form part of a specially produced control package which provides all of the controls necessary once activated by the pressure and flow limit switches attached to the enclosure (see Section 11.5 of this chapter).

Internal release of flammable material

Unlike static pressurization, flammable materials may be brought into the enclosures with pressurization by leakage compensation, provided the pressurization is with inert gas. The reason air is not permitted is that if the enclosure is other than very badly sealed the pressurizing gas flow into it will be small; indeed that is the objective. In such circumstances, if air were to be used the interior of the enclosure would rapidly become filled with an explosive atmosphere if a leak occurred because the air inside the enclosure would be almost static, and the amount of flammable gas in the mixture inside the enclosure would increase at the rate of its leakage and would rapidly exceed the lower explosive limit.

The incursion of the flammable material from the containment system into the enclosure produces additional problems even if an inert gas is used, as there may be oxygen in the released flammable material. To allow for this, the purge time determined for the enclosure when no leakage is considered needs to be increased, and a figure of 1.5 times that figure is considered as appropriate when the internal release is taken into account. In addition, there must be no more than 2 per cent oxygen in the contained flammable gas mixture permitted to enter the enclosure if this type of pressurization is to be used.

Pressurization with leakage compensation is not considered as acceptable when release is a normal part of operation in the containment system within the enclosure as, in such circumstances, the enclosure would always contain flammable material and would require that the containment be cleared and the enclosure purged before it could be opened. This is considered as too cumbersome a control procedure to be acceptable (see Table 11.1).

It must also be recognized that the release from the enclosure, either by leakage or by purging, will contain a flammable gas or vapour in times of internal leakage and an explosive atmosphere may surround the enclosure due to this. While this is normally not a problem because the enclosure is usually in an area made hazardous by the same materials as those leaking, in some exceptional cases the apparatus may contain reagents and similar materials which are more hazardous than those in the surrounding area. Therefore, the surrounding area may change to a more onerous sub-group, affecting other apparatus in the area.

11.2.3 Pressurization with continuous dilution

Pressurization with continuous dilution (or gas flow after purging) is the most expensive form of pressurization and is only necessary where leakage is such that continuous flow of gas is necessary to keep the enclosure pressure above the 50 N/m^2 differential required, or where dilution of internal releases are present. The technique requires purging of the enclosure before operation to ensure that the interior is free from explosive atmospheres before electrical energization but is different in that a continuous significant flow of gas continues after energization. As with previous methods of pressurization, the situation of possible entry of explosive atmosphere into the enclosure on pressurization failure has to be taken into account and the same procedures are appropriate.

No internal release of flammable material

The only two reasons for using this technique where there is no release of flammable material are: first, where leakage is great, in which case it is merely a limiting case of pressurization with leakage compensation and as such need not be addressed here; and, second, where personnel enter, but as the only situations where this is likely are analyzer houses and rooms (both excluded from BS/EN 50016[6]) this approach is not necessary where no release occurs inside the apparatus.

Internal release of flammable material

Where there is a limited release of flammable material under fault conditions, the continuous flow of pressurizing gas through the enclosure may be either air or inert gas. The purging approach in these cases is different, in that account is taken of the release from the containment in both the purge and the later continuous dilution. Where the purge gas is inert, air at the maximum rate of internal gas leakage rate possible from process is injected into the enclosure throughout the purge test in addition to initially filling the enclosure with air. The purge time again becomes the time taken for the outlet gas to reach a point where it contains less than 2 per cent oxygen. Where air is the purge gas the injection is one or both of the test gases (i.e., helium or argon/carbon dioxide) and the purge time is the time required to reach the limit of less than 1 per cent helium or 0.25 per cent argon/carbon dioxide. The helium/carbon dioxide flow into the enclosure equal to the maximum at which gas can leak into the enclosure in service.

Dilution flow rates are also determined in the same way, with the maximum leak rate of flammable material. The object is to maintain the maximum outlet oxygen level for inert gas purging at less than 2 per cent and the maximum outlet concentration of flammable gas or vapour at less than 25 per cent of lower explosive limit if the dilution gas is air.

Where there is a deliberate normal release of flammable material into the enclosure it must be quantifiable, and is treated as for the limited fault release except that the dilution and pressurization gas must be air to ensure that the majority of the mixture inside the enclosure is always non-explosive, even when the enclosure is opened. Likewise, where the upper explosive limit of the released gas or vapour is more than 80 per cent, only dilution with air is possible as, even with the low air concentration of 2 per cent required for inert gas dilution, the situation is not considered as sufficiently safe.

In the case of unlimited releases (caused by release of liquid which then vaporizes) air is not considered as suitable for a purge and dilution gas as it is difficult to achieve the 25 per cent lower explosive limit figure with sufficient confidence. Therefore, inert gas must be used and the criterion of less than 2 per cent oxygen must be met in the worst case. This presupposes that the maximum release rate of oxygen from the containment must be quantifiable even where the release contains more than 2 per cent oxygen.

11.3 Purge and dilution gases

Supplies of gas used for purging pressurization, leakage compensation and dilution may be supplied from fans, compressed gas mains or cylinders. In all cases it should be ensured that the gas is clean and free from significant quantities of moisture, by filtering if necessary. In line with the general situation it should be at a temperature of between −20 and +40 °C, but within that range it is acceptable for it to be used as a heating or cooling medium. Where inert gas is used it must be made clear to those involved in application of the apparatus that a significant asphyxiation risk may exist in the proximity of the apparatus, particularly where continuous dilution is used.

Under no circumstances may significant flammable constituents be included in the gas.

11.4 Flammable materials imported into enclosures and their containment

11.4.1 Flammable materials imported into enclosures

The flammable materials entering pressurized enclosures may be gases, vapours, mists or liquids which are above their flashpoints and can, therefore, form an explosive atmosphere in air. It is necessary to know the maximum vaporization rate of liquid pools forming inside the enclosure as these have an effect on the airflow required. If the liquids which enter the enclosure do not have a vaporization rate which can be easily shown to prevent build up of liquid in the enclosure, attention is necessary to the method of draining such liquids to ensure that the enclosure does not fill with flammable liquid. Draining should be to safe containment, such as a receiver designed for the purpose which will contain the liquid and not adversely affect the specification of the hazardous area in which it is located. An approach similar to that used on sampling points may be appropriate.

There are limits within which the specification of any flammable material must fall if it is to be acceptable. For pressurization with leakage compensation it must not have more than 2 per cent oxygen in its gas/vapour-phase mixture under any conditions, and for pressurization not more than 21 per cent. This latter figure is intended to prevent with continuous dilution of oxygen enrichment and is necessary as there is only 21 per cent oxygen in air. It is common to all types of protection that they are not intended for explosive atmospheres containing more than 21 per cent oxygen.

11.4.2 Containment of flammable materials within enclosures

Where there is a flammable material transported into the enclosure, other than the pressurization medium, it will be in some type of containing transport mechanism. Typical of such systems are piping, and cells with optical viewports (such as those used in optical analysers), or piping and controlled release systems (such as those used in chromatographs). There are effectively three types of these for the purposes of this protection concept.

Where the containment can leak it is necessary to consider the situation where, although the electrical circuits within the enclosure are isolated by pressurization failure, there are items within the enclosure which remain ignition capable due to retained charge or high temperature. In these circumstances the devices which identify the loss of pressurization must also cut off the flow of flammable material to the containment.

Infallible containment

If the flammable material can be effectively contained within the pressurized enclosure so that there is a very high level of confidence that in all normal usage it cannot be released, then the containment may be described as infallible. Such containment may not rely on such things as metal or elastomeric compression seals, which may fail, but must be achieved by methods such as welding, brazing or glass-to-metal seals formed by fusion or similar processes to achieve the required confidence. Even low temperature sealing methods, such as soldering, are not considered to be sufficiently secure for the purpose of infallible containment. In addition, the fact that some of these techniques produce brittle seals (e.g., glass-to-metal fusion seals) mechanical considerations need to be carefully considered. The seals must be secure against the drop and impact normally required by BS/EN 50016[6] but, in addition, assembly stresses and temperature changes in use need to be considered to ensure they do not cause sufficient stress on the joints produced which may cause fractures. There are no specific tests for these possible situations associated with use in explosive atmospheres alone, but normal engineering practice is appropriate to determine their suitability.

Infallible containment is not considered to release flammable material and so, for the purposes of Pressurization, any enclosure where the containment of flammable materials which enter is deemed infallible, it may be treated as an enclosure without entry of flammable material.

Containment with limited release capability

Where containment systems inside pressurized enclosures contain, for example, compression seals and threaded joints, release is possible. and To be considered as limited release, the flow of released flammable material must be controlled to a known maximum value. Unless the size of leak can be accurately identified, the only way to achieve this is to include a specification for a flow-limiting device to be installed outside the enclosure by the installer, or to place such a controller inside the enclosure – in which case the containment up to and including the controller itself must be infallible. Alternatively, where such joints as metal/metal compression joints, or screwed joints, etc., are used it may be sufficient to specify the pressure of the flammable material entering the containment and calculating the release rate at the maximum pressure for the purposes of defining the limited release (see Chapter 4).

In addition to limited release caused by leaks, there are cases, such as those in chromatographs, where flammable material is deliberately released. In such cases it should be relatively easy to define the maximum release rate in the worst operating conditions. It should be noted, however, that further restrictions exist where the release is deliberate where the only form of pressurization acceptable is pressurization with continuous dilution using air.

The volume of air required to ensure that the gas mixture leaving the enclosure is less than 25 per cent lower explosive limit can be calculated if the volume of gas released is known together with the percentage of flammable material in that gas. The formula for this is:

$$Q_1 = Q_2 \times (Y_1/100) \times (100/Y_2) \times (100/F) \qquad \text{m}^3/\text{hour}$$

where
- Q_1 = Minimum flowrate of protective gas — m^3/hour
- Q_2 = Maximum release rate of gas or vapour — m^3/hour
- Y_1 = Volumetric percentage of flammable material in the release — % v/v
- Y_2 = Volumetric lower explosive limit of the flammable material in air — % v/v
- F = The percentage lower explosive limit required (25 per cent in this case) — % v/v

Where there is more than one flammable material in the released mixture, the amount of air should be calculated for each component individually and then the quantities added to give the required minimum airflow.

Containment with unlimited release

This description addresses containment that, if it released gas or vapour would be called containment with limited release, releases flammable liquid which can evolve flammable vapours at rates which cannot be quantified with confidence.In such cases, obviously, while the liquid release rate can be defined the rate of vaporization is not so easy to specify. Therefore it is not possible to effectively dilute the vapour produced with confidence.

Where this occurs there may also be oxygen entrained (usually as air) in the release and the use of inert gas pressurization with continuous gas flow, which is the only option acceptable here, must ensure that the mixture leaving the enclosure does not contain more than 2 per cent oxygen by volume. The mixture of vapour and oxygen at the point of release must not contain more than 21 per cent oxygen. The objective of this latter requirement is to allow only entrained air in the release, as any gas entrained with a higher level of oxygen could cause this criterion not to be met if vaporization rates of the liquid were low.

Calculation of the minimum flow of inert gas to reduce the oxygen content of a release to the required 2 per cent may be carried out in the same way as the air dilution already discussed:

$$Q_1 = Q_2 \times 100/Y_1 \qquad \text{m}^3/\text{hour}$$

where Q_1 = Minimum flowrate of inert gas — m^3/hour
Q_2 = Volume of oxygen in the release — m^3/hour
Y_1 = Percentage oxygen permitted in outlet from enclosure (2 per cent in this case) — %v/v

11.5 Enclosures, ducting and internal components

11.5.1 Enclosures

The enclosures used for pressurized apparatus are required to be sufficiently strong to withstand normal use without damage, in common with other protection concepts, and may be manufactured of metallic or non-metallic materials provided that, if non-metallic, the material of construction is not adversely affected by either the pressurization medium or any flammable material released in the enclosure. The strength of enclosures must also be such that they are not damaged by the maximum pressure which can occur in service. While an easy method of achieving this is to specify a maximum pressure and then leave it to the installer to ensure that it is not exceeded, such an approach is not practical. In many cases it is easier to install an over-pressure relief device in the enclosure so that if there is any unwanted pressure elevation in service the enclosure is automatically safeguarded.

A requirement for the enclosure to be weather proof is not necessary as the pressurization requirements will effectively prevent the ingress of moisture. Prevention of entry of solid foreign bodies, however, remains necessary as these may still enter due to their nature and, unlike moisture, will not be easily removed by purging if they enter prior to energization. A requirement is for the enclosure to have an integrity of not less than IP40 in accordance with BS/EN 60529[8] in the absence of the pressurizing gas. In the case of rotating machines where IP-ratings are defined slightly differently, due to the nature of such apparatus, the Standard used is EN 60034-5, which is published in the UK as BS 4999, Part 105.[9]

When considering the IP-rating of the enclosure, the deliberate apertures for inlet and outlet of the purge gas may be ignored. These, however, must be sited to ensure adequate purging and the avoidance of dead spots where any flammable gas or vapour may dwell even after purging. This may only require careful siting of single apertures in each case but may, where enclosure shapes are complex or components create divisions in the enclosure, need several inlet and outlet apertures. The choice is one which can only be made individually but it is not likely that multiple apertures will be the norm.

Where outlet apertures are fitted to enclosures which are pressurized by static pressurization or pressurization with leakage compensation, these must be arranged so that they can be closed or sealed after purging by devices which form part of the apparatus.

It is recognized that the apparatus will, in common with other types of apparatus, be fitted with doors and covers which permit access to the interior of the enclosure. The ideal method of dealing with these in the case of pressurization with leakage compensation, and pressurization with continuous dilution, is to utilize an interlock which isolates the electrical supplies and any other electrical connections (see Fig. 11.2) when the door or cover is opened. Because this would limit the opportunity for adjustment it is possible to introduce an interlock defeat system (see Fig. 11.3) which would permit competent persons to open the enclosures, under a system of control, for adjustment and similar purposes without electrical isolation. After such work, when the enclosure is reclosed it is important that the system goes through its full purge cycle to remove any gas which has entered, although it is not necessary to isolate the electrical supplies during this period.

Where a tool or key is required to open doors or remove covers isolation is not necessary, but the purge cycle needs initiating after reclosure. In this case it will have to be done manually. A device can be fitted which recognizes opening or removal, and isolates electrical supplies with an override as already described. The tool or key requirement in this case does not indicate any requirement for 'special fasteners' or the like (see Chapter 8).

In the case of static pressurization, doors and covers will not be provided for adjustment after pressurization due to the nature of the approach. All

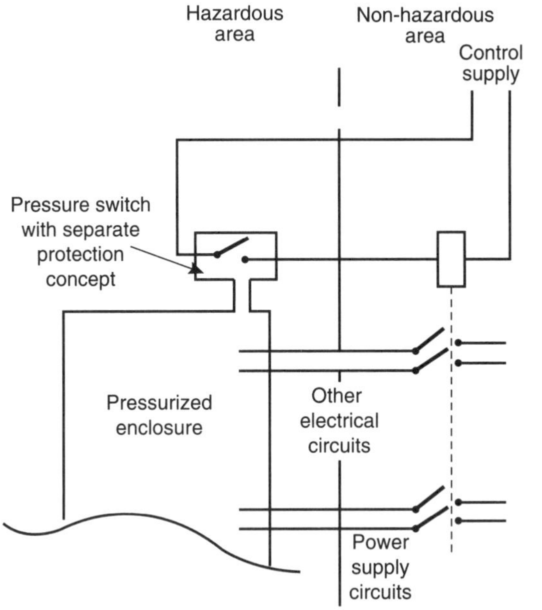

Fig. 11.2 Disconnection of electrical supplies and circuits on pressure failure

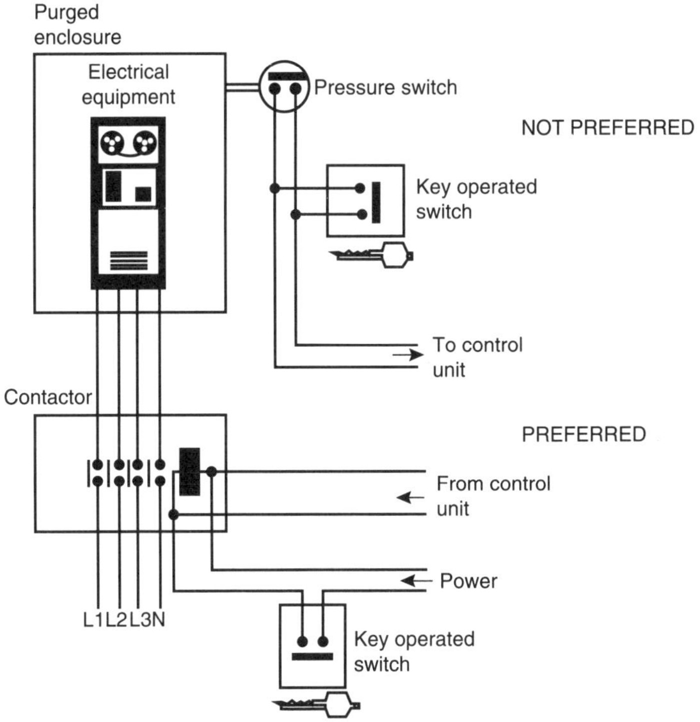

Fig. 11.3 Defeating of control system. *Note*. The preferred method ensures the repurge of the enclosure after reinstatement of pressure.

that is required is for any doors or covers to need a tool or key for them to be opened or removed. Once again, the requirement for a tool or key does not indicate a requirement for the 'special fasteners' described in Chapter 8.

11.5.2 Ducting

As the ducting forms part of the enclosure it needs to satisfy the same requirements as those for enclosures. With the use of compressed gas, this is no problem as the ducts will be short, being only in the area of the enclosure (see Fig. 11.4) – the supply of gas to that point normally being compressed gas piping, and the outlet ducting being short as it discharges into the hazardous area. (It is not possible to permit the exit ducting to exhaust into a non-hazardous area, as to do so would make it a hazardous area). Therefore, in these cases, all piping and ducting will be at a pressure above atmospheric pressure and the ducts can form a part of the apparatus.

Where the protective gas is air, and fan supplied (not normally possible for inert gas), then there are two possibilities. First, the fan and immediate ducting may form part of the enclosure and be under the control of the manufacturer. The air must, however, be obtained from a non-hazardous area resulting in a considerable length of ducting. This, then, becomes an installer problem. Which makes matters very difficult because the pressure

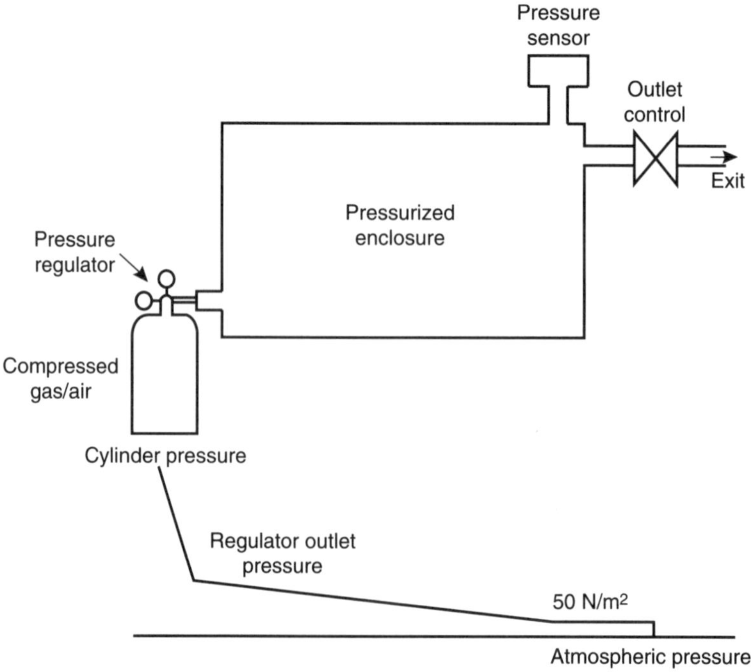

Fig. 11.4 Pressurization using compressed gas

in the supplying duct will be below atmospheric pressure (see Fig. 11.5) and, as the ducts must pass through a hazardous area, any leak will permit the possible entry of an explosive atmosphere into the enclosure. This first approach is not, therefore, recommended and the alternative of the remote fan with pressurized ducting is preferred (see Fig. 11.6).

Where the exhaust ducting is short and discharges into a hazardous area any incandescent sparking inside the enclosure can, in certain circumstances, cause the ejection of incandescent particles into the hazardous area. A device to prevent such ejection is normally necessary when the apparatus produces ignition-capable sparking which can give rise to such particles or contains some other mechanism (for example, a flame ionization chromatograph), which can in normal operation, and the exhaust duct discharges into any hazardous area and when even though the apparatus does not itself produce such particles in normal operation but the exhaust ducting exhausts into a Zone 1. This latter is to cover the

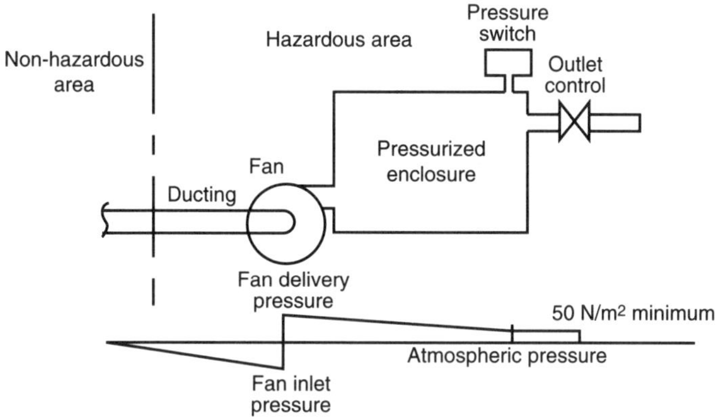

Fig. 11.5 Fan pressurizing with fan at enclosure inlet

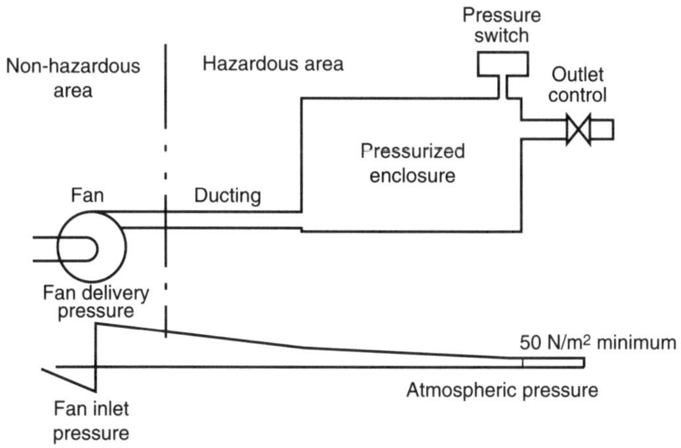

Fig. 11.6 Fan pressurizing with fan in non-hazardous area

situation where internal electrical fault can cause the incandescent particles. Table 11.2 produces this in tabular form.

Table 11.2 Requirements for spark and particle barriers

Zone into which purge gas exhausts	Necessity for spark/particle barrier	
	Apparatus sparks in normal operation	Apparatus does not spark in normal operation
Zone 0	Exhaust not permitted	Exhaust not permitted
Zone 1	Barrier required	Barrier required
Zone 2	Barrier required	Barrier not required
Non-hazardous	Barrier not required	Barrier not required

(from BS/EN 50016)

Spark-arresting devices are usually labyrinthine devices or, for example, steel wool (see Fig. 11.7).

Finally, it must be noted that the exhaust ducts provide a route for explosive atmosphere entry in periods when no pressurization is present. Therefore, some method of preventing or slowing down entry of such atmospheres is necessary as part of the procedure for restricting the rate of entry of explosive atmosphere on pressurization failure or electrical isolation.

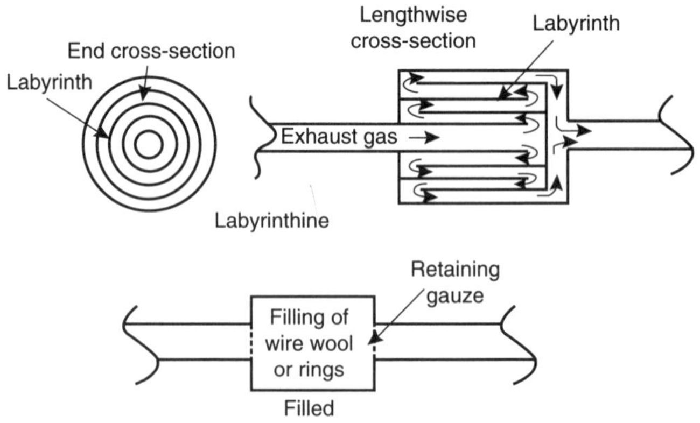

Fig. 11.7 Spark and particle arresters

11.5.3 Internal electrical components, etc

As the internal parts of the enclosure are protected by pressurization, the requirements for them are normally only those which would be required for normal industrial use. There are some special conditions however.

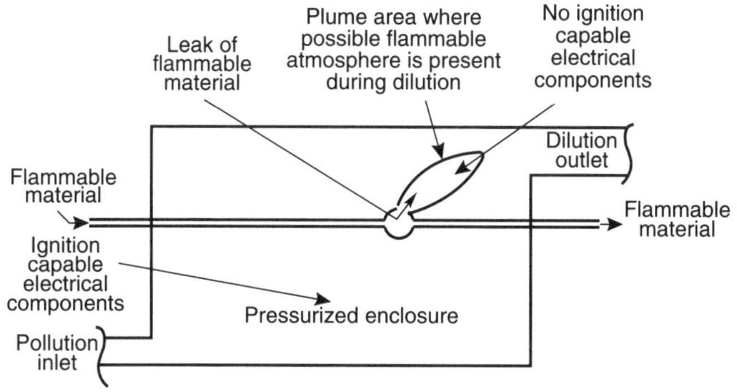

Fig. 11.8 Internal release of explosive atmosphere

Where the pressurized enclosure contains other enclosures such as those normally fitted to the enclosed equipment (e.g., relay cases, television monitor cases, etc.) it is possible that these could fill with an explosive atmosphere and not be effectively purged. For this reason the inner enclosures should either be removed or have large holes cut in to ensure that the purge is effective. The easier way is normally to remove the internal enclosure. This is not necessary when the inner enclosure is effectively sealed by some means. Elastomeric seals in addition to fusion seals are considered adequate for this purpose.

There is a further possible problem in that where an internal release of flammable material occurs an explosive atmosphere may occur in the region of the release before complete dilution of the release has taken place by the continuous flow of protective gas (if that gas is air or if oxygen is contained in the release itself). In these circumstances all electrical components, other than those which are rendered non-ignition capable by another protection concept, should be kept well away from the dilution area (see Fig. 11.8). This is normally achieved by ensuring that no unprotected electrical components are near the line of sight from the release to the enclosure exit aperture. This can be assured by siting the possible source of leakage between the electrical components and the exit aperture. This does not apply, of course, to deliberate ignition sources such as flames in flame ionization chromatographs and their ignitors.

11.6 Safety provisions and devices

It is clear that the security of this protection concept relies to a very large extent upon the monitoring and control devices which ensure that purging is effective and pressurization is maintained. As in all cases, except those associated with pressure maintenance in static pressurization, these are not always provided by the manufacturer. It appears at first sight to be somewhat incongruous that a formal Standard is written for a protection concept which is less controlled by the manufacturer than others. This is not, however, true as a close look at any installation using any protection concept will show that much of its safety is determined by installation matters (e.g., what electrical protection provisions are made,? what cables are used?, etc.). Therefore, the situation where the purge and pressurization sensing devices and their associated control devices are only controlled by specification is acceptable.

Pressure and purge rate detection devices should, as far as possible, be sited at or near the enclosure outlet to avoid incorrect identification of the purge/pressure situation occurring (e.g., a gas leak at the input of the purge gas causing identification of correct purge when, in fact, gas is leaking before it enters the enclosure, or identifying correct over pressure when inlet to enclosure is blocked). In addition, small bore connections to such devices should be avoided as far as possible to prevent blockage.

The sequences for purging should be as follows for all three applications of the technique:

1. Detectors should identify that minimum pressure and flowrate is achieved before timing of purge is commenced.
2. If pressure or purge flowrate falls below the specified minimum specification during the purge, the purge should cease and the control circuits should recommence purge when the minimum conditions have been restored.
3. After purging, in the case of pressurization with leakage compensation or with continuous dilution, the control system should close purging exit valves and continue to monitor pressure and, in the case of continuous dilution, gas flow.
4. On failure of either pressure, or in the case of continuous flow, gasflow provision must be made for an alarm to be sounded or complete electrical isolation the choice being made by the user.
5. If the enclosure is opened, even if alarm or isolation action is overridden by maintenance control circuits, the apparatus must go through its entire purge cycle on reclosure as soon as the purge conditions have been established.

It is possible to pressurize several enclosures from the same source but care must be taken in so doing. If they are pressurized in series, it is likely that failure of pressure in any one enclosure will cause failure in all downstream enclosures. In this case the corrective action on any single failure must apply to all affected enclosures. Even if this is not the case any single failure will initiate the repurging of all enclosures. Where the common pressurization source is pressurizing the enclosures in parallel, this situation does not occur and, provided the failure of any one enclosure can be uniquely identified, it is only necessary to repurge that one enclosure after correction.

The reliability of the purge and pressurization control devices is fundamental to the security of the protection concept. A European Standard

(EN 954)[10] is in preparation and will concern itself with the reliability of safety related circuits and devices, but until this is available there is no European Standard which can be effectively applied. General safety approaches (e.g., fail to safety) should govern the design of systems and if there is any doubt in a particular case, duplication of components or circuits should be considered.

References

1 CP 1003	Electrical Apparatus and Associated Equipment for use in Explosive Atmospheres of Gas or Vapour Other Than Mining operations. Part 2 (1966). Methods of Meeting the Explosion Hazard Other Than by the Use of Flameproof and Intrinsically Safe Equipment.
2 NEC 70 (1990)	National Electrical Code (USA). Article 500, hazardous (Classified) Locations.
3 76/117/EEC (1975)	Council Directive on the Approximation of the Laws of Member States Concerning Electrical Equipment for Use in Potentially Explosive Atmospheres. December.
4 CENELEC	Centre Européen de Normalization Electrique.
5 BS 5501	Electrical Apparatus for Potentially Explosive Atmospheres. Part 3 (1977). Pressurized Apparatus 'p'.
6 BS/EN 50016 (1996)	Electrical Apparatus for Potentially Explosive Atmospheres. Pressurized Apparatus 'p'.
7 BS/EN 50014 (1993)	Electrical Apparatus for Potentially Explosive Atmospheres. General Requirements.
8 BS/EN 60529 (1991)	Specification for Degrees of Protection Provided by Enclosures (IP Code).
9 BS 4999	General Requirements for Rotating Electrical Machines. Part 105 (1988). Specification for Degrees of Protection Provided by Enclosures for rotating Machinery.
10 EN 954	Safety of Machinery – Safety Related Parts of Control Systems (in Preparation).

— 12 —

Apparatus with protection concept increased safety 'e'

(BS/EN 50019 (1994))

The protection concept (type of protection) of increased safety is one intended for use in Zone 1 and less hazardous areas. It is a German development (erhohtesichereit) which explains the use of 'e' as its concept symbol. Increased safety did not figure significantly in UK thinking before 1970 and only became important then because of the effect on UK attitudes produced by the increasing importance of the European dimension emerging at the time of the European Free Trade Association (EFTA), of which the UK was a member prior to its entry into the European Union (EU). It gained further importance in UK thinking with the UK's entry into the EU itself.

It is a type of protection where, even though the ingress of an explosive atmosphere into the enclosure is not prevented, the apparatus does not spark, arc or become excessively hot in normal operation and, in addition, is of such quality that it is unlikely to become faulty in a way which would make it ignition capable. This security from fault is further increased by enclosure protection from its environment, reducing the risk of environmental conditions adversely affecting its operation. The protection, however, is much more sensitive to electrical protection devices (fuses, circuit breakers, etc.) than the other types of protection so far considered as any fault (e.g., internal short circuit, connection failure, etc.) is likely to make it ignition capable. Therefore part of the protection depends upon the length of time for which such a situation can exist prior to the protective devices operating.

There were many misgivings in the UK concerning the adoption of increased safety as a protection concept suitable for Zone 1 and less hazardous areas, particularly for such things a rotating machines and luminaires, as the requirements for the protection concept in the German National Standard (VDE 0171) did not, to many, appear to offer a significant increase in the requirements applied by British Standards to Standard industrial equipment of these types in UK. There is still considerable concern in respect of rotating electrical machines and this is dealt with later in this chapter.

Despite this reservation it was accepted that increased safety would become a standard protection concept in Europe and the world at large and to exclude it in the UK for what were, to the majority in the UK, unconvincing technical reasons (no real evidence existing at the time of its level of protection being too low, rather than historic UK approaches being too high) would merely damage UK manufacturing industry. It was also noted that an International Standard (IEC 79–7 (1969)[1]) was likely to be accepted by most countries of the world.

12.1 The situation in regard to standardization

The UK accepted the protection concept of increased safety and a National Standard was produced in 1973 (BS 4683, Part 4[2]). This Standard was rapidly overtaken by BS 5501 Part 6 (1977)[3] (which was the first edition of a European Standard, EN 50019) and both of these Standards have now been overtaken by BS/EN 50019 (1994)[4] which is the second edition of the European Standard and will, in effect, be the Standard to which future apparatus will be constructed. This chapter will therefore be based upon the requirements of BS/EN 50019.

12.2 Basic construction requirements

The basic security of increased safety apparatus is in the construction of the apparatus itself and the limitations of the types of apparatus to which the protection concept is applicable. These limitations are:

1. The apparatus must not arc or spark or produce ignition capable hot surfaces in normal operation
2. No apparatus operating at a supply voltage of more than 11 kV rms, or which internally produces voltages in excess of this, can be protected within this protection concept.
3. Apparatus where component construction cannot be defined in a way which will permit compliance with the requirements of the protection concept, or which cannot comply by virtue of their construction (e.g., semiconductor devices) cannot be dealt with in this protection concept. Therefore, increased safety is not normally applicable to instrumentation.

The above means that the protection concept finds its greatest application in such apparatus as connection boxes, luminaires, rotating machines, transformers, batteries, resistance heating devices and measuring instruments (basic meters, etc.).

12.2.1 Construction of enclosures

Enclosures need to comply with the general hazardous area requirements (see Chapter 8) but because of the nature of this protection concept they must satisfy additional requirements.

As previously stated, the protection concept relies to a high degree on the exclusion of the external environment (keeping out the weather but not gas) and to this end the enclosures must have a degree of protection of at least IP54 in accordance with BS/EN 60529[5] (As elsewhere, the method of determination of IP-rating for rotating electrical machines is slightly different and BS 4999 part 105[6] is used in place of BS/EN 60529[5] for such machines). Where the enclosure contains only insulated conductors and components, rather than bare live parts, this enclosure integrity may be reduced to IP44. Further reductions are permissible if breathing or draining holes are necessary for the reliable operation of the apparatus. In these circumstances IP44 is acceptable for enclosures containing bare live parts, and IP24 for enclosures containing only insulated conductors and components. In these latter cases, to utilize the lower IP-ratings, the position of the holes is critical and the apparatus will be subjected to installation conditions which minimize the possibility of ingress of liquid or solid foreign bodies in its installed location.

The requirements become more complex when this protection concept is used in conjunction with intrinsic safety (see Chapter 13 which discusses intrinsic safety) as is sometimes the case when it needs internal monitoring devices (e.g., temperature sensors in rotating machine windings) to ensure that early isolation takes place in case of fault. It is clear that the actual construction of the apparatus must be such that the intrinsic safety is not compromised but there is a particular point where outside influences can produce such a compromising effect. This is where the external connections are made for the increased safety part of the apparatus in the same place (terminal box, etc.) as the intrinsic safety external connections. In these circumstances an inner cover of at least IP30 is necessary for the increased safety connection facilities and a warning is necessary to ensure that this cover is not removed when the outer cover is off and the increased safety terminations energized or the intrinsically safe circuits are connected to external circuits. The inadvertent application of the levels of voltage in most increased safety apparatus could damage an intrinsically safe installation in a way which would not be apparent and which may cause danger, not only in the particular installation but in other intrinsically safe installations using facilities in common with it.

These enclosures and covers need to be fixed by special fasteners as described in Chapter 8.

12.2.2 Terminals and connection facilities

All electrical connections, both those within the apparatus and those to permit connection of external electrical conductors, are important in this concept as any failure, even partial, of a connection can give rise to sparking.

Of the possible electrical connections for external conductors themselves, only terminals are specifically addressed with specific detailed requirements which have to be satisfied to ensure they are reliable. The general use of plugs and sockets is not specifically mentioned in any Standards for this protection concept but, although this may be thought as precluding their use, a relaxation in respect of the general requirements for plugs and sockets in the case of battery assemblies, (see BS/EN 50014[7] and Chapter 8) indicates that they are acceptable provided they meet the requirements of BS/EN 50014, and that the connection facilities which they provide for conductors satisfy the requirements of increased safety (either as terminals or as internal connections when the plug and/or socket is supplied with a fixed cable).

It will be remembered that the general requirements for plugs and sockets are that they should either be interlocked, so that any attempt to separate them isolates their electrical supplies, or that they are secured together by special fasteners and suitable warnings are supplied on the apparatus against separation while energized. It will be remembered that for operational currents not exceeding 10 A rms ac or dc, at voltages of less than 250 V rms ac or 60 V dc, foregoing requirements may be removed, provided that the part of the coupling remaining energized after separation is the socket; the circuit is broken before the plug pins separate from the socket to ensure that any arc is extinguished before total separation, and the combination remains flameproof in accordance with BS/EN 50018[8] during the arc extinguishing period. In addition, the socket contacts which remain energized need to be protected to prevent ignition. This latter requirement is normally achieved by arranging the socket so that it is a flameproof enclosure after the plug has been removed, or that it forms an increased safety enclosure in such circumstances. In both cases automatically moving parts will need to be fitted to the socket to complete the enclosure after plug removal.

Terminals for either internal or external connections, including those permitting connection of conductors to plugs and sockets, need to be constructed so that they are: sufficiently well fixed to ensure that stresses (such as those produced by tightening screws) do not adversely affect the connection of the terminal to internal circuits and components are not able to damage the external conductors being connected to them by such things as direct connection to the screw providing the connection pressure or any sharp surfaces on their parts and are able to satisfy these requirements even when connecting stranded conductors. Crimped ferrules are permitted in the case of stranded conductors and screws of terminals may impinge directly on the ferrule but this is not permitted in the case of a stranded conductor without a ferrule.

When more than one conductor is terminated in one terminal (an unusual situation which should be avoided as far as possible), the maximum number of conductors which may be terminated in a single terminal needs to be specified in each case. Figure 12.1 gives an example of a terminal which is acceptable for a single conductor and Fig. 12.2 for a multiple conductor terminal. The intermediate pad between the screw and the conductor is not necessary when the conductor is fitted with a crimped ferrule.

In addition to using the means described for external connection internal connections may be made by:

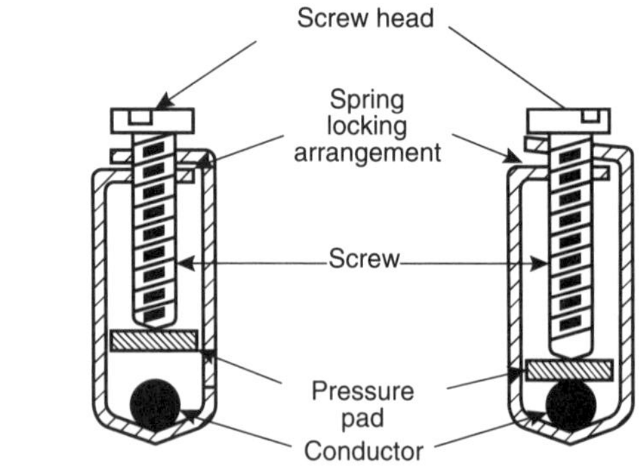

Fig. 12.1 Typical single conductor terminal. *Note*: The pressure pad is not necessary if the conductor is crimped in a suitable ferrule

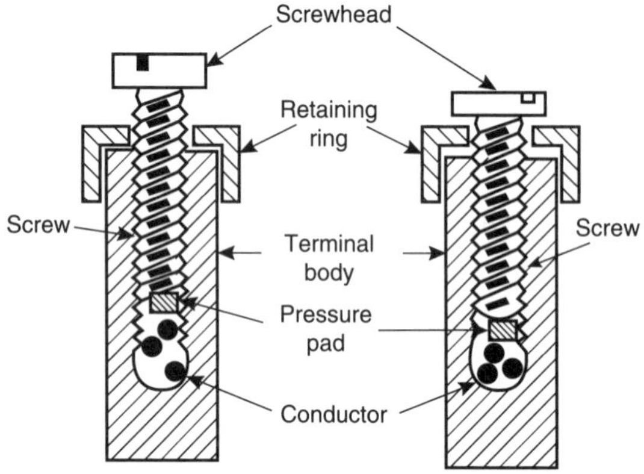

Fig. 12.2 Typical multi-conductor terminal. *Note*: The pressure pad is not necessary if the conductors are individually crimped into suitable ferrules

1. any form of screwed or bolted connection which does not damage the conductor, provides good electrical connection, and is locked against loosening (see Fig. 12.3);
2. crimped connections such as those using a crimped ferrule where the conductors are either placed in the ferrule together and secured by a single crimping action or separately at each end and each is secured by a separate crimping action, (see Fig. 12.4);
3. brazed or welded connections;
4. soldered connections where the joint is not supported by the solder in view of the lower level of physical strength of such joints.

12.2.3 Separation of conducting parts

As the enclosure is not sealed against the ingress of the outside air which may contain moisture impurities and, of course, flammable gases,

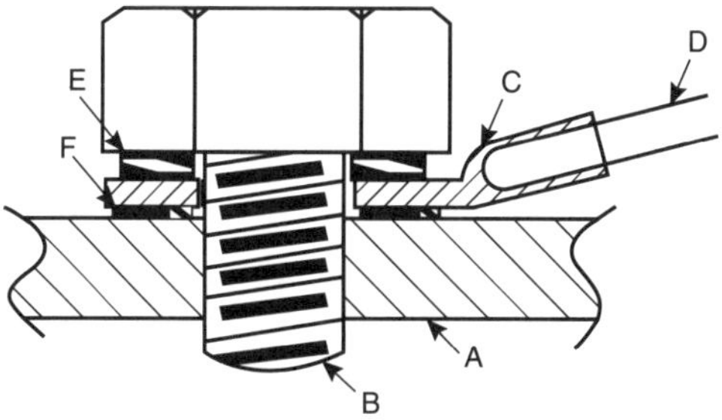

A = Conducting part of apparatus
B = Connection screw
C = Spade or eylet termination or similar
D = Conductor crimped, soldered, welded or brazed to termination
E = Spring washer to prevent loosening
F = Star washer (if necessary to ensure good electrical connection)

Fig. 12.3 Typical spade/eylet termination

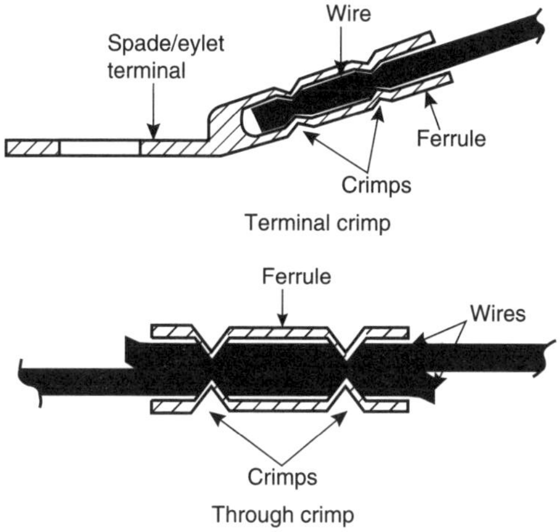

Fig. 12.4 Typical crimped connections

vapours and mists, there is the possibility of breakdown of the air between separate bare conducting parts or the breakdown of the surface of any insulating material separating and/or supporting the conductors. To avoid this possibility, bare live conductors are required to be separated by certain minimum distances in air and these are called clearances. In addition where the bare live parts, and these may be just the bare end of an insulated wire where it is connected into a terminal, are separated by the surface of an insulating material, the insulant must be of a certain quality, and the distance along its surface must be of at least a specified minimum value which is called a creepage distance. The insulation quality is determined by measurements of the comparative tracking index (CTI), in accordance with BS 5901 (1980)[10] which is a measurement identifying the capability of the insulating surface to retain its properties in the presence of contaminants.

As the breakdown of insulation is usually more likely than the breakdown of air, the creepage distance figures are normally greater than those for clearance (see Table 12.1). The working voltage figure in Table 12.1 is the highest figure of voltage which can occur across the conductors in question, either with recognized supply and load variations or with open circuits applied in the apparatus where these give worse conditions. Transient voltages are ignored as these do not normally influence tracking. Fig. 12.5 shows the basic difference between creepage distances and clearances.

Table 12.1 Minimum creepage and clearance distances

Working voltage U (rms)	Minimum creepage distance (mm)			minimum clearance (mm)
	Material Group I[1]	Material Group II[2]	Material Group IIIa[3]	
$0 < U \leq 15$	1.6	1.6	1.6	1.6
$15 < U \leq 30$	1.8	1.8	1.8	1.8
$30 < U \leq 60$	2.1	2.6	3.4	2.1
$60 < U \leq 110$	2.5	3.2	4.0	2.5
$110 < U \leq 175$	3.2	4.0	5.0	3.2
$175 < U \leq 275$	5.0	6.3	8.0	5.0
$275 < U \leq 420$	8.0	10.0	12.5	6.0
$420 < U \leq 550$	10.0	12.5	16.0	8.0
$550 < U \leq 750$	12.0	16.0	20.0	10.0
$750 < U \leq 1100$	20.0	25.0	32.0	14.0
$1100 < U \leq 2200$	32.0	36.0	40.0	30.0
$2200 < U \leq 3300$	40.0	45.0	50.0	36.0
$3300 < U \leq 4200$	50.0	56.0	63.0	44.0
$4200 < U \leq 5500$	63.0	71.0	80.0	50.0
$5500 < U \leq 6600$	80.0	90.0	100.0	60.0
$6600 < U \leq 8300$	100.0	110.0	125.0	80.0
$8300 < U \leq 11000$	125.0	140.0	160.0	100.0

(from BS/EN 50019)
1 = Material Group I has a CTI of at least 600
2 = Material Group II has a CTI of at least 400
3 = Material Group IIIa has a CTI of at least 175

While the above deals effectively with the situation where the insulating surface is even, as shown in Fig. 12.5, it does not adequately cover many normal situations where there are grooves in the insulation, or where there are ribs which separate conductors, both of which situations often occur in terminal blocks. In these circumstances, additional problems can sometimes occur. Grooves can be partially filled with dirt which may conduct, and ribs can act as barriers allowing dirt to build up in the right angle between themselves and the insulation. For these reasons, in all cases where ribs

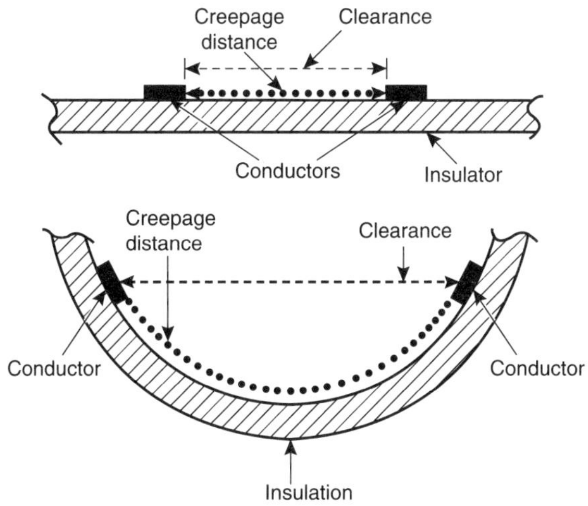

Fig. 12.5 Basic creepage distances and clearances

or grooves are used to increase creepage distances those distances will need to be larger than those which occur on flat insulation to give the same assurance of security. This is achieved by using the figures for the group of insulation with the adjacent lower CTI value to that in question for determination of minimum creepage distances. This means that for materials of Group I (CTI >600) with grooves or ribs, the minimum creepage distances will be taken from the column of Table 12.1 appropriate to insulating materials of Group II (CTI 400–600). This effectively excludes Group IIIa insulating materials where any grooves or ribs are used to enhance creepage distances. Such materials may of course, be used provided the added separation given by the rib height or the groove depth is ignored. Figure 12.6, 12.7 and 12.8 show how creepage distances are measured in the presence of grooves and ribs, and where fixing screws are included in grooves.

To be considered as a groove for the purposes of measuring creepage distances, a groove must be at least 2.5 mm deep and 2.5 mm wide if it has square sides and bottom. If it is not of such regular shape, however, as is the case when the bottom is, for example, radiused, then any part of the separation where the plane distance is less than 2.5 mm is ignored (see Fig 12.6). Where the voltage difference is such that less than 3 mm of creepage distance is required (approximately 150 V for materials of group 1 and 50 V for materials of Group II) the groove width may be reduced to 1.5 mm because of the lower level of criticality at such low voltages. Where such grooves contain screws, the situation is shown in Fig. 12.8, which shows the same effective considerations are applied.

To be considered as a rib for the purposes of measurement of creepage distances, the rib must be at least 2.5 mm high. The minimum thickness of a rib for this purpose is 1 mm, but any rib must be sufficiently rigid to avoid being pushed aside or damaged by any legitimate activity associated

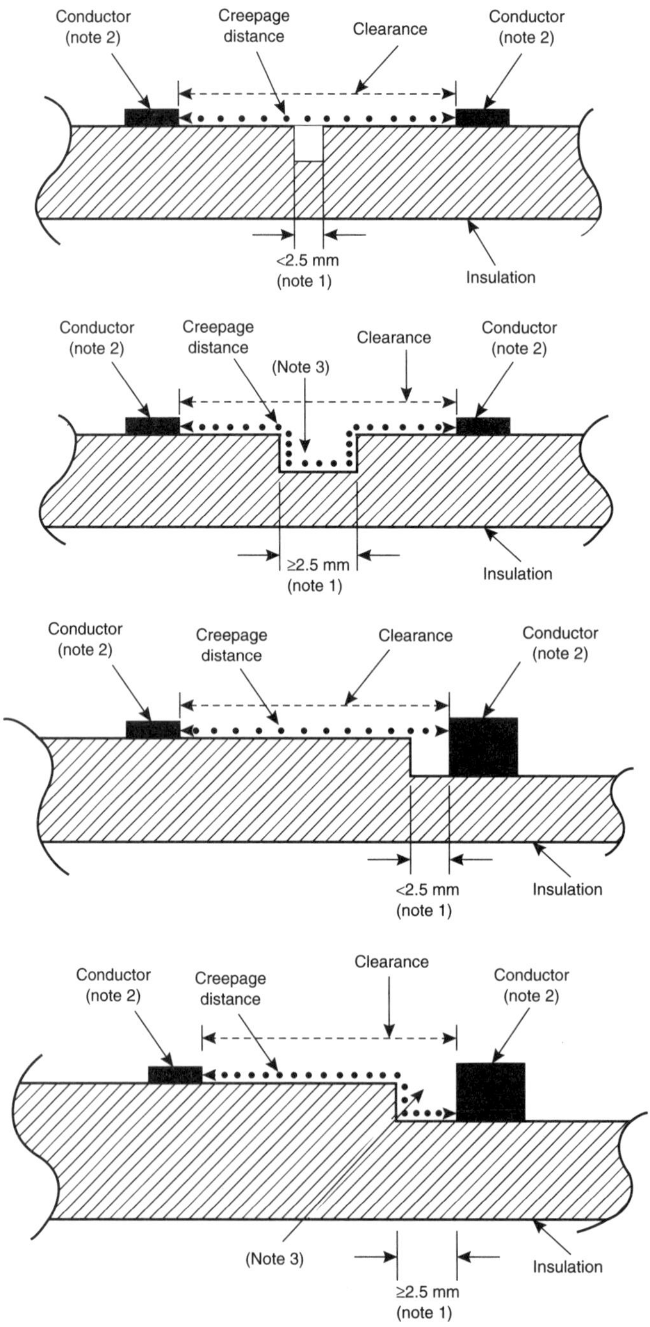

Fig. 12.6 Creepage distances and clearances in the case of slots (Figure continued on p. 305). *Notes*: (1) Where total creepage distance required is less than 3 mm this dimension may be reduced to 1.5 mm. (2) Conductors may be current conductors or isolated conduction, but see also Fig. 12.9. (3) Where the effective slot depth is less than 2.5 mm the slot is ignored for creepage distance measurement.

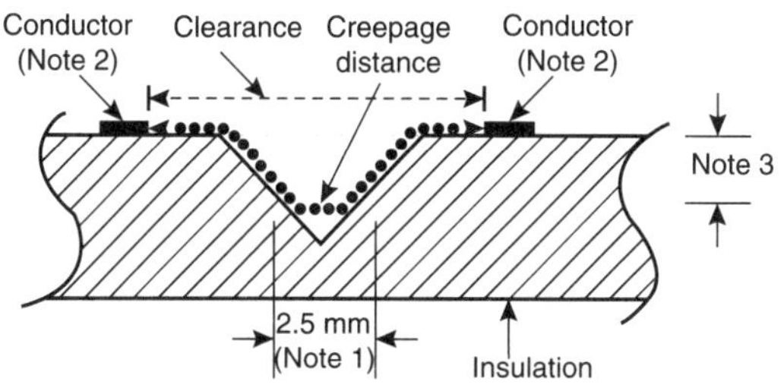

Fig. 12.6 (*continued*)

with the rib, such as terminating conductors. This does not mean that it must have similar strength to the enclosure, but that it must have adequate strength for the use to which it is put. Ribs may be either an integral part of the insulation moulding or may be cemented into the insulation, provided that the entire interface between the rib and the insulation is cemented. Where this is not so, the creepage distance will be assumed to be under the rib if this is shorter (see Fig. 12.7).

There are only two variations to the above. The first is where the conducting parts are associated with connection facilities for external conductors. In these cases there is an absolute minimum creepage distance and clearance of 3 mm. This is considered as the minimum necessary to ensure that connections can be made without risks of short circuit and is therefore a physical limitation.

The second variation relates to screw lamp caps and holders (the only type of lampholder/cap combination recognized as increased safety without having to be tested to ensure they do not transmit flame as a result of sparking during removal or fitting). In this case there are Standards already in existence governing their construction and those Standards give slightly different figures than is the case for increased safety equipment in general. To avoid having the necessity to develop a special series of lamp for screw lampholders, the different figures given in Table 12.2 are used for both the insulation on the screw cap of the lamp and in the lampholder. These are the figures from the appropriate industrial Standard and give sufficient confidence to be used without change in this case. The CTI of the insulation is, however, required to be of Group I.

To give some idea of the types of material falling into the various CTI levels Table 12.3 is included. This is for indication only and does not seek to be exhaustive, as many materials of a particular type can, if treated in certain ways, have a CTI quite different from that in the table. The table does, however, give some idea of the types of insulation to be sought for a particular use.

12.2.4 Insulation

Insulation within apparatus is basically of two types, namely that used on conductors and that used in such things as terminal blocks or as a layer

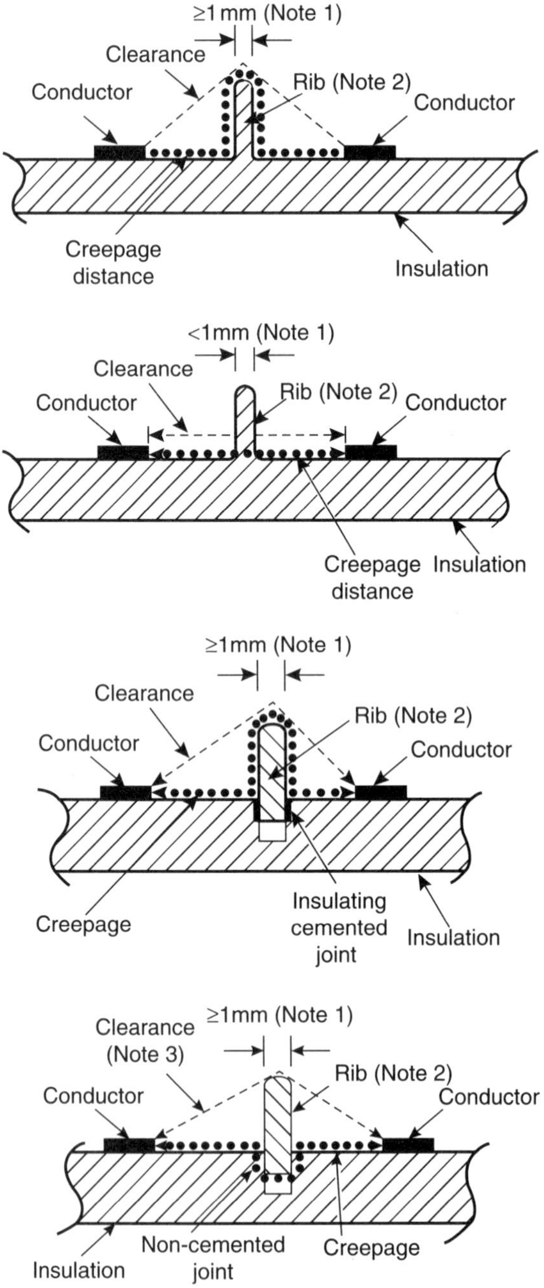

Fig. 12.7 Creepage distances and clearances in the case of ribs (continued on p. 307). *Notes*: (1) In addition to a minimum of 1 mm the rib must be sufficiently wide to be mechanically sound. (2) The rib must be 2.5 mm minimum height or it will be discounted and creepage distances and clearances measured directly across the horizontal surfaces. (3) If creepage distance is shorter than clearance then clearance will be measured under barrier and be equal to creepage distance.

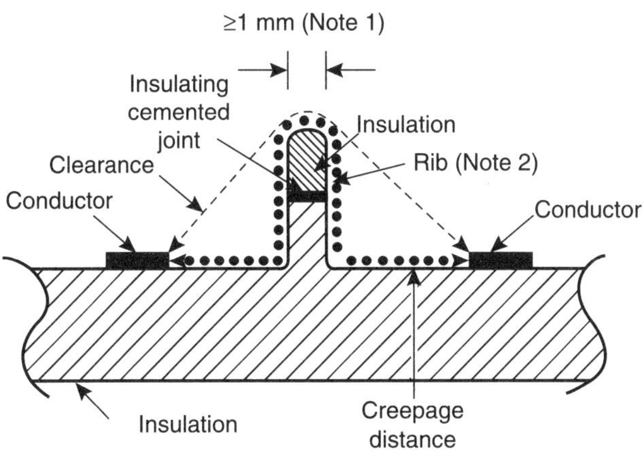

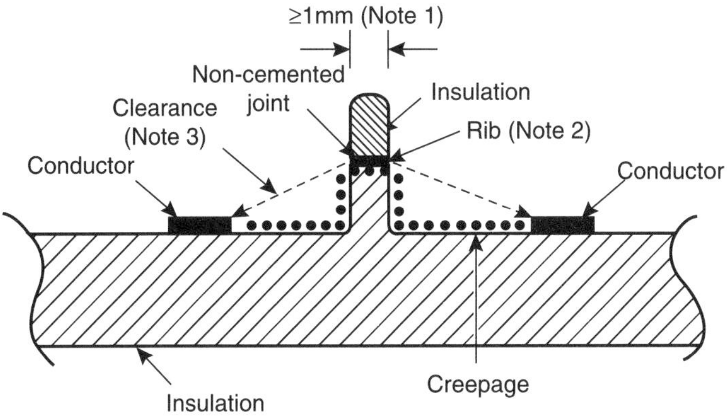

Fig. 12.7 (*continued*)

between conducting parts. With insulation used on conductors there is no special requirement for either the plastic or elastomeric insulation used on wires or varnishes which are typically used as insulation on winding wires when cured. All that is required is that they remain functional at the maximum temperature achieved in rated service (the service conditions specified which do not include faults). This means that their specified maximum operating temperature needs to be in excess of the maximum temperature which they achieve in the apparatus. Insulating parts, such as solid sheets and moulded blocks do, however, need a safety factor as they not only insulate but have a functional support role to play. They must remain viable at a temperature of at least 20 °C higher than the maximum temperature which they achieve in service, with a minimum upper temperature limit of 80 °C. The derivation of the 80 °C is fairly arbitrary but nonetheless reasonable as it coincides with the maximum operating temperature of such things as PVC and, because of this, excludes such materials as waxes, celluloid and shellac. It is important to note that

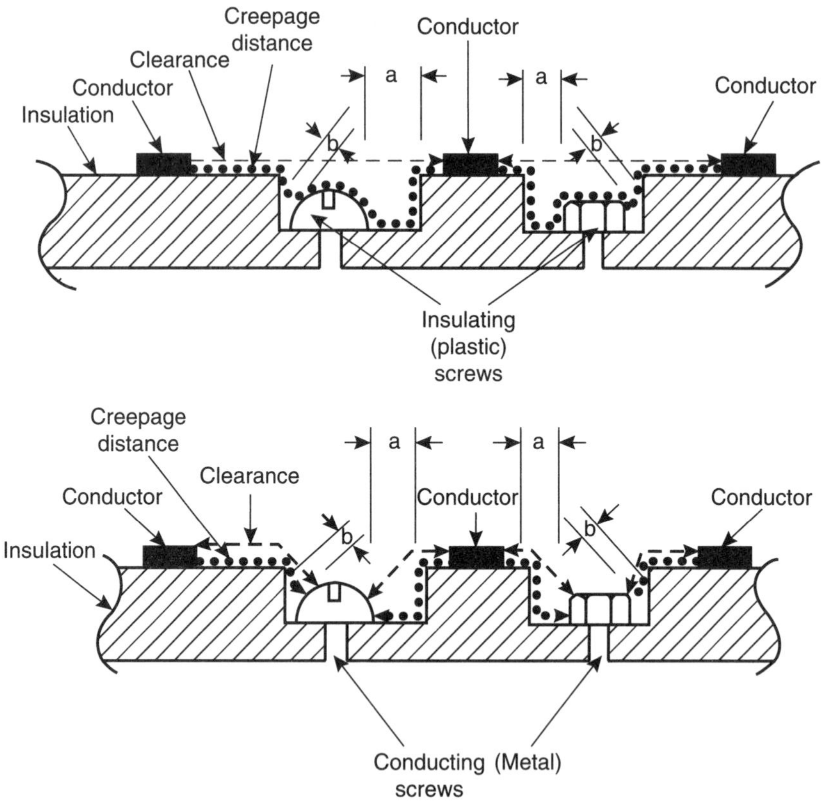

a = Separation equal to or greater than 2.5 mm (1.5 mm if total creepage distance required is equal to or less than 3 mm)
b = Separation equal to or less then 2.5 mm (or 1.5 mm if total creepage distance required is equal to or less than 3 mm)

Fig. 12.8 Effects of screws and bolts on creepage distances and clearances

Table 12.2 Creepage and clearance distances for screw lampcaps and lampholders with insulation having a CTI of ≤600

Working voltage V (rms)	Creepage distance and clearance (mm)
0< U ≤60	2
60< U ≤250	3

(from BS/EN 50019)
Note: For lamps of over 250 V Table 12.1 applies

Table 12.3 Typical CTI values for material families

Family of material	Approximate CTI limits
Polycarbonate (e.g., makrolon)	80–100
Phenolic laminates (e.g., tufnol)	80–150
Resin bonded materials (e.g., fibreglass)	100–140
Epoxides (e.g., PCB material)	150–300
Nylon (e.g., maranyl)	200–600
Polyvinyl Chloride (PVC)	300
Polystyrene	250–300
Polyesters (e.g., permaglass)	200–700+
Polyethylene	700+

if the CTI of solid insulation is reduced by machining or similar activities, the situation may be recovered by using coatings of varnishes, etc. with the required CTI. Such materials should not need to satisfy the 80 °C minimum limit as they do not carry out a supporting function.

12.2.5 Windings

Windings are recognized as a particular source of danger and have additional requirements applied. The wires of which they are made, if enamelled, need to comply with HD 555[11] which is an international specification for enamelled winding wires. They should comply with grade 2 of that Standard. They may also be acceptable if they only comply with grade 1 but, in addition, have breakdown voltages appropriate to grade 2 and satisfy an enhanced security requirement when breakdown tested. The detail of the additional requirements for grade 1 wires are given in BS/EN 50019. Wires not complying with HD 555 may be insulated with plastics or similar insulation or may be covered with insulating varnish. In all such cases, however, the insulation must be adequate for the voltage involved and there must be two complete layers of such insulation.

To avoid the risk of wire movement causing insulation failure, windings are normally required to be fully impregnated by a means which precludes the formation of voids within the assembly. For this reason, coating with impregnation material is not normally sufficient and a method such as vacuum impregnation is likely to be necessary. Where solvents are used to make the impregnation material fluid, the impregnation operation needs to be carried out at least twice, the second time to ensure that any voids created by the later evaporation of solvent after the first process, are filled. Variations to this requirement are possible in the case of windings which are intended for fitting into the slots of machines or similar locations and are not accessible after fitting. In these cases their impregnation, or suitable alternative insulation and consolidation procedure, may be carried out before fitting for windings operating above 1100 V rms Below this figure it is not considered likely that this problem will arise.

No wires of conductor diameters of less than 0.25 mm are considered sufficiently robust to be secure against breakage and such wires are not permitted for increased safety windings. This would exclude the windings of resistance thermometers which are often used to prevent the winding from overheating and this is not the intention. Therefore, resistance thermometers are absolved from the necessity of satisfying the size limitation. It should be noted, however, that the performance of such devices is affected by their proximity to the winding being protected and that they need to be effectively impregnated with the windings. This is especially so in the case of rotating machines where they need to be in the slots with the windings to ensure efficient operation.

While needing to comply with the basic requirement (i.e., that no part of the apparatus to which an explosive atmosphere has access may exceed the limiting temperature of the temperature class for the apparatus, and no part of the apparatus may exceed the maximum temperature for which its material and assembly is designed, even if the explosive atmosphere does not have access) there are further limits of temperature with which windings must comply to ensure reliability and these are given in Table 12.4. These need to be satisfied even when physical faults occur (e.g., a locked rotor in the case of a rotating machine), and if the winding alone cannot satisfy these requirements then the temperature sensing devices already referred to must, together with associated devices, ensure temperature limitation or electrical isolation so that the limits are not exceeded.

Table 12.4 Limiting temperatures for windings

Criteria and winding type measurement	Method of temperature measurement	Maximum winding temperature (°C)				
	(note 3)	Thermal material insulation class (notes 1 and 2)				
		A	B	E	F	H
Single layer windings. (maximum temp)	R or T	95	110	120	130	155
Other windings (maximum temp)	R	90	105	110	130	155
	T	80	95	100	115	135
Rotating machines (temp at t_e time)	R	160	175	185	210	235
	T	N/P	N/P	N/P	N/P	N/P

Notes:
1 Insulation classes in accordance with BS 2757.
2 These figures are included on a temporary basis pending the inclusion of figures in BS 2757.
3 R indicates measurement by the resistance thermometer method and T by the thermometer method. The thermometer method is not acceptable where the resistance thermometer method is usable and never for rotating machines

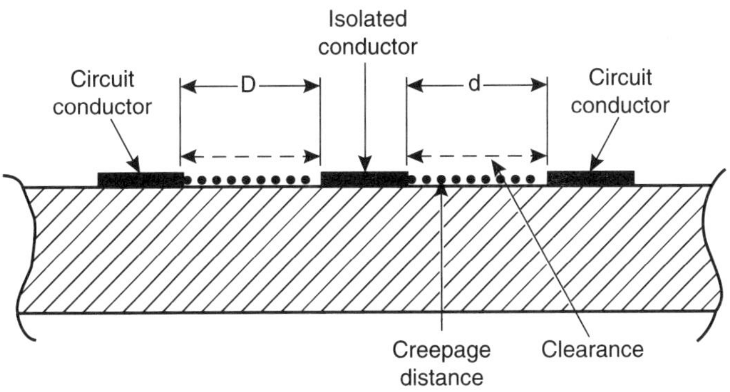

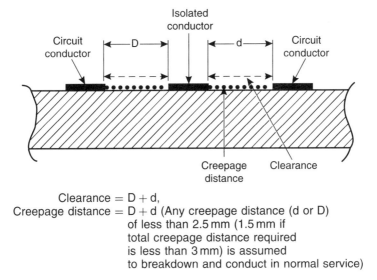

Clearance = D + d,
Creepage distance = D + d (Any creepage distance (d or D) of less than 2.5 mm (1.5 mm if total creepage distance required is less than 3 mm) is assumed to breakdown and conduct in normal service)

Fig. 12.9 Effect of isolated conductors on creepage distances and clearances

12.3 Additional requirements for specific types of apparatus

In addition to the basic requirements for increased safety already identified, there are specific variations necessary in the case of particular types of apparatus such as terminal enclosures, mains luminaires, cap lamps, measuring instruments including transformers, secondary batteries, electric heating apparatus, and rotating machines. Other specific types of apparatus may require additional specific constructional requirements but these are not specified in detail. The Standard (BS/EN 50019) requires that, where appropriate, the constructional requirements which follow should be applied to other types of apparatus in addition to the general constructional requirements necessary for increased safety as appropriate.

12.3.1 Terminal enclosures

It is normal to give a degree of flexibility to increased safety terminal boxes as to the number and types of terminals fitted. This can cause problems in that the connection of a wire to a terminal has a finite resistance, as does the amount of wire inside the enclosure. Wiring outside the enclosure may generally be ignored because of the enhanced cooling which is normally apparent in this case, but that within the enclosure cannot. Power will be dissipated in both internal conductor and terminal which will give rise to temperature elevation and, where several terminals are fitted in close proximity, adjacent terminals also have an effect. In addition, the ambient temperature in the enclosure will also be affected by the total internal power, which can be dissipated within the enclosure by all terminals and wiring therein. In order to determine the worst case for any terminal box it is therefore necessary to identify the worst terminal intended for use therein. This is the terminal which achieves the maximum surface temperature when connected to a conductor of its maximum specified size which has, inside the terminal, box a length equal to the diagonal dimension of the terminal box (e.g., 1.4 m for a 1 m × 1 m terminal box). The box is then fitted with the maximum number of such terminals of that type for which it is designed which are wired in series (see Fig. 12.10). As conductors within the box will often be loomed together, the conductors used for this purpose are loomed together, in sets of six and then the maximum rated current is then applied to the circuit produced. It is then necessary to identify the maximum temperature reached within the box and this will be the temperature which determines the temperature classification of the box. The power used in this evaluation can also be calculated once the wire and wire/terminal connection resistance is known, and this will then constitute the maximum power dissipation permitted for the box. When in service the box may then be used for any number of the worst case terminals or other less limiting terminals, provided the maximum power figure is not exceeded and no terminal operates at more than its rated current. The parameters of all intended terminals then need to be quoted so that the permissible combinations are easy to determine.

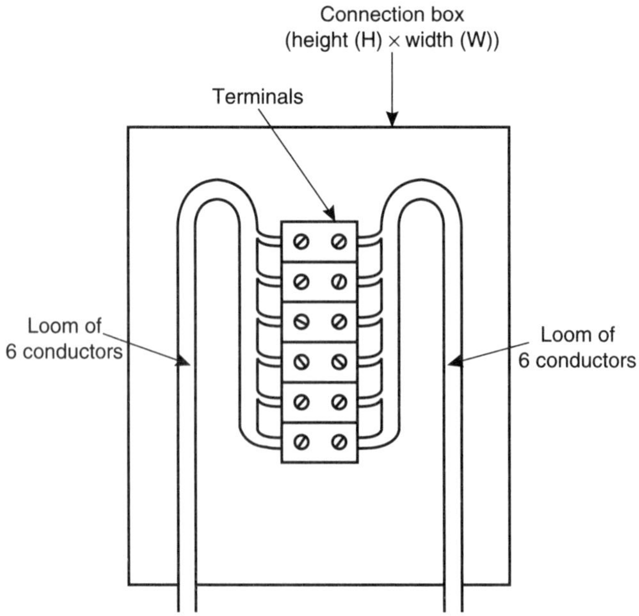

Fig. 12.10 Arrangement for temperature measurement in terminal enclosures. *Note*: Length of each conductor is half of diagonal box dimension ($\sqrt{H^2 + W^2}$) inside the box

As a result of this the temperature classification can be specified as either the classification achieved by specific combinations of terminals, or by any combination of specific types of terminal which together do not dissipate more than the specified power limitation.

12.3.2 Mains powered luminaires

Although it is obviously possible to utilize any type of lamp in which no temperature will be ignition capable, even that inside the lamp glass itself when the lamp is broken, this is not a real flexibility as most lamps have incandescent filaments or operate at high temperature and would not satisfy this requirement. The only type of lamp which will normally be acceptable in such circumstances is the cold cathode (fluorescent) type where internal temperatures are always within those limits. Other than that, the use of lamps must be very specific as breakage could lead to ignition, or specific constructional requirements exist in the case of such things as lamp connection arrangements. It is normally necessary to specify from the following list:

1. tungsten filament lamps in accordance with both BS 5971 (1988)[12] and BS 161 (1990);[13]
2. mixed light (tungsten and mercury fluorescent) lamps type MBTF. (These are high pressure types as the content of the lamp is lower than for low pressure (MTAF) lamps, thus reducing problems on breakage);
3. cold starting fluorescent lamps in accordance with EN 60061 (1993)[14] (this is not the same as IEC 61–1). It will be remembered from Chapter 10 that these lamps have a single pin for use in 'flameproof type' lampholders.

In general, all lamps and their lampcaps are required to form enclosures which, at the time of contact separation, pass the flame transmission tests specified for flameproof enclosures (see BS/EN 50018[13] and Chapter 10) or be arranged so that separation occurs in a separate flameproof enclosure complying with this standard prior to separation of the lamp contacts. This is not necessary if the connection is made by contacts which can be assumed to be non-sparking (e.g., multiple contacts with sufficient pressure), removal of the lamp is prevented while the luminaire is energized (e.g., by having an isolating switch interlocked with the outer cover of the luminaire), and ensuring that the lamp cannot work loose (e.g., by the use of a locking device to prevent unscrewing in the case of a screw lamp or to prevent end-cap float in the case of a fluorescent). While these latter situations are not specifically addressed in the case of luminaires, they are in the case of plugs and sockets and will be equally valid for luminaires. The main problem in their application is that the contacts made in a plug and socket which are not considered as sparking are made in two or more places by design. This is not normally the case in respect of lamps which usually only have one connection and do not lend themselves to this approach. It has, however, been used in the case of fluorescent tubes which have bi-pin bases and are normally used with hot cathodes. In these cases it has been shown that such tubes can work with cold cathodes and for the purposes of connection the endpins, connected as they are by a low resistance heater, can be effectively used in parallel to achieve the required security of connection, provided their lamp cap is modified to increase the security of connection.

In normal circumstances the above approach is not possible and it is necessary to allow for sparking on lamp disconnection. This is done either by using the lampcap/lampholder assembly as a sort of flameproof enclosure which needs to satisfy some or all of the requirements of BS/EN 50018 (See Chapter 10) which are specified for lampcap/lampholder combinations in clause 18 of that Standard, or by an arrangement so that the electrical circuit is broken in a separate flameproof enclosure (see Fig. 12.11) before

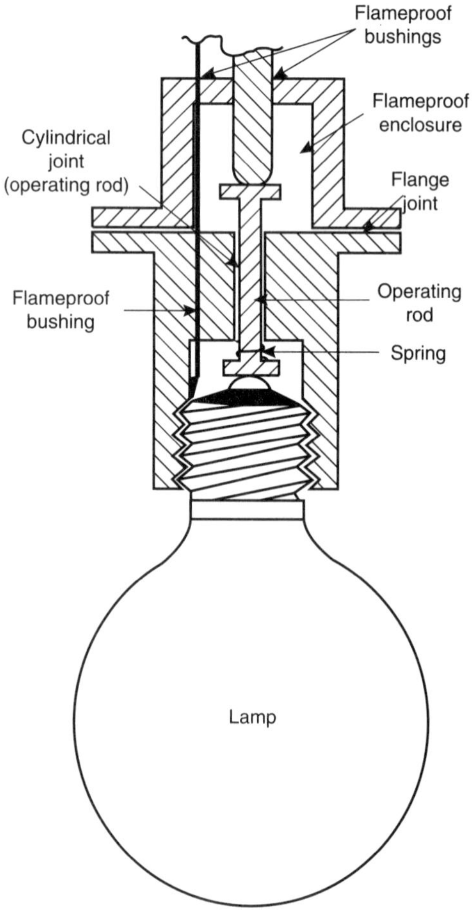

Fig. 12.11 Example of indirect lamp isolation. *Note*: If final connection to external supply is not within flameproof enclosure then it should be in an additional increased safety enclosure

the connection between the lampcap and lampholder is broken. In either case the assembly must be suitable for sub-group IIC.

In all cases the electrical connection to the lamp needs to be secure to ensure that no sparking occurs when the lamp is fully inserted. While this may be considered as too great a requirement, as the assembly is shown not to transmit flame, it must be remembered that there is a difference between occasional sparking during removal and continuous sparking due to loosening or bad contact. Security of contact is assured by one of the following means. First, the spring contacts used in the case of cylindrical pin contacts, such as those used in fluorescent tubes, need to have a contact force of 10 N when the lamp is fully engaged. Second, the spring contacts of cylindrical plug-in lamps, such as bayonet fitting lamps, need to have a contact force of 10 N when the bayonets are fully engaged. Third, in the case of screw caps, the end-spring contact should have a force of at least 15 N when the lamp is fully home and the thread contact should be made through at least two full threads or, alternatively, through spring side contacts having a force of 30 N. In cases where the lamp connection is broken in a separate flameproof enclosure during removal of the lamp from the lampholder, before the lamp contacts are broken, the minimum required force of any spring contact elements is reduced to 7.5 N.

There is a particular problem in the case of a screw lamp in that it is not normally positively secured against loosening, and as a result there needs to be some measure used to demonstrate its security against this problem. To achieve this a test may be applied. The lamp may be inserted into the lampholder with a specific torque and then unscrewed by 15°. The torque necessary to achieve further unscrewing must then be above a certain minimum value. Table 12.5 indicates the necessary torque values and the necessary security may, if desired, be achieved by the use of a locking device to prevent lamp removal.

Lamps (except those used in fluorescent fittings) are normally extremely hot and, to minimize the risk of the cover of the luminaire suffering damage due to heat and to allow good air circulation around the lamp, the separation between the lamp and luminaire cover needs to be above a

Table 12.5 Torque tests for screwed lamps

Lamp cap size	Insertion torque Newton Metres	Minimum removal torque Newton Metres
E10	see note	see note
E14	1.0 ± 0.1	0.3
E27	1.5 ± 0.1	0.5
E40	3.0 ± 0.1	1.0

(*from BS/EN 50019*)

Note: No test is considered as necessary for this small size of lamp.

specified minimum figure. This figure is given in Table 12.6 for all except fluorescent lamps. For fluorescent lamps, where there is less heat a more simple solution may be adopted and a 5 mm minimum is applied. This is further reduced to 2 mm where the cover is effectively an additional tube around the fluorescent tube.

Table 12.6 Separation between lamp envelope and cover

Lamp power (P) (Watts)	Minimum lamp/cover separation (mm)
0< P <60	3
60≤ P <100	5
100≤ P <200	10
200≤ P <500	20
500< P	30

(from BS/EN 50019)

The confined space inside luminaires has an effect upon the ignition of contained explosive atmospheres, probably due to processes such as convection, causing gas movement from hot parts of the luminaire to cooler parts resulting in causing heat loss. This effect can be used by filling a particular luminaire with the most easily ignited mixture of a particular flammable gas and air, and determining the lamp temperature at which ignition occurs. By this means a lamp can be permitted which exceeds the class, maximum for a given temperature class, provided its maximum temperature is 50 °C lower than the minimum ignition temperature measured for that luminaire and that explosive atmosphere. This relaxation is, however, only permitted where individual tests have proved its efficacy in particular luminaires, and the list of explosive atmospheres for which the relaxation is validated by tests in each case needs to be specified for the particular luminaire.

Many luminaires utilize control equipment (e.g., chokes, capacitors and starting arrangements) for fluorescent luminaires. These present specific problems which require attention, particularly as lamp failure (but not envelope fracture) is considered as normal operation.

In the case of fluorescent luminaires the following approach is usual. The normal switch starter which is used in fluorescent lamps contains a switch which, although usually hermetically sealed, is not acceptable in the type 'e' concept. To overcome this, type 'e' fluorescents are usually switchless (semi-resonant) starting. This is more expensive to use but removes the need for as starter. If a switch starter was to be used it would need to be flameproof (see Chapter 10) which would make it more expensive than the switchless-start approach and, for this reason, it is seldom used. Generally, when a fluorescent tube fails, the choke in the fitting will overheat. This is not acceptable in type 'e' as it could both cause the fitting to heat to above its temperature classification, and the choke itself to fail. Either would not be acceptable. In case of tube failure the choke must not heat either beyond its material rating or the fitting temperature classification. This can be achieved by choke design or by utilizing the increase in choke current when the lamp fails to operate electrical protection. Capacitors used in fluorescent fittings cannot comply with type'e' requirements because of their construction in having two layers of foil very close together, and therefore not being able to satisfy the separation requirements of type 'e'. To overcome this, such capacitors need to be otherwise protected. Typical ways in which this is done are to arrange the capacitor in a flameproof enclosure (see Chapter 10) or use powder filling (see Chapter 9).

12.3.3 Caplamps

These are normally battery-operated devices and have a separate battery pack. While increased safety is also used for lamps in such things as torches, it is not usual to use the technique in any but the most powerful of such devices, or in conjunction with another protection concept (e.g., intrinsic safety – see Chapter 13).

The requirements for caplamps are relatively simple as the lamps, if screwed in, are normally E10 or less, and so no insertion torque requirements exist. The lamp needs a protective cover and if this has less than a 50 cm^2 surface area, which is the more likely case, then all that is required is a guarding rim of at least 2 mm height. Should the surface area exceed this figure, however, a full guard satisfying BS/EN 50014[7] is necessary. The batteries need to satisfy the requirements of this protection concept or another (e.g., Intrinsic Safety – See Chapter 13) and the switch needs to either be interlocked to prevent its separation in a Hazardous Area or be otherwise protected (e.g., Flameproof – see Chapter 10).

12.3.4 Measuring instruments and transformers

The requirements for such devices of increased safety are aimed at voltage and current measuring devices, the latter using current transformers, and normal electrical voltage transformers. No electronic measuring devices are envisaged and, because of the fragility of connection springs, no moving coil devices are presumed to be capable of complying with the requirements for increased safety.

Normal voltage or current transformers need to comply with the requirements for windings and their temperature rise for selection of insulation grade, and temperature classification is determined at rated load. Their temperature rise may be limited by either an integral protective device or an external device, provided that, if external, the device is fully specified. Where the transformer load is external to the apparatus, the required degree of control cannot be exercised and the temperature rise, again with protective devices in circuit, is measured with the secondary short circuit in the case of voltage transformers, or open circuit in the case of current transformers also and, if a more adverse external condition can be identified, it must also be taken into account.

Where such transformers are within instruments and become 'instrument transformers' they must, additionally, withstand without damage 1.2 times their maximum-rated current or voltage. If deemed current transformers they must, in this case, be capable of suffering the thermal and dynamic stresses produced by the application of the specifically safety-factored currents I_{th} (a safety factored rms current used to determine thermal stresses and temperature rise) and I_{dyn} (a safety factored peak current for dynamic stress evaluation) given in Table 12.7. In the case of I_{dyn} two safety factors are used. The first is 1.25 and is intended to give a general safety factor for dynamic stresses with normal variations and the second is 2.5 and is intended to give an safety factor to allow for waveforms other than sinusiodal. I_{th} is the current used for determination of maximum operating temperature in these cases, and apart from that temperature having to be within the limit specified by the insulation and temperature classification, an overall limit of 200 °C is applied in these cases. It is possible that current transformers may exit a piece of apparatus, and in such cases it is necessary to identify this and ensure that users are aware of the need to prevent open circuits occurring.

Measuring instruments are similarly treated, in that they should be capable of withstanding 1.2 times their rated voltage or current indefinitely, and not exceed the maximum permissible temperature determined by

Table 12.7 Proof against damage by short circuit currents

Test current	Safety factors to be used as multipliers for determination of test current using short circuit current (I_{sc}) as a base	
	Basic safety factor	Safety factor for waveform variation
I_{th}(note 1)	1.1	1.0
I_{dyn}(note 2)	1.25	2.5

Notes:
1 I_{th} is the current to be used for temperature rise determination.
2 I_{dyn} is the current to be used for dynamic stress testing.
3. The maximum values of I_{sc} in any waveform configuration are I_{th} /1.1 rms and I_{dyn}/1.25 peak.

insulation requirements and temperature classification. They must also satisfy the thermal and dynamic stability requirements at I_{th} and I_{dyn} and the 200 °C overall limit.

These requirements are significantly different to those in BS 5501, Part 6[3] which were based on rated current, rather than short-circuit current and thus were less realistic. The figures in that Standard assumed that short-circuit currents were a maximum of 100 times rated-current rms for current transformers, reducing to 50 times for measuring instruments, and 250 times peak-rated current for current transformers, reducing to 125 times for measuring instruments. There was only a safety factor of 1 for I_{th} and 1.3 for I_{dyn} in these cases also. The more recent figures are therefore much more closely related to reality.

12.3.5 Secondary batteries

Batteries cannot be switched off like external power supplies and although batteries comprising both primary and secondary cells are permitted tacitly by the inclusion of cap lamps, there are specific additional requirements for batteries comprising secondary cells. However, the basic requirements of the protection concept apply to the external parts of all cells and batteries. In the case of batteries containing secondary cells there are several additional requirements, particularly because of the possibility of their regeneration capability by charging.

First, all secondary cells must be of the lead/acid, nickel/iron or nickel/cadmium type construction and no other chemical type of constructions are permitted. In addition, for larger batteries (if the battery comprised of secondary cells has a capacity of greater than 25 ampere hours when discharged at the 5 hour rate) several additional constructional requirements apply. The cells of these larger batteries need to reach a basic quality of construction to prevent short circuits caused by plate movements, electrolyte slurry build up and corrosion. To this end the following requirements need to be addressed:

1. The cell plates shall be positively secured to prevent movement, and constructed together with their lugs and busbars so as to prevent significant corrosion at lowest electrolyte level for the expected life of the cell.
2. Where it is necessary to top up an electrolyte from time to time, cells must have a clear indication of maximum and minimum levels of electrolyte acceptable.
3. Seals should be provided between each pole and the lid of the cell to prevent electrolyte leakage, and the cell lid should be sealed to the outer cell case for the same reason. There will also have to be sufficient volume inside the cell to ensure that expansion of electrolyte, due to expected heating, does not cause overflow of electrolyte from the filling plugs.
4. Filling plugs for electrolyte replenishment will need to be of a design which prevents ejection of electrolyte when the electrolyte in the cell

is within specification and the cell operating conditions are also within specification.

5. The space provided at the bottom of the cell should be sufficiently large to prevent build up of slurry from short circuiting the plates in the expected life of the cell.
6. The insulation between any poles and the outside of the cell container should have a resistance of at least 1 MΩ when the battery is new. If one pole is connected to the cell case and the insulation resistance between the outside of the cell case and that pole is less than 1 MΩ then it will be necessary to provide additional insulation in the battery container (as opposed to the cell container) to ensure that the pole is effectively insulated from other conducting parts using the 1 MΩ criterion.

A typical cell construction is shown in Fig. 12.12.

The containers of these larger batteries likewise have additional requirements applied to them and these are basically as follows:

1. Battery containers may be of metal or plastics, or indeed other suitable materials, provided they produce a rigid container and, where of conducting material, are manufactured with their internal surfaces fitted with bonded insulating material to ensure cell insulation. This applies to

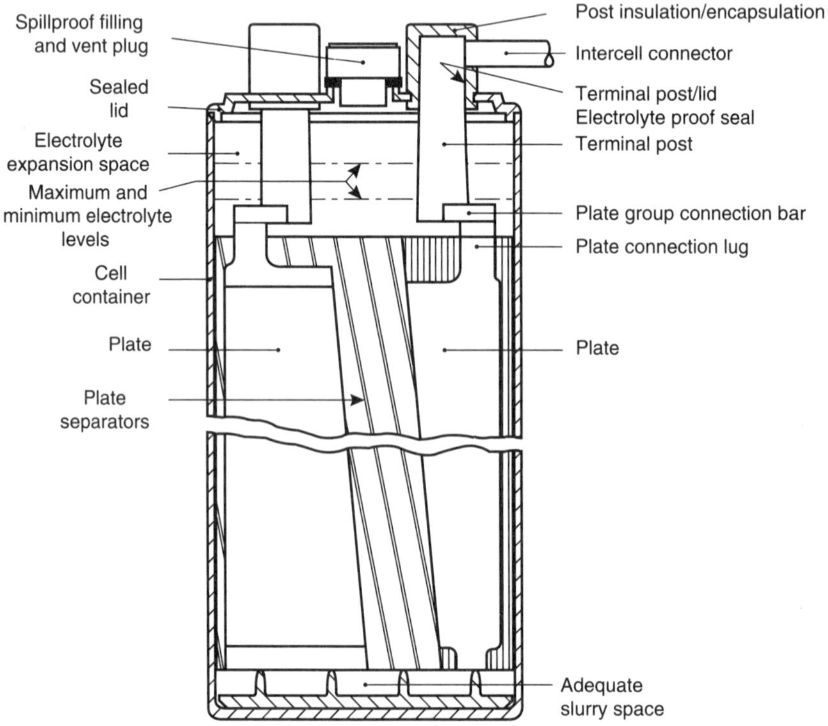

Fig. 12.12 Typical increased safety cell construction

covers also but here it is sufficient to use insulating paint because of the lower likelihood of contact with cells.

2. Battery containers need to be of sufficiently strong construction to withstand any mechanical stress to which they may be subjected in service, and must be resistant to attack by the cell electrolyte. To achieve the necessary strength, partition walls may be fitted between cells but must be insulated in the same way as the enclosure, the lid relaxation not being appropriate here.
3. Insulating barriers (which may be insulated partition walls) need to be fitted to ensure that no section of the battery in one compartment of the enclosure exceeds 40 V. (This is a very common limitation often also used in normal batteries to prevent significant electric shock). The height of these insulating barriers needs to be at least two thirds of the cell height and the creepage distances necessary between conducting parts (described in Table 12.1) must not utilize any distances around slots produced by such barriers, whatever the dimensions of the slot (the creepage distances must be line of sight).
4. The creepage distance between poles of adjacent cells (the connection points) and between these poles and the battery container (insulated or otherwise) need to be at least 35 mm where the voltage between the poles is 24 V or less, and this distance needs to be increased by 1 mm for every 2 V by which this voltage exceeds 24 V. These distances are to ensure safe connecting and disconnecting.
5. No single container or part of a container separated from other parts of an insulated barrier, as already described, must contain sufficient cells to permit the voltage in that container or section to exceed 40 V immediately the voltage has stabilized after charging.
6. Battery enclosures may have a lower ingress protection limit than normal enclosure to permit dispersion of any gas produced during charging and IP23 to BS/EN 60529 is the lower limit. The enclosure must, however, be sufficiently well ventilated to ensure that when the maximum amount of hydrogen is released from the cell vent plugs, the general atmosphere within the battery box does not exceed 2 per cent hydrogen. This can be shown by releasing hydrogen from the vent plug of each cell at a rate determined by the formula;

$$H_2 \text{ rate } = \text{cell capacity (A H)} \times 5 \times 10^{-6} \text{ m}^3/\text{hr}$$

Battery containers should also allow any liquid which collects within them for whatever reason to drain away. This will not normally be acid as the acid is contained in a manner which should prevent release. If this cannot easily be done then the container should be arranged so that the liquid can be removed without disturbing the cells. This latter approach is. however, not ideal as it requires regular inspection of the container in service to ensure that no liquid has collected, and a removal procedure where it has.

The connections between cells and between the battery and the remainder of the apparatus also needs to meet specific requirements to ensure freedom from sparking and inadvertent contact. All cell connectors must be capable of carrying the maximum current which could flow without overheating and, if the maximum current cannot be specified, they must carry the current from the battery which relates to that flowing in a one hour discharge situation. Connectors also need to be protected from the possibility of corrosion by electrolyte (e.g., this will mean that they will need coating with lead for lead/acid batteries). In addition, connectors need to be insulated to avoid inadvertent electrical contact when the container lid is removed.

Where flexible connections are used they may be welded or soldered on to the cell terminal posts, provided the precautions required for general soldered joints are applied in that case, or, where copper conductors are used, they may be crimped into a copper terminal post or terminal screwed to a terminal post. In the latter case, the connection to the terminal post must have at least the same contact area as the conductor connection.

Where plugs and sockets are used to connect the battery to the remainder of the apparatus they do not need to comply with the general specifications for plugs and sockets, provided they can only be separated by a tool and are not intended to be separated in the hazardous area. It is worthy of note here that all of the foregoing requirements are not sufficient to cover the recharging situation and thus it is assumed that batteries are not recharged in a hazardous area.

12.3.6 Heating devices

Increased safety heating devices may be heating resistance elements such as cartridge heaters, heating cables which are protected by design in that at maximum voltage the heater cannot exceed a particular temperature in service unless a fault occurs, heating cables which have temperature control devices to limit the temperature and self-limiting heating cables and tapes. Thus the heating is by defined apparatus, and not by merely applying a current to the process fluid or pipeline and using its resistance to create the heating effect or by production of eddy currents.

The basic heating element which may be a resistance (and here the requirements for windings are not applied to such resistances) or a resistance cable wound round the object to be heated will normally continue heating until equilibrium is reached. The temperature achieved will be that of the heater outside insulation at the insulation/heated object interface and, if this can exceed the heater materials operating limits or permit the required temperature classification to be exceeded, a device to prevent this needs to be fitted. Such a device must not perform a normal temperature control function, and if normal temperature control is necessary a separate device must be used. The heater temperature rise is obviously affected by its mode of use, and the required mode of use must be specified in all cases including such things as the temperature of its surroundings including the workpiece, any flowing fluid, etc., and the heat transfer characteristics of the heater. Protective devices need to either sense the temperature of the heater or its immediate surroundings, the temperature plus other conditions such as flow in heated pipes, etc., or sense parameters other than temperature which have significant bearing on temperature. The objective is always to prevent the temperature class being exceeded and the material of construction of the heater from exceeding a temperature of 20 °C less than the limiting temperature for that material. Heater insulating materials must prevent access of the explosive atmosphere to the heater elements and therefore quartz, sand and similar materials will not be suitable.

As a result of their nature most resistance heating cables, and some units, may be subjected to mechanical stress particularly during insulation. To ensure their suitability these devices are subjected to being crushed by a steel rod of 6 mm diameter with a 1500 N force applied and subjected to being bent through 90° on the mandrel shown in Fig. 12.13 at its lowest operating temperature. These actions should not damage either the heater or its insulation. Devices intended for use under water or other liquids will also be tested immersed to ensure that no leakage occurs.

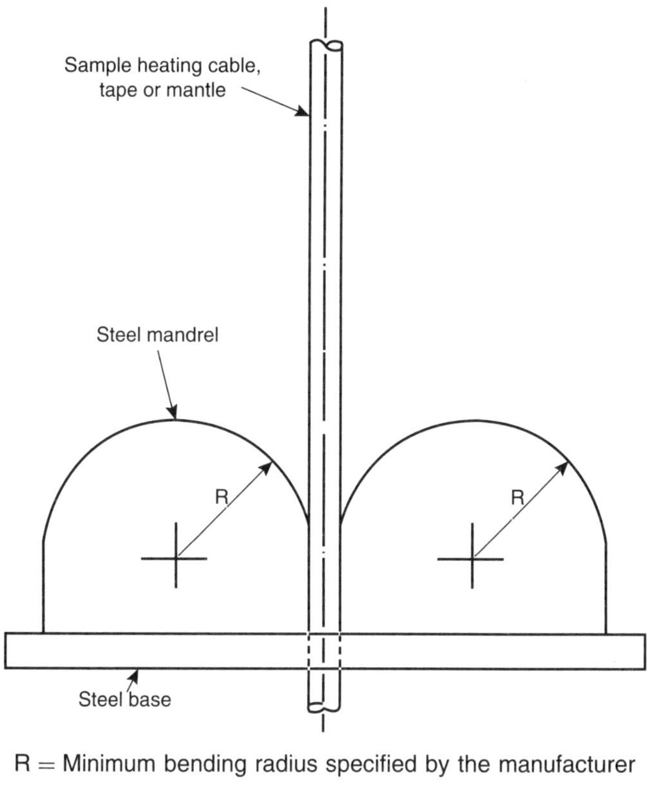

Fig. 12.13 Test apparatus for resistance heat devices subject to bending stresses in service

Increased safety heating devices are, as all other increased safety devices, based upon the fact that the enhanced constructional requirements make failure very unlikely and if failure does occur then isolation follows rapidly. Heating devices, and heating cables particularly, cover fairly large areas and the most suitable type of electrical protection for insulation failure is the residual current circuit breaker, ideally one which operates at a leakage current of 30 mA although operating currents up to 300 mA are acceptable. The rate of operation of the device is, however, important given that the failure of insulation may be in the hazardous area and a maximum of 5 s at minimum rated operating current falling to 0.15 s at five times that current is required. These are, of course, not usable where the supply is IT (its neutral is connected to earth at source through an impedance) and in such cases (which are unusual in the UK) an insulation monitor is necessary. This monitor should operate when the insulation falls to less than 50 Ω/V of rated voltage (e.g., 12,500 Ω at 250 V rated supply voltage).

Wires connecting the heating elements to the device terminals need to exceed 1 mm to ensure reliability and, where the heating device is covered with a conducting sheath to assist in operation of earth fault devices, the sheath should have a significantly lower resistance than the heater to ensure it does not produce additional heating unless it is prevented from so doing by the over temperature protective device. The conductive covering must also extend over at least 70 per cent of the heater surface to ensure correct operation.

12.3.7 Rotating machines

Rotating electrical machines, together with terminal boxes, constitute the most common use for increased safety as the construction of the machine is much easier than its flameproof counterpart and the resulting machine is much lighter. There are problems, however, since the machines include bearings and relative movement of parts is likely. As this could lead to such problems as stator/rotor clashes, the construction must try to minimize their possibility. In addition, machines operate at much greater currents during starting and the possibility of ignition from such devices must take account of several different conditions.

Increased safety machines are generally induction machines with squirrel cage rotors as, with this construction, there is no necessity for electrical connections to the rotor which are not possible within the concept of increased safety. Increased safety machines with wound rotors which are permanently short circuited are also possible but, in general, when a machine rotor is wound electrical connections to that rotor are operationally required for such reasons as limiting of starting torque and speed control (by control of slip). In these cases, the connections to the rotor are by rotating spring contacts or brushes which constitute sparking contacts and are not possible in the increased safety context. Where these are present, therefore, they need to be protected by another protection concept and are usually flameproof giving a composite form of protection to the machine.

Rotor/stator clearances

The first necessity is to prevent rotor/stator clashes as far as possible in all operating conditions, and the stresses created by those conditions. This is done by specifying a minimum clearance between rotor and stator when the machine is at rest which is the worst case as any 'sag' of the rotor, due to its mass, will be present. This minimum clearance is derived from a formula which at first glance appears complex and is as follows:

$$\text{Air gap} = \{0.15 + [D - 50/780][0.25 + (0.75 \times n/1000)]\} \quad \text{mm}$$

where D = rotor diameter in mm (subject to a minimum of 75 mm and a maximum of 750 mm)
n = machine speed in revs/min (frequency × 50/pole pairs per phase)

The above figure is multiplied by a figure derived from core length (mm)/1.75 × core diameter (mm) where this exceeds 1 and further multiplied by 1.5 where sleeve, rather than rolling element bearings, are used. This calculation looks much more complex than that used in the first edition of the European Standard (BS 5501, Part 6) but, in effect, does not significantly affect the clearance requirements, giving on average a figure which is lower than the figure which would previously have been necessary but normally within around 10 per cent of that figure.

Insulation of stator and rotor conductors

The normal insulation requirements apply to both stators and wound rotors but, in the case of machines, the magnetic stresses will mean that special attention must be given to ensuring the security of windings to prevent insulation damage due to movement. Where squirrel cage rotors are used the rotor bars are not insulated from the rotor magnetic base and, in addition to the necessity to ensure secure interconnection between the bars themselves, the contact between the bars and the rotor core needs to be extremely firm to ensure that sparking does not occur between rotor bars and between rotor bars and the core, particularly during starting when stresses are at their maximum. To achieve this the squirrel cage including its end rings, is normally either cast as a single unit or the rings and bars are brazed or welded together. Their tightness of fit in the rotor slots is achieved by casting them in the slots with aluminium but supplementary slot lining, wedging or keying are also acceptable methods. Figure 12.14 shows a typical simple squirrel cage.

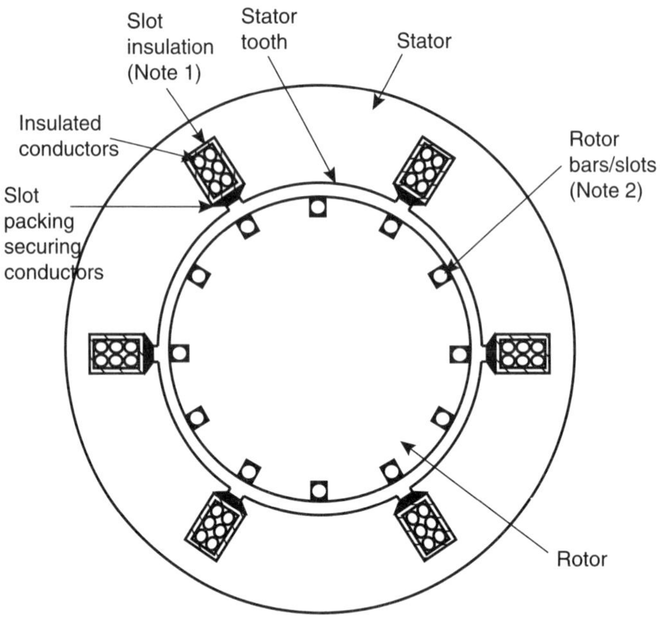

Fig. 12.14 Typical three-phase squirrel cage machine. *Notes*: (1) Stator temperature limiting devices fitted inside slot insulation at rear of slot. These need to be adequately insulated themselves. (2) Rotor bars secured in slots by conductive packing or aluminium casting

Machine temperatures

No temperature within the machine should exceed either the maximum temperature for the temperature class or the limiting temperature for the materials used in the machine, and there is an overall upper limit of 300 °C even if these figures exceed that temperature. The conditions which need to be taken into account are starting and running under full load with recognized overloads, including locked rotor conditions. With a normal machine such as a squirrel cage machine there is no way of measuring the rotor temperature in service, and temperature limitation must be achieved by detecting the stator temperature or monitoring the current drawn by the machine, the relationship between the stator and rotor temperature being confirmed in the design of the machine.

For machines which are only started infrequently and do not have arduous starting conditions (e.g., being started on full load for instance) temperature control can be achieved by a normal direct on-line starter with a thermal overload release device (inverse time delay overload protection). This is acceptable provided the device not only monitors starting current and disconnects if this is excessive, but also disconnects the machine if the rotor is stalled, before the temperature of any part of the machine exceeds the maximum temperature of operation of the insulation, or the temperature class limit is reached. This latter is achieved by measurement of the time taken for the machine to reach the limiting condition if, when it has been operating at its maximum ambient temperature and at rated load until its temperature has stabilized, the rotor is stalled. This time is called the t_e time (see Fig. 12.15.). Because of the possible rate of rise of temperature in the stalled rotor condition, minimum figures are set for this time dependent upon the ratio of stalled (starting) current (I_a) to rated running current at full load (I_n) and these are shown in Fig. 12.16. Reduction of t_e time is only possible if it can be shown that the particular protective device used isolates the machine within the time specified, and in no circumstances is a t_e time of less than 5 secs considered as acceptable because of the rate of temperature raise which this infers. The specification of t_e time is not necessary where a machine is protected by thermal sensing devices in the stator windings which isolate the machine before the limiting temperature is reached.

Where a machine is subjected to arduous starting conditions, either by being started on full load or at regular intervals (duty cycle operation), it is considered that only temperature sensing within the stator is acceptable as a means for temperature limitation because the temperature rise is at its greatest or the machine is already at elevated temperature when started. In these circumstances, t_e time is not relevant. The inclusion of sensing elements in stator windings must, of course, satisfy the requirements for temperature sensors in windings in general. A method of determination of what are called arduous conditions in relation to starting load (but not duty cycling) is to determine the time for the machine to reach full speed. This should not exceed 1.7 t_e. Duty cycling is where a machine is started

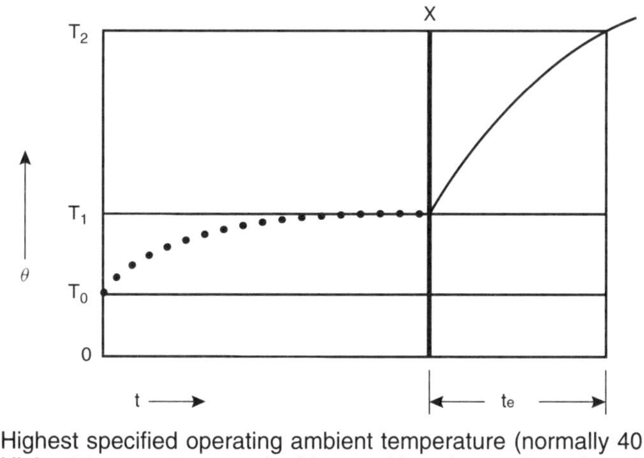

T_0 = Highest specified operating ambient temperature (normally 40 °C),
T_1 = Highest temperature reached by machines in rated service at T_0,
T_2 = Limiting temperature,
θ = Temperature,
t = Time
t_e = t_e time
X = Rotor stall point

Fig. 12.15 t_e time determination

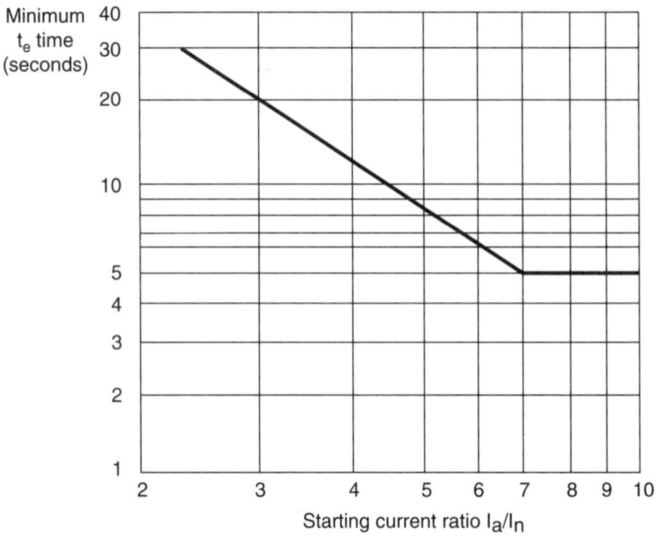

Fig. 12.16 Minimum permissible t_e times for I_a/I_n ratios *Note*: Minimum acceptable t_e time in any case is 5 second

regularly as part of its designed use and such repeat startings are likely to occur where the machine, after stopping, is likely to be restarted before it has cooled to ambient temperature. Such a cooling time is often in excess of one hour and to be secure, any machine which is started more frequently than once every two hours should be assumed to be on a duty cycle.

Starting/stalled rotor current

As a final requirement it is not acceptable for any machine to have a stalled rotor (starting) current of more than ten times its full load running current as again this would indicate a very high rate of temperature rise.

Discharges in rotating machines

Notwithstanding these requirements, there has been considerable concern expressed at the use of increased safety machines, particularly those operating at high voltages because of several ignitions of explosive atmospheres by such machines under starting conditions. Work carried out by ERA Technology Ltd[15] at the behest of the Health and Safety Executive showed that there was a real risk of ignition due to sparking in both the rotor and the stator. The sparking occurring in the stator end windings in starting conditions is, in many cases, ignition capable and this has led the Health & Safety Executive to issue a warning[16], against the use of machines operating at line voltages in excess of 3000 V. Investigations into this problem are ongoing but it would be wise to consider the alternative of flameproof machines at least for those operating at more than 3000 V until this problem has been fully resolved. It may, of course, be wise to use only flameproof machines for all installations until resolution of the problem as the current understanding of it is not complete.

12.3.8 Other types of apparatus

Increased safety is in principle applicable to other types of apparatus than those discussed. To apply it, however, the apparatus must be fully specifiable and the requirements used will need to be chosen from those basic requirements appropriate to the type of equipment and those appropriate from the additional requirements for the types of apparatus discussed. It is not possible to apply increased safety to apparatus using semiconductor and similar devices as these do not have clearly defined physical design criteria to which increased safety could be applied.

The heating of rotating machines is also affected by their supply waveform. While this is not normally a problem, as the waveform is that of the supply, it can become so in the case of variable speed machines. These are often run from inverters which generate ac at a varying frequency to achieve speed variation. The output of these devices is not nearly so predictable as normal mains supplies and they often contain significantly more harmonic content (which does not assist the drive but dissipates heat in the machine). Where such invertors are used with increased safety machines therefore, the machines must be shown to retain their increased safety properties when used with the particular inverter in question. It is important to note that the particular type of inverter used is not just one of the same range, or a similar one.

References

1 IEC 79-7	Electrical Apparatus for Explosive Gas Atmospheres. Part 7 (1969) Increased Safety.
2 BS 4683	Specification for Electrical Apparatus for Explosive Atmospheres. Part 4 (1973) Type of Protection 'e'.
3 BS 5501	Electrical Apparatus for Potentially Explosive Atmospheres. Part 6 (1977). Increased Safety 'e'
4 BS/EN 50019 (1994)	Electrical Apparatus for Potentially Explosive Atmospheres. Increased Safety 'e'.
5 BS/EN 60529 (1989)	Specification for Degrees of Protection Provided by Enclosures (IP Code).
6 BS 4999	General Requirements for Rotating Electrical Machines. Part 105 (1988) Classification of Degrees of Protection Provided by Enclosures for Rotating Machinery.

7 BS/EN 50014 (1992) Electrical Apparatus for Potentially Explosive Atmospheres. General Requirements.

8 BS/EN 50018 (1995) Electrical Apparatus for Potentially Explosive Atmospheres. Flameproof Enclosure 'd'

9 BS 2757. (1986) Method for Determining the Thermal Classification of Electrical Insulation.

10 BS 5901 (1980) Method of Test for Determining the Comparative and Proof Tracking Indices of Solid Insulating Materials Under Moist Conditions.

11 HD 555 (1992) Specification for Particular Types of Winding Wires. Part 3, Polyester Enamelled Round Copper Wire, Class 155. Part 7, Polyimide Enamelled Round Copper Wire, Class 200. Part 8, Polyesterimide Enamelled Round Copper Wire, Class 180.

12 BS 5971. (1988) Specification for Safety of Tungsten Filament Lamps for Domestic and Similar General Lighting Purposes.

13 BS 161 (1990) Specification for Tungsten Filament Lamps for Domestic and Similar General Lighting Purposes. Performance Requirements.

14 EN 60061–1 (1993) Lamps and Holders Together with Gauges for the Control of Interchangeability and Safety. Part 1, Lampcaps Part 2, Lampholders.

15 92–0474 The Incendivity of Electrical Discharge Activity in Rotating Electrical Machines. ERA Report, Bartels, A.L. and Bradford, M.

16 HSE 498/12 (1992) High Voltage Types Ex 'N' and Ex 'e' Explosion Protected Motors Operating in Potentially Explosive Atmospheres. HSE Information Document.

13

Apparatus and systems using protection concept intrinsic safety 'i'

(BS/EN 50020 – Apparatus)

(BS 5501, Part 9 – Systems)

Intrinsic safety is unique among the protection concepts in its mode of operation. All other concepts rely on prevention of sparking and hot surfaces, the exclusion of explosive atmospheres from such ignition sources, or containment of any explosion produced. Intrinsic safety is quite different in that no attempt is made to prevent sparking and no attempt is made to exclude explosive atmospheres. Safety is achieved by limiting the power and energy (apart from limited cases where stored energy is concerned and specific measures are taken to prevent or limit its rate of release as a spark or arc) in the hazardous area to levels below those which can cause ignition.

As hydrogen, for example, can be ignited by around 20 μJ in ideal circumstances the energy fed to and used in a hazardous area is severely limited and intrinsic safety is only really practicable for such things as intelligence gathering, analysis, and limited operating functions. The technique depends, almost uniquely, on the effective limitation of the energy which can be fed to a hazardous area, as well as the performance of the apparatus in the hazardous area itself. It is therefore, a 'system concept', where the detail of the apparatus in the hazardous area, in a non-hazardous area with which it is interconnected, and the means of interconnection are equally important in achieving safety. Likewise, because it acts by limiting available energy and restricting storage or release of stored energy, it relies on the circuits within the apparatus themselves, rather than applying enclosures or other additional means to achieve safety. This has the advantage of freeing the apparatus from the limitations produced in many of the other types of protection (i.e., if sparking which occurs is not ignition capable, the isolation required in other types of protection for connection/disconnection purposes becomes unnecessary). It does, however, make the protection concept somewhat more complex in construction and use. Notwithstanding this, the advantages far outweigh the complexity problems as evidenced by the fact that all normal installations in Zone 0 and almost all instrument installations in Zone 1 are intrinsically safe. Its use in Zone 0 is significant as no other standard protection concept is accepted as a matter of normal practice in Zone 0. This is because, by its nature, the level of security in an intrinsically safe system can be varied depending upon the hazardous area risk, so that in Zone 0 (where the risk is greatest) the level of security can be increased to a much higher level than is possible for any of the other single standard types of protection.

Intrinsic safety is second only to flameproof enclosure (Chapter 11) in age, having been developed in the coalmining industry to cover the simple signalling systems used in that industry (typically, leclanche cell/bell circuits) which were suspected of causing ignition in at least two explosions, one of which was the worst which ever occurred in the UK.

13.1 The situation in respect of standardization

Although used widely in the UK for such things as signalling systems, public address systems, solenoid valves and sensors, no definitive National Standard existed until 1977, probably because the applications prior to that date were relatively simple. A British Standard, BS 1259,[1] had existed from 1958 but was significantly lacking in detail and with the rapid expansion of the use of the protection concept for reasons described earlier, there was a significant lack of detailed constructional requirements by the late 1960s. Because a European Standard was being produced it was not considered as appropriate to produce a National Standard and this resulted in EECS/BASEEFA,[2] being the only national certification/approvals body in the UK at that time, producing their own document, SFA 3012,[3] in 1972 which remained in force until the publication of the European Standard as BS 5501, Part 7[4] in 1977 (the UK publication of EN 50020.[5]) Thus, from the rapid increase of the use of the protection concept which came on the heels of the equally rapid introduction of the transistor to replace the thermionic valve, and the equally rapid expansion of the requirements for sophisticated monitoring and control of complex processes, until the publication of SFA 3012[3], arbitration on what was intrinsically safe had to be by EECS/BASEEFA[2] against essentially unpublished rules. A similar situation existed elsewhere and the Physicalisch Technische Bundesanstalt (PTB[6]) in Germany had a similar role. SFA 3012 was not produced by EECS/BASEEFA in isolation but was derived from an International Standard being produced by the International Electrotechnical Commission (IEC[7]) as IEC 79-11[8]. This document was also used as a basis for BS 5501, Part 7[4] by the European Standards body CENELEC[9].

Even so, the technology of intrinsic safety was still very much in its infancy in the new more complex scenario which ensued where semiconductors were applied causing many discussions and developments in BS 5501, Part 7, as witnessed by the number of papers and articles produced in journals and at conferences on the subject and the discussion which these led to. All of this discussion produced rapid development of the protection concept and led to interpretive documents which were issued in the UK to clarify problems encountered with the application of BS 5501, Part 7 – some 38 between 1981 and 1992. These interpretation sheets, together with those produced by other CENELEC member countries, resulted in the publication by CENELEC of no less than eight amendments to the Standard and 20 interpretation sheets to clarify the meaning of the Standard – a far higher number than for any of the other European Standards in the range. All of these amendments and interpretations are now included in BS/EN 50020 (1995),[10] the second edition of the European Standard. (An interpretation sheet does not amend a Standard but only clarifies its meaning, unlike an amendment which may do either or both).

BS/EN 50020[10] and its predecessor, BS 5501, Part 7[4] carry specifications for intrinsically safe and associated apparatus only. As already noted, the protection concept is unique in that it is a system concept and it is necessary to determine the safety of a system in all cases. Because of the complexity involved this cannot be done by an installation Code in all cases, and a further European Standard exists to define how items of apparatus and interconnecting cabling can be combined to form intrinsically safe systems. This is BS 5501, Part 9 (1982).[11]

13.2 Basic application of the concept

As previously stated, intrinsic safety is a system concept relying for its security upon the detailed design of both the apparatus in the hazardous area, the apparatus in the non-hazardous area which is interconnected with it, and the interconnections between the two. This is unlike most other forms of protection where only the electrical protection circuits in the non-hazardous area are important as, in those protection concepts, the apparatus in the hazardous area is designed to maintain safety or minimize danger during isolation which automatically follows an equipment failure. There are, therefore, several elements which need to be considered when defining an intrinsically safe system.

13.2.1 Intrinsically safe apparatus

This is defined as 'Apparatus in which all the circuits are intrinsically safe'. This apparatus is intended for installation in a hazardous area and will be designed so that, when fed from appropriate apparatus (associated apparatus) in a non-hazardous area (associated apparatus) it will not produce incendive arcs, sparks or hot surfaces, either when it is operating normally or when faults occur in the electrical circuits and components within it and its interconnecting cables. The use of faults within the apparatus and its interconnecting cables is the method by which it derives its level of safety. These circuit or component faults have a particular statistical likelihood of occurrence and (as when one has occurred the likelihood of another independent fault occurring is considerably lower) the overall security of the apparatus is determined by the number of such faults occurring. To give a level of security of faults occurring which is acceptable, the entire apparatus is subject to detailed specification as to the quality of its component parts. Therefore, the possibility of faults occurring is defined and repeatable. Figure 13.1 indicates the position of intrinsically safe apparatus within an intrinsically safe system.

13.2.2 Associated apparatus

Associated apparatus is defined as apparatus which contains both intrinsically safe and non-intrinsically safe circuits, designed so that the non-intrinsically safe circuits cannot adversely affect the intrinsically safe circuits within it and to which it is connected. Such apparatus is not intended to be installed in the hazardous area but is intended to define the electrical power and energy constituting the input to the intrinsically safe apparatus to which it is connected. Its role is to define the voltage, current, power and energy (input) to such apparatus and to ensure that even when faults occur those levels are not exceeded. Again, faults in the components and circuits within the associated apparatus are considered in the equation and the number of these taken into account allows the determination of the level of safety achieved. As with intrinsically safe apparatus, requirements are applied to the quality of component parts to ensure a definable, repeatable level of safety. Figure 13.1 shows the position of the associated apparatus in an intrinsically safe system.

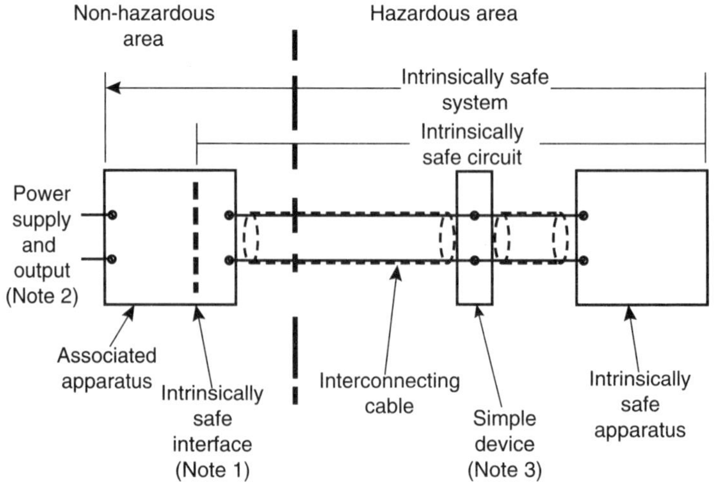

Fig. 13.1 The intrinsically safe system. *Notes*: (1) The intrinsically safe interface (the point beyond which voltages, currents, power and energy are controlled to an intrinsically safe level) is normally within the associated apparatus, not at its terminals. (2) Power supplies to associated apparatus and readouts etc., are normally assumed to be at mains potential. (3) Items defined as simple devices may be added in intrinsically safe circuits with little additional evaluation

13.2.3 Interconnections

The interconnections between intrinsically safe apparatus and associated apparatus are also important for two reasons. First, they are normally cables and are capable of storing energy when electrical currents are passed through them due to their inductance and capacitance. Second, as it is common to use multicircuit multicore cables for interconnection, there is the possibility of faults within such cables which could give rise to the interconnection of separate intrinsically safe circuits whose interconnection could give rise to a composite circuit which is ignition capable. Although these cables are not as dangerous as those containing, for example, mains circuits their construction must reach a minimum level to avoid problems, particularly where multicore cables are involved.

13.2.4 Simple apparatus (devices)

It is recognized that some devices, such as switches and terminal boxes and similar items of simple construction, do not contribute to the energy available for sparking or heating as they are essentially inert and their parameters can easily be defined because of their simplicity. These are called simple apparatus and the definition is that such apparatus will be a component or assembly of components of simple construction having well-defined electrical parameters. This would include thermocouples (but not thermopiles), resistance thermometers, switches, terminals and similar devices, and their use in intrinsically safe circuits is given a great degree of freedom because of their simplicity. Unfortunately, many attempts have been made to extend the use of this type of defined apparatus to cover complicated assemblies of components on the basis of the fact that no inductance or capacitance is present in such assemblies. Such an approach should be resisted as it would almost certainly lead to errors which could have disastrous results. It should be remembered that the original definition of such apparatus in BS 5501 Part 1 (1977)[12] was 'devices in which, according to the manufacturers specifications, none of the values of 1.2 volts, 0.1 amps 20 μJ or 25 mW were exceeded'. Clearly the initial intent was to limit the relaxations to devices (components) and it was only when it was recognized that some assemblies of components (e.g., terminal boxes) could fit the same limitations that device was replaced by apparatus. The intent, however, remains the same and the relaxations in the protection concept for simple apparatus are intended only to apply to devices and very simple assemblies.

13.2.5 The intrinsically safe circuit

The intrinsically safe circuit is the basic intrinsically safe block. It is, unlike the other protection concepts, that part of the intrinsically safe system where the energy levels are intrinsically safe – that is, all of the circuit downstream of the components in the associated apparatus which define the voltage, current, power and energy fed to the hazardous area. The intrinsically safe circuit normally comprises of the intrinsically safe apparatus, the interconnecting cables, any simple apparatus fitted to the circuit, and those parts of the associated apparatus downstream of the limiting components. This is, in fact, the basic building block of intrinsic safety, rather than the intrinsically safe apparatus (unlike the case of the other protection concepts).

13.2.6 The intrinsically safe system

The intrinsically safe system is the entirety of the installation including all parts which have an effect on intrinsic safety. It includes all parts of the associated apparatus, unlike the intrinsically safe circuit which does not.

13.3 Levels of intrinsic safety

As already stated, intrinsic safety is the only single standard protection concept which is normally acceptable in Zone 0 and in its most secure form it offers a much higher level of security than do the other standard protection concepts. Recognizing this, it is also obvious that the standard of intrinsic safety which is suitable for Zone 0 (and hence all Zones) will probably be overly expensive and complex for systems intended for Zone 1 and less-hazardous areas. To overcome this potential problem, two grades of intrinsic safety are recognized, that called 'ia' (which is intended for all Zones) and that called 'ib' (which is intended for Zones 1 and 2 only). The grade can apply to: an item of intrinsically safe apparatus, which is assumed to be connected to associated apparatus with specific output parameters and has all the requirements of the particular grade of Intrinsic Safety applied within it; to an item of associated apparatus, where the output parameters are defined with all the conditions appropriate to the grade of intrinsic safety applied within it; or to an intrinsically safe system where the conditions appropriate to the grade of intrinsic safety are applied to the intrinsically safe system as a whole, rather than to the items of apparatus in isolation. Applications to items of apparatus in isolation is the most common approach as this allows parameters of apparatus to be defined in the worst case and determination of the safety of the interconnection is then much easier. It does, however, often lead to a higher level of overall security than is absolutely necessary.

13.3.1 Intrinsic safety category 'ia'

This is the higher grade of intrinsic safety intended to permit its intrinsically safe circuits to enter Zone 0, and apparatus and systems in this category are required to be incapable of causing ignition of an explosive atmosphere by arcs, sparks and hot surfaces in all of the following conditions.

1. with no 'countable faults' applied and with the worst combination or combinations of 'non-countable faults applied. (A safety factor of 1.5 is applied to voltage or current – or combination of both as appropriate – which is available in these conditions to cause an arc or spark but no safety factor is applied to that causing hot surfaces.);
2. with any one of the possible 'countable faults' applied together, in each case, with the worst combinations of 'non-countable faults' applied. (The safety factors applied in these conditions are as in 1 above.);
3. with any two of the possible 'countable faults' applied together, in each case, with the worst combinations of 'non-countable faults' applied. (In these conditions no safety factor is applied to voltage or current, or the combination thereof.)

Clearly, if no countable faults are possible the apparatus can be 'ia'. If the worst combinations of possible non-countable faults do not cause an incendive arc or spark with the 1.5 safety factor applied, or produce an ignition-capable hot surface with no safety factor, the apparatus or circuit can be considered as 'ia'. Likewise, if only one countable fault is possible the apparatus may be considered as 'ia', provided it remains non-incendive with the worst combinations of non-countable faults applied in both normal operation, and with the one countable fault applied, and the safety factor of 1.5 applied for arc or spark ignition.

13.3.2 Intrinsic safety category 'ib'

This is the lower grade of intrinsic safety and the most hazardous area into which its circuits are intended to enter is Zone 1. Its performance in both normal operation and with any possible single countable fault should be exactly as specified in (1) and (2) as applied to category 'ia' but, there is no need to address any situation in which two countable faults occur. In cases where no countable faults are possible it is treated in the same way as category 'ia'.

13.4 Countable and non-countable faults

Faults, be they countable or non-countable, are failures of components conductors and any other failures which are possible within the apparatus or system. There are three situations within apparatus relating to faults, and the situation in interconnecting cables is governed by cable design. Details of specifications for components, connections, cables etc., will be detailed later in this chapter. Any part of the apparatus or system which does not comply with the requirements of the protection concept is assumed to be capable of fault as of normal operation (non-countable fault), and those which comply are mostly considered as still capable of fault (countable fault).

13.4.1 Non-countable faults

A non-countable fault is a failure of any component, assembly or interconnection within the apparatus which occurs in any of those which do not comply with the basic requirements of the protection concept. Where only partial non-compliance is present, the fault is only related to the effect of that non-compliance (e.g., where a bare conductor complies with the requirements but its separation from other bare conductors does not, then short circuits will be considered as non-countable faults but open circuit of the conductor will not).

13.4.2 Countable faults

A failure of any component, assembly or interconnection which complies with the basic constructional requirements of the protection concept (which in most cases include rating safety factors) is called a countable fault.

The Standard also contains enhanced specifications in addition to its basic specifications and where the component, assembly or interconnection complies with the basic requirements of the protection concept and, additionally, complies with the enhanced requirements, any facet of its operation which so complies will not be considered as becoming faulty. (For example, a separation of conductors which meets the additional requirements of the protection concept will not be considered as a possible short circuit, whereas the conductors themselves will be considered as going open circuit if they only comply with the basic requirements).

13.4.3 Effects of other faults

Where a component interconnection or assembly satisfies the basic requirements of the Standard when no countable faults are applied elsewhere in the circuit, but ceases to do so when one (or in the case of 'ia' two) countable faults are applied elsewhere, then that component, interconnection or assembly ceases to be considered as a countable fault when that fault (those faults) are applied and is considered to be a non-countable fault which may be applied if it adversely affects intrinsic safety.

Where a component, assembly or interconnection complies with enhanced specifications of the protection concept in normal operation, but ceases to do so when appropriate faults are applied elsewhere in the circuit within the scope of the Standard, then that component, assembly or connection is likewise reduced to being considered as a countable or non-countable fault, depending upon the conditions in which it operates in those fault conditions.

Component, assembly or interconnection faults are only important insofar as they increase the risk of danger and, therefore, if they have the reverse effect (e.g., a short circuit fault on the output of an associated apparatus) they are not applied.

13.4.4 Infallible component, assembly or interconnection

Where any component, assembly or connection satisfies the additional requirements of the protection concept discussed in Sections 13.4.3 and 13.4.4, which enable it to be considered not subject to fault it will be called infallible. It will only, however, be viewed as infallible in the mode where the additional requirements are applied (e.g., a resistor of specific construction may be considered as infallible as far as failure to a value of resistance lower than its specified value, but will still be assumed to be capable of open circuiting). Likewise, it will only be considered as infallible provided the conditions at its point of connection into the circuit remain the same. If they change so that it is subjected to, for example, higher voltages or currents then it may cease to be infallible in those circumstances.

13.5 Confirmation of intrinsic safety in respect of arc and spark ignition

Confirmation of intrinsic safety is by ensuring that no arc or spark is ignition capable, either in normal operation or after applying the various fault scenarios specified in Section 13.3 above.

The ignition capability of any part of an intrinsically safe circuit (i.e., intrinsically safe apparatus interconnecting cables and that part of associated apparatus within the intrinsically safe circuit – see Fig. 13.1) needs to be shown to be incapable of causing an ignition by any arc or spark occurring where such an arc or spark is considered possible, which is normally in such places as between conductors, in series with a conductor, at terminals, etc., unless the construction of the apparatus gives confidence that such sparking cannot occur (where construction endows infallibility). The parts which form the electrodes between which sparking occurs will vary widely and, as the incendivity of a low energy spark depends to a considerable extent on the geometry of these electrodes a basic yardstick is necessary to ensure repeatability. For this reason a special spark test apparatus has been developed to simulate sparking which may occur and this is shown in Fig. 13.2 and 13.3. This spark test apparatus (called the breaklash in the UK) is more sensitive than any typically expected practical electrode configuration, using as it does very small tungsten wire contacts which are more springy than copper as one electrode, thereby giving confidence that if no ignition occurs in a test in which it is employed then no ignition will occur

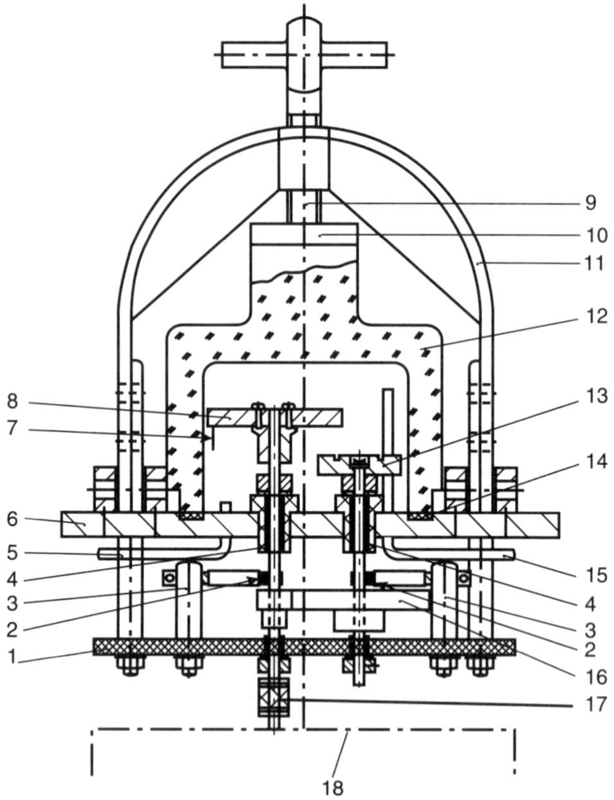

Fig. 13.2 Typical spark test apparatus. 1 Insulating plate, 2 Current connection, 3 Insulated bolt, 4 Insulated bearing, 5 Gas outlet, 6 Base plate, 7 Contact wire, 8 Contact holder, 9 Clamping screw, 10 Pressure plate, 11 Clamp, 12 Chamber, 13 Contact disc, 14 Rubber seal, 15 Gas inlet, 16 Gear wheel drive 50 : 12, 17 Insulated coupling, 18 Drive motor with reduction gears 80 rev/min

in any practical situation. The use of cadmium for the lower disc of the device is to cover the situation where cadmium, zinc, magnesium or, to a lesser degree, titanium is included in the materials within the apparatus to be tested and which may form the actual sparking electrodes. This is because it is known that these materials enhance the incendivity of electrical sparks (probably by the release of free radicals) and render ignition much easier. An energy of approximately 40 μJ released efficiently in a spark will ignite an ideal mixture of hydrogen/air in the presence of cadmium, whereas approximately 130 μJ is necessary where neither cadmium or the other metals are present. Cadmium is used because it is the most sensitive of the metals in question. In addition, cadmium and zinc plating is so common in the engineering industry that it is considered highly likely that, even if these materials were excluded during manufacture, servicing would introduce them in service by replacement of screws, etc., and a control system to prevent this is not considered as practicable.

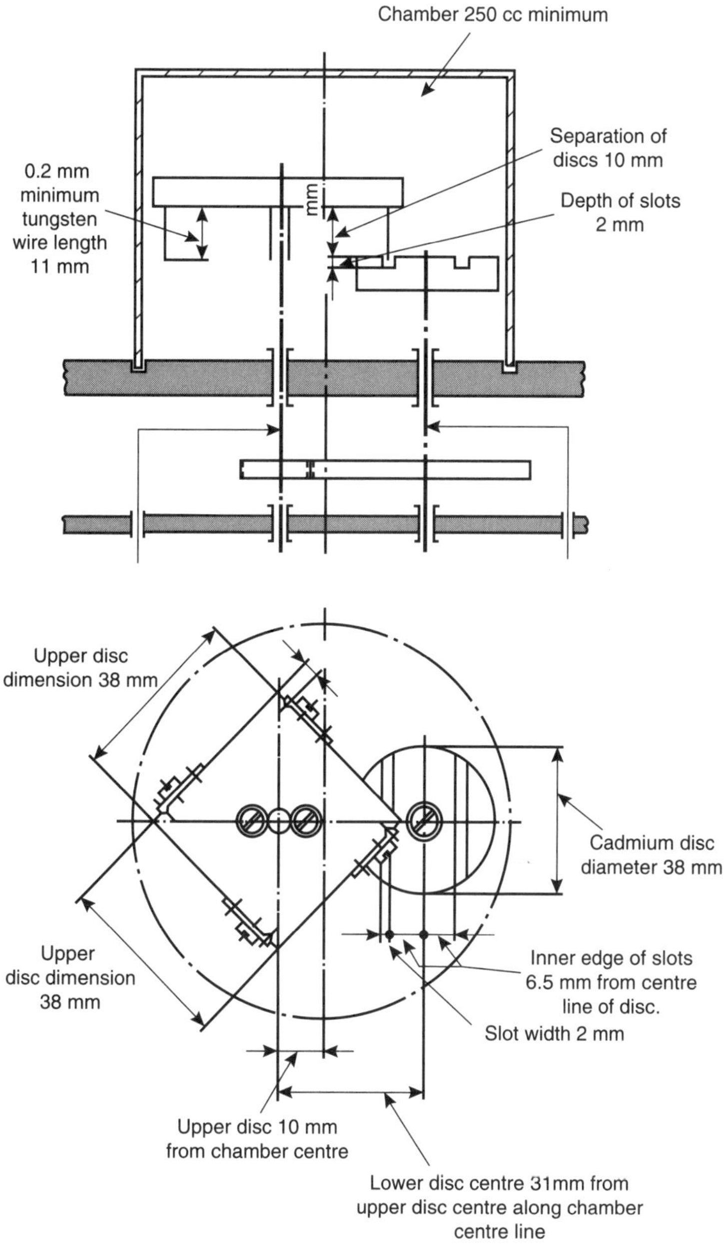

Fig. 13.3 Typical spark test apparatus dimensions

The mode of operation is to fill the enclosure of the apparatus with the test gas appropriate to the sub-group for which the apparatus is intended (the appropriate test gases are given in Table 13.1). The apparatus is then standardized by switching it on so that sparks are produced by the contra-rotation of the two discs which contra-rotate at 80 rpm for the disc holding

Table 13.1 Test mixtures and ignition currents/energies (normal tests – with electrical safety factors)

Sub-group	Hydrogen (% VV)	Ethylene (% VV)	Propane (% VV)	Calibration current (mA)	Calibration energy (μJ)
IIA	N/A	N/A	5.25 ± 0.25	100	475
IIB	N/A	7.8 ± 0.5	N/A	65	201
IIC	21 ± 2	N/A	N/A	30	43

(*from BS/EN 50020*)

the wires, and 19.2 rpm for the cadmium disc. The discs are then fed with the standardizing electrical supply current shown in Table 13.1, derived by placing a resistor in series with a 24 V dc power supply or battery so that the current is the short circuit current on the outboard end of the resistor. This current is fed to the test apparatus through a 95 mH air-cored series inductor and an ignition must occur within five minutes (400 revolutions of the upper disc) to confirm that the apparatus has reached its minimum sensitivity. It should be noted here that no maximum sensitivity calibration is carried out and the sensitivity of each test can vary. Although it is possible for significant variation in sensitivity to occur (up to 40 per cent is often quoted as possible, although this cannot be confirmed), the minimum sensitivity gives sufficient (although not total) confidence that ignitions will not occur in practical circumstances. The sensitivity variation is therefore an inconvenience rather than a safety problem.

After calibration the apparatus is refilled with the same gas/air mixture and its two discs connected, each to one of the points between which sparking is considered as possible, after applying the fault requirements for the protection concept and the necessary safety factors described in Sections 13.3.1 and 13.3.2. The apparatus is then energized and allowed to operate for 5 minutes (400 revolutions of the upper disc) for a dc circuit or 12.5 minutes (1000 revolutions of the upper disc) for ac circuits. If no ignition occurs and the gas/air mixture within the enclosure is then caused to explode by once again applying the calibration supply to the discs for 5 minutes, the test is considered as successful.

The reason for using 1000 revolutions in the case of an ac circuit is because it is not always possible to arrange the spark at the peak of a cycle and thus, to maximize the possibility of so doing, the length of the test is increased. In the case of a dc circuit, the test is normally stopped at 2.5 minutes and the polarity of connection reversed to ensure that any polarity effects in the circuit being tested are taken into account. With capacitive circuits and, to a lesser extent, inductive and resistive circuits, it is necessary to ensure that the circuit can return to its open circuit condition between sparks and this may not be possible when using a standard test apparatus. This problem is overcome by removal of wires from the upper disc to allow more recharging time. When this is done the number of rotations for both standardization and test must be increased (e.g., if the two opposite wires are removed leaving two wires, the time for testing and calibration needs to be doubled).

13.5.1 Achievement of safety factors

The safety factors of 1.5 where specified as necessary (see Section 13.4) are normally achieved by modification of the apparatus being tested to give the required factor. If this is not convenient or possible the circuit may be simulated for testing purposed by a specially constructed circuit, although great care is necessary in such circumstances to ensure that the simulated circuit is indeed identical to the actual circuit. For this reason it is always preferable to operate on the actual circuit. These safety factors are always in addition to any adjustments made to allow for such things as mains variations. All testing has to be carried out in (at least) the following conditions. First, the mains supplies to the apparatus must be increased to 110 per cent of their nominal value (it is assumed that mains tolerance will not exceed this). Second, any other power supplies and voltage-limiting circuits, and devices such as zener diodes, must be increased to give the maximum voltage which will occur at the worst combination of component tolerances with any mains supply to them at 110 per cent of its nominal value. Third, batteries shall be arranged or simulated to give the voltages specified in Table 13.6 on page 362.

The above actions need to be taken in all cases but, in addition, where the safety factor of 1.5 is required, the following actions must also be carried out before the test is commenced. First, for resistive circuits the current which would flow into a short circuit should be increased to 1.5 times its normal maximum value by the reduction of such things as current-limiting resistors, or if this is not possible by increasing the voltage in the circuit although this gives a more onerous test. This needs to be done even with power supplies which have crowbar protection, although in this case it must be arranged so that the supply recovers between short circuits created by the test which may require both wire removal from the test apparatus and alteration of the crowbar circuit.

Second, for inductive circuits the current through the inductance needs to be increased to 1.5 times its value achieved when all supplies are at the maximum of their maximum values, as already specified by the methods defined for resistive circuits, although care needs to be taken to ensure that the resistive circuit does not itself become incendive by this means and give a misleading test result. Third, for capacitive circuits the voltage across capacity of the circuit needs to be increased to 1.5 times the maximum which it achieves in the worst condition taking account of tolerances etc., and, it needs to be ensured that the circuit does not become resistively ignition capable and give a misleading result.

The above methods of determination of test conditions are applicable to simple inductive, capacitive or resistive circuits. In most practical cases, circuits will contain at least two of the parameters (e.g., resistive power and capacitive energy, resistive power and inductive energy, or both inductive and capacitive energy). In cases where this occurs or the circuit contains all three it is often necessary to test with the safety factor developed by increase of current, and repeat the test with it produced by increase in voltage to cover all possibilities.

Where increases in current or voltage are not considered to be convenient as an acceptable alternative, the test gases may be altered to give the required safety factor. The factored gas mixtures for the various sub-groups are given in Table 13.2 along with the reduced calibration currents for these gas mixtures. The test currents are derived by placing a limiting resistor in series with a 24 V dc supply so that the current is actually the short circuit current and the feeding this current to the test apparatus via a series 95 mH air-cored inductance.

Table 13.2 Test mixtures and ignition currents/energies (gas mixtures providing safety factors)

Sub-group	Hydrogen	Oxygen	Air	Calibration	
				Current	Energy
	(% VV)	(% VV)	(% VV)	mA	μJ
IIA	48 ± 2	None	52 ± 2	67	211
	85 ± 2	15 ± 2	None	67	211
IIB	38 ± 2	None	62 ± 2	43	89
	75 ± 2	25 ± 2	None	43	89
IIC	30 ± 2	17 ± 2	53 ± 2	20	19
	60 ± 2	None	40 ± 2	20	19

(*gas mixtures from BS/EN 50020*)

Note: These mixtures provide safety factors equivalent to a 1.5 safety factor on current or voltage.

13.5.2 Assessment of circuits

In order to assist in design of circuits and to simplify the process of confirming intrinsic safety, a set of curves has been produced to identify the minimum sensitivity of the test apparatus and which may be used in cases where the circuits are simple and can be defined with confidence. The curves used are intended for circuits that are simple, in that the capacitive curves are concerned with capacitive sparks only, the inductive circuits with inductive sparks only, and the resistive circuits with resistive sparks only. Practical circuits, however, seldom achieve this degree of purity and so there are limits on the use of the curves. The situation is helped, by the nature of the sparking which is different for the different sources (e.g., inductive, capacitive or resistive).

Inductive circuits

The inductive sparking mechanism is usually a break spark produced when the contacts break and a high, back emf is generated by collapse of the magnetic field (see Fig. 13.4). As the spark is not created by a short circuit (as there is little or no inductive stored energy when that occurs) but by the breaking of an inductive circuit when the back EMF seeks to perpetuate the current flow, it rises to high levels, sustaining a spark or arc, until all of the energy is dissipated. Inductive sparks are the most efficient in releasing energy into sparks and, in the test apparatus, the following energies are sufficient to ignite the test gases for the three sub-groups.

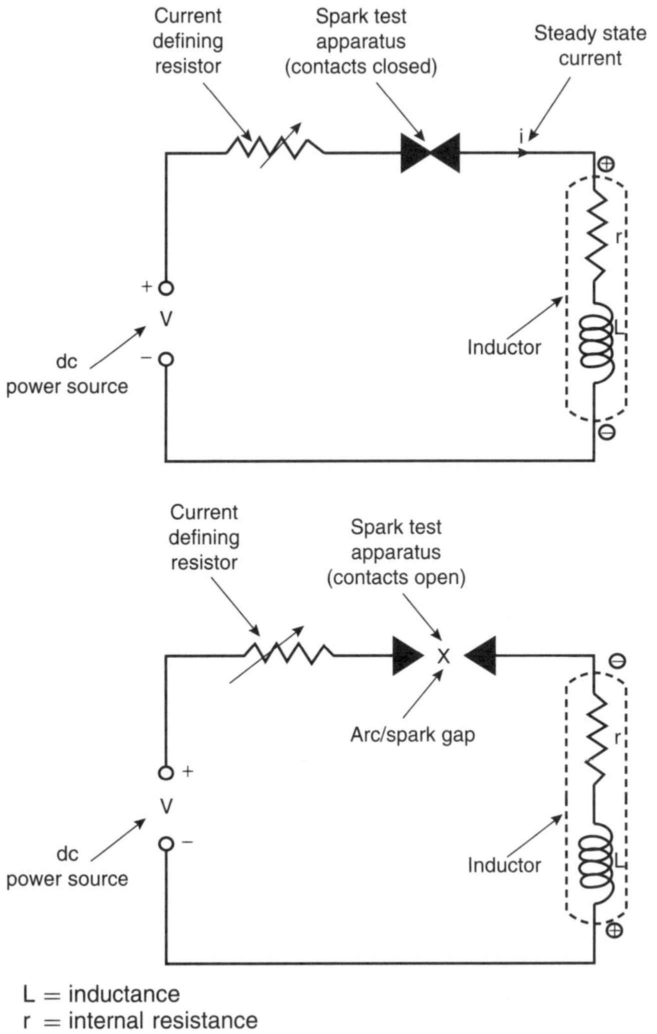

Fig. 13.4 Inductive spark production

$$IIA = 320\,\mu J$$

$$IIB = 120\,\mu J$$

$$IIC = 40\,\mu J$$

Figure 13.5 shows the minimum inductance levels for ignition at 24 V and various currents from the type of source shown in Fig. 13.4, and Fig. 13.6 shows the same information for lower voltages. (At voltages above 24 V the information in Fig. 13.5 is appropriate). These values are worst case as they refer to air-cored inductors and, as most inductors have magnetic cores of iron or other solid magnetic materials which are less efficient from a discharge point of view, they can be used with confidence in general.

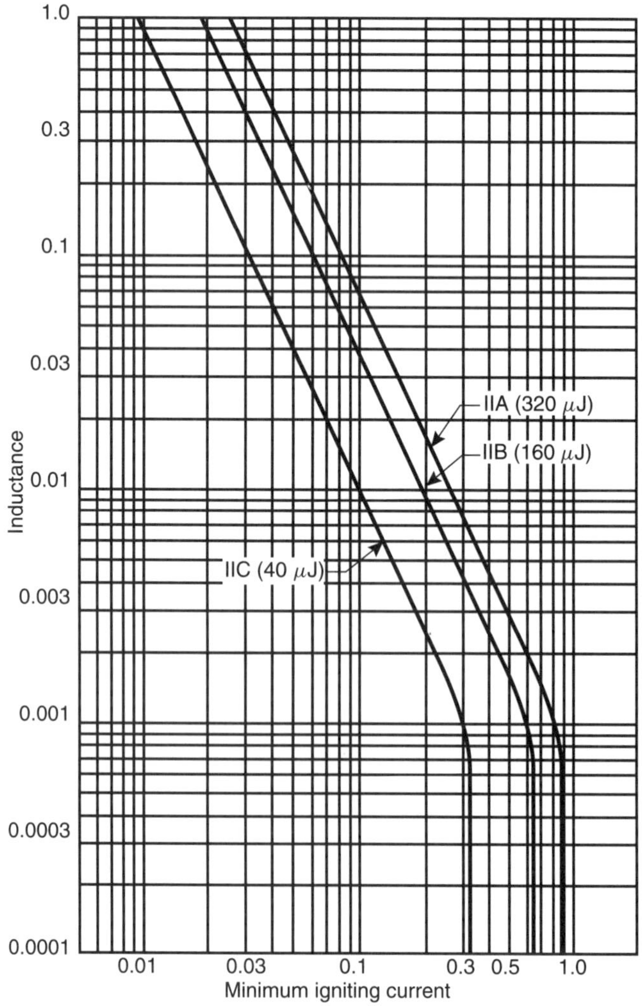

Fig. 13.5 Ignition threshold/inductive circuits at 24 V and above. *Note*: Ignition threshold for inductive circuit shown in Fig. 13.4 with V = 24 V

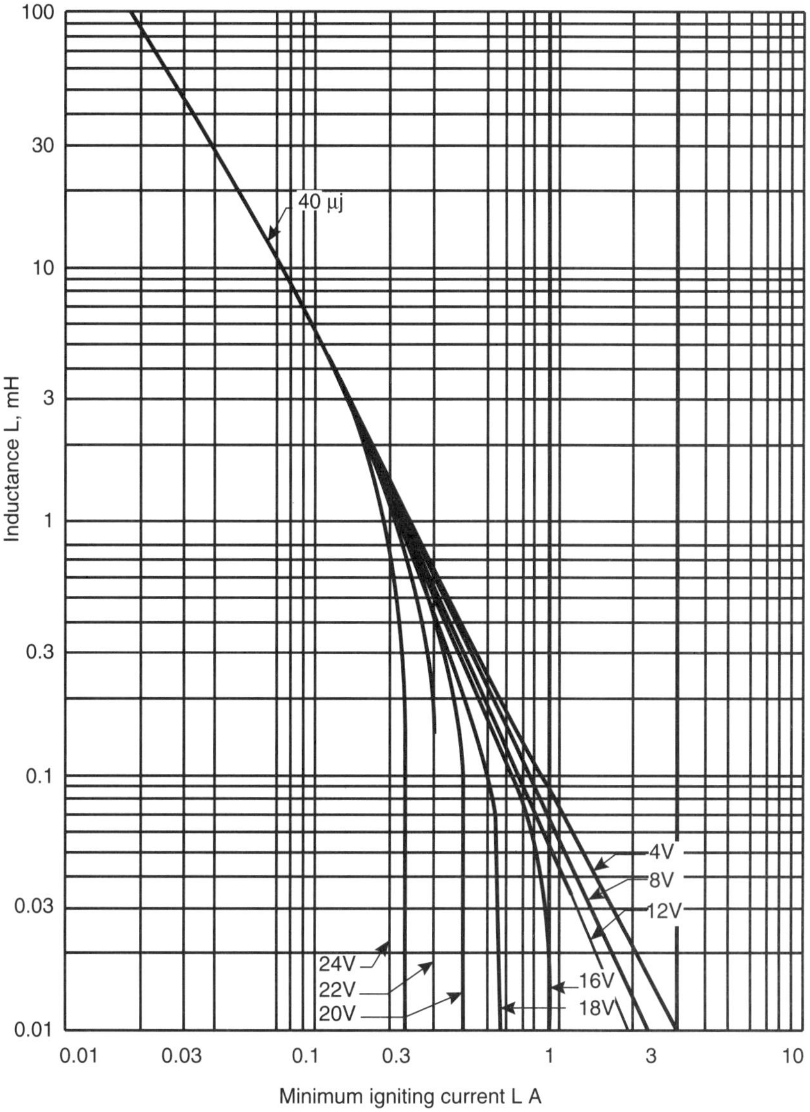

Fig. 13.6 Ignition threshold/inductive circuits at <24 V. *Note*: Ignition thresholds for inductive circuit shown in Fig. 13.4 for values of less than 24 V

Capacitive circuits

The capacitive sparking mechanism is usually a make spark occurring when the contacts have been separated for sufficiently long for the capacitance to charge to the open circuit voltage, and not when the contacts open for, at that time, the capacitance to be effectively discharged. The spark is not normally an arc as the voltage in most intrinsically safe circuits is not sufficient to break down an air path, but is a spark occurring when the first contact is made and only present because of the paucity of that contact (i.e., if the contact were made very firmly and completely at very high speed then almost no spark would occur). The voltage across the spark begins at the voltage across a charged capacitor and decays with charge. Thus energy discharge is not so efficient as in the inductive case and typical energy values are as follows:

$$\text{IIA} = 4.0\,\text{mJ (at 20 V)} - 1.25\,\text{mJ (at 100 V)}$$

$$\text{IIB} = 1.0\,\text{mJ (at 20 V)} - 500\,\mu\text{J (at 100 V)}$$

$$\text{IIC} = 200\,\mu\text{J (at 20 V)} - 50\,\mu\text{J (at 100 V)}$$

$$(240\,\mu\text{J (at 20 V)} - 110\,\mu\text{J (at 100 V)})$$

The IIC figures in brackets are the figures from BS 5501, Part 7[4] showing a significant reduction in permissible capacitance in BS/EN 50020[10].

Unlike the situation with inductance, the voltage across the spark tends to fall rapidly as the energy is released thus inhibiting the release of energy into the spark and, therefore, energy release is not as efficient, particularly at low voltages. Figure 13.7 shows the mechanism used for determination of effective spark ignition energy and Fig. 13.8 shows typical values for the three sub-groups.

Again, the curves in Fig. 13.8 are based upon capacitors with very efficient electrolytes and are much more sensitive than would be the case for such things as electrolytic capacitors. They can therefore be used with some confidence.

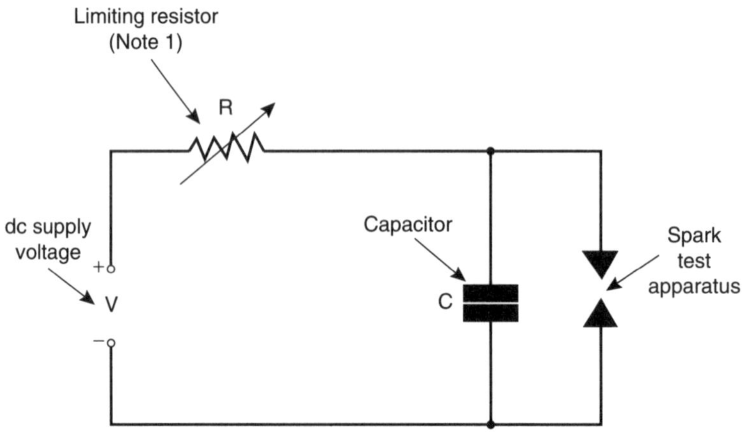

Fig. 13.7 Capacitive spark production. *Note*: Value of R must always be such that current does not exceed 0.5, the threshold current for resistive circuits – see Fig. 12.11. Alternatively, R may be replaced by a switch which opens before the spark test apparatus sparks (make spark)

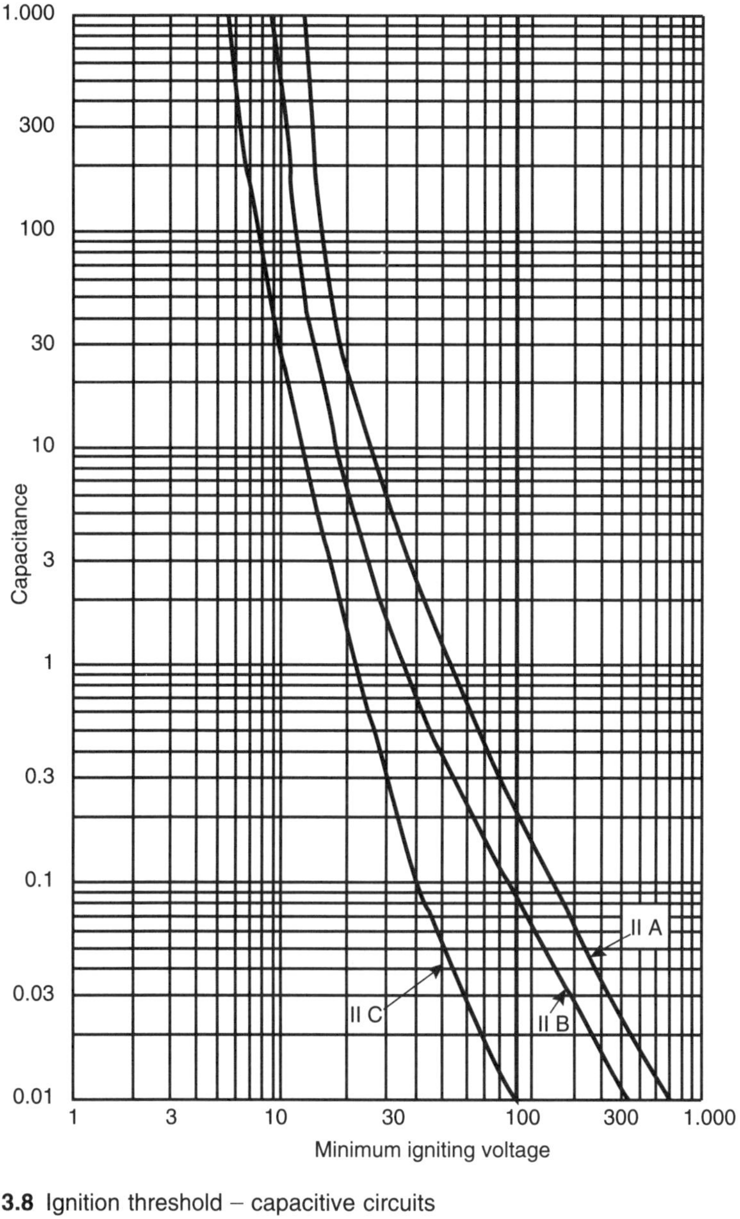

Fig. 13.8 Ignition threshold – capacitive circuits

Resistive circuits

Resistive circuits have, unlike their inductive and capacitive counterparts, limited voltages and currents. The sparks produced are usually less intense than the sparks produced by the discharge of an inductance or capacity but occur repeatedly as the wires scrape across the lower disc surface. The ignition mechanism for these is not as well understood as that associated with a single application of energy as occurs during the spark in the inductive and capacitive case.

Figure 13.9 shows the resistive circuit and constant current voltage limited circuits used to produce minimum ignition current curves and Figures 13.10 and 13.11 show the curves themselves for the three sub-groups. The constant current voltage limited circuits come from a proposal made by the HSE to the British Standards Institution (BSI) for inclusion in BS/EN 50020[10] and passed to the European (CENELEC) committee but not yet acted upon. As already mentioned, the energy released is not clearly definable and power transfer capability is the important parameter in this case. This is typified by the following power capability for ignition threshold circuits of this type:

$$\text{IIA} = 2.5\,\text{w to } 8\,\text{w (at 20 V)} - 2.1\,\text{w to } 2.6\,\text{w (at 50 V)}$$

$$\text{IIB} = 2.2\,\text{w to } 6.5\,\text{w (at 20 V)} - 1.5\,\text{w to } 1.9\,\text{w (at 50 V)}$$

$$\text{IIC} = 0.95\,\text{w to } 2.5\,\text{w (at 20 V)} - 0.65\,\text{w to } 0.8\,\text{w (at 50 V)}$$

Resistive circuits are therefore shown to be more ignition capable as the voltage rises.

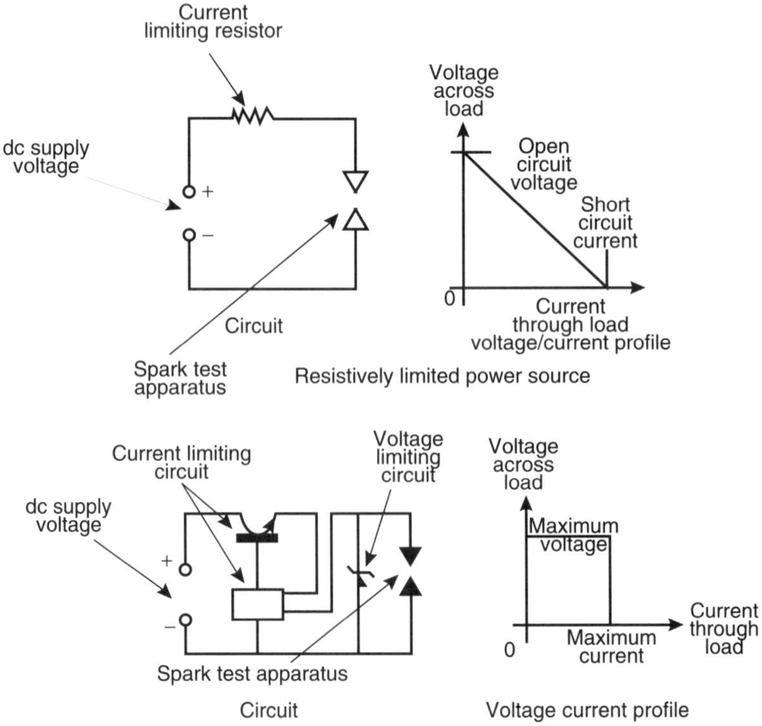

Fig. 13.9 Ignition threshold – resistive and voltage limited constant current circuits

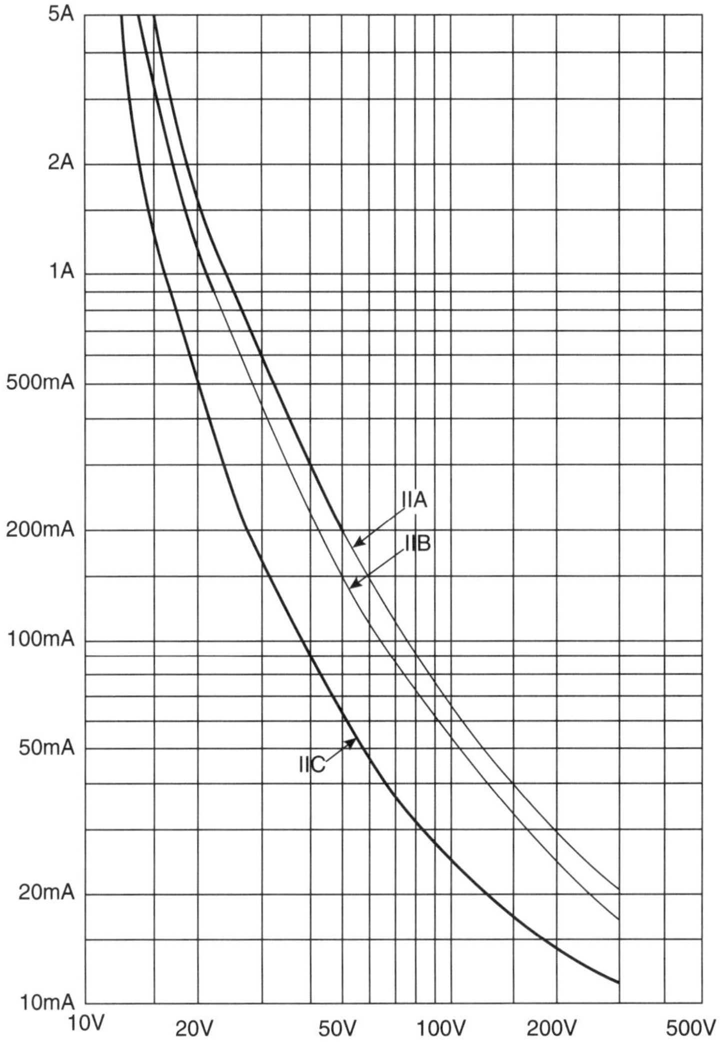

Fig. 13.10 Open circuit voltage/short circuit current threshold profile for resistive circuits

Composite circuits

Most practical circuits contain some of all three types of power or energy and these coexist normally because the fault conditions which give them the maximum risk condition are different in each case. This means that when one parameter is at its limit the others are well away from theirs. Practical testing historically has shown this to be the case and this can be confirmed by examination of the various ignition curves in Fig. 13.5, 13.6, 13.8 and 13.10. These figures show that the effect of the differing methods of sparking mean that the energies produced are not additive directly and

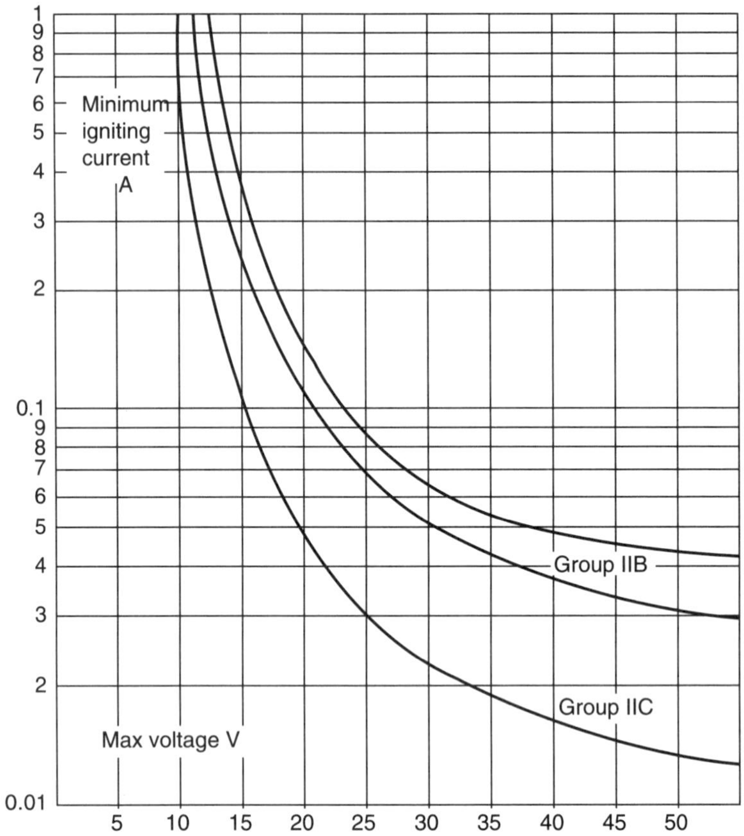

Fig. 13.11 Open circuit voltage/short circuit current profile for constant voltage current limited circuits

the effect of having inductive sparking, together with resistive sparking, is less ignition capable than would be expected from a direct addition. This leads to the possibility of using the curves for more composite circuits where those sparking parameters, other than the one being evaluated, are significantly less than the limiting parameters. Historic application of the curves has shown that the addition of energies is much less than would be expected and, although no firm confirmation exists, a derivation from the inductive circuits and curves (Fig. 13.4 and 13.5) shows that, provided the inductance present is less than 80 per cent of that permitted at the short circuit current available from a resistive circuit complying with Fig. 13.10, it is unlikely that an ignition would result from the presence of that inductance in a composite circuit. As a design guide, therefore, it is possible to use the curves where all but one of the parameters in question (e.g., inductance, capacitance and resistive limitation) give figures less than 80 per cent of their limiting figures in isolation. This may not exclude the necessity for later testing but will give a high degree of confidence that the circuits will prove to be intrinsically safe on any later test.

Crowbar protected circuits

Crowbar-type circuits, where voltage is arranged to collapse when overloads are applied, present particular problems when tested. The crowbar removes the voltage on the initial short circuit in the test apparatus and, depending upon the recovery of the circuit sparking, is inhibited for some time after that. The circuit must be tested with the spark test apparatus but, to ensure that the situation where that apparatus does not produce the most onerous condition, it must be shown not to deliver more than the following maximum energy during the crowbar operation:

$$\text{IIA} = 160\,\mu\text{J}$$

$$\text{IIB} = 80\,\mu\text{J}$$

$$\text{IIC} = 20\,\mu\text{J}$$

These figures are approximately half of those for ignition in inductive circuits and even less in the case of capacitive circuits. As the sparking mechanism is different to that for an inductive circuit, where the addition is more important, it is possible in design to ignore additive effects with confidence that any test will be passed.

13.6 Confirmation of intrinsic safety in respect of hot surface ignition

As already stated, there are no safety factors applied to voltages and currents in respect of hot surface ignition. Like the other protection concepts, however, a basic safety factor of 5 °C is applied in the case of temperature classes T3 to T6 and 10 °C in the case of T1 and T2, by requiring that maximum surface temperature is below the class limit by that amount. This requirement in BS/EN 50020[10] represents a change for that in BS 5501, Part 7[4] which, by wording in its exclusion clauses, did not require the 5 °C or 10 °C difference. The maximum surface temperature is, of course, measured in all cases in the appropriate worst case conditions specified for 'ia' and 'ib' and, the fault conditions which need to be taken into account may well be different to those used for spark ignition evaluation.

As intrinsic safety is typically an instrumentation concept using small electronic components, the normal requirements for maximum temperature are very onerous, particularly as they are in fault conditions and it is known that it is more difficult to ignite explosive atmospheres by small components. Considerable work done by the Safety in Mines Research Establishment (HSE) in the UK has led to a situation where considerable relaxations are permitted for small components. For T5 temperature classification it is permissible for typical components with a total surface area of less than 10 cm^2 (excluding any lead-out wires forming part of the component) to reach a measured temperature of 145 °C without causing ignition, whereas for larger components the figure is 95 °C (these figures representing elevations over the maximum ambient temperature permitted plus the ambient itself). For T4 classification, where the normal maximum measured temperature should not exceed 120 °C, the situation is more flexible and Table 13.3 indicates the relaxations permissible.

There is also the possibility that wiring in intrinsically safe circuits may be a source of ignition and to this end specific requirements are applied to ensure that this is not so. Maximum currents are specified for the various types of wiring encountered to ensure that these do not exceed the limiting temperature for the required temperature class. Figures for copper wire

Table 13.3 Temperature relaxations for small components and wiring

Total surface area (excluding wires)	Requirement for T4 rating
$<20\,mm^2$	Maximum permitted surface temperature = 275 °C
$\geq 20\,mm^2 - <10\,cm^2$	Maximum permitted surface temperature = 200 °C
$\geq 20\,mm^2$	Maximum power dissipation: – at 40 °C Ambient = 1.3 watts – at 60 °C Ambient = 1.2 watts – at 80 °C Ambient = 1.0 watts

Table 13.4 Current/temperature classification relationship for copper wire at 40 °C ambient temperature

Diameter of circular wire (mm)	Cross-sectional area of any wire (mm^2)	Maximum permissible rms wire current for temperature classification at 40 °C ambient (Amps)		
		T4	T5	T6
0.035	0.000962	0.53	0.48	0.43
0.05	0.00196	1.04	0.93	0.84
0.1	0.00785	2.1	1.9	1.7
0.2	0.0314	3.7	3.3	3.0
0.35	0.0962	6.4	5.6	5.0
0.5	0.196	7.7	6.9	6.7

(*from BS/EN 50020*)

Note: While the diameter of the wire only refers to circular solid wires the cross-sectional areas apply to wire of any cross-section form including stranded and flat conductors. They do not apply, however, to printed circuit tracks and similar situations.

Table 13.5 Minimum printed wiring widths for copper conductors of various thicknesses on insulating boards

Minimum track width (mm)	Maximum permissible current for temperature classification shown (Amps)								
	T4			T5			T6		
	A	B	C	A	B	C	A	B	C
0.15	0.8	1.2	1.56	0.67	1.0	1.3	0.6	0.9	1.1
0.2	1.2	1.8	2.3	0.97	1.45	1.88	0.87	1.3	1.69
0.3	1.87	2.8	3.64	1.5	2.25	2.92	01.3	195.0	2.53
0.4	2.4	3.6	4.68	1.94	2.9	3.77	1.67	2.5	3.25
0.5	2.94	4.4	5.72	2.34	3.5	4.55	2.01	3.0	3.9
0.7	3.81	5.7	7.41	3.08	4.6	5.98	2.74	4.1	5.33
1.0	5.02	7.5	9.75	4.05	6.05	7.86	3.61	5.4	7.02
1.5	6.56	9.8	12.7	5.42	8.1	10.5	4.02	6.9	8.97
2.0	8.04	12.0	15.6	6.49	9.7	12.6	5.62	8.4	10.9
2.5	9.04	13.5	17.5	7.7	11.5	14.9	6.43	9.6	12.4
3.0	10.7	16.1	20.9	8.77	13.1	117.0	7.7	11.5	14.9
4.0	13.0	19.5	25.3	10.7	16.1	20.9	9.58	14.3	18.5
5.0	15.2	22.7	29.5	12.6	18.9	24.5	11.1	16.6	21.5
6.0	17.2	25.8	33.5	14.6	21.8	28.3	12.6	18.9	24.5

(from BS/EN 50020)
A = 18 μm copper tracks
B = 35 μm copper tracks
C = 70 μm copper tracks

Notes:
1 Where the pcb is at least 0.5 mm and is less than 1.6 mm thickness divide the above current figures by a factor of 1.2.
2 Where the board is double-sided, divide the figures in the table by a factor of 1.5 and where the board is also of the lower thickness of Note 1, divide the figures in the Table by a factor of 1.8 instead of 1.5.
3 Where the board is a multilayer board divide the figures in the Table by a factor of 2 and the board layers also have a lower thickness as described in Note 1, divide the figures in the Table by 2.4 instead of 2.
4 Divide the result of applying the Table and Notes 1, 2 and 3 by a further factor of 1.5 where the printed circuit track passes under a component dissipating 0.25 watts or more.
5 Divide the result of applying the Table and Notes 1, 2, 3 and 4 by a further factor of 2 if the track is additionally used to terminate a component dissipating 0.25 watts or more. Alternatively, widen the track at the point of termination and up to 1 mm from that point to 3 times that determined from Table 13.2 after the application of Notes 1, 2, 3 and 4 as appropriate.

and copper printed circuit board tracks are given in Tables 13.4 and 13.5 respectively. No figures are given for higher temperature classes (T1, T2 and T3) as experience has shown that these are not normally required.

There is also a calculation procedure possible to cover unusual circumstances such as these cases and conductors of other metals such as ligaments in moving coil meters etc. The current limit for any temperature limit can be defined by:

$$I_{max} = I_f\{t(1 + \alpha T)/T(1 + \alpha t)\}^{0.5} \text{ amps}$$

where I_{max} =	maximum permissible current	Amps
I_f =	current at which the wire melts	Amps
t =	temperature class limit (−5 °C or 10 °C)	°C
T =	temperature at which wire melts	°C
α =	temperature coefficient of resistance for wire material (α for copper is 0.004265/°C)	/°C

The above formula will again give a worst case scenario as the wires in question will be connected to termination components which will have significant mass and therefore the actual temperature can be expected to be lower due to the thermal shunting effect of such devices, unless the wire is very long which is not normally the case in apparatus.

If this approach does not give the desired result there is a final approach which may be taken but this is based upon a test and applies only to T4. The component to be evaluated is placed in a chamber filled with a mixture of air and diethyl ether in the ratio 72% ± 2% air and 28% ± 2% diethyl ether. The component is then energized with the maximum power which it can dissipate in fault conditions and the temperature of the gas mixture raised by 25 °C above the maximum desired ambient temperature of operation. No ignitions or cold flames (blue coronas) should occur. Ignitions can be determined by measurement of sudden temperature elevation with a thermocouple in the gas or by visual or other methods, but cold flames are likely only to be identified by visual methods. To ensure repeatability these tests should be repeated on at least five samples of the components in question. As an alternative to raising the gas temperature to achieve the 25 °C above maximum ambient, the temperature of the component can be similarly raised.

The temperature of windings of transformers and coils are sometimes difficult to measure directly and an indirect method of measurement is acceptable for these items. The method used is the resistance variation method and relies upon measurements of the resistance at ambient temperature with the coil de-energized and then a further measurement taken after the coil has been energized for sufficient time for the temperature to stabilize. No figure for this time is given but it should be sufficient to utilize a time where the current in the coil does not change by more than one per cent per hour after taking account of the change in supply voltage at constant temperature. Measurement of the initial voltage/current relationship and the final relationship will give two values for resistance – one cold and one at heated equilibrium provided a dc supply is used. If the supply is ac, the cold resistance will need to be measured, and the hot resistance immediately after isolating the ac supply. The temperature rise can then be calculated from:

$$t = \{R(k + t_1)/r\} - (k + t_2 - t_1)$$

where	t = temperature rise	°C
	t_1 = initial ambient temperature (when r is measured)	°C
	t_2 = final ambient temperature (when R is measured)	°C
	R = measured final resistance (after energization)	Ohms
	r = measured initial resistance (before energization)	Ohms
	k = constant (234.5 for copper) (This constant is the α, inverse of the temperature coefficient of resistance)	

This formula takes into account any variation of ambient temperature between the time when the cold resistance of the winding is measured prior to its energization and that when its temperature is again measured after it has been energized and its temperature has stabilized at its maximum value.

13.7 Basic component and construction requirements

13.7.1 Safety factors on component rating

Components and connectors need to be operated at no more than two thirds of their relevant maximum rated operating voltage, current and power in their conditions of use if their failures are to be considered as countable faults. This criterion needs to be true in both normal operation of the intrinsically safe circuit and with the appropriate countable and non-countable faults applied elsewhere in that circuit (this criterion is normally determined by confining faults to within the apparatus itself and defining maximum supply or external circuit parameters which the rest of the intrinsically safe circuit must not exceed in the worst case of the entire fault count and associated non-countable faults elsewhere in the system). Clearly such a requirement does not make sense in the case of such things as fuses, relays, thermal trips, transformers and similar devices as these operate differently.

Components not subjected to the 1.5 rating factor

Fuses

The specification for such fuses is concerned with their ability to interrupt current at a specific level and applying the rating factor above would produce a more dangerous condition as more current would be let through before they ruptured.

Thermal trips

Thermal trips are intended to operate at specific temperatures and no temperature rating reduction is specified. Also, if they are current operated any attempt at applying rating factors could cause them to be less effective.

Relays

Applying a safety factor to voltage or current to a relay would prevent operation of the device as their specification is to operate at a specific voltage.

Transformers

Again, application of safety factors to transformers is inappropriate as they would achieve nothing other than to damage the efficiency of the device.

Switches

As switches do not dissipate power then no safety factor is necessary provided the physical construction of the switch is such that its failure is a countable fault.

Components which are subject to the 1.5 rating factor

In general, all other components are subjected to the rating safety factor unless, as already stated, the application of that factor produces a reduced level of security. As the rating factor is large, its calculation can be done in a relatively simplistic way to avoid the necessity for long and tortuous calculation which will do little to add to the security of the protection concept. Typical of the procedures adopted are the following.

Resistors

Resistors will have their power dissipation calculated at the maximum value including manufacturers tolerances normally quoted, and at the maximum ambient temperature in which they are to be used to the manufacturers specifications. The power so calculated will be the power subjected to multiplication by the rating factor.

Semiconductors

Semiconductors need to have their maximum current, voltage and power dissipation calculated. These are done using manufacturers information by determining the power which would give the maximum acceptable junction temperature in the mounting conditions. Maximum current is not seriously affected by the temperature as it is only limited by the fine connections between the semiconductor material and the outgoing wires and will not, in any event, be exceeded if the power is defined. Semiconductor breakdown voltage is temperature sensitive due to semiconductor activity and this must be specified in the conditions of mounting. It is these parameters which are subjected to the two thirds rating limitation.

Zener diodes

The voltage across these, which also determines the power which can be dissipated, will be the manufacturers specified voltage in dynamic test conditions at the maximum ambient temperature in the mounting conditions used, with the manufacturers tolerance added. Voltage elevation due to junction temperature elevation need not be considered. It is this power to which the rating factor is applied not, for obvious reasons, the voltage.

Capacitors

The rating factor for capacitors is applied to the maximum voltage for which the capacitor is rated and the maximum ac current.

13.7.2 Specific requirements for particular components

Fuses

The exemption of rating factors for fuses has already been discussed but there are several requirements appropriate to fuses concerned with their protection of other circuits and their installation in a hazardous area. The fuses used are normally cartridge-type fuses or similar, and rewirable fuses are not normally acceptable. Fuses should be mounted inside any enclosure for the apparatus, except that mains fuses in associated apparatus may be accessible from the front of the apparatus if they use proper holders designed for that purpose. As fuses of the acceptable type are normally commercial plug-in assemblies, they do not need to comply with the creepage and clearance requirements of the protection concept which are described later in this chapter unless they are encapsulated for use in a hazardous area, but they do need to comply with a recognized Standard for fuses such as EN 60127 (1991).[13]

First, the fuse will be assumed to continuously let through 1.7 times its rated current (I_n), and the circuits which it protects should be evaluated on that basis. In addition, the rupturing time/current characteristic of the fuse is important in that it determines the size of any transient let through during the rupturing time. If this can be obtained the circuits protected by the fuse need to be evaluated in regard to their performance in the presence of these transients to ensure that they do not damage the components therein. If this information is not available then it is necessary to test ten samples of any component protected by the fuse by subjecting it to pulses at the fuse supply voltage, with a source resistance equal to the cold resistance of the fuse plus any other infallible resistance in the circuit in the condition where the fuse blows, to ensure no damage occurs.

The fuse itself must have a voltage rating of at least that of the voltage against which it is protecting circuits, and a prospective current rating sufficient to ensure that it will rupture (the prospective current is the current which the supply can provide into a short circuit continuously as, if the fuse is not rated for this, the arc produced on rupture may not extinguish and current may continue to flow). Where the prospective current rating of a fuse is not sufficient the current it ruptures can be limited by the inclusion of an infallible resistor (see later in this chapter) which has the following specification:

$$\text{voltage rating} = \text{maximum supply or circuit voltage } (U_m, U_i)$$

$$\text{current rating} = 1.5 \times 1.7 \times I_n \text{ (The fuse current rating)}$$

$$\text{power rating} = 1.5 \times (1.7 \times I_n)^2 \times \text{value of resistance}$$

The prospective current requirements for mains fuses are normally 1500 A.

Where the fuse is in a hazardous area the rupture of the fuse element itself could be a source of ignition and therefore the explosive atmosphere must be excluded from the fuse element. The fuse must be encapsulated to prevent explosive atmosphere access and the method of carrying out such encapsulation is described later in this chapter. The problem with encapsulation is that if it enters the fuse it can affect its operation. For this reason it is necessary to ensure the fuse assembly is sealed before any encapsulation is commenced.

Cells and batteries

Both primary cells (those not subject to charging) and secondary cells are permitted within intrinsic safety provided they do not exhibit particular unwelcome parameters. Lithium cells, for example, can explode, overheat, or vent in conditions where a current flows into them from another power source, or they are subjected to short circuit or overheating. Where these conditions can occur lithium batteries should not be used. Guidance is given in HSE Guidance Note GS 43.[14] Likewise, nickel cadmium cells can suffer polarity reversal if deeply discharged, and may then explode on charge. Where these conditions can appear in a way which adversely affects intrinsic safety, such cells and batteries are not permitted. It should be noted this is not an invitation for their use elsewhere as other safety issues are present.

Cells are normally ill defined as to their interiors as manufacturers are continually improving their performance by altering the internal construction. For this reason it is normal to consider each cell as a sealed component and consider only the sparks and hot surfaces which occur outside it for the purposes of ignition capability. In addition, the reliability of a cell is considered as sufficient to consider an internal short circuit as a countable fault. There are limits to this approach, however, and cells or batteries which are not sealed by compression of plastics, washers or similar, not sealed by moulded plastic enclosures, or not fusion sealed are not considered as sealed. This limit mainly affects batteries (assemblies of cells, rather than the cells themselves) and means that where battery enclosures are only held together by metal swageing or adhesion between parts which are not clearly gas tight, the interior of the battery needs to be considered as far as ignition possibilities are concerned. Acceptable methods of cell or battery construction are: sealed (gas tight) cells or batteries; sealed (valve regulated) cells or batteries; and sealed cells and batteries not having pressure relief valves.

In addition to satisfying the above requirements such cells and batteries have limits applied to their construction in that they need to be in an enclosure which is spun or moulded in one piece apart from the end cover or covers which must be either fused to the enclosure, stuck to it with appropriate adhesive ensuring the joint is gas tight, or sealed by swageing over the end of the enclosure and compressing an insulating washer is so doing (see Fig. 13.12).

There is no specific prohibition on the leakage of electrolyte from cells and batteries but if electrolyte is released either in short circuit conditions (when the cell is subjected to the maximum input or charging current specified by the manufacturer whatever the battery condition, and where the cell or battery is charged with one cell fully discharged including reversal of a single cell where this occurs when the cell is discharged) the battery needs to be fitted in an enclosure which prevents the leaked electrolyte from damaging the intrinsically safe circuits. (Sealed gas-tight and sealed valve-regulated cells and batteries are not considered to release electrolyte.)

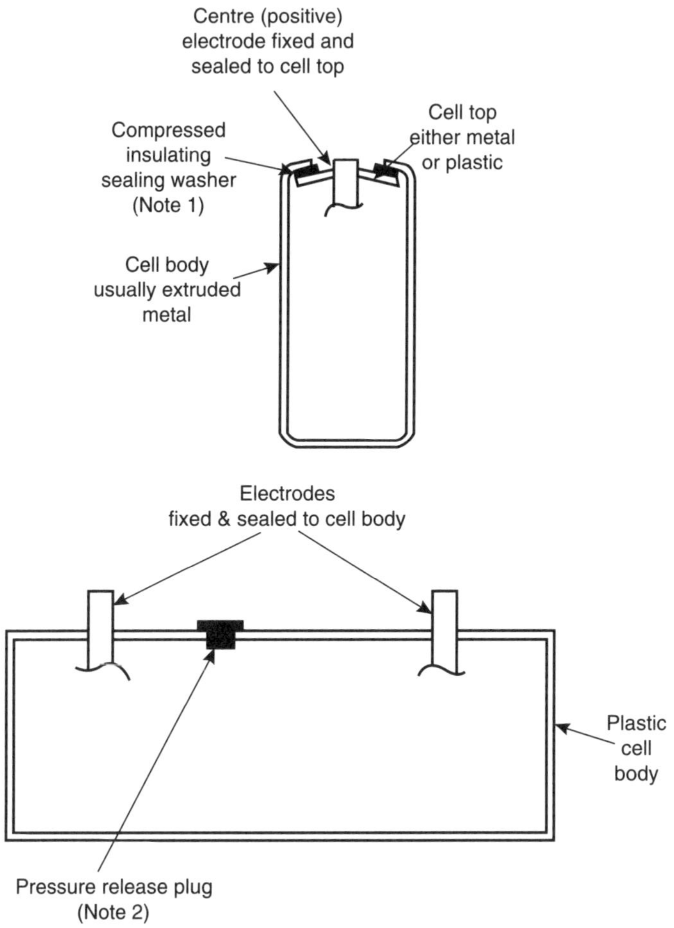

Fig. 13.12 Typical cell construction. *Notes*: (1) In case of excessive pressure in cell, release is via compressed washer. (2) In case of excessive pressure, release is via specially fitted release plug.

Where cells and batteries can vent gases (hydrogen, etc.) which is most likely in cases where they are chargeable cells, the battery container should be arranged to vent the released gases directly to the outside of the apparatus. The amount released if handled in this way is unlikely to create any significant amount of explosive atmosphere inside the enclosure and, as significant charging is normally done in a non-hazardous area because otherwise the charging circuit would need to be an intrinsically safe circuit, release is not likely to affect the hazardous areas in which the batteries are used.

Cells of particular chemical configuration will give different voltages and these can vary from cell to cell in some cases. In addition, the voltage relevant to spark ignition will often be different to that appropriate for hot surface ignition as one is transient and the other has to exist for considerable lengths of time to cause heating. To avoid confusion, therefore, the maximum voltages relevant in the two cases for a range of cell types are given in Table 13.6.

Table 13.6 Output voltages of cells of various types to be used for evaluation of circuits using batteries

IEC type Code	Cell type (chemical)	Peak o/c voltage for spark ignition (V)	Nominal voltage for hot surface ignition (V)
K	Nickel Cadmium	1.5	1.3
–	Lead Acid (Wet)	2.67	2.2
–	Lead Acid (Dry) (See Note 1)	2.35	2.2
L	Alkaline – Manganese	1.65	1.5
M	Mercury – Zinc	1.37	1.35
N	Mercury – Manganese Dioxide–Zinc	1.6	1.4
S	Silver – Zinc	1.63	1.55
A	Zinc – Air	1.55	1.4
C	Lithium – Manganese Dioxide	3.7	3.0
–	Zinc – Manganese Dioxide	1.735	1.5
	(Zinc – Carbon Leclanche)	1.725	1.5
–	Nickel – Hydride	1.6	1.3

(from BS/EN 50020)

Notes:

1 Dry Lead/acid cells are those with paste electrolytes which do not need electrolyte addition during their lives.

2 Rechargeable cells such as nickel/cadmium or lead/acid may not achieve their maximum voltages on initial charge and thus may not achieve these voltages. They will, however, after two or three charges, and so if tests are carried out the cells should be cycled first.

While the internal short circuiting of cells and batteries satisfying the foregoing requirements is not considered to be within a hazardous area for spark ignition purposes, external short circuiting is. It is necessary to ensure that the current which flows is intrinsically safe and the method of doing this is to ensure that the separation of cell or battery terminals is infallible, or not considered as subject to fault, and then to introduce current limiting devices in series with one or both of the terminals limiting the short circuit current to an intrinsically safe level. These current limiting devices need to be enclosed or encapsulated with the cell or battery if it is intended to be changed in a hazardous area or, where this is not so, the cell or battery needs to be in an enclosure fastened with special fasteners as described in Chapter 5, and warnings are then necessary to ensure that it will only be changed in a non-hazardous area. Charging terminals for rechargeable cells or batteries must be enclosed to IP20 (BS/EN 60529[15] and in these circumstances the recharging must take place in a non-hazardous area. Alternatively, the charging terminals can be protected by diodes (two for 'ib' and three for 'ia') which prevent removal of current from them, or by an infallible resistor which forms an intrinsically safe circuit. Where, in these circumstances, charging is carried out by a charger whose output is not intrinsically safe, the diodes or resistor must be protected by a fuse which prevents excess current flowing during charging and, if the fuse carries current normally (i.e., is in the discharging circuit as well as the charging circuit), it should be encapsulated to prevent access of the explosive atmosphere to its element. Where the charger output is not intrinsically safe charging should only be carried out in the non-hazardous area.

Semiconductor devices (diodes, zener diodes, thyristors, transistors, integrated circuits etc.)

Failure of properly rated semiconductor devices is normally considered as a countable fault but because of their nature they must be shown to be proof against transients. In the case of associated apparatus, where this is fed from or otherwise connected to the mains supplies, the transient currents which occur are determined by the mains and such currents will, at worst, be the peak value of the mains voltage divided by any infallible series resistance present in the circuit between the mains and the semiconductor device. Thus the semiconductors must be capable of suffering significant voltage and current transients without damage, even when an infallible transformer is included in the circuit to provide a low voltage from which to derive the intrinsically safe circuit. This is an onerous requirement but it is only applied to those semiconductor devices upon which intrinsic safety depends, such as shunt voltage limiting devices, etc. Once out of the associated apparatus transients can be ignored as it is assumed that they will be suppressed to a large extent in the associated apparatus and what remains will not cause problems.

Apart from the three diodes permitted for blocking in 'ia' circuits, semiconductors used for series limiting are restricted to 'ib' circuits because of their transparency to transients which would be of very great concern in circuits which entered Zone 0 because of the permanent presence of an explosive atmosphere and the possibility of their passing of a brief ignition capable transient, which would in that case coincide with the presence of the explosive atmosphere, unlike the case in Zone 1 where coincidence is much less likely.

Where semiconductors are used as shunt voltage limiting devices they can only include diode connected transistors (e.g., those connected so that they are either fully on or fully off), thyristors, zener diodes and similar devices. They must have a forward current rating of 1.5 times the maximum current which can flow including fault conditions if they were short circuited. This requirement is also applied to zener diodes and is determined by consideration of the current limit when the diode is used in the forward diode direction (the opposite polarity to the zener direction). Zener diodes need also to operate at no more than two thirds of their rated zener maximum power dissipation when operated in the circuit as zener diodes with faults applied in the circuit.

The use of controllable semiconductors, such as transistors, voltage regulators and thyristors is generally restricted to 'ib' circuits, except in situations where both input and output circuits are intrinsically safe, or where it can be shown that transients from the power supplies do not occur. In such circuits two parallel devices are considered as infallible, even in 'ia' circuits. In addition, even where transients can occur three shunt thyristors are acceptable in 'ia' circuits if they can handle the transients and their let-through energy is limited to the following when they operate:

$$\mathrm{IIA} = 160\,\mu\mathrm{J}$$

$$\mathrm{IIB} = 80\,\mu\mathrm{J}$$

$$\mathrm{IIC} = 20\,\mu\mathrm{J}$$

Internal connectors (terminals, plug-in cards, plugs and sockets, etc.)

In general there are no requirements for the quality of the connecting elements of internal connectors which are additional to those required for normal industrial use, and failure of connecting elements to high resistance or open circuit are considered as a countable fault. In failure to high resistance there will obviously be a potential heating problem but the requirements for the protection concept in BS/EN 50020[10] specifically state that a temperature classification of T6 is to be applied to such devices and therefore no evaluation in this regard is necessary. The reason for this lies in the fact that experience of failures in such connectors is that such failure is to open circuit or to a very high resistance, and the possibility of significant power dissipation in such connector is considered to be extremely small.

Where there is a connector in an item of apparatus, the arrangement must be such that it cannot be reverse connected if such connection adversely affects intrinsic safety. The required security is normally achieved by keying the connector so that it will only fit one way and most commercial plugs and sockets are configured in such a manner. With printed circuit connectors keying is normally by replacing one of the connectors with a slot in the board and blocking one of the receptacle positions in the socket (see Fig. 13.13). Obviously if such is not the case then reverse connection is not important except for operational reasons, but these would probably require the same precautions in any event. Where the apparatus contains more than one connector interchangeability between connectors must not be possible where it could adversely affect intrinsic safety. Keying or a similar approach is the optimum approach both for incorrect connection of a single connector and inadvertent interchange between connectors. It is recognized that such an approach is not always economic and the identification of connectors to make incorrect connection obvious, for example, by some form of colour coding, is regarded as an alternative.

Where connectors carry earth connections which are necessary for the provision of intrinsic safety, the contacts need to be duplicated for 'ib'

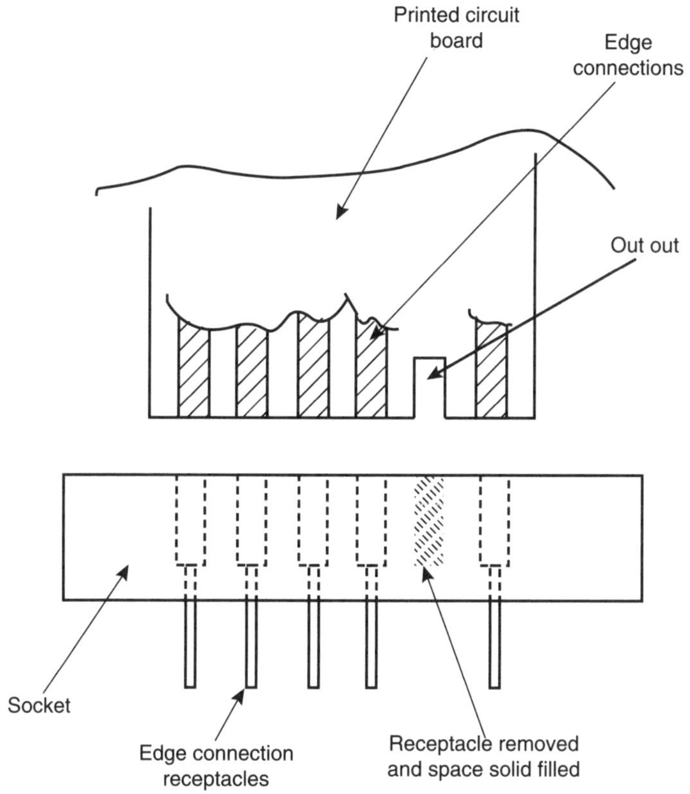

Fig. 13.13 Typical keyed edge connector

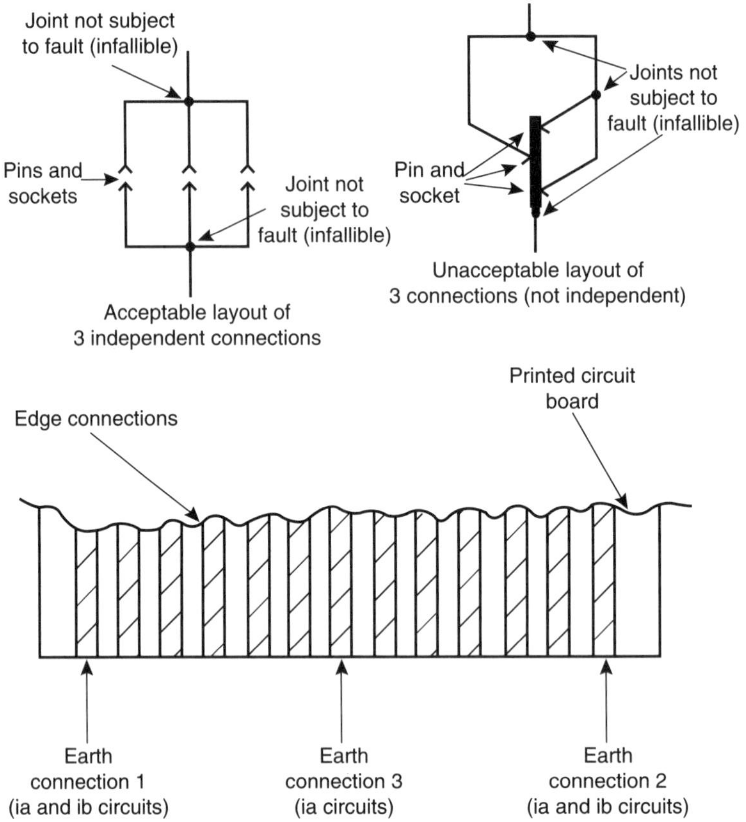

Fig. 13.14 Layout of connections on in-line plugs and sockets

and triplicated for 'ia' in a manner which achieves the objectives shown in Fig. 13.14. In addition, in the case of in-line connectors such as those used for printed circuit boards, where withdrawal could be at an angle, the connections need to be distributed along the connector to ensure that at least one of them remains in contact until the connector is fully removed. This requires one connection at (or very close to) each end of the connector.

Terminals need not comply with any requirements other than those applied for industrial use and, like connectors, they will be considered to fail to a very high resistance or open circuit as a single countable fault. Therefore, they will be considered in respect of temperature classification in the same way as connectors and will be T6.

Soldered joints

There are no specific requirements for soldered joints and normal soldered joints will be considered only to fail as a countable fault. Temperature classification of such joints will, as for terminals and other connectors, be considered as T6. Where a wire becomes detached as a result of the failure of a soldered joint connection of that wire to any other conducting part within its resultant range of movement, it will, as with other disconnected wires, be considered as a second countable fault.

Connectors for external connections (terminals, plugs and sockets, etc)

Terminals for connection of external circuits must comply with the requirements for those used internally and must, in addition, comply with the following requirements. First, they must have a separation between each other and between them and any earth connection of at least the figures given for creepage, clearance and separation needed so that interconnection can be ignored.

Second, they must be separated from one another by at least 6 mm and from earth by at least 3 mm (the distance in question being measured as shown in Fig. 13.15) when all circuits in question are intrinsically safe circuits, and by at least 50 mm from non-intrinsically safe circuits.

Third, any partitions used to assist in separation must be at least 0.9 mm thick if made of insulating material and 0.45 mm thick if made from metal. In both cases the partitions must pass a test which applies a lateral force of 30 N to determine their rigidity and, if metallic, must be earthed or of sufficient thickness that it can be demonstrated that burn through will not occur in case of fault. Also, their earth connection must be such as to preclude loss of earth. If this is achieved by an earth connection rather than their forming part of an earthed frame the connection must satisfy the requirements for infallible connections.

Finally, where partitions are used the 50 mm separation may be waived if the partitions used are arranged so that the separation between their extremities are within 1.5 mm of the walls and cover of the enclosure.

The burn-through problem is not a real problem for most circuits as their power consumption is so low as to make the minimum thickness quoted sufficient. It must, however, be carefully considered in circuits which use high energy, such as those associated with some relay output contacts in associated apparatus.

The terminals themselves must satisfy the normal industrial requirements but must also satisfy additional requirements when used for connection of earths important to intrinsic safety. They need to be free of any sharp edges which could damage or sever any connected wires and not rely on insulating materials to transmit the pressure necessary to ensure conductor clamping. When stranded conductors are used without crimped ferrules it is necessary to introduce a pressure plate between the terminal screw and the wire to ensure good connection without damage to the strands, and if they have a maximum allowable conductor size below 4 mm^2 they must be arranged so that they can effectively clamp smaller conductors also.

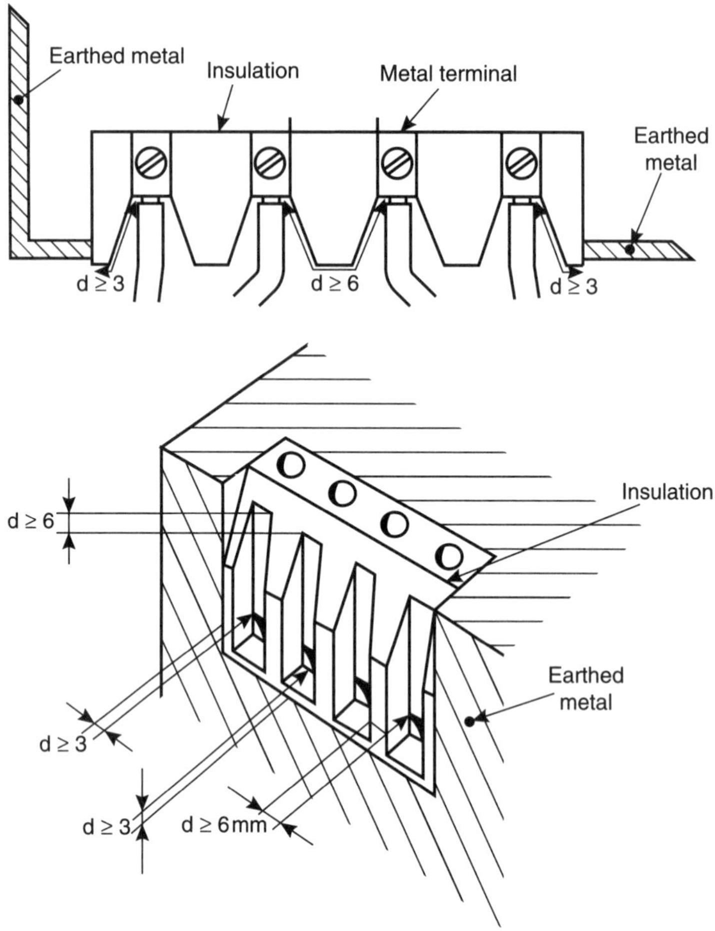

Fig. 13.15 External terminal spacing. *Note*: For separation between intrinsically safe and non-intrinsically safe terminals the ≥ 6 mm distance is increased to ≥ 50 mm

Plugs and sockets need to comply with the same requirements as internal plugs and sockets for construction and interchangeability and, in addition, the facilities for wiring to the plugs and sockets should comply with the same requirements as terminals unless special precautions are taken in terminating the wires in the plug or socket, or the cable is attached during manufacture.

Piezo electric devices

Piezo electric devices are relatively unique in that they have the ability to translate mechanical stresses into electrical signals. Because of this they can add to the electrical energy in an intrinsically safe circuit. The possible electrical energy can be measured by subjecting external parts of the apparatus into which they are fitted to the impact tests usually used for strength determination (see Chapter 8), and noting the maximum voltage generated in the device during such impact testing. If the capacitance of the devices is then measured the maximum output energy can then be calculated from:

$$e = 0.5\,CV^2x \qquad \mu j$$

where	e =	energy generated	j
	C =	capacitance	μF
	V =	maximum voltage generated	V

This energy must not exceed the following maximum values:

$$IIA = 950\,\mu J$$

$$IIB = 250\,\mu J$$

$$IIC = 50\,\mu J$$

Guards may be fitted to reduce the effects of impacts in this regard but they must not be damaged in a way which reduces their effectiveness by the impact if so used. Also, in special circumstances, the apparatus may be deemed to be free of such impacts but in such circumstances it is essential that users are clearly informed of what must be achieved by any installation to achieve this.

Relays

The construction of relays is important when they are used to separate parts of the same intrinsically safe circuit, separate intrinsically safe circuits, or intrinsically safe circuits and non-intrinsically safe circuits. Interconnections between coils and contacts and contacts and other contacts can be important and are dealt with in Sections 13.6 and 13.7. There are, however, design limits in the case of relays where the coils are in intrinsically safe circuits and the contacts in non-intrinsically safe circuits, or where the relay has two sets of contacts one in each type of circuit. These are determined by the need to ensure that ionization arising from sparking is not a problem and are as follows. First, the contacts in non-intrinsically safe circuits should not normally switch circuits operating at more than 250 V rms with a rating of more than 100 VA and the switched current should not exceed 5 A rms.

Second, these figures may be increased to 10 A rms and 500 VA, but, where breakdown must not occur the spacings between the coil and contacts or the two sets of contacts must be increased over those in Table 13.7 by a factor of 4.

Table 13.7 Creepages, clearances and separations considered as not subject to fault (infallible)

Maximum peak (V)	Creepages, clearances and separations (mm)					CTI values Note 1	
	Clearance	Creepage		Separation			
		Air	CTG	CC	SI	'ia'	'ib'
10	1.5	1.5	0.5	0.5	0.5	Note 2	Note 2
30	2.0	2.0	0.7	0.7	0.5	100	100
60	3.0	3.0	1.0	1.0	0.5	100	100
90	4.0	4.0	1.3	1.3	0.7	100	100
190	5.0	8.0	2.6	1.7	0.8	175	175
375	6.0	10.0	3.3	2.0	1.0	175	175
550	7.0	15.0	5.0	2.4	1.2	275	175
750	8.0	18.0	6.0	2.7	1.4	275	175
1000	10.0	25.0	8.3	3.3	1.7	275	175
1300	14.0	36.0	12.0	4,6	2.3	275	175
1575	16.0	49.0	13.3	5.3	2.7	275	175
3.3 kV	Note 3	Note 3	Note 3	9.0	4.5	N/A	N/A
4.7 kV	Note 3	Note 3	Note 3	12.0	6.9	N/A	N/A
9.5 kV	Note 3	Note 3	Note 3	20.0	10.0	N/A	N/A
15.6 kV	Note 3	Note 3	Note 3	33.0	16.5	N/A	N/A

(from BS/EN 50020)
CTG = Conformal coating
CC = Casting compound
SI = Solid insulation

Notes:
1 CTI refers only to quality of insulation providing the creepage path in air.
2 CTI is not considered as important at these low voltages.
3 No values are given for these voltages and thus it is considered that separation by creepages or clearances alone is not sufficient.

Third, if the figures of 250 V rms or 10 A rms or 500 VA are exceeded in normal operation, then the different circuits on the relay (coil and contacts and, where appropriate, separate sets of contacts) need to be separated by the techniques used to separate intrinsically safe circuit external connection facilities from those for non-intrinsically safe circuits (which are detailed earlier in this section).

13.8 Component and circuit failure modes

Failures of components and circuit connections need to be identified in the fault count unless they are not considered as subject to fault by virtue of additional constructional requirements described later in this chapter. The fault modes which need to be taken into account depend upon the component in question.

13.8.1 Wire and printed circuit tracks

Wires or printed circuit tracks may be considered to become disconnected or break and in either case the action will be considered as a single countable fault, provided that they only carry two thirds of their maximum rated current (the 1.5 safety factor is applied). Where wires are involved, rather than printed tracks, it is possible for them to move and in doing so they may contact other uninsulated conductors in the apparatus. This possibility must be considered and any such interconnection will be considered as a second countable fault and not part of the first one (i.e., the wire break). Thus the interconnection described by wire movement is only important in the case of 'ia' circuits. Wires which are crimped together are not considered as a single wire but as two wires which are connected together.

13.8.2 Connections

Failure of connections of any type other than plugs and sockets (e.g., terminals, crimps, soldering, etc.), provided that they are properly made and, are not operated at more than two thirds of their ratings (the 1.5 safety factor), are considered to fail to open circuit only as a single countable fault. They are not considered to fail to a higher resistance, as is the case for plug and socket elements, as such connections are assumed to have a greater degree of permanence to those made by a plug and socket where wear on the connecting parts, due to multiple removals and insertions, adds a wear element to the consideration not present in the case of other connection systems.

13.8.3 Capacitors and inductors

Capacitors and inductors operated at not more than two thirds of their appropriate ratings (again the 1.5 safety factor) are considered to fail to open circuit, to short circuit, or to lower values of inductance or capacitance. This is because of their construction where the reactance value of both is usually governed by wound lengths of wire or foil. In the case of inductors, it is a wire winding and the inductance cannot increase without increasing the number of turns. All that can happen, therefore, is a reduction of the number of turns which will reduce the inductance and, as in most cases, it will be by short circuit of some turns – the inductor will have a short circuit turn which will dramatically reduce the inductance to the leakage inductance value defined by the efficiency of the coupling between the remaining part of the inductor and the short circuit turn. In the case of capacitors, the capacitance is determined by the length of two parallel wound plates of foil and cannot be increased, except by increase of length.

13.8.4 Resistors

Resistors can fail to any value higher or lower than their specified value. Again this is because of their construction. While this is varied in both materials and detail the worst case has to be assumed. For example, a carbon composition material used in preference to pure carbon in many cases contains impurities which are known to have the possibility to allow failure to reduced resistance. In addition, it is possible for erosion to reduce dimensions of resistance tracks within a resistor. Thus the general situation has to be failure to higher or lower resistance. Failure of a resistor to a particular value is considered as a single countable fault in any fault-counting exercise, providing rating factors are honoured, and once the failure has been assumed further change is not assumed to occur.

13.8.5 Semiconductors

Semiconductors have relatively complex modes of failure which depends upon their construction.

Diodes and zener diodes

Diodes and zener diodes which are not operated at more than two thirds of their maximum current or power ratings (the 1.5 safety factor) can, for example, be assumed to fail to open circuit, short circuit and to a matched condition. The former two modes are usually most important when power transfer to, or protection of, other components is involved but the matched condition is usually the most important where the surface temperature of the diode or zener diode is concerned. Open circuit, short circuit or failure to another resistance value is considered as one countable fault.

Transistors

The situation in regard to transistors operated at no more than two thirds of their maximum current, voltage and power ratings (again the 1.5 V safety factor) is different in that they normally have three leads. Short circuit of any one of those to any one of the others (or both of the others) needs to be considered, together with their interconnection, in a manner which gives the maximum power transfer to other components, for evaluation of the intrinsic safety of the apparatus. The transistor also needs to be considered for temperature classification on the basis of the maximum power available to it being dissipated within it. Once having applied a fault (e.g., a short circuit) the transistor cannot then be assumed to fail in another mode within the same fault evaluation but all modes of failure need to be considered in the various fault-count exercise undertaken (e.g., open circuit as part of the one fault train, short circuit as part of another, etc.).

Integrated circuits

Integrated circuits, while being treated in the same way as transistors, are even more complex as they have a multiplicity of fault possibilities. For the purposes of temperature classification the fault considered is that which will cause all the available power to be dissipated in the unit. The single countable fault will also be considered as interconnections of any combination of pins and open circuits of any number of pins all occurring simultaneously (e.g., in a ten pin circuit all pins can be considered, several interconnections between one or more of them, and total short circuit between them all are valid parts of the single fault). Again resistance interconnection between pins is not considered for evaluation of the circuit outside the integrated circuit in such cases but is considered where device temperature is concerned.

Components which exceed their ratings

If any component or assembly or connection method does not satisfy the rating requirements (two thirds operational safety factor on appropriate parameters) then any of the failures described here are considered as non-countable faults; that is, they are applied in addition to the countable faults required by the grade of intrinsic safety ('ia' or 'ib'). Where they do comply in normal operation, but cease to do so when any permissible countable or non-countable fault or faults are applied elsewhere in the circuit, their failure is considered a part of that or those other faults and is not separately counted.

Application of the test apparatus for spark ignition

Testing for Intrinsic Safety is by insertion of the spark test apparatus. This is placed between points in the circuit where sparking may be considered to occur. It can be placed between any conductors and components, or in series with any components, where partial or total short or high resistance/open circuit failure is considered as a non-countable fault after the appropriate faults have been applied. In addition, the spark test apparatus can be placed in similar situations where failure would be considered as a countable fault, and in such cases the placement and use of the test apparatus will not be considered as an additional countable fault. This position is taken because, although the failure in question would be considered as countable, a transient problem caused by partial disconnection or partial short circuit could cause sparking here for a considerable time and coincide with other fault modes which would make the spark incendive.

13.9 Apparatus construction requirements

In addition to the requirements for components there are minimum requirements for their assembly into items of apparatus to ensure that intrinsic safety is maintained. These requirements include requirements for enclosures, wiring, connections, creepages, clearances and separations.

13.9.1 Enclosures

The requirements for enclosures for intrinsically safe and associated apparatus are that such an enclosure need only exist when necessary to protect bare conductors or infallible separations from being degraded by external influences, such as access. In these cases enclosures need only to have a degree of protection IP20, in accordance with BS/EN 60529[15], which is effectively the degree of protection necessary to prevent live parts being touched. In general, however, apparatus is fitted with an enclosure of a much higher integrity for other reasons, for example, as weatherproofing. What this means is that, except in very special circumstances, the apparatus enclosure will be determined by industrial reliability and basic safety requirements, rather than those of intrinsic safety. This means that requirements for enclosures which are necessary for the other protection concepts for the following reasons are *not* applied in the case of intrinsic safety:

- enclosure opening delay to allow discharge of energy storing devices;
- specific requirements for plastics material to ensure adequate performance (excluding static charge capability);
- specific requirements for threaded holes in plastics and light metal (aluminium, etc.) enclosures;
- requirements for construction of bushings, interlocking devices and fasteners;
- requirements for cementing materials and actions;
- requirements for connection facilities, terminals and terminal compartments;
- impact testing requirements for enclosures to ascertain their strength.

With the exception of drop testing for portable apparatus, therefore, the only requirements in such cases are those which are specified within the Standards related to the protection concept itself. This is because the protection is within the enclosed components and assemblies themselves, and not the enclosure. Thus exposure of the circuits will not lead to a dangerous condition as the circuits remain intrinsically safe. A situation where there was no enclosure because of damage would not be tolerated for long periods as the possibility of environmental attack causing maloperation of the apparatus could not be tolerated, even though it remained intrinsically safe.

Unlike other protection concepts intrinsic safety permits, in special circumstances, apparatus to be in more than one enclosure provided the two parts of the apparatus can be shown to be unique in their interconnection. This is because of the use of the technique in such things as portable radio transceivers and similar devices. Later in this chapter intrinsically safe systems will be discussed and there will be seen to be some similarity between these and the portable radio transceiver with a hand microphone on a short lead. To use the system concept for such equipment, where the two parts are manufactured and supplied together, would be excessively cumbersome and therefore they can be said to fall within the definition of apparatus for intrinsic safety. There may well be other similar situations but it must be stressed that they are exceptional and there must clearly be little possibility of interchange between different parts of different composite apparatus of this type.

13.9.2 Internal layout (wiring, printed circuit boards, etc)

Wiring and tracks on printed circuit boards can, in principle, be uninsulated (bare) conductors. If this is so they may come into contact with one another and create faults. This is not a great problem with printed circuit tracks as they are rigidly placed, but normal conductors or conductors on flexible printed wiring substrates are not. In addition, there is the possibility that insulated wires or tracks may also come into contact and in such cases the quality of the insulation is important. Insulation normally means a plastic or elastomeric coating on the conductor, and varnishes are specifically identified as not being considered as insulation.

The insulation on wires of intrinsically safe circuits and non-intrinsically safe circuits also has to meet certain minimum requirements where its failure could adversely affect intrinsic safety and its thickness is not in accordance with Tables 13.7 and 13.8. If no fault between wires can be tolerated the insulated wires of either the intrinsically safe circuit or the non-intrinsically safe circuit must be within a screen which is earthed, and sufficiently robust to carry any current which may flow from either circuit during the operating time of protection devices such as fuses. If no such screen exists an alternative is to insulate the intrinsically safe wires with insulation which will withstand an rms ac test voltage of at least 2000 V. This latter solution is only acceptable in 'ib' circuits. It is often necessary to include an additional insulating sleeve over the wire to achieve this.

There are certain minimum values (see Table 13.8) below which failure of separations will be considered as a non-countable fault, such separations being measured with possible movement of conductors being chosen to give minimum values. The situations which need consideration are as follows.

Clearance

This is the shortest distance between two uninsulated conductors measured through air. It is not necessarily a line-of-sight measurement as it could be around an insulating barrier which must be at least 0.9 mm thick and sufficiently rigid to withstand a lateral pressure of 30 N. Figure 13.16 shows how clearance is measured. Where an earthed metallic barrier is placed between two conductors it is not necessary to measure the clearance between them, but where the metallic barrier is isolated it is and the thickness of the barrier should be deducted from the value obtained.

Creepage

Creepage distances are measured in a similar way to clearances but here the distance must be along an insulating surface (e.g., the surface of a printed circuit board or a terminal block. The Comparative Tracking Index (CTI, see BS 5901[16]) of the insulating surface is important here as it must reach a minimum value to ensure sufficient insulation quality, except where the voltage between the two conductors is below 30 V as at such low voltages it is considered that CTI is much less important. If the insulating material and the conductors are all covered by an insulating coating, this protects the insulation from degradation and CTI ceases to be important and, because of the protection from the environment provided by the coating, the creepage distances can be significantly reduced. Where, however, the insulating materials and/or the conductors exit the coating, such reductions are not permitted and the insulating material and/or the coating must have the minimum required CTI. The coating must be a conformal coating which adheres to and completely covers the conductors and insulation to which the relaxation is applied. If the coating is brushed on, produced by dipping the assembly into the coating, or produced by vacuum impregnation only one coat is necessary. Where it is applied by other methods, such as spraying, then two separate coats need to be applied. If a solder mask is applied and is not damaged during the soldering operation, only one additional coat is required whatever the method of application. The method of measuring creepage distances is shown in Fig. 13.17, 13.18 and 13.19.

Separation

Separation distances are the distances which must be achieved between bare live conductors, either through solid insulation or encapsulation separations through solid insulation, being less than that through encapsulation reflecting the higher quality of insulation which is normally the case. The method of measurement of separation distances is to measure the shortest distance between the two conductors through the insulation. Insulating partitions are not relevant in the case of those embedded in solid insulation but in the unlikely case of an insulating partition embedded in encapsulant, the effects of the partition can be taken into account. Methods of measurement are shown in Fig. 13.16.

Table 13.8 gives the minimum values of clearances, creepage distances and separations which need to be achieved, so that breakdown between

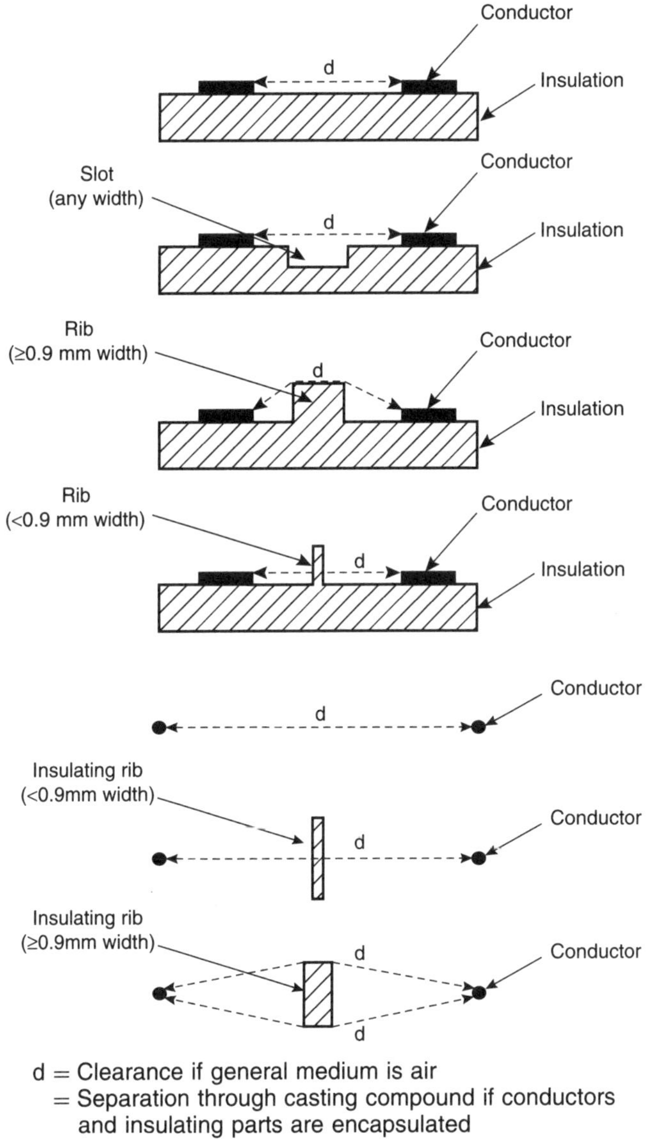

Fig. 13.16 Measurement of clearance and separation distance

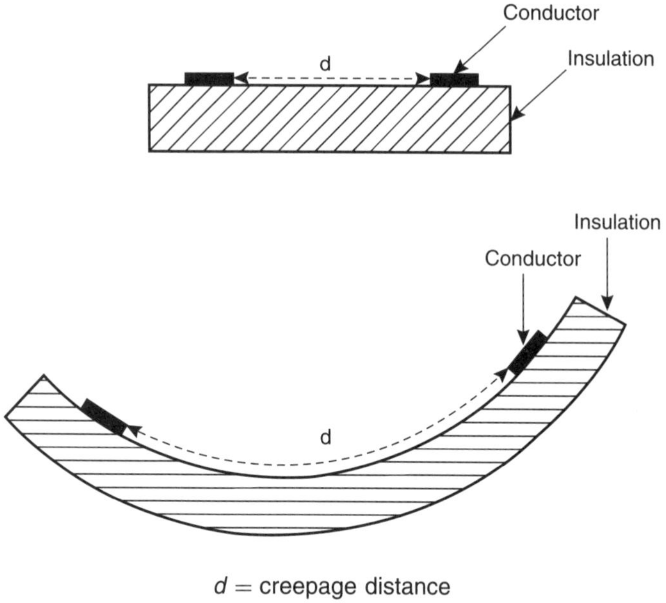

Fig. 13.17 Basic measurement of creepage distance.

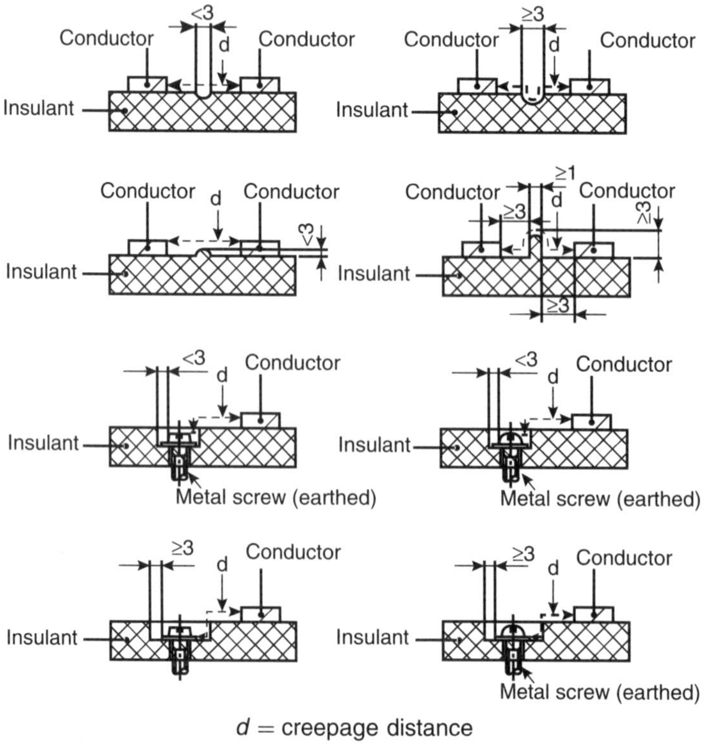

Fig. 13.18 Effect of slots on creepage distance.

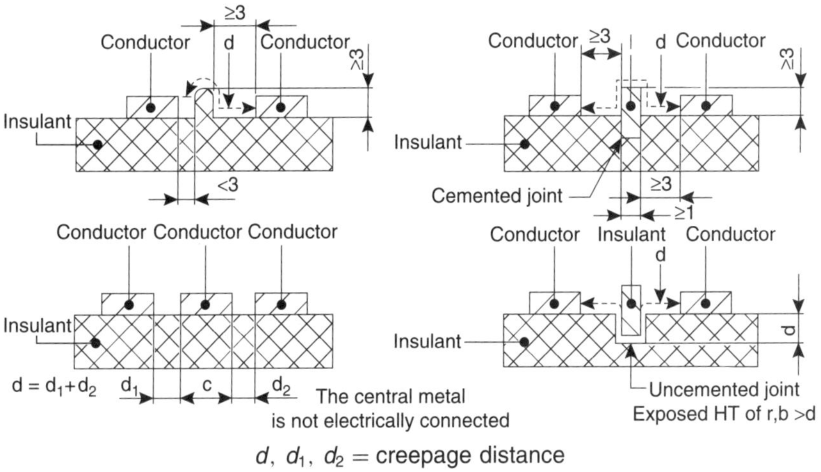

Fig. 13.19 Effect of ribs on creepage distance.

Table 13.8 Creepages, clearances and separations (countable faults)

Maximum peak (V)	Clearances, creepages and separations (mm)					CTI value	
	Clearance	Creepage		Separation		Category	
		Air	CTG	CC	SI	'ia'	'ib'
10V	0.5	0.5	0.17	0.17	0.17	Note 1	Note 1
30V	0.67	0.67	0.24	0.24	0.17	100	100
60V	1.0	1.0	0.34	0.34	0.17	100	100
90V	1.34	1.34	0.44	0.44	0.24	100	100
190V	1.67	2.67	0.87	0.57	0.27	175	175
375V	2.0	3.34	1.1	0.67	0.34	175	175
550V	2.34	5.0	1.67	0.8	0.4	275	175
750V	2.67	6.0	2.0	0.9	0.47	275	175
1000V	3.34	8.34	2.77	1.1	0.57	275	175
1300V	4.67	12.0	4.0	1.54	0.77	275	175
1575V	5.34	16.34	4.44	1.77	0.9	275	175
3.3KV	Note 2	Note 2	Note 2	3.0	1.5	N/A	N/A
4.7KV	Note 2	Note 2	Note 2	4.0	2.0	N/A	N/A
9.5KV	Note 2	Note 2	Note 2	6.67	3.34	N/A	N/A
15.6KV	Note 2	Note 2	Note 2	11.0	5.34	N/A	N/A

CTG = Coating
CC = Casting compound
SI = Solid insulation

Notes:
1 CTI is not considered as important at these low voltages.
2 No values are given for these voltages and thus it is considered that separation by clearance or creepage is not sufficient in such circumstances.

the conductors will be a countable fault and Table 13.7 gives values where they will not fault. If these are not achieved any such breakdown which leads to a less secure condition will be considered a non-countable fault, and applied as appropriate to give the worst condition in both normal operation and the appropriate countable fault scenario. If the distance between the two conductors is comprised of a mixture of clearance and/or separation distance it is possible to add the distances, provided that all component spacings to be added are at least one third of the minimum given in Tables 13.7 and 13.8 for the type of spacing required if that type of spacing existed alone at the voltage between the two conductors in question. The addition is referred to one of three possibilities (clearance, separation through encapsulant, or separation through solid insulation) by the use of the multipliers specified in Table 13.9 (based upon Fig. 13.20) for the voltage between the conductors. Where part of the creepage distance is coated with a conformal coating, the composite creepage is calculated in much the same way but using the multipliers in Table 13.10, based upon Fig. 13.21. In the case of creepage, no minimum is applied to either of the two constituents.

The clearances, creepage distances and separations given in Table 13.8 apply between conducting parts in any intrinsically safe circuit where

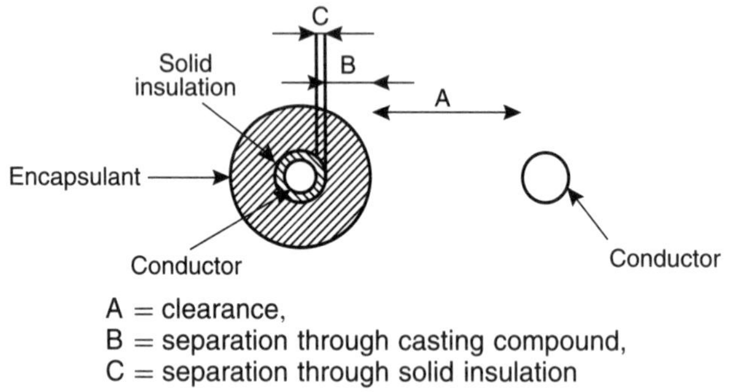

Fig. 13.20 Composite clearance/separation criteria.

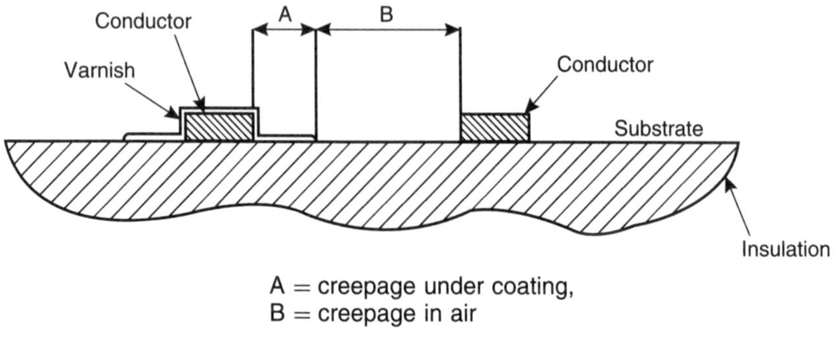

Fig. 13.21 Composite creepage distance criteria.

Table 13.9 Multiples used in calculation of composite spacings

Type of spacing	Peak voltage (Volts)		
	0< U ≤10	10< U ≤30	30< U ≤1575
		Ref: Clearance	
Clearance	1.0	1.0	1.0
Separation through CC	3.0	3.0	3.0
Separation through SI	3.0	4.0	6.0
		Ref: Separation Through CC	
Clearance	0.33	0.33	0.33
Separation through CC	1.0	1.0	1.0
Separation through SI	1.0	1.33	2.0
		Ref: Separation Through SI	
Clearance	0.33	0.33	0.33
Separation through CC	1.0	0.75	0.55
Separation through SI	1.0	1.0	1.0

CC = Casting compound
SI = Solid insulation
Note: Clearance alone is not considered as sufficient above 1575 V and thus composite clearances and separations are not possible. Composite separations through casting compound and solid insulation are, and the relationships between those two are still valid up to 15.6 KV.

Table 13.10 Multiples used in calculation of composite creepages

Type of spacing	Peak voltage (V) 0< U ≤1575
Ref: Creepage Distance in Air	
Creepage in air	1.0
Creepage under conformal coating	3.0
Ref: Creepage Under Conformal Coating	
Creepage in air	0.33
Creepage under conformal coating	1.0

failure is required to be a countable fault, such as across the connections of a diode and between any two separate intrinsically safe circuits where interconnections at countable fault level have been evaluated and shown not to produce an unsafe condition. In addition, the figures apply between an intrinsically safe circuit and a non-intrinsically safe circuit if the addition of the non-intrinsically safe circuit does not cause an unsafe condition when it becomes part of the intrinsically safe circuit. This occurs, typically, in 'ia' apparatus, when such a failure at countable fault level only short circuits part of the current limiting resistance, and hence is acceptable because of the lower safety factor permitted after the second countable fault, and between a conductor of an intrinsically safe circuit and any earthed metal.

The voltages used to apply Tables 13.7 and 13.8 are the peak voltages which occur between the two conductors. These are derived as follows, first, in parts of the same circuit the voltage is the maximum peak voltage which can be measured between the two parts of the circuit if both voltages come from the same source or the numerical addition of the two peak voltages if they come from different sources, except if one of these voltages is less than 20 per cent of the other it can be ignored. For dc voltages the polarity is taken into account but the spacings are also required to be acceptable when the lower of the two voltages is absent. In ac circuits numerical values are chosen which removes the necessity of determination of phase angles. In these cases obviously the situation when one voltage is absent it is less onerous than when both are present. Second, in separate circuits the voltage is always the numerical addition of the two voltages, for both ac and dc, unless one is less than 20 per cent of the other as in this case polarities of dc supplies cannot be guaranteed.

Voltages used are the maximum peak value which can occur in an item of apparatus in either normal or acceptable fault conditions when any electrical supplies are at their maximum declared values (U_m or U_i – see BS/EN 50020), except that any mains supplies will be considered without the addition of their supply tolerance. Transiently higher voltages (such as those which occur during fuse operation and are thus one-offs) are ignored, but if a transient can occur repeatedly with some degree of regularity it must be taken into account. In addition, any conductors which are present in the apparatus need to be secured if insulated to prevent movement causing chafing or cutting of insulation, and must be moved as far as they can be to give minimum spacings before spacing measurement. It is accepted that manufacturing tolerances can further reduce spacings because of manufacturing tolerances, particularly in the case of printed circuit boards. Provided these tolerances are less than 10 per cent they may be ignored and the manufacturers nominal figures taken.

13.9.3 Earth conductors and connections (including terminals)

Earthing is often used in intrinsic safety as a method of ensuring separation of conductors and parts which would damage intrinsic safety if they came into contact. The need for earthing includes the necessity of earthing conductors, screens, enclosures and safety barriers (these are dealt with later in this chapter).

Conductors within the apparatus which connect parts to earth need to use connection methods which are not subject to fault (infallible). The conductors themselves must also be capable of carrying, without overheating or damage, the maximum current which could flow in them in both normal operation and in possible fault conditions.

Connectors which carry such earthed connections need to be arranged so that they do not have the possibility of a disconnection occurring. As normal plug and socket connections are considered to be countable faults, then there needs to be redundancy in the connector. This results in a requirement for two connecting pins for 'ib' and three for 'ia' connected in parallel. Figure 13.14 shows how that can be achieved including the necessary layout in such devices as edge connectors, which can possibly be removed at an angle. Permanent connections to the item requiring earthing for conductors transferring such earth connections through plugs and sockets need to be separate from one another for the same reason, or must be such that they are not considered to fail. The latter type of permanent connection is dealt with later in this chapter.

Terminals in particular need special consideration if they are to be assumed not to fail to open circuit and need to satisfy the following requirements:

1. They must effectively clamp the conductor being terminated to prevent it from slipping from its intended location, even with temperature changes expected (normally −20 °C to +40 °C).
2. They must maintain effective electrical connection of the conductor throughout the range of temperature expected.
3. In cases where multistrand conductors are used without first being crimped in a ferrule there must be an additional clamping plate in the clamping mechanism (e.g., between the screw and the conductor) to ensure proper clamping of all strands.
4. Terminals which are intended for conductors of maximum cross sections of 4 mm^2 or less must be capable of effectively clamping cross sections smaller than the maximum for which they are designed. It is probably not necessary to cover cross sections less than 0.000962 mm^2, which is the minimum for which a maximum permissible current for temperature classification is given (see Table 13.4).
5. There must be no sharp edges on terminals which could damage the conductors being terminated.
6. Terminals must not twist or become deformed when normal screw tightening torques are applied.
7. The transmission of pressure to the parts which ensure contact must not be via any insulating materials.

An easy way of complying with all of these requirements is to select terminals for this use, and for any other use where security from disconnection is required (infallibility) from ranges complying with the requirements for increased safety 'e' (BS/EN 50019) (see Chapter 12).

13.9.4 Encapsulation

Encapsulation can be used for two reasons. It may be necessary to enlarge the surface area of a component in intrinsically safe apparatus to lower the surface temperature where the energy within the encapsulant is intrinsically safe, or it may be used to exclude an explosive atmosphere from a component from an intrinsically safe circuit where energy levels are incendive (e.g., the connection between an inductor and its suppression components). The minimum requirements for the encapsulant are the same in both cases but, in the case of temperature limitation, the amount and thickness of the encapsulant must be such as to achieve the necessary temperature limitation if this requires thicker encapsulant.

The encapsulant must satisfy the following requirements in both intrinsically safe apparatus and in associated apparatus, although in this latter case encapsulant would only be used to maintain spacings. First, it must adhere to the components and/or circuits being encapsulated where they exit the encapsulant. This is necessary because creepage distances are not measured within encapsulant on the basis that contamination cannot enter, and if the encapsulant did not adhere to the encapsulated parts in such cases the contamination could enter which is not acceptable.

Second, where bare conductors exit the encapsulant the encapsulant must have the necessary CTI to protect the creepage distances across its surface.

Third, the encapsulant must also have an operating temperature range specification which ensures that it is not damaged by temperatures reached during operation in both normal and possible fault conditions through the temperature range for which the apparatus is designed (normally $-20\,°C$ to $+40\,°C$). Alternatively, if the encapsulant is shown not to be damaged within this temperature range by tests then it will be acceptable, even if it is operated outside its specification.

Fourth, where the surface of the encapsulant forms part of the outer enclosure of the apparatus it must be a hard (rigid) encapsulant, such as epoxy resin.

Fifth, where the encapsulant has no enclosure, its minimum thickness between any encapsulated component and assembly and its free surface (see Fig. 13.22) must satisfy half of the minimums specified for the voltage of the component or assembly with a minimum of 1 mm.

Finally, where the encapsulant is within an enclosure there is no minimum thickness of encapsulant if the enclosure is of insulating material, but if the enclosure is of conducting material the thickness is determined by that required to prevent any earth connection which could damage intrinsic safety.

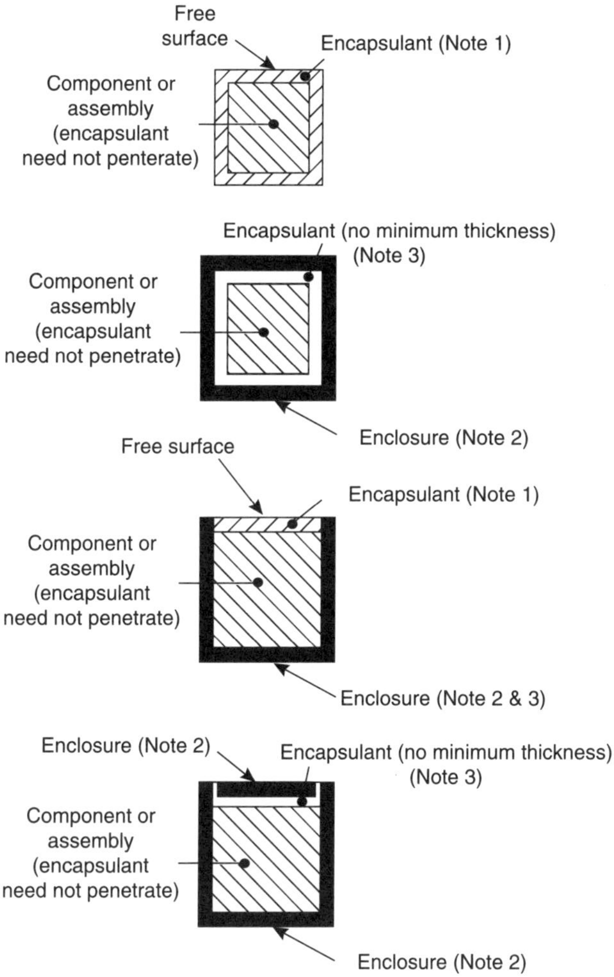

Fig. 13.22 Encapsulation procedures. *Notes*: (1) Encapsulant must be half of the thickness required for separation purposes (Table 13.7) with a 1 mm minimum. (2) Enclosure may be metal or insulating material. Metal has no minimum thickness but insulating material must conform to the thickness for separation purposes (Table 13.7). (3) Where enclosure is metal and can be earthed, thickness of encapsulant inside metal must conform to Table 13.7 or 13.8 as appropriate if earthing adversely affects intrinsic safety

13.10 Infallible components, assemblies and construction elements

As is by now clear, intrinsic safety includes, in its evaluation, failures of components and other circuit elements in two ways, where such failures reduce security. Those which reach a specific level of construction excellence are considered to fail only as part of a limited fault count and those which do not reach this level are considered to fail in any event if such failure makes the circuits more ignition capable. There is a third level to be considered which is that level where construction and rating is of such a high level that failures can be ignored. In components, assemblies of components, and connection elements this level of excellence warrants the award of the title of infallible component, assembly or connection. Such things as separations can also reach a level where failure need not be considered (see Table 13.7) but in this case they are termed as 'not subject to fault' and Infallible is not used. In any event, the results are the same and when carrying out a fault-counting exercise specific failure modes in any of these components, assemblies, wiring, connections and separations need not be considered.

In all cases the infallibility of such components, assemblies, wiring, connections and separations is limited to the particular mode of failure which their construction permits to be ignored (e.g., the separation of a pair of printed circuit tracks may make them such that connections between them can be assumed not to occur, but it will not have any effect upon consideration of their breakage).

While it is confusing to have the two terms 'infallible' and 'not subject to fault' applied to particular failure modes of components and other circuit elements, the use of either term is understood to impart the same information and no danger should result.

Infallible components, assemblies and arrangements which are considered as not subject to particular fault conditions need to comply with specific requirements which are additional to the basic constructional requirements of the protection concept which give countable fault status (see Sections 13.7 and 13.8).

13.10.1 Infallible transformers

Clearly, mains transformers, used in associated apparatus to reduce voltage to the normal low levels used in intrinsically safe circuits, are important as failure of the windings associated with that circuit to the mains winding or other auxiliary windings on the transformer associated with other intrinsically safe circuits or non-intrinsically safe circuits, would lead to a situation where intrinsic safety was compromised. Such a transformer needs to be infallible against such interconnections both in normal operation and in failure conditions. In addition, where failure of windings associated with the intrinsically safe circuit to the core of the transformer, which is normally earthed, could produce an ignition-capable condition, the transformer must be infallible against that failure also. The requirements for such transformers are as follows.

Mains transformer construction

Several modes of construction are envisaged for mains transformers in BS/EN 50020 and are given type numbers. The simplest of these is the

Table 13.11 Minimum dimensions for wire or foil used for transformer screens

Rating of protective fuse or circuit breaker Amps	Thickness of foil forming screen (Note 1) mm	Diameter of wire forming layers of screen (Note 1) mm
0.1	0.05	0.2
0.5	0.05	0.45
1.0	0.075	0.63
2.0	0.15	0.9
3.0	0.25	1.12
5.0	0.3	1.4

(from BS/EN 50020)

Note: 1 The above figures for wire and foil dimensions are nominal figures and a tolerance of up to 10% manufacturing tolerance is permitted provided that in all cases the variation in dimension may not exceed 0.1 mm.

type where the transformer is permitted to exceed its insulation ratings but a failure between non-intrinsically safe circuit windings and other windings is prevented by an earthed metal screen of thickness complying with Table 13.11. This is termed a 'Type 2b transformer and its principles of construction are shown in Fig. 13.23.

Type 2b transformer

The Type 2b transformer is normally a 'shell type' transformer (see Fig. 13.23) with its windings over one another on a single bobbin, or without a bobbin, but consolidated in both cases on a single core so that any separations are reliable and repeatable. The screen must be the full width of the winding area to ensure that no possibility exists for interconnection across the screen except at the outer edge of the windings where Table 13.7 applies. In either case the insulation or other separation between the windings associated with intrinsically safe circuits and the core, the screen and the other windings must ensure that the transformer satisfies the following as a minimum:

1. The composite separation between the winding mass of the separate windings around the screen must satisfy the requirements of Table 13.7. (In most cases this will require a composite calculation of separation distance – see Figs. 13.20 and 13.21).

2. The screen must be of either a single layer of foil which comprises at least one turn and overlaps but is insulated so that the ends of the screen cannot become interconnected, or of two layers wound in insulated (varnished) wire. For a foil screen this requirement is to avoid the screen ends becoming

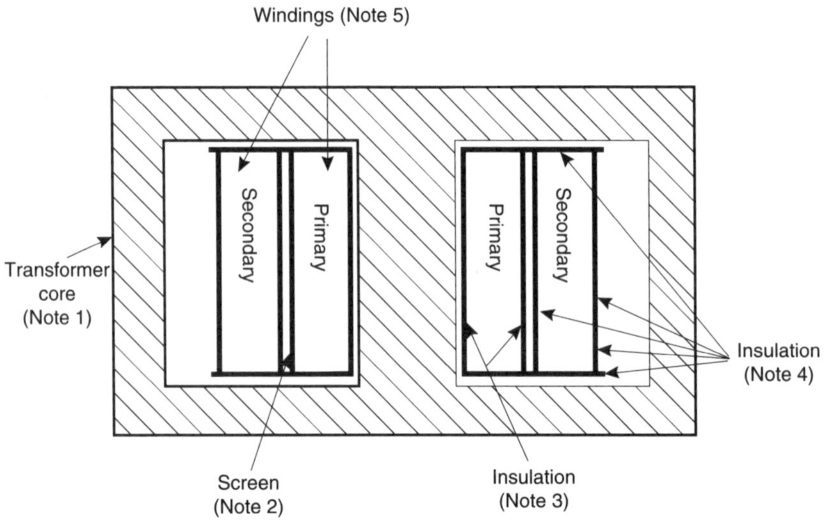

Fig. 13.23 Type 2b transformer. *Notes*: (1) Core to be provided with earth connection (interleaved in laminations if appropriate) unless core material is non-conducting. (2) Screen to be provided with two earth connection wires if foil; both layers to have one end brought out if wire layers. (3) Insulation to normal industrial requirements. (4) Insulation to withstand 500 V test unless earth faults not acceptable when Table 13.7 applies, as appropriate. (5) Windings to be consolidated

connected to form a short circuited turn which will cause the transformer to fail. For a wire screen, insulation between each turn of wire and between the two layers is necessary for the same reason. Because of this, the only insulation requirement between layers is that the insulation will not fail when subjected to an insulation test at an applied voltage of 500 V rms ac or 700 V dc. The voltage is applied by raising the applied voltage steadily so that the specified value is attained after 10 seconds and then maintaining that value for 60 seconds. The leakage current should be less than 5 mA and must be constant or reducing as any increase will be assumed to be advance warning of insulation failure.

3. The transformer must not create a condition where the winding/s associated with a particular intrinsically safe circuit become connected to other windings. To prove this a test is applied where one (any one) of the output windings of the transformer is short circuited and then all other output windings are subjected to a load which will produce maximum rated current from that winding at rated voltage. The transformer then is subjected to application of its rated voltage at the input winding or such smaller voltage, as will give $1.7I_n$ into the transformer. This condition is applied for 6 hours or until the transformer fails. The criteria for insulation is that when a voltage of twice the transformer rated voltage (U_n) plus 1000 V with a minimum of 1500 V is applied between the windings in question, the current which flows should not exceed 5 mA and should be

constant or falling. The transformer may fail during this test but must not burst into flames as burning may introduce further consequent failures.

4. Where failure to earth may cause problems for the intrinsically safe circuit, failure of the transformer must not occur and the transformer must not exceed its temperature rating during the above test. This can be achieved by the use of in-built thermal trips as already described or by the inclusion of a limiting resistor to limit current in the transformer. Where automatically resetting trips are used, rather than non-resetting trips, the test is extended to 12 hours to allow for repeated trip operations. Where a resistor is fitted it will be mounted in the input circuit of the transformer and must satisfy the separation requirements of Table 13.7, be of adequate rating (see earlier in this chapter), and be infallible as described later. The separation of the winding/s supplying the intrinsically safe circuit and other windings and the screen must in this case satisfy Table 13.7. The possible effect of failures to earth is shown in the example in Fig. 13.24.

5. Where the screen is of two separate layers of winding each layer should be individually connected to earth and provision made for this on the transformer. Where the screen is a foil it must have two separate wires connected to it to allow the same security of earth connection and care is necessary to ensure that connection of these wires does not introduce a partial short circuit turn on the transformer.

6. The core of the transformer must also be earthed and its construction should allow for this. This is usually done by interleaving a conducting strip in the laminations and then providing a terminal on it where it exits the laminations. Some transformer materials, such as ferrites, may be insulating in themselves and in such cases the earth connections are not necessary. It would not be acceptable, however, to insulate a conducting core and not earth it unless the insulation thickness satisfied Table 13.10 and the transformer was prevented from overheating as previously described.

7. The separation of the connection facilities should also comply with the requirements of Table 13.10 to prevent interconnections at the termination points.

Type 1a, 1b and 2a transformers

The other types of transformer envisaged are the Type 1a transformer, the Type 1b transformer, and the Type 2a transformer. The Type 1a transformer has its windings wound side by side on one limb of the transformer and the Type 1b transformer follows the same construction but has the separate windings on separate limbs of the transformer, but still as separate entities (not one over the other).

The Type 1b transformer is more common as it uses a 'shell type' core where one limb goes through the winding and the two other limbs surround it, rather than the Type 1a transformer which normally has a 'core type' core with one limb through each winding and usually no surrounding limbs.

The Type 2a transformer is similar to the Type 2b transformer, but in this case there is no screen with the windings being on top of one another and having insulation between them. The insulation must, of course, be the full width of the winding area (see Fig. 13.24) to prevent the presence of a path through it except around the outside edge of the winding where Table 13.7 applies.

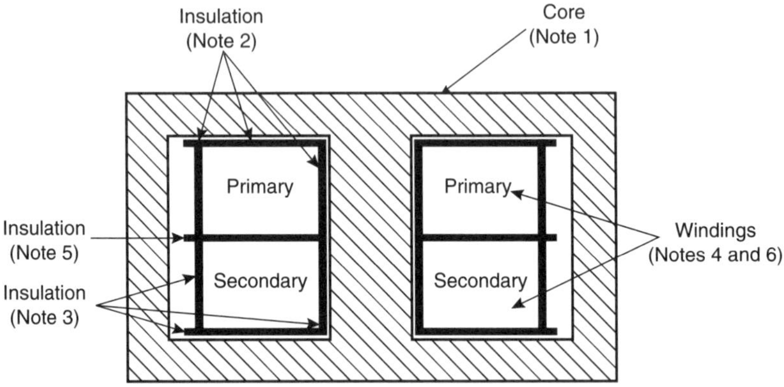

Fig. 13.24 Type 1a transformer. *Notes*: (1) Core to be provided with earth connection (interleaved in laminations if appropriate) unless core material is non-conducting. (2) Insulation to normal industrial standards. (3) Insulation to withstand 500 V test unless earth faults are not acceptable when Table 13.10 applies. (4) If necessary to prevent overheating, thermal trip embedded in either primary or secondary (as appropriate). (5) Insulation to Table 13.10. (6) Windings to be consolidated

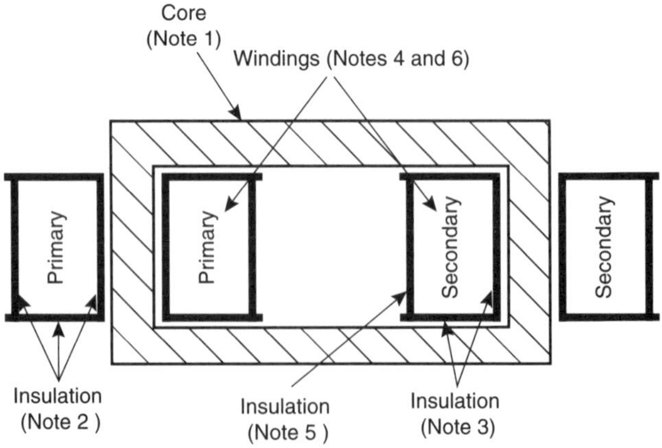

Fig. 13.25 Type 1b transformer. *Notes*: (1) Core to be provided with earth connection (interleaved in laminations if appropriate) unless core material is non-conducting. (2) Insulation to normal industrial standards. (3) Insulation to withstand 500 V test unless earth faults are not acceptable when Table 13.7 applies. (4) If necessary to prevent overheating, thermal trip embedded in either winding (as appropriate). (5) Insulation to Table 13.7. (6) Windings to be consolidated

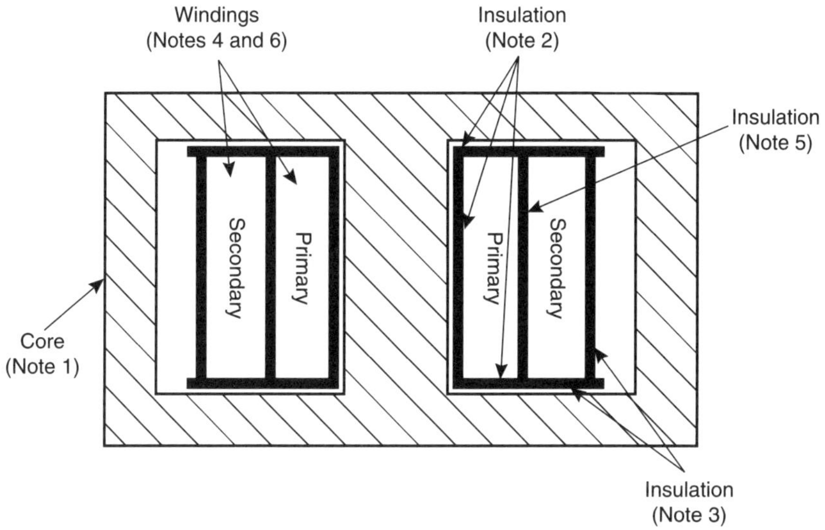

Fig. 13.26 Type 2a transformer. *Notes*: (1) Core to be provided with earth connection (interleaved in laminations if appropriate) unless material is non-conducting. (2) Insulation to normal industrial standards. (3) Insulation to withstand 500 V test unless earth faults are not acceptable when Table 13.10 applies. (4) If necessary to prevent overheating thermal trip embedded in primary or secondary winding (as appropriate). (5) Insulation to Table 13.10. (6) Windings to be consolidated

In all these cases the transformer must have its windings consolidated and must not fail when subjected to type tests described for Type 2b transformers, which almost invariably means that a thermal trip or limiting resistor is needed as in the case of most Type 2b transformers. The thickness of insulation between each winding and others, or the earthed core of the transformer (if earthing causes a problem) must satisfy Table 13.7. Detail of the construction of Types 1a, 1b and 2a transformers are shown in Fig. 13.24, 13.25 and 13.26.

As transformers being wound and generally assembled components are subject to a higher degree of variability than other more critically controlled components a routine test is necessary and this test is described in Table 13.12.

Construction of transformers which are not mains transformers

Within intrinsically safe circuits it is common to use transformers for other purposes (e.g., to produce galvanic isolation between parts of the circuit). Such transformers must be constructed in accordance with the mains transformer requirements except that the 5-hour test need only be done at rated transformer load. Where such transformers are connected between

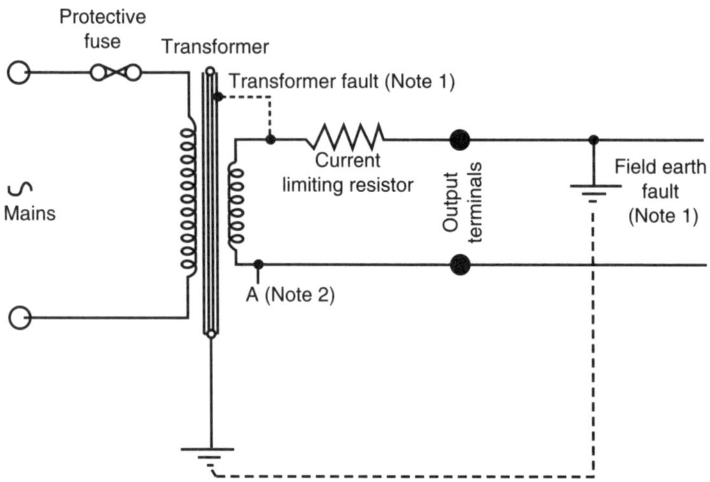

Fig. 13.27 Effect of transformer winding/core or screen faults. *Notes*: (1) Field earth fault can be expected as *normal operation* and thus secondary/frame fault in transformer (either as single countable fault or non-countable fault) will bypass current limiting resistor destroying intrinsic safety. (2) If this point is infallibly earthed transformer fault shown will merely blow protective fuse leaving intrinsic safety intact

Table 13.12 Routine test voltages for mains transformers

Application points	rms applied voltages
Between the mains input winding and all secondary windings	$4\,U_n$ or 2000 V rms
Between all the windings (both input and secondary) and the transformer core.	$2\,U_n$ or 1000 V rms
Between the Intrinsically Safe circuit winding(s) associated with a particular intrinsically safe circuit and all other secondary windings.	$2\,U_n + 1000$ V rms with a minimum of 1500 V rms

Note: The criteria for the test is a current of less than 5 mA which is steady or falling during the test which is applied for 60 seconds the voltage having been raised steadily to the test value in 10 seconds.

intrinsically safe and non-intrinsically safe circuits there is, however, a further problem in that the non-intrinsically safe circuits are not evaluated and it must be assumed that mains can break through to the transformer. In such cases it is necessary to introduce measures to prevent this causing damage to the transformer. Such precautions could be those applied to mains transformers of the same type or, alternatively, by placing a shunt zener diode across the affected winding and then protecting the diode with a suitably rated fuse to ensure that the mains breakthrough is removed before the transformer or zener diode can be damaged. The requirements of Table 13.7 need to be applied to this fuse/zener combination to ensure it cannot be by-passed.

Transformer protection

To ensure that no failures occur it is essential that the transformer cannot be operated in such a way as to allow those failures. This necessitates protection of the transformer in a way which allows its worst case conditions to be defined. All mains transformers have to be supplied with an input fuse to remove the mains supplies if failures occur either in the transformers themselves or the connected circuits.

The basic level of protection is to fuse the input circuit so that the maximum design operating conditions of the transformer specified during its design cannot be exceeded. As the transformer can handle these without causing problems in the intrinsically safe circuit, it can be considered as infallible.

The fuse must comply with the requirements already described in Section 13.6.2 for fuses mounted in associated apparatus, which means that the maximum current which the transformer can continuously draw is, with the presence of such a fuse, considered as 1.7 times the rated fuse current (I_n). A suitably rated circuit breaker may be used in place of a fuse and the circuit breaker need only comply with a recognized standard of construction for such circuit breakers. The 1.7 I_n figure is retained and in this case is 1.7 times the rated current at which the breaker will operate. Therefore, the transformer must be capable of withstanding this current without damage, which could adversely affect intrinsic safety.

The basic requirements of circuit breakers is that they comply with a recognized Standard which normally is taken to mean a European Standard, a harmonized International Standard or, failing the presence of either of these, a National Standard.

The use of the fuse or circuit breaker described above is usually sufficient for transformers of Type 2b construction unless winding faults between the transformer windings and core or screen are not acceptable when, in common with Types 1a, 1b and 2a transformers, the current which the fuse will pass (1.7 I_n) must not additionally allow the winding temperatures to exceed their insulation rating. In circumstances where this can occur a thermal trip will be necessary to ensure this does not occur.

Where such a thermal trip is used to disconnect the transformer from its supplies before winding temperatures are exceeded it must not be accessible. It must be embedded, in or consolidated with, the windings so that confidence is present that it will reliably disconnect before any winding or other insulation within the transformer exceeds its rated limit. The trip may be non-resettable or automatically self-resetting but not manually reset as this implies external intervention which would not be acceptable as it would permit resetting before the transformer could cool, and the possibility exists of the temperature limits of the construction being exceeded. Only one such device is necessary.

The constructional requirements for such a thermal trip are that it should be to a recognized Standard for such devices. (Recognized Standard in this context usually means a European Standard where one exists, a harmonized International Standard or, failing either of these, a national Standard).

Where the transformer is possessed of a suitable earthed screen it is not essential to ensure that insulation temperature limits are not exceeded if earth faults within the transformer do not cause problems. It must be remembered that, in the UK, the normal mains supplies are earthed as a matter of policy for personnel protection by connection of the neutral pole of the supply to earth at the point of supply origination. This means that in the case of a fault in the transformer any supply pole could be earthed. To ensure that the supply is effectively isolated on such failures all non-earthed electrical supply conductors must have a fuse or circuit breaker satisfying the already specified requirements.

In cases where it is not considered necessary to include transformer winding/earth faults in the fault scenario and the power supply is not referenced to earth (which is the case in some other countries), only one protection device in the input circuit may be necessary as failure to earth of a single supply conductor does not cause the same type of problem as it may where the supply is referenced to earth. An evaluation of the possible fault scenarios shows that, even if the fault combination envisaged within the intrinsic safety concept does not include a situation of by-passing protection devices, the more remote possibility of this occurring is enough to produce a recommendation that all non-earthed supply conductors have a protective device, regardless of the type of transformer used and its supply.

13.10.2 Damping windings

Damping windings are used to minimize the effects of inductance in cases such as relays. They are effectively short circuit turns and reduce the apparent inductance to the leakage inductance which represents the inverse of the efficiency of coupling between them and the main winding. If such windings are used to minimize inductance for the purposes of intrinsic safety, they must be reliable so that they can be considered as infallible against open circuit failure. The typical way to ensure this is to use uninsulated copper tubes or wires which are continuously short circuited by soldering or welding. Any winding used for this purpose needs to achieve this level of security against open circuiting.

13.10.3 Current limiting resistors

Current limiting resistors are typically used to limit short circuit current to a hazardous area, to limit the current which can be fed to an inductor, to limit current to a component for temperature classification purposes, or to limit discharge rates of otherwise ignition capable capacitors. These resistors need to be infallible against failure to a lower resistance value but may increase in resistance or become open circuit. In order to achieve this the resistors must be of particular types of construction as follows. First, carbon or metal film type, where the resistance element is effectively an insulated layer of pure carbon or metal deposited on a substrate which is normally ceramic or similar insulating material, helically etched to give the required resistance, and then protected by insulating enamel or varnish to prevent external contact with the element; second, wound in wire on a ceramic former or a former of similar material and then consolidated by enamelling, varnishing, etc., to prevent the wire from unwinding on breakage or being contacted from the outside of the resistor; and third, printed resistors used in hybrid circuits where the resistor is printed on an insulating substrate using conducting inks, produced by metal deposition, or constructed in a similar manner and then covered with an insulating conformal coating or encapsulated.

The commonly available carbon composition resistors are not suitable for this use as experience has shown they can fail in a way which produces lower resistance values due to the impurities introduced into the carbon in their construction.

13.10.4 Blocking capacitors

Where capacitors are used to prevent the transmission of dc and are required to be infallible it is possible to use only two capacitors in 'ia' circuits to achieve this, provided the capacitors are of sufficient reliability. This effectively excludes electrolytic and tantalum types and restricts the choice of capacitor to those with solid dielectrics such as ceramic, paper, polyester and similar materials. Where two capacitors of acceptable types of construction are connected in series they are considered as infallible and the effective capacitance will be that present if either of them fails to short circuit. Thus a single capacitor failure is equated to two countable faults. Apart from their construction type each of the two capacitors needs also to be proof against the following situations.

First, each capacitor must withstand, without breakdown, a 50 Hz rms ac and dc voltage of $2U + 1000\,V$ with a minimum of 1500 V. The test is applied as previously described for withstand tests (i.e., raising the voltage steadily over 10 seconds and then maintaining it over 60 seconds) and also, as previously, the maximum current which may flow is 5 mA which must be either falling or stable during the 60 seconds of the test. For the ac test the current passing will, of course, be dependent on the reactance of the capacitor but increases during the test are taken as a sign of failure.

Second, where the capacitors are connected between the intrinsically safe circuit and earth, or separate intrinsically safe circuits, and failure to earth could create an unsafe condition by, for example, by-passing safety components, the test voltage above should be reduced to 2 U with a minimum of 500 V.

In both of the above cases the mounting of the capacitors must be such as to comply with Table 13.10 if the assembly is to be considered as infallible against direct interconnection of the two circuits separated by the capacitors.

The voltage U, specified in the electric strength tests above, is the maximum voltage which can appear across the capacitor combination in service in the case of capacitor combinations.

13.10.5 Shunt safety assemblies

A shunt safety assembly is one which typically limits discharge of inductors (using normally reverse biased diodes) or limits voltage across parts of intrinsically safe circuits so as to ensure safety. Such limiting action must be infallible and such assemblies are considered as infallible against open circuit failure. The mounting and connection of such assemblies needs to be such that open circuit of connections can be ignored (see Section 13.10.6).

Shunt safety assemblies are limited to semiconductor devices as it is necessary to have confidence that the devices themselves have a low rate of failure to open circuit and, almost uniquely, the mode of failure of a semiconductor junction is a short circuit or lower resistance as it results from degradation of the junction in the semiconductor. This permits the number of elements of the shunt protection to be reduced from three to two in 'ia' circuits.

The particular use of thyristors presents a problem due to their operating time and resultant let-through energy. Where such devices are used as safety shunts this let-through energy must not exceed the following limits:

$$\text{IIA} = 160\,\mu\text{J}$$

$$\text{IIB} = 80\,\mu\text{J}$$

$$\text{IIC} = 20\,\mu\text{J}$$

Shunt safety assemblies which limit voltages within intrinsically safe circuits

Shunt Safety Assemblies which limit voltage are those which are interposed between power supplies and intrinsically safe circuits, between other circuits (e.g., output receptors) and intrinsically safe circuits, or used to further limit voltages within an intrinsically safe circuit where the principal supply voltage has already been defined. In the two former cases the external circuits must be assumed to contain transients unless their power supplies are fed from the mains via an infallible transformer or are batteries. Where the voltage limiter in question is not the prime voltage limiter (e.g., it has a further infallible voltage limiter between it and the external circuit or power supply) it can also be assumed that transients do not occur.

Voltage regulator assemblies, thyristors diodes, zener diodes, and similar devices are permissible provided the circuits in which they occur are free from transients as described above. (Clearly this is not the case where such elements are connected on the output side of mains transformers or used to limit voltages entering the intrinsically safe circuits from other circuits as the lack of definition and control of such supplies and circuits makes it impossible to identify freedom from transients.) In such cases there need to be two parallel shunt paths which normally means two of the shunt components or assemblies in parallel. Each shunt component, assembly or path needs to be able to withstand not only the maximum voltage with which it is supplied and the maximum power which it may dissipate in operation, but needs to be able to carry the current which would flow through it if it failed to short circuit (the normal mode of failure for semiconductors). This is particularly important in the case of semiconductors and similar devices, as the internal leads connecting the semiconductor material to the leads are usually very fine and excessive current could fuse them which would mean that a short circuit failure would inevitably lead to an open circuit failure. Because of the requirement for the absence of transients, these components or assemblies are normally to be found carrying out such functions as limiting the voltage which can occur across a capacitor within an intrinsically safe circuit, providing a lower voltage supply in such a circuit where the principal voltage has already been defined by other components or assemblies, or limiting power supply voltages in power supplies using infallible transformers to provide mains isolation. The reason for this is that devices such as transistors and thyristors and voltage regulators using such devices do not effectively quench transients and sparking associated with such transients could occur. In Zone 0, where 'ia' circuits enter, there will be an explosive atmosphere for much of the time and this is not acceptable.

Where the shunt safety components or assemblies are used to define voltages in situations where transients are possible, such as within power supplies not fed from infallible transformers where mains-borne transients can occur, transistors, voltage regulators and thyristors cannot be used in 'ia' circuits and the only effective options left are diodes and zener diodes. Again two components or assemblies are considered as infallible but in such cases the elements used have to withstand any transients which may occur. In some cases this can be determined by comparing the component specification with the fuse/time characteristic to determine the size and duration of transients and the ability of the shunt component to deal with them without damage. Where this is not the case, however, it is necessary to test the devices. This is done by determining the maximum current which can flow from the mains or other power source by dividing its maximum voltage by the minimum value for the cold resistance of the fuse and any other infallible series resistance present. The device is then subjected to five current pulses of that amplitude, each 50 μs wide (or if the fuse pre-arcing time at that current is longer the pre-arcing time) at intervals of 20 ms. The voltage of the device after that test must not have risen by more than 5 per cent.

Circuit protection and component energy safety shunts

In general, these devices do not operate normally but only in case of a fault elsewhere. This does not necessarily mean that they do not normally conduct or perform an operational function but only that their intrinsic safety function is not called upon in normal operation. Again, two devices are acceptable with the restriction as for voltage limiting shunts where transients may occur and the assumption of transients as already specified. Transients are not considered in this case when such components and assemblies are used to limit discharge of inductors or voltage appearing across capacitors in intrinsically safe circuits.

13.10.6 Internal wiring and connections

It has already been discussed how properly constructed screw terminals may be assumed not to allow disconnection of their conductors and the requirements which such terminals must satisfy. These terminals can, of course, also be used for internal connection and will be considered as not subject to fault (infallible). Likewise, the need for redundancy in plugs and sockets for earth connections has shown that such connections cannot be considered as infallible and need to be subjected to the normal fault count. Internally the normal wiring and connection arrangements need addressing as to their reliability. Both wires (and printed circuit tracks) and their end connections can be made infallible by reaching a minimum standard of construction.

Wires and printed circuit tracks

The necessary requirements for wires to achieve infallibility are as follows. First, an interconnection of two wires in parallel is considered as infallible provided that they reach normal standards of construction. This means that there must be no obvious movement or sharp edges which could be expected to reduce their reliability and increase the risk of their breaking. The precautions taken in this regard are no more than would be expected in good industrial practice. In this case each wire will be rated for current carrying capacity assuming the other has failed.

Second, the connection may be reduced to one wire for infallibility where the wire has a single conductor of at least 0.5 mm diameter, is secured adjacent to each point of connection to avoid stresses at the connection point, and has no unsupported length (unsecured length) which exceeds 50 mm.

Third, a single stranded wire subject to the same fixing requirements as a single wire with a single conductor without any minimum size of strand is accepted as infallible, provided the total conductor cross sectional area (the addition of the cross sectional area of all of the strands) is greater than 0.125 mm^2 (equivalent to a 0.4 mm single conductor). This area is less than would be expected for a single conductor as stranded wires are more flexible and less prone to conductor breakage.

The requirements for printed circuit tracks are a little different as such tracks are not subject to movement in the same way. It is true that flexible printed circuit tracks can flex but these must be accepted as similar to wiring and the requirements for wiring will apply to these. For rigid printed circuit boards the following requirements are necessary for infallibility. First, a minimum thickness of deposited copper forming the track is necessary and this minimum is 35 μm. Tracks of less than this thickness will be considered to fail as a single countable fault if properly rated.

Second, two tracks of at least the above thickness, each having a minimum width of 1 mm, are considered as infallible. In this case each track needs to be rated to carry the current which would flow if the other track were broken.

Third, a single track of at least the above thickness is considered as infallible if it has a width of at least 1 per cent of its length, with a minimum of 2 mm.

The wires and tracks require to be rated in the conditions stated above assuming the required range of faults (both countable and non-countable) have occurred in the apparatus and the 1.5 safety factor needs to be applied. This means that in the case of a two parallel conductor configuration, the current through each conductor will be determined in all possible fault conditions and then multiplied by 1.5 to determine the necessary rating for the conductor.

Connections and connectors

As wires are deemed to be infallible in certain circumstances the end connections of these wires must also have that credibility or the infallibility of wires would be pointless. As already stated, plugs and sockets cannot attain this level of security and a normal fault count is applied to these requiring three parallel connections. For more stable connections infallibility is possible and, to achieve this, the following requirements need to be met.

First, two permanent connections in parallel, such as two screwed connections, two soldered joints or two wire wrapped connections are always considered as infallible provided they satisfy the normal requirements of good industrial practice. This matches up well with the situation where two parallel wires or printed circuit tracks are used and the connection must be rated for the maximum current which could flow in it, assuming the other connection has become open circuit. Second, a single welded, brazed or crimped joint is accepted as infallible.

Third, and alternatively, a single soldered joint is considered as infallible, provided it is additionally mechanically secured against separation. For wires this offers little advantage as the methods of additional securing, such as crimping, are infallible in themselves but for printed circuit joints considerable advantage exists. If the wire is inserted through a plated-through hole in the printed circuit board and then bent over on the other

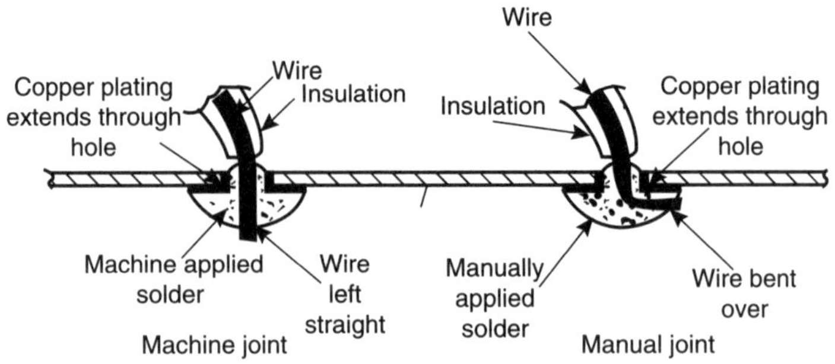

Fig. 13.28 Infallible soldered joints

side (see Fig. 13.28), when it is soldered the solder will penetrate the hole to a degree and give much more security of joint together with the larger volume of solder used on the bent conductor. Where a high reliability and repeatability form of soldering, such as machine soldering, is used then bending over the wire is not necessary.

A single screwed type joint (terminal joint) is also acceptable, provided that it satisfies the requirements for earth connection terminals described earlier in this chapter.

As before, each joint needs to be rated to carry the maximum current which would flow in the recognized conditions of fault with a safety factor of 1.5. This applies to each joint where two parallel joints are used.

13.10.7 Galvanic separation

Galvanic separation (galvanic isolation) is often required between intrinsically safe and non-intrinsically safe circuits to prevent breakthrough of unacceptable voltages and currents, between separate intrinsically safe circuits for the same reasons, and between separate earths. This latter requirement may be considered as somewhat surprising but it must be borne in mind that in cases of electrical fault heavy electrical currents can flow in earth connections, and the voltage at one so-called grounded point can be different to that at another. As intrinsic safety relies upon control of energy in the hazardous area, a circuit which is connected to earth at more than one point may, due to different voltages existing at its points of connection, have added into it an unknown and essentially uncontrolled voltage. Thus circuits are earthed at only one point or not at all, although the latter is not common due to the problems associated with charging of isolated circuits.

Galvanic separation from earth by insulation

Unless more than one earth can by-pass a safety component when the normal insulation and separation requirements of the concept apply, it is only necessary to insulate an intrinsically safe circuit so that it will withstand an ac insulation test voltage of at least twice the circuit voltage with a minimum withstand of 500 V rms. Where safety components may be by-passed, the requirements of Tables 13.7 must be applied.

Galvanic separation between separate intrinsically safe circuits

Separation between separate intrinsically safe circuits may be achieved by insulation or separation between them using such elements as transformers, relays, optocouplers, capacitors, etc. Where the separation is required to be infallible, the physical separation must comply with Table 13.7 or infallible components or assemblies must be used. In other cases, the normal requirements of the concept apply and failure is taken as non-countable or a countable fault according to the construction or separation.

Optocouplers are also used for galvanic separation and are subject to the two thirds rating reduction. They will not have to satisfy Table 13.7, however, if they withstand a voltage test of 2U + 1000 V rms with a minimum of 1500 V rms between their separate parts. In this case, U is the highest manufacturers voltage rating for the device.

Galvanic separation between intrinsically safe and non-intrinsically safe circuits

Separation by transformers has already been dealt with in consideration of infallible transformers. Separation by relays has been partially dealt with in that the coil contact requirements for relays have already been considered. It is necessary, however, to remind ourselves that Table 13.7 applies to the separation between any two elements of the relay (e.g., coil/contact or contact/contact to achieve galvanic separation). Where the contacts of the relay are in the non-intrinsically safe circuit, the voltage considered is already the normal mains voltage and the circuit to which the contacts are connected will, if satisfying the maximum VA contact requirements in normal operation, in all probability have suitable fault protection so that these ratings are not exceeded in fault conditions. It must also be noted that the use of such things as increased separations or barriers for higher VA ratings will apply where the separation is between separate contacts, as well as between coil and contacts. Also, where any doubt exists as to the maximum VA rating of the contacts in conditions of fault in the non-intrinsically safe circuits to which they are connected, protection such as fusing will be necessary in the contact circuits.

Separation by blocking capacitors is also a possibility but again the capacitors must satisfy the requirements for infallibility and the external separations must satisfy the requirements of Table 13.7.

Optocouplers are used for the purposes of galvanic separation but are usually in low voltage circuits. As there is a possibility of the non-intrinsically safe circuit being at mains potential because it is not evaluated, some form of protection for the optocoupler will be necessary in addition to the separation of its two parts having to meet Table 13.10 requirements. This is normally achieved by using a shunt zener diode across the non-intrinsically safe connections and protecting it with a suitable rated fuse. The fuse/zener diode combination is chosen in the same way as for safety shunts to ensure that the fuse will always clear before the zener diode is damaged.

13.11 Diode safety barriers

Developed in the late 1960s the diode safety barrier (or shunt zener barrier as it also known) provided a tool which revolutionized intrinsic safety as a technique. The device was designed to fit at the hazardous area/non-hazardous area interface of an intrinsically safe circuit and be proof against breakthrough of dangerous voltages into the hazardous area. When one is fitted, therefore, the maximum voltage and current which needs to be considered is the let-through voltage and current of the barrier device whatever the apparatus connected on the non-hazardous area side of the device. Thus, for the first time, it was not necessary to use specially constructed associated apparatus and almost any normal industrial apparatus was usable resulting in great increases in flexibility and decreases in cost. The only problem was the necessity for the devices to have safety earths which dictated the point at which the intrinsically safe circuit was earthed, but this was only a problem in a small minority of cases (such as some public address systems) and in these special associated apparatus could be constructed.

The barrier device in its earliest form relied on the characteristics of the zener or avalanche diode which, although a normal diode in the forward direction was specially constructed so that it suffered recoverable avalanche breakdown in the reverse direction (see Fig. 13.29. These devices were assembled, as shown in Fig. 13.30, to form an assembly which was proof against mains breakthrough (or breakthrough of the supplies to the apparatus on the non-hazardous side) into the hazardous area and define the maximum open circuit voltage, short circuit current, and let through power available to the circuit in the hazardous area. The operation of the device is as follows:

1. The voltage is controlled by two shunt zener diodes, Z1 and Z2 in Fig. 13.30, forming a shunt voltage limiting network. Because of the sensitivity of such devices and their usual ultimate encapsulation, the diodes are routinely subjected to a 150 °C storage test for 2 hours and then the pulse test for shunt voltage limiters.
2. To allow confidence in the action of the diodes they need to be protected by a fuse, F1 in Fig. 13.30, offering the same protection as the fuse described for shunt voltage limiters.

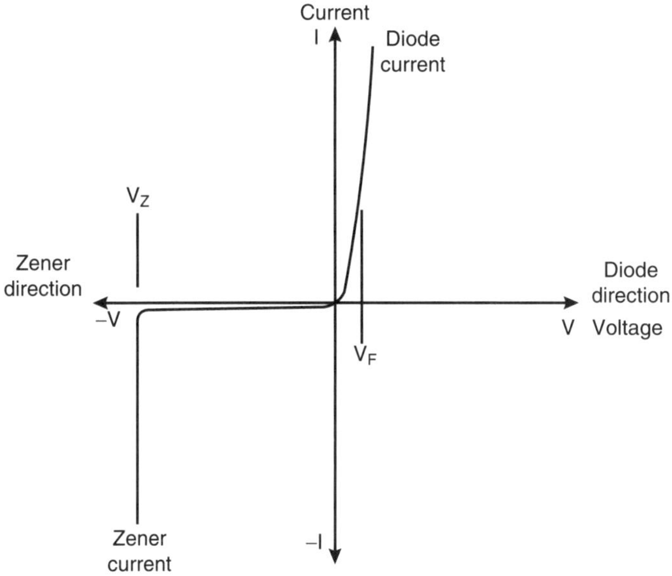

V_F = Forward diode voltage (usually 0.5–0.8 V),
V_z = Zener or avalanche breakdown voltage (3–100 + V)

Fig. 13.29 Typical zener (avalanche) diode characteristics

3. A resistor, R1 in Fig. 13.30, is placed between the diodes so that after assembly, when they cannot be accessed, it is still possible to test for their presence.
4. A final resistor, R2 in Fig. 13.30, is then placed after the zener diodes to limit the short circuit current to the hazardous area to a safe level at the maximum zener diode voltage

The whole is then encapsulated or enclosed by some other means which ensures that access to the components will not be possible without destroying the barrier. The assembly needs to be fitted with an earth connection which is effectively infallible (either a single infallible connection or two connections in parallel) which is used to earth the barrier only. Any circuit conductors which are at earth potential may not share this connection but must have other separate connection facilities. Mounting systems for barriers need to make it impossible for them to be reverse mounted or make such mounting so obvious that it can be assumed not to occur. Typical of such methods is asymmetrical mounting using the earth connection facility to effect mounting on the earth bar (the most common method – see Fig. 13.31) or keying such as used for terminal rails where it is only possible to mount in one orientation.

Barrier devices are now available in a wide variety of formats (see Fig. 13.32) and a wide range of voltages to cater for most possible requirements. The problem is that once the barrier has acted in its protective

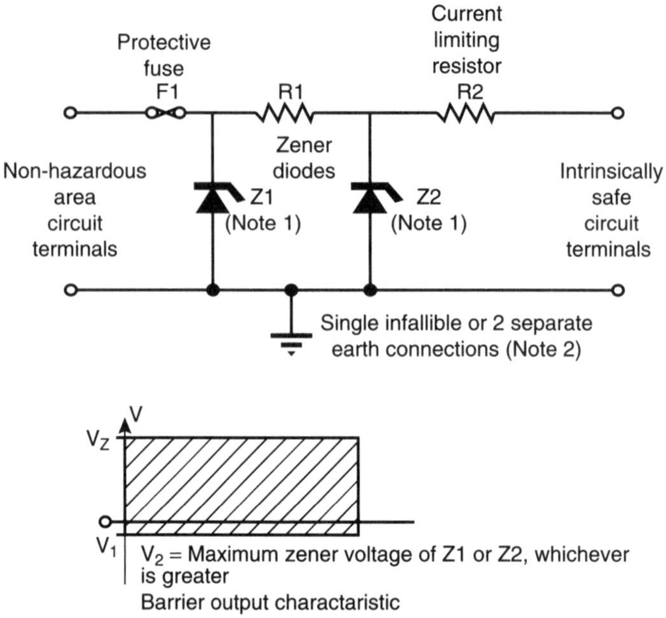

Fig. 13.30 Typical zener barrier configuration. *Notes*: (1) Both *Z*1 and *Z*2 are chosen so that they will not suffer damage during fuse pre-arcing period when maximum (mains) input voltage is applied. (2) If earth connection is a wire it must be of at least 4 mm^2 conductor cross section

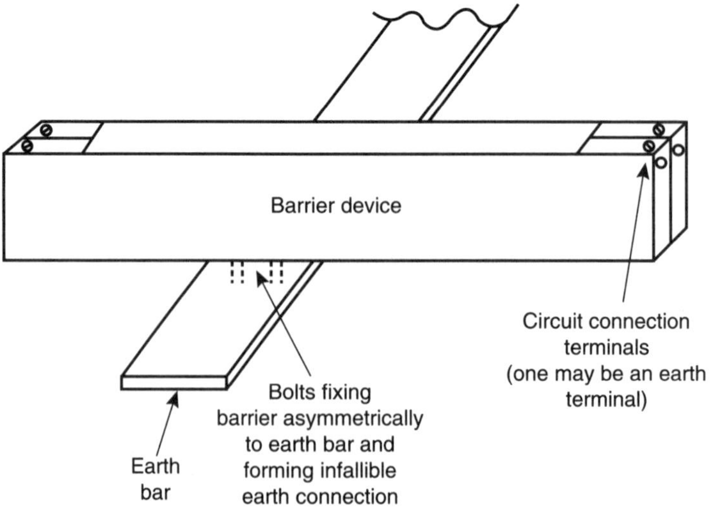

Fig. 13.31 Typical barrier mounting system

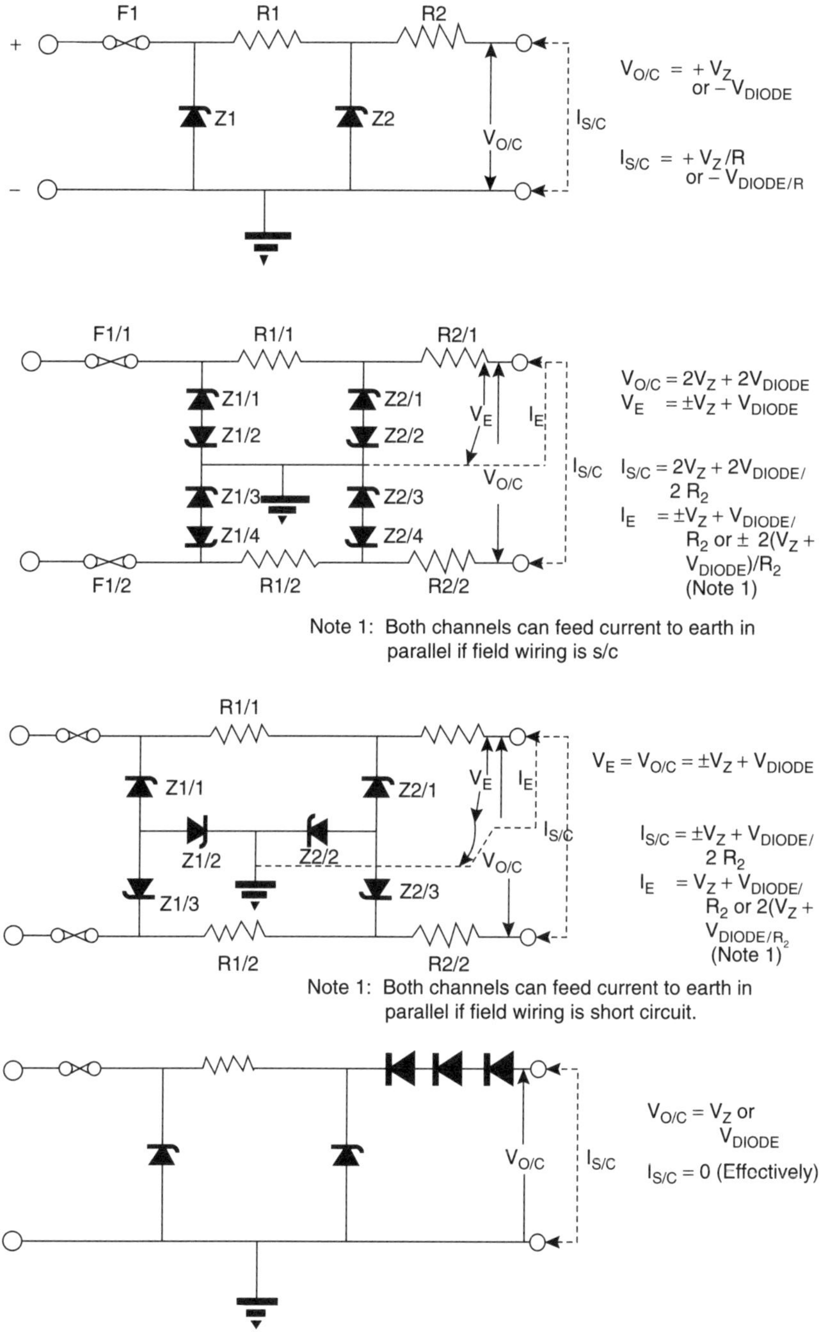

Fig. 13.32 Typical zener barrier configurations

mode, it is a throw-away item as its fuse will have operated and thus it will be open circuit. To prevent this it is perfectly acceptable to insert a fuse of lower rated rupturing current in series with the barrier on the non-hazardous area side so that it will rupture before that in the barrier.

Barrier devices offering galvanic isolation and many other more complex functions are also available, and almost all of the intrinsically safe installations now used utilize barrier devices which confirms their value and the revolution which they produced.

13.12 Input and output specifications

Due to of the wide range of intrinsically safe equipment it is necessary to identify that which can be interconnected. To this end items of apparatus have specifications which accompany them and are required to be identified on their labels if possible, but in any event to accompany them. These differ for associated apparatus (including barriers) and intrinsically safe apparatus.

Associated apparatus

The important parameters for associated apparatus are as follows:

[ia] or [ib]

This identifies the level of intrinsic safety and the square brackets indicate that the apparatus is for connection to intrinsically safe apparatus but is not intended for hazardous area mounting. It may be hazardous area mounted if, however, it is protected by another method (e.g., by being placed in a flameproof enclosure).

IIA, IIB or IIC

This indicates the sub-grouping and is common with all other types of protection.

U_m

The supply terminals and output terminals of associated apparatus will be marked with U_m which is the maximum voltage which may be connected to them without violating intrinsic safety. This is normally considered to be the maximum supply voltage to the apparatus to which they are connected, and is normally assumed to be the mains.

U_o

This is the maximum open circuit voltage which the associated apparatus can supply to the intrinsically safe apparatus with which they are interconnected. It determines the maximum capacitance which will be permitted in the intrinsically safe circuit.

I_o

This is the maximum short circuit current which the associated apparatus can supply to the hazardous area and will determine the maximum inductance acceptable in the intrinsically safe circuit.

P_o

This is an indication of the maximum power which the associated apparatus can deliver into the hazardous area. It also goes some way to identifying the type of source represented by that apparatus (e.g., resistively limited or constant current voltage limited).

L_o

This specifies the maximum inductance which can be connected to the intrinsically safe circuit terminals of the associated apparatus, and hence the maximum inductance acceptable for the combination of cable and intrinsically safe apparatus.

C_o

This specifies the maximum capacitance which can be connected to the intrinsically safe circuit terminals of the apparatus, and hence the maximum acceptable capacitance of the combination of interconnecting cable and intrinsically safe apparatus.

These parameters allow the maximum facility for interconnection of associated and intrinsically safe apparatus without carrying out complex calculations. The only other parameter which is of interest is a parameter called Inductance/Resistance ratio (L_o/R_o) which is a measure of the maximum inductance per unit of resistance which may be connected to the power source. This is valuable because it is known that as cable length increases so does its resistance and current will fall, which means the permitted inductance will rise. For a resistively limited source (and these comprise most of the sources used in intrinsic safety) it can further be shown that the maximum stored energy occurs when the external resistance equals the source resistance (see Fig. 13.33) and, if this is safe, then any other situation is also safe. If this is applied to cable, therefore, no limit of cable length which would otherwise be imposed by inductance per unit length is necessary. For any situation the L_o/R_o can be calculated (see Fig. 13.34) and this ratio is given by:-

$$L_o/R_o = \{8e\,R_x + (64e^2R_x^2 - 72U^2eL_x)^{0.5}\}/4.5U \qquad \text{H}/\Omega$$

where R_x = The circuit resistance excluding the cable (R_s or $R_s + R_i$, whichever gives the worst case) — Ω

U = The open circuit voltage of the power source — V

L_x = The total value of lumped inductance in the circuit (L_s or $L_s + L_i$ whichever gives the worst case) — H

e = The minimum ignition energy — J

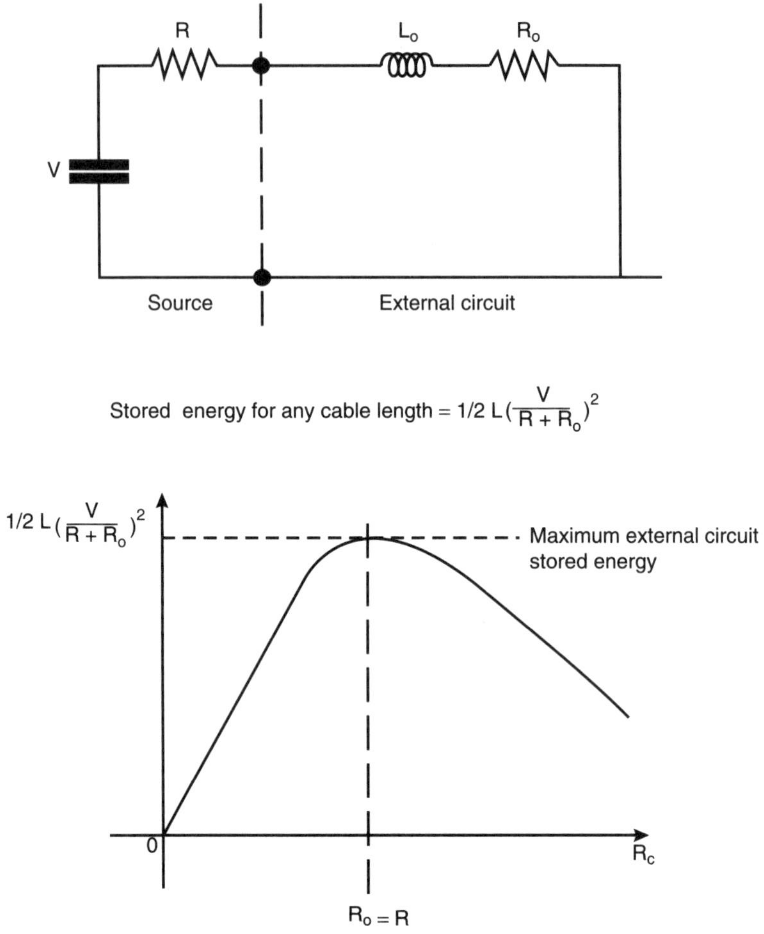

Fig. 13.33 Cable stored energy characteristic

For the purposes of this calculation the minimum energy is derived from the curves (see Figs. 13.35 and 13.36) and is as follows:

$$\text{IIA} = 320 \times 10^{-6} \quad \text{J}$$

$$\text{IIB} = 160 \times 10^{-6} \quad \text{J}$$

$$\text{IIC} = 40 \times 10^{-6} \quad \text{J}$$

Where there is no lumped inductance in either the associated or the intrinsically safe apparatus this formula simplifies to:

$$L_o/R_o = 3.56eR_x/U \quad \text{H}/\Omega$$

Regrettably there is no similar method of identifying capacitance, although clearly the cable resistance will have an effect of reducing the

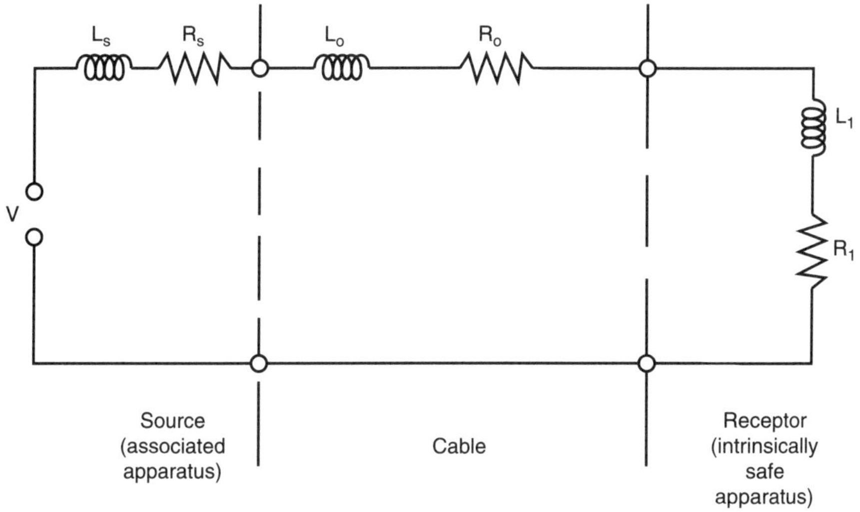

L_s = Source lumped inductance (fixed)
L_i = Reception lumped inductance (fixed)
L_o = Cable capacity (varies with length)
R_s = Source resistance (fixed)
R_i = Reception resistance (fixed)
R_o = Cable resistance (varies with length)
V = Source voltage

Fig. 13.34 Calculation of L/R ratio

rate of capacitive discharge. The problem here is that the cable comprises a set of series resistors and shunt capacitors which is much more difficult to analyse than is the inductive case, where all components are in series. Thus in most cases the limit on cable length will be the cable capacitance, although experience has shown that with normal cables the problem of cable length only becomes real in the case of sub-group IIC installations as the capacitance for IIA and IIB for all circuits below 30 V, where most intrinsically safe circuits are concentrated, is large enough to accommodate any reasonable length of cable required.

Where voltage limited constant current supplies are concerned the calculation of L/R is on the face of it more difficult. By using a tangent line as shown is Fig. 13.35 it can, however, be calculated and, although the result is somewhat limiting, it is often useful to have.

Intrinsically safe apparatus

In the case of intrinsically safe apparatus the required parameters in most cases are those within the apparatus, as the apparatus is connected to a power source. What is necessarily marked on or referred to for the apparatus is:

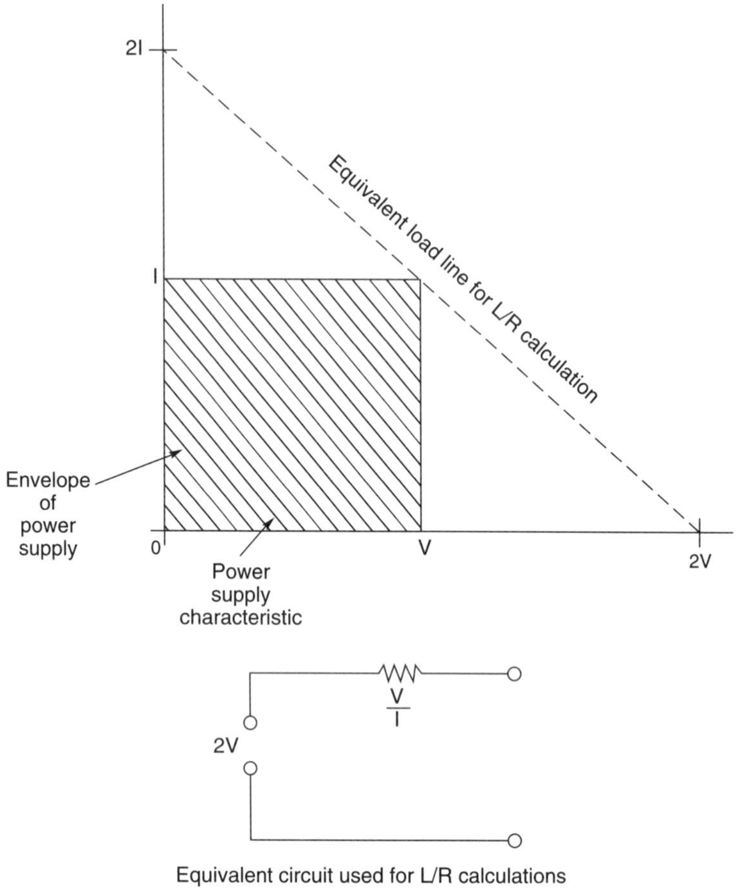

Fig. 13.35 Calculation of L/R for constant current voltage limited power supply

U_i – the maximum voltage which a power source may deliver to the apparatus;

I_i – the maximum short circuit current which any power source connected to the apparatus may deliver;

P_i – the maximum power delivery capability of any source connected to the apparatus;

L_i – the maximum inductance within the apparatus which appears on the input terminals;

C_i – the maximum internal capacitance which appears on the input terminals of the apparatus;

The internal inductance can be additionally stated as an L/R ratio and this sometimes assists in connection. Also, where the apparatus is something such as a temperature transmitter and is connected to a primary element in addition to its connection to a power source, U_o, I_o and P_o may also need

Acme Products plc
Controller type ×R2
Serial No × 2643
EEx [ia] IIc

$U_m = 250$ V rms	$L_o = 22$ mH
$U_o = 30$ V dc	$C_o = 0.1\,\mu$F
$I_o = 0.1$ A	$L_o/R_o = 25\,\mu$H/ohm
$P_o = 0.75$ W	

Typical associated apparatus label

Exelsior Transmitters Ltd.
Temperature transmitter type TR6
Serial No. 2
EEx ia IIC T6

$U_i = 30$ V	$L_i = 22$ mH
$I_i = 0.1$ A	$C_i = 0.1\,\mu$F
$P_i = 0.75$ W	

Typical intrinsically safe apparatus label

Fig. 13.36 Typical apparatus labels

to be specified insofar as its terminals connected to their primary element are concerned.

Typical labels for associated and intrinsically safe apparatus are shown in Fig. 13.36.

13.13 Examples of fault counting in apparatus

Fault counting for production of information to be placed on apparatus labels has to be all within each piece of apparatus.

Associated apparatus

This is apparatus which feeds intrinsically safe apparatus but which is not itself intended for installation in a hazardous area. Figure 13.37 shows a typical power source which feeds a voltage to the hazardous area comprising an infallible mains transformer, followed by a rectifier and a capacitor for smoothing purposes. These are then followed by three resistors, R1 having a value of 700 Ω minimum in place to limit the current to Z1 in no load conditions, R2 having a value of 30 Ω minimum in place to provide the necessary separation for individual zener diode testing, and R3 having a value of 300 Ω minimum in place to provide further current limiting. All components are assumed to have adequate ratings.

For 'ib' apparatus it is only necessary to consider one fault, failure of one of the zener diodes. This will give an open circuit maximum voltage output of 30 V limited by Z1. If the output terminals are short circuited the current which flows is 38 mA (39/R1 + R2 + R3). At this current the voltage across Z1 will be 12.5 V and the voltage across Z2 will be 11.35 V. Thus the zener diodes will be switched off and not play any part in short circuit current determination. Likewise, if a load of 1030 Ω (a matched load) is connected across the output terminals, the voltage across Z1 will be 17.35 V and across Z2 will be 17 V. Again, at a matched load situation both Z1 and Z2 will be switched off and not affect the power transfer. Maximum output power will therefore be 0.37 W ($39^2/4\times$ R1 + R2 + R3). There is

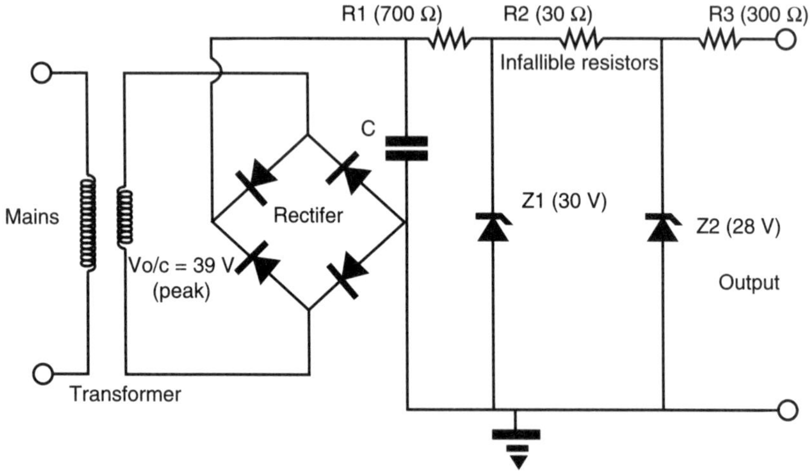

Equivalent power source

[ib] $V_o = 30\,V\ (V_{Z1})$
$I_o = 39/1030\,A\ (V_{o/c}/R_1 + R_2 + R_3)$
$P_o = 0.37\,W$
$L_o = 0.22\,mH$ (from Fig. 13.5 – no internal inductance)
$L_o/R_o = 96\,\mu H/ohm$ (from formula – no internal inductance)
$C_o = 0.067\,\mu F$ (from Fig. 13.8 no internal capacitance)

[ia] $V_o = 39\,V\ (V_{o/c})$
$I_o = 39/1030\,A\ (V_{o/c}/R_1 + R_2 + R_3)$
$P_o = 0.37\,W$
$L_o = 0.22\,mH$ (see above)
$L_o/R_o = 96\,\mu H/ohm$ (see above)
$C_o = 0.033\,\mu F$ (see above)

Fig. 13.37 Fault counts in associated apparatus

no effective capacitance in the circuit as C is placed across the transformer output voltage and separated from the output terminals by R1, R2 and R3 in series. It thus looks just like a voltage supply and not like a capacitor.

If 'ia' is considered the only change is the failure of Z1, which allows the output open circuit voltage to rise to 39 V. Output short circuit current, and output power remain the same as the zener diodes are not used in their formulation, as do capacitance and inductance. The parameters on the label will therefore be:

[ib]	– output open circuit volts (V_o)	30 V
	output short circuit current (I_o)	38 mA
	maximum output power (P_o)	0.37 W
	maximum external inductance (L_o) (from Fig. 13.35)	0.22 mH
	maximum external inductance/resistance ratio (R_o/L) (from formula)	96 μH/Ω
	maximum external capacitance (from Fig. 13.8)	0.067 μF

For [ia] the figures all remain the same with the exception of the open circuit output voltage (V_o) which rises to 39 V reducing external capacitances to 0.035 μF maximum. In both cases, there is no effective internal inductance or capacitance (L_i or C_i) but this is not normally recorded on the labelling. Should there be any internal inductance, however, it is necessary that it be recorded to permit calculation of the L/R ratio for interconnecting cables.

Intrinsically safe apparatus

This is the apparatus which does go into the hazardous area and is powered from associated apparatus, such as that shown in Fig. 13.37. A typical item of intrinsically safe apparatus is shown in Fig. 13.38. As this apparatus is not powered itself, the main interest lies in its internal parameters so that an assessment of its safety when connected to a power source can be made. Once again a presumption is made that all components are properly rated for analysis purposes. The only slightly unusual problem here is the presence of R1. It will be seen that the resistor is in series with a variable resistor and this is often necessary as the power dissipation can be in one small part of the variable resistor track if it is set to a low value. It is normally assumed that only 10 per cent of the track is present for temperature classification purposes and, as many variable resistors are very small, this gives rise to very high temperature rises which are often minimized by the insertion of a series resistor as shown.

If one makes the assumption that the apparatus is suitable, from a power dissipation point of view, for connection to a supply of 39 V with a short circuit current of 38 mA and a power delivery capability of 0.37 W, then no condition of the power source shown in Fig. 13.37 can overload it.

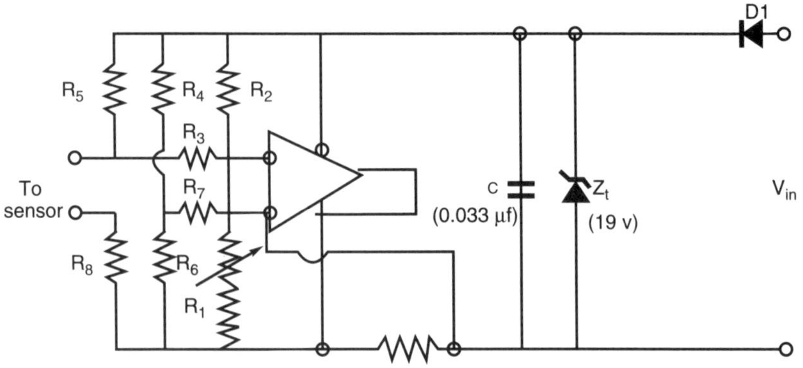

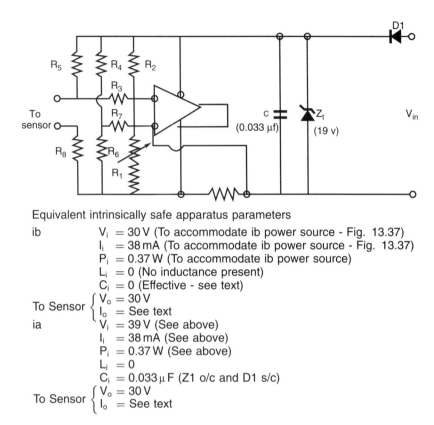

Equivalent intrinsically safe apparatus parameters

ib V_i = 30 V (To accommodate ib power source - Fig. 13.37)
I_i = 38 mA (To accommodate ib power source - Fig. 13.37)
P_i = 0.37 W (To accommodate ib power source)
L_i = 0 (No inductance present)
C_i = 0 (Effective - see text)
To Sensor { V_o = 30 V
I_o = See text
ia V_i = 39 V (See above)
I_i = 38 mA (See above)
P_i = 0.37 W (See above)
L_i = 0
C_i = 0.033 µF (Z1 o/c and D1 s/c)
To Sensor { V_o = 30 V
I_o = See text

Fig. 13.38 Fault counts in intrinsically safe apparatus

For 'ib' considerations the maximum voltage from the power source is 30 V and can be used for evaluation of this apparatus in the 'ib' mode. In the 'ib' mode only one fault needs to be considered and that can be the failure of D1 or Z1. As either D1 or Z1 is always present in these circumstances there is no possibility of direct connection of the capacitance, C, to the input terminals of the apparatus when it can be charged to more than 19 V. If C does charge to more than 19 V on failure of Z1 then it is intrinsically safe, even if it can charge and discharge into a spark within the intrinsically safe apparatus, because the maximum voltage of the power source is 30 V as already stated. As the capacitance cannot be placed across the output terminals and charged to more than 19 V, and the maximum permissible capacitance is 0.258 µF at 19 V, no problem exists because the maximum cable capacitance, must be calculated at 30 V. Therefore, the total capacitance in the 19 V situation is 0.132 µF, well below the 0.258 µF limit even with the maximum 30 V cable capacitance added. Parameters for the apparatus are:

ib	– maximum input voltage (V_i)	30 V
	maximum input current (I_i)	38 mA
	maximum input power (P_i)	0.37 W

effective terminal inductance (L_i)	0
effective terminal capacitance (C_i)	0.033 μF

The value of C_i is because of the possibility that the cable capacitance can add internally to the apparatus and this restricts cable capacitanc to 0.034 μF. This is normally dealt with by specifying C_i as 0.033 μF even though this is not the actual terminal capacitance.

The only other important information is the voltage out to the sensor which can be up to 30 V, and the current and power to the sensor which are controlled by resistors R1, R2, R3, R4, R5, R6, R7 and R8. As the sensor is usually very close to the intrinsically safe apparatus the capacitance of the connection is very small and the current to the sensor is usually small, also making inductance no problem. It is not usually necessary to identify these parameters on the label but one should be aware of the total situation nonetheless.

When considering the apparatus for 'ia' matters are very different as 2 faults are applied in 'ia' circuits. Thus if D1 fails to short circuit and Z1 to open circuit, the capacitor is across the terminals. This gives a C_i figure of 0.033 μF which at 30 V still allows for 0.034 μF in the cable. To allow connection to the described power source, however, V_i is now increased to 39 V.

ia	– maximum input voltage (V_i)	39 V
	maximum input current (I_i)	38 mA
	maximum input power (P_i)	0.37 W
	effective terminal inductance (L_i)	0
	effective terminal capacitance (C_i)	0.033 μF

This means that as the power supply in Fig. 13.37 supplies 39 V in the 'ia' situation it is only suitable for connection to this intrinsically safe apparatus in the 'ib' situation as permissible cable capacitance for ia is reduced to 0.001 μF (an unacceptably low figure – <10 m for a typical screened cable). The situation in respect of the output to the sensor remains unchanged from the 'ib' situation.

13.14 Intrinsically safe systems

As previously stated, intrinsic safety is a system concept in which the total installation has to be considered. The construction and specification of apparatus as previously described is used as a tool to make the evaluation of a system easier but is not intended to be excessively limiting. The production of intrinsically safe systems is described in BS 5501, Part 9 (1982)[11] (the UK text of EN 50039). There are two ways of producing an intrinsically safe system, the first being to apply the fault counts to each item of apparatus individually, and the second to additionally apply the count to the system as a whole. The latter approach shows intrinsic safety can be achieved in situations where it is not possible to identify this from the apparatus parameters produced, as discussed earlier in this chapter. It must be remembered that the objective is to achieve intrinsic safety with up to two countable faults, plus appropriate non-countable faults applied to the system, either in one of the items of apparatus forming it or divided among all of them.

The easy way to ensure intrinsic safety is to compare the output parameters of associated apparatus with the input parameters of intrinsically safe apparatus and, if the following is the case, intrinsic safety is ensured very simply. The comparison of parameters should be carried out as follows (and see Fig. 13.39):

associated apparatus		*intrinsically safe apparatus*
output voltage (V_o)	$\leq$	input voltage (V_i)
output current (I_i)	$\leq$	input current (I_i)
output power (P_o)	$\leq$	input power (P_i)
external inductance (L_o)	$\geq$	effective terminal inductance plus cable inductance ($L_i + L_c$)
external capacitance (C_o)	$\geq$	effective terminal capacitance plus cable capacitance ($C_i + C_c$)

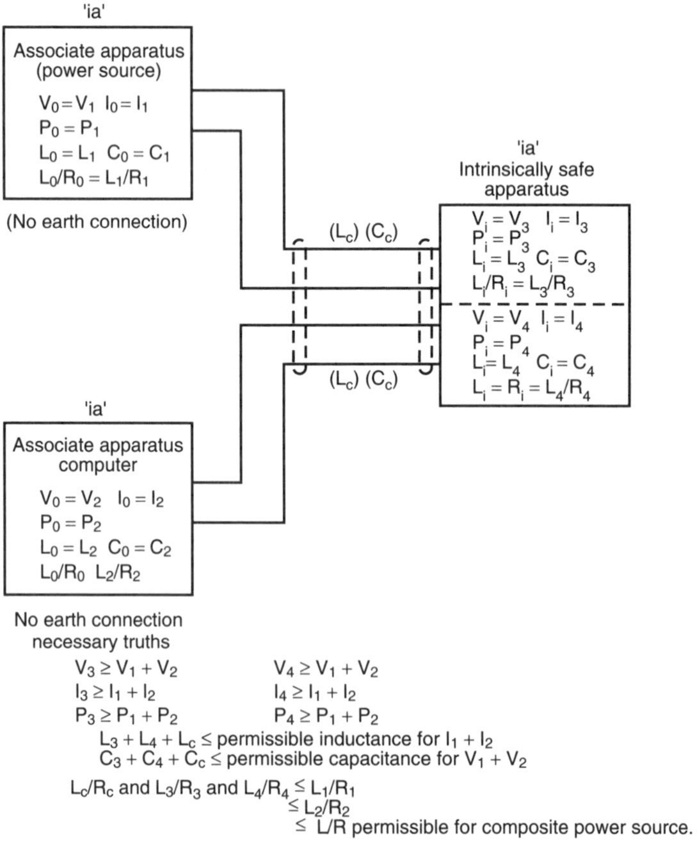

Fig. 13.39 Assessment of systems on the basis of input and output definitions for apparatus (based on assessment of each item of apparatus alone). *Note*: If L/R requirements are met the inductance requirements need not be

Where the cable inductance to resistance ratio (L_c/R_c) has been calculated (see earlier in this chapter), taking account of the lumped inductance (L_i) in the circuit, it is not necessary to add the cable inductance to the lumped inductance provided that the cable has an L/R ratio equal to or less than L_c/R_c.

As previously stated, an item of 'simple apparatus' may be added into the intrinsically safe system provided that its temperature does not exceed the limiting temperature of the temperature class without further detailed consideration. The temperature must, however, be confirmed as not doing so. While a single item of simple apparatus may be added it is not acceptable to add several items unless a detailed study of the total addition of energy to the intrinsically safe system has been carried out because of the possibility of energy addition.

The items of intrinsically safe apparatus and associated apparatus may be either all 'ia' or 'ib' or may be a mixture of 'ia' and 'ib' apparatus. The resulting system will, however, be 'ib' unless all items of apparatus are 'ia'.

The above approach covers most practical situations but in a few cases it would not permit a configuration which was manifestly intrinsically safe. An alternative is the system fault count (see Fig. 13.40). If, for example, we were to take the two items of apparatus in Fig. 13.37 and 13.38 intrinsic safety would be achieved if the following were the case:

associated apparatus	*intrinsically safe apparatus*
2 Faults	no Faults
1 Fault	1 Fault
no Faults	2 Faults

Application of the above criteria to the apparatus shown in Figs. 13.37 and 13.38 shows clearly that interconnection of the two items of apparatus comprises an intrinsically safe system, whereas comparison of the output and input parameters of the two items of apparatus indicates the contrary. This system fault count, however, requires considerable knowledge of the detail of the two items of apparatus and can only be carried out at the apparatus design stage. It also can be very restrictive on the items of apparatus as it will identify the other apparatus with which each item of apparatus can be interconnected, rather than the parameters only which are easy to compare. It is thus not often used but can be of significant assistance in complex systems such as public address systems.

Another problem is the possibility of interconnection of separate intrinsically safe circuits in field wiring. To understand this it is necessary to identify the normal procedure for installation of intrinsically safe systems. Because these are basically normally instrumentation systems, usually for intelligence transmission or low power operating systems, the cables which they use in the normal industrial context are not as robust as those used for power circuits. It is one of the objectives of intrinsically safe circuits that this situation be maintained and, as sparking produced by breaking,

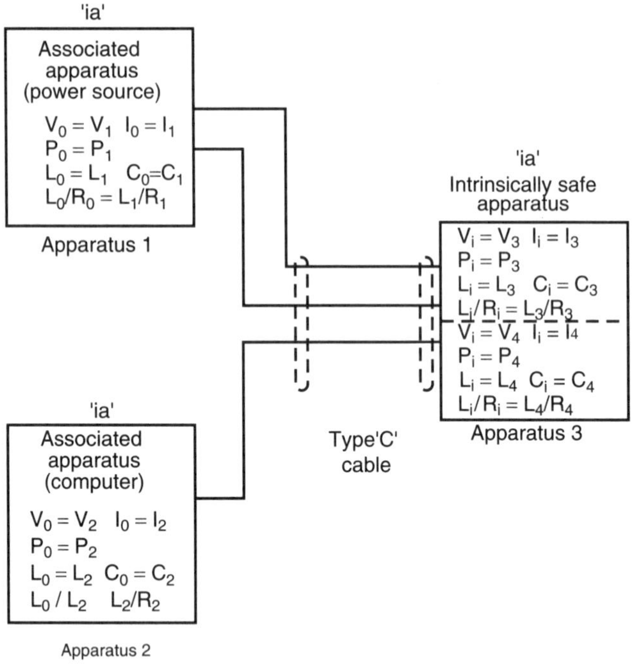

	Fault count Apparatus 1	Apparatus 2	Apparatus 3
Case 1	2	0	0
Case 2	1	1	0
Case 3	1	0	1
Case 4	0	1	1
Case 5	0	2	0
Case 6	0	0	2

Fig. 13.40 System fault counting. *Note*: The above means that only in cases 1, 5 and 6 are any of the parameters specified for the apparatus necessarily true, rather than restrictive, and only the set for one piece of apparatus is appropriate to each case

short circuiting, or earth faults in such cables will not produce ignition capable sparks from the power in intrinsically safe circuits, it is possible to do so. The problem lies in the fact that it is normal to use multicore cables each containing several instrumentation circuits, as, for example, in telephone systems. These cables are then locally terminated to the point where sensors, etc., occur and individual cables used for the latter part of the run (see Fig. 13.41). The use of such multicore cables does, however, create the possibility that interconnection between individual intrinsically safe circuits can occur. It is often very difficult to carry out a detailed evaluation of such interconnected circuits and it is better if such interconnections cannot occur. There are several ways of doing this.

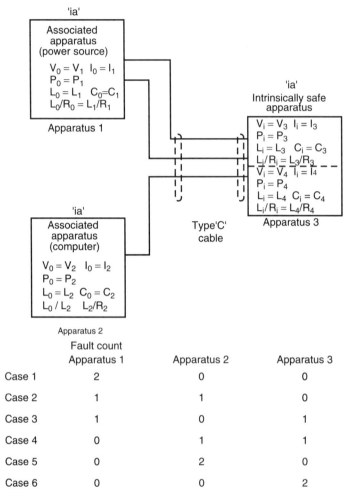

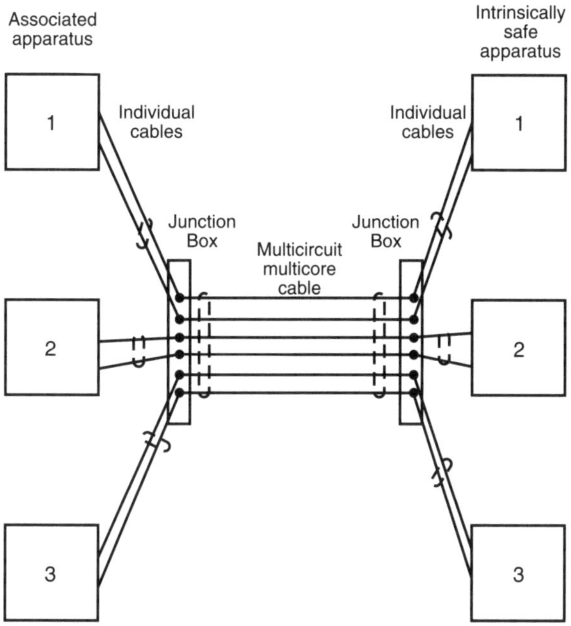

Fig. 13.41 Typical use of multicore cables

13.14.1 Interconnecting cable systems

Separate cables

The easy way to prevent interconnection is to use separate cables for each individual intrinsically safe circuit. This solves the problem but is both expensive and cumbersome. Very large numbers of cables are required at considerable extra cost and termination becomes a problem in that many individual cables may need to enter one connection box, or many connection boxes may be necessary.

Multicore cables

To overcome this there are several approaches which will allow the use of multicore cables containing several intrinsically safe systems.

Type 'a' cable

The first of these is a Type 'a' cable. In this cable the conductors of each intrinsically safe circuit are contained in an individual screen and the cable will contain many screened groups of conductors. This is a fairly general type of cable principal often used for instrumentation systems to prevent crosstalk in the cable. The presence of such screens means that, although faults to the screen can occur in each intrinsically safe circuit, provided the screens are earthed there is no likelihood of circuits becoming interconnected. The problem with this type of cable is that the screens are often not isolated from the another and this creates a problem for intrinsic safety. If the screens are earthed at different places there could be voltage between them when power faults occur in the general installation of which the intrinsically safe systems are a part. Unless, therefore, all of the installations are earthed at the same point, the screens must be insulated one from another so that they will withstand a test voltage of 500 V rms. Likewise, where the intrinsically safe circuits which they contain are also earthed, the screens must be earthed at the same effective point as the contained circuits. This is because faults in the circuit within the screen are assumed to occur and, if the circuit and screen are earthed at different points, there is again the possibility of invasion of the intrinsically safe circuit by currents due to faults in associated power installations.

The conductors themselves are required to be insulated in the same way as their normal industrial counterparts are and this requires around 0.2 mm thickness of insulation for polyethylene or PVC, as below this thickness it is considered that, unless special precautions are taken, it is difficult to ensure a reliable continuous insulation cover.

All cables are required to have a sheath of the quality normally associated with industrial installations using this type of cable, but they are not required to have any particular type of sheath offering increased protection such as armouring or cross-linked polyethylene, as in other protection concepts. One of the principal requirements for this sheath is to ensure that conductor relative positions are fixed enabling inductance and capacitance to be quoted with confidence.

These cables are considered as suitable for installation in 'ia' systems, which enter Zone 0, even when mixed with 'ia' or 'ib' systems which do not.

Type 'b' cable

The second type of cable used is the Type 'b' cable in which individual intrinsically safe circuit screens are not fitted. The cores of the cable are, as for type 'a' cable, required to have adequate insulation on the cores and this normally means 0.2 mm minimum thickness for polyethylene or PVC. In addition, for the same reasons as in Type 'a' cable they are required to have a suitable overall sheath, although no additional requirements for this are necessary other than those which would normally be applied in an industrial installation.

These cables are assumed to be proof against faults between cores if they are installed in a way which minimizes the risk of damage by, for example, being led on a cable tray fixed at high level and protected from damage from above, or being run in the web of plant support girders so that they are unlikely to be struck by objects being carried around the plant. This type of cable is probably the most common type of cable used and is normally used to carry a group of circuits from locations such as control rooms to particular locations on a plant or in a factory. They need not be screened but may be, provided all of the circuits within the cable are earthed at the same point (if earthed), and the screen is earthed at that point also.

The fitting of cables with a steel wire or braid armouring is not considered as effective for the purposes of protection against mechanical damage as it does not prevent the cable being crushed which could lead to interconnection between systems. For operational reasons, however, cables are often armoured as it gives some protection against damage and thus, although that protection is not considered as enough for intrinsic safety purposes, it does increase reliability of operation and is used for that purpose.

One consideration which must be borne in mind, however, is that the security of such cables is not considered as sufficient to allow intrinsically safe circuits, which enter Zone 0, to pass through them.

Type 'c' cable

A Type 'c' cable is one of exactly the same construction as a Type 'b' cable but installed in a way which does not effectively protect it from mechanical damage. Thus damage has to be considered but, because of its robust construction, the damage is limited to the following: first, up to two short circuits between cores of different intrinsically safe circuits will be considered to occur coincidently; second, at the same time as the short circuits, any number of open circuits of cores may occur. This has the effect of permitting a variety of interconnections in intrinsically safe circuits, the limits of which are three power sources in series, or parallel connected, to a single item of intrinsically safe apparatus (see Fig. 13.42) or three items of intrinsically safe apparatus in series, or parallel connected, to a single associated apparatus power source (see Fig. 13.43). There are many other possible combinations between these limits which also need consideration, and this makes the use of this cable very difficult unless it forms part of a specifically designed system. An analysis based upon the output and terminal parameters of apparatus would almost certainly in most cases identify the result as non-intrinsically safe.

To overcome this, detailed knowledge of all apparatus is necessary to allow a system fault count and this knowledge is usually only known to the manufacturer. In limited cases this is not necessary as in the case of three identical polarity power sources, each identically earthed. Using output parameters for the power sources, a composite power source of similar voltage but three times the short circuit current of one can be envisaged, but not three series power sources. Thus provided the resultant current remains intrinsically safe and, provided the cable and other inductances and L/R ratios are suitably reduced, intrinsic safety of the composite can be simply deduced. Due to this difficulty such cables are not normally specified except in the case of single intrinsically safe systems which contain multiple intrinsically safe circuits, such as public address systems, in which the manufacturer can carry out a detailed evaluation of the entire system.

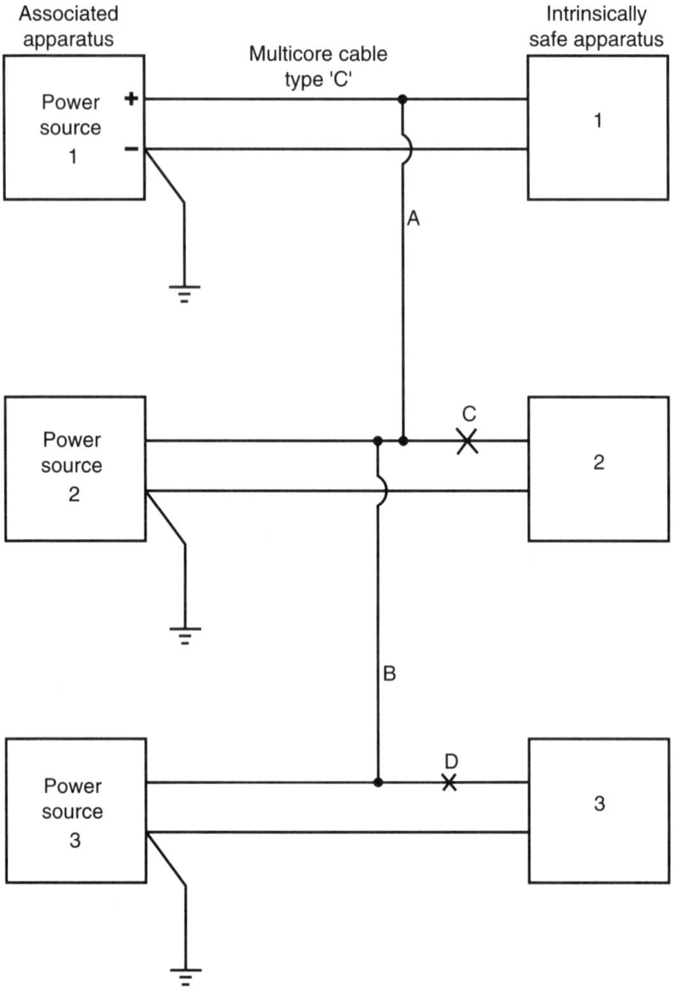

A = Short circuit fault 1
B = Short circuit fault 2
C = Open circuit fault
D = Open circuit fault.
Power supplies 1, 2 and 3 connected in parallel to intrinsically safe apparatus

Fig. 13.42 Effects of faults in multicore cables

Type 'd' cable

In Type 'd' cable no specification of insulation and sheathing for the purposes of intrinsic safety are applied and it may not meet any of the requirements of Type 'a', 'b' or 'c' cables. Any number of simultaneous core/core faults with any number of simultaneous open circuit faults are considered as possible. The limitations of Type 'c' cable apply even more to this type of cable and it has little general use.

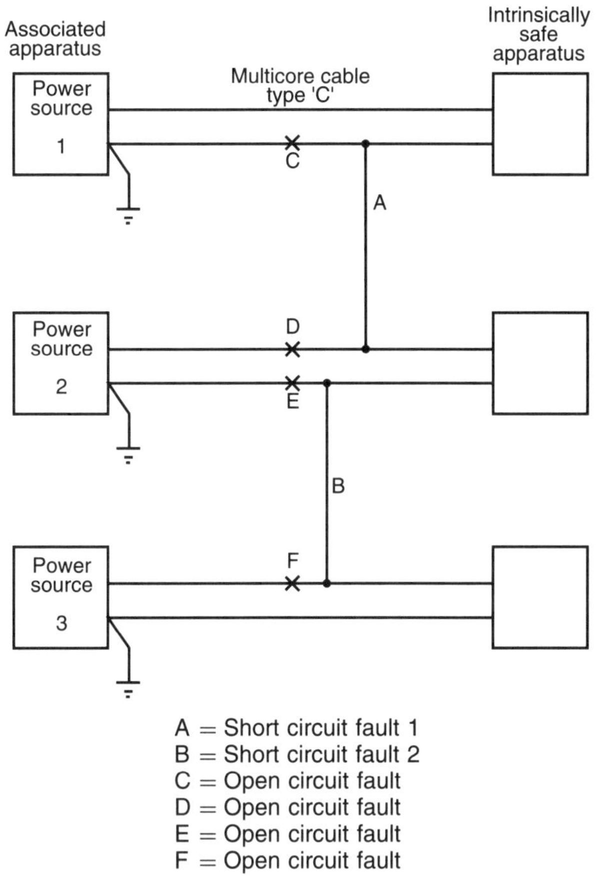

Fig. 13.43 Effects of faults in multicore cables

Screen short circuits in multicore cables

The connection of circuit conductors of any intrinsically safe circuit to the screen is considered as normal operation in all of the above types of cable but does not adversely affect intrinsic safety, provided that both of the screens are earthed at the same point in Type 'a' cable (this constitutes two parallel connections) or, in the case of Type 'b' cable, the screen conductor is a sufficient size to be infallible (see earlier in this chapter) and its earth connection is also infallible. If this is not so in Type 'b' cables, the screen must be insulated from the body of conductors to the same level as the conductors are insulated from one another so that faults can be ignored within the cable.

This is not true for Type 'c' and 'd' cables and in these cases multiple screen/conductor connections must be considered from the standpoint of the effects of multiple earths and interconnections. This is a further reason for avoiding such cables if possible.

13.14.2 Cable parameter measurement

Calculation of cable parameters of inductance and capacitance is somewhat complex due to the fact that the configuration of a cable is not that of a classic inductor or a classic capacitor (for inductance it is a long narrow single-turn coil, and for a capacitor it is two plates of far from ideal dimension). For this reason it is far more effective to measure these parameters on a specific length of cable. They can then be extrapolated on to longer lengths with confidence due to the regular nature of cable construction. It must be remembered that the core/core and core/screen parameters are both important.

Cable capacitance

Cable capacitance becomes a problem where sub-group IIC circuits have significant open circuit voltages. A typical instrumentation cable may have a capacitance between cores, or a core and the screen, of as little as 50 picofarads/metre but this figure may rise to in excess of 100 picofarads/metre in some cables, and between a core and the screen. It is usually necessary to know what the capacitance of a particular type of cable is. If the core/core or core/screen capacitance were 200 pF/m, for example, then for IIC circuits at 30 V open circuit output the maximum cable length would be restricted to 330 m for an unscreened cable, but may be less than 115 m for a screened cable as two parallel capacitances are involved in this latter case (see Fig. 13.44). While this may appear to be an adequate length, it must be remembered that because of the necessary deviation in cable runs these distances are equivalent to much smaller distances as the crow flies.

In any case of doubt it is easy to measure the cable capacity of a 10 m length of a particular cable using a normal capacitance bridge, and extrapolate as capacitance is proportional to length, or obtain the manufacturers specification.

Cable inductance

Cable inductance can be measured using an inductance bridge on a short length of cable and extrapolating for longer lengths, as inductance is proportional to length. If the resistance of that length is also measured the L/R ration of the cable can also be obtained and this is, of course, independent of length. Accurate measurements are necessary, however, as a standard instrumentation cable is typically 1 μH/m and 0.1Ω/m (10 μH/Ω).

The position with inductance is somewhat better than capacitance as the stored energy in inductance is related to current and not voltage. Placing conductors in parallel has the effect of dividing the current (see Fig. 13.45) and where each inductor is separate, halving the stored energy. This reduction is not practically likely but it shows that the effect of core/core or core/screen interconnection in cables is to reduce stored energy and not increase it.

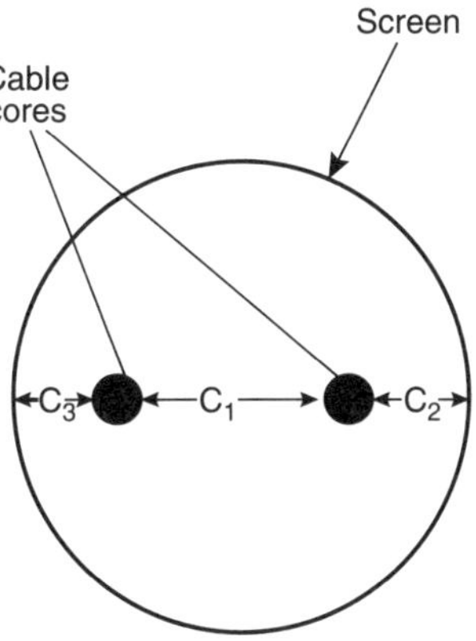

Capacitance between cores at worst

$C_T = C_1 + C_2 \times C_3/C_2 + C_3$

If $C_2 = C_3$

$C_T = C_1 + 1/2C_2$

Fig. 13.44 Effects of screen on cable capacitance C_T

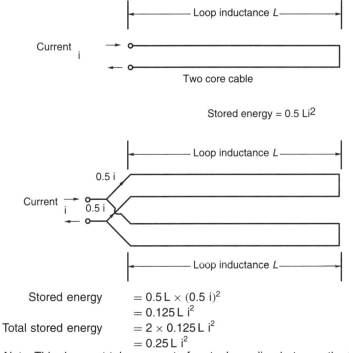

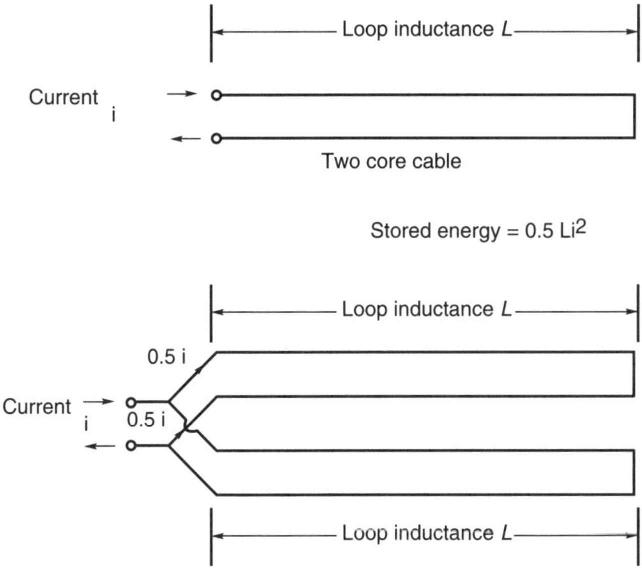

$$
\begin{aligned}
\text{Stored energy} &= 0.5\,L \times (0.5\ i)^2 \\
&= 0.125\,L\ i^2 \\
\text{Total stored energy} &= 2 \times 0.125\,L\ i^2 \\
&= 0.25\,L\ i^2
\end{aligned}
$$

Note: This does not take account of mutual coupling between the two loops but does indicate the effects of current division.

Fig. 13.45 Effect of short circuit cable faults on inductive stored energy

L/R is not usually a problem as the vast majority of intrinsically safe circuits are designed to have permissible L/R figures of above 25 μH/Ω, which is much greater than the typical instrumentation cable.

References

1 BS 1259 (1958)	Intrinsically Safe Electrical Apparatus and Circuits for use in Explosive Atmospheres.
2 EECS/BASEEFA	Health and Safety Executive – Electrical Equipment Certification service. British Approval Service for Electrical Equipment in Flammable Atmospheres.
3 SFA 3012 (1972)	BASEEFA Certification Standard Intrinsic Safety.
4 BS 5501.	Electrical Apparatus for Potentially Explosive Atmospheres. Part 7 (1977). Intrinsic Safety, 'i'.
5 EN 50020 (1977)	Electrical Apparatus for Potentially Explosive Atmospheres. Intrinsic Safety 'i'.
6 PTB	Physicalisch Technische Bundesanstalt.
7 IEC	International Electrotechnical Commission.
8 IEC 79–11.	Electrical Apparatus for Explosive Gas Atmospheres. Part 11 (1984). Construction and Test of Intrinsically Safe and Associated Apparatus.
9 CENELEC	Comite European de Normalization Electrique.
10 BS/EN 50020 (1995)	Electrical apparatus for Potentially Explosive Atmospheres. Intrinsic Safety 'i'.
11 BS 5501	Electrical Apparatus for Potentially Explosive Atmospheres. Part 9 (1982). Intrinsically Safe Systems 'i'.
12 BS 5501	Electrical Apparatus for Potentially Explosive Atmospheres. Part 1 (1977). General Requirements.
13 BS/EN 60127 (1991)	Miniature Fuses. Part 1, Definitions for miniature fuses and general requirements for miniature fuse links. Part 2, Specification for Cartridge Fuse Links. Part 3, Specification for Sub-Miniature Fuse Links.
14 HSE GS43 (1987)	Lithium Batteries.
15 BS/EN 60529 (1991)	Specification for Degrees of Protection Provided by Enclosures (IP).
16 BS 5901 (1980)	Method of Test for Determining the Comparative and the Proof Tracking Indices of Solid Insulating Materials Under moist Conditions.
17 BS/EN 50019 (1985)	Electrical Apparatus for Potentially Explosive Atmospheres. Increased Safety 'e'.

14

Apparatus using protection concept 'N' ('n')

(BS 6941 (1988))
(IEC 79-15 (1987))

Unlike the protection concepts already described, protection concept (type of protection) 'N' is intended for installation only in Zone 2 areas. In such areas the risk of an explosive atmosphere occurring is so much less than in Zone 0 and 1 that historically it has been considered that the installation of 'high quality' industrial equipment, which does not spark or produce ignition-capable hot surfaces in normal operation is sufficient for this risk. The use of the term 'high quality' did not imply special equipment but was used to ensure that installers did not cut corners and use equipment not really intended for the industrial environment. Historically, any non-sparking equipment which was specifically designed for the industrial environment and had no special features demanding higher than the normal level of maintenance was acceptable. For equipment which did spark or become hot enough to cause ignition in normal operation, the Zone 1 compatible protection concepts would, have to be used.

This situation continued until 1972 when a British Standard which, for the first time introduced the possibility of apparatus which could create arcs or sparks, was published. This Standard suggested several methods of avoiding ignition from such sparking based upon those approaches used for Zone 1, but with lower security to reflect the lower possibility of the presence of an explosive atmosphere.

14.1 The situation in respect of standardization

The approach to selection and use of apparatus for Zone 2 was described initially in BS/CP1003, Part 3[1] (use) and, in BS 4137[2] which was produced to give detail upon selection of non sparking-industrial apparatus for Zone 2 use. This approach has continued up to the present day and the use of 'selected industrial apparatus' is still recognized but now in BS 5345, Part 1[3] there is a specification of the required qualities of those who select such apparatus and these are: first, that they must be familiar with the requirements of any relevant Standards and Codes of Practice including their interpretations. (This requirement is clearly intended to ensure that they are to a degree expert in the construction and installation of explosion-protected apparatus); second, they must have access to all the necessary information so that they can carry out the selection. (This will mean that they will need to know the detail of the apparatus design and intended use); and third, that if any tests are necessary these must be done using test apparatus and procedures similar to those used by recognized third-party test laboratories. (This means that the facilities and knowledge available to those who select apparatus must be similar to what is available to 'Notified Bodies' under Directive 76/117/EEC[4] or 94/9/EC[5]).

The above requirements make it quite clear that the selection of industrial equipment on the basis of it being non-sparking and not becoming hot enough to cause ignition is not, and never was, intended to be a relatively relaxed approach used by all installers, but rather a relatively formal approach and, while used by other than third party certification/approval bodies, was intended to include the level of detail similar to that which would be involved if a third party certification/approval body had been used.

The selection situation was never fully satisfactory and led to the position where industry sought some form of third party approval for the apparatus which they intended to use and, not surprisingly, turned for this to HM Factory Inspectorate, the body which regulated industry other than coalmining. Because there was no specific Standard and thus no detailed set of rules to which to approve such apparatus, the Factory Inspectorate could not approve apparatus but could identify that it had no sparking contacts, no hot surfaces and no other peculiarities which would make it unacceptable in the light of knowledge available at the time. This was done by the issue of a 'Letter of no objection' which was taken as approval, but was not in fact that. It was what it said – an identification that the Factory Inspectorate knew of no reason why it should not be installed in Zone 2. The letter would, unlike most certificates which continue in validity even after requirements have changed providing there is no evidence of imminent danger, become invalid if an increase in knowledge identified problems.

The situation, apart from the UK peculiarities of the 'Letter of no objection', was almost identical to the Zone 2 situation in most other developed countries – Germany, for example, having selection requirements in their installation document VDE 0165, and the United States of America in Article 500 of the National Electrical Code.

As industry developed there was a considerable demand for sparking Zone 2 apparatus as it was recognized that the Zones 0 and 1 requirements, which had hitherto been applied, were overly restrictive for Zone 2 and, as in all other fields, the advent of the transistor had introduced much more complexity into the field causing much more hazardous area mounted apparatus. In addition, there was an increasing demand for definitive constructional requirements for Zone 2 apparatus to remove the 'judgement' element present in the selection procedures. This led to the publication of the first British Standard for the production of apparatus for Zone 2 which was called 'Apparatus with Type of Protection 'N' and was BS 4683, Part 3 (1972)[6]. This Standard began the process of translating the criteria for apparatus selection into requirements for construction, and opened the door for full third-party certification.

International interest in construction requirements for apparatus for Zone 2 increased during this period also and an IEC[7] committee was formed to produce an International Standard for this type of apparatus using the international coding 'n' (the UK Standard used 'N' to show that the protection concept was a national concept and not an international one). The IEC committee, not surprisingly as this was the first attempt to internationalize a situation which had been national until this time and included a wide range of national ideas not accepted or even understood by some other countries, had considerable difficulties in coming to an agreement.

At the same time the limitations of BS 4683, Part 3, in the light of further progress, were becoming evident and there was considerable support for replacing it by a more detailed Standard which would include all of the ideas in the IEC[7] committee with which the UK agreed (which were all essentially the same except for the Swiss developed restricted breathing concept). This Standard was published in 1988 as BS 6941[8]. This Standard also addressed particular types of equipment, such as Type 'N' electric motors (addressed also in BS 5000, Part 16 (1972)[9]) and luminaires with Type 'N' protection. (Addressed also in BS 4533, Part 2, Section 2.1 (1976)[10]).

The IEC committee ultimately produced their document as IEC 79–15 (1987)[11] but, because of the divergence of opinion in the IEC[7] the document was produced as a report rather than a Standard. The fact, however, that BS 6941[8] followed almost exactly IEC 79–15[11] text (with the exception of the restricted breathing concept) makes the use of that Standard a valid basic approach for the technical requirements of type of protection 'N'.

The IEC and CENELEC[12] are now producing a Standard which will be both European and international, based upon IEC 79–15[11] which adds further weight to the requirements in BS 6941[8].

Notwithstanding the fact that a detailed construction standard now exists, the flexibility of selecting apparatus for Zone 2 with no absolute requirement for third-party approval still remains both nationally in the UK and in Directive 94/9/EC[5] in the EU. The rules against which this selection takes place, however, will now by those exist in BS 6941[8] and its European and international successor.

14.2 Basic requirements of the protection concept

The definition of Type 'N' (n) apparatus is that it will not be capable of causing the ignition of an explosive atmosphere in normal operation and that a fault making it so capable is unlikely to occur. Now that sparking is accepted as part of the protection concept, this basic definition may be expanded to cover this as follows: first, the apparatus must not produce an arc or spark in normal operation which can cause ignition of an explosive atmosphere, unless that arc or spark is prevented from so doing either by current limitation or by some other means which are defined as being capable of prevention of such ignition; and second, that the apparatus must not produce a surface temperature capable of igniting an explosive atmosphere, unless that surface temperature is prevented from causing such an ignition by containment or some other suitable means.

While the 'General Requirements' identified in Chapter 8 do not, in general, apply to apparatus of Type 'N', some are appropriate – for example, sub-grouping into IIA, IIB and IIC which is carried out for sparking apparatus. Likewise, the method of surface temperature classification used in other protection concepts is also appropriate to Type 'N' apparatus.

The apparatus is also expected, in common with other protected apparatus, to have additional features where it is used in environments which are more onerous than normal outdoor environments, such as those where solvent vapours may occur and where plastics enclosures may not be appropriate. These additional requirements are, as in the case of other protection concepts, agreed in particular cases in relation to particular risks, such as additional exposure to mechanical damage or chemical damage, unusually moist environments, etc..

14.3 General constructional requirements

The general constructional requirements are those which apply to all types of Type 'N' apparatus and address environmental protection, mechanical strength and electrical connections.

14.3.1 Environmental protection

Because Type 'N' apparatus is assumed to include electrical circuits which can contain incendive energies, the entry of the environment is assumed to be able to cause internal faults which would allow those energies to be released. For this reason, as with other forms of protection exhibiting this phenomenon, the enclosure of the apparatus is required to provide a suitable degree of protection against entry of liquids and solids present in the external environment. The degree of protection necessary in this regard is as follows: in the case of general use, IP54 is necessary where the apparatus contains bare live parts reducing to IP44 where all internal live parts are covered with insulation, encapsulant or similar protection; in the case of equipment intended for installation in areas where the risk of entry of solid foreign bodies or liquids is prevented by other means, such as indoor installation in a clean environment, the protection afforded by the enclosure can be reduced to IP4X for bare live parts reducing to IP2X where live parts are covered by insulation, encapsulant or similar protection. (The X indicates there is no basic requirement for exclusion of liquids).

The standards appropriate to the determination of IP rating are BS 5490[13] in the general case, and BS 4999[14] in the case of rotating machines. These enclosures are only necessary where ingress is possible and could cause an ignition-capable situation. In cases such as resistance thermometers, strain guages and similar low energy devices where ignition-capable sparking can be precluded, the above degrees of enclosure do not apply and, likewise, in some cases identified in the protection concept a higher degree of protection is required. It should also be stressed that the IP-rating is that which is necessary to ensure the correct operation of the apparatus and not only that necessary to avoid ignition-capable situations.

14.3.2 Mechanical strength

The apparatus enclosure is required to be proof against mechanical damage and this is shown by subjecting it to the mechanical impact test described in Chapter 8. However, due to the reduced likelihood of the presence of an explosive atmosphere in Zone 2 and the likelihood that a reasonable inspection routine is likely to identify damage before such an atmosphere occurs, the strength test is reduced to the figures given in Table 14.1. These would clearly mean that in many cases the Standard impact device at 1 Kg would require a height of 20 cms or less which would make the test less easy to define. For this reason the test may, be carried out with reduced mass testing devices in accordance with Table 14.2.

This test may chip the apparatus or may cause deformation of the enclosure but in either case neither the degree of protection (IP-rating) of the enclosure nor the correct operation of the apparatus must be adversely affected.

Table 14.1 Impact testing of enclosure parts

Part of apparatus	Impact energy (J)	
	Normal damage risk	Low damage risk
All parts of enclosures including guards and fan hoods, excluding light transmitting parts	3.5	2.0
Light transmitting parts which do not have a guard	2.0	1.0
Light transmitting parts which are guarded (These are tested with their guards removed)	1.0	0.5

(from BS 6941)

Table 14.2 Use of smaller impact tester masses for testing

Impact energy (J)	Impact test mass (K)	Impact test height (m)
3.5	1.0	0.35
2.0	0.25	0.8
1.0	0.25	0.4
0.5	0.25	0.2

(from BS 6941)
Note: For the purposes of this Table, g_n (the acceleration due to gravity) in the formula, height of fall = energy (mass × g_n) is taken as 10 m/s^2 for convenience, rather than the more accurate figure of 9.81 m/s^2.

14.3.3 Wiring and internal connections

Wiring

The internal wiring of Type 'N' apparatus need only comply with the requirements for normal industrial apparatus except that additional care needs to be taken to avoid damage by rubbing against metallic parts or sharp edges. This is normally achieved by securing internal wiring where it comes into contact with other parts of the apparatus to prevent movement and damage, and ensure there are no sharp edges inside the apparatus.

Internal connections

The wiring may be connected to components and other metallic parts by the following means all of which are considered as non-sparking:

1. screwed or bolted connections including pinching screws where conductors are not damaged by the screws or bolts or connection method;
2. crimped connections;
3. soldering;
4. brazing;
5. welding;
6. pressure-type wire connectors where connection is made by inserting the wire in between two pieces of metal which are sprung together and provide a pressure on the inserted conductor, preventing its movement;
7. machine wrapping of conductors around a post (more normally known as gun wrapping) but in this case the technique is limited to conductors which carry 1 A or less in normal service;

8. plugs and sockets, provided their separation requires the application of a force of at least 15 N and they are either arranged so that incorrect connection is not possible or is obvious by some form of arrangement or identification.

Other forms of connection and plugs and sockets not complying with the above must be considered as normally sparking.

14.3.4 External connection facilities

These are normally plugs and sockets or terminals unless the apparatus is fitted with a flying lead (permanently connected cable).

In addition to the requirements for internal plugs and sockets those for external connection need to be arranged so that sparking is unlikely to occur due to inadvertent energized separation. This can be achieved by interlocking them so that isolation occurs if separation is attempted while the combination is energized, or by securing them together by fasteners with a warning label to specify pre-separation isolation. It is also important that the fixed part of the plug and socket combination does not adversely affect the degree of protection of the enclosure (IP) when the moveable part has been removed and that accumulations of dust, liquids and other foreign bodies do not occur while the plug and socket are separated. This is most likely to be a problem in relation to the socket where the accumulation will not be so obvious.

Terminals for external connection need to satisfy similar requirements to those used for Zone 1 types of protection (see Chapters 8 and 12) but, in this case, terminal security may be achieved by friction alone.

Cables can enter Type 'N' enclosure via cable glands or conduit but in either case the degree of protection (IP) of the enclosure must be maintained. This is particularly true where conduit is used as a stopper box needs to be used to seal the end of the conduit. In the case of cables the normal types of cable gland for outdoor use will usually be adequate. It is important that, in the case of cable glands, the gland provides mechanical clamping of the cable to prevent stress on the terminals.

The normal types of cable used will be polyethylene or PVC insulated and sheathed. For this reason, apparatus which generates heat could raise the cable temperature above its maximum operating temperature. For this reason where the temperature at the point of fitting of the gland exceeds 70 °C, or that at the point where the conductors separate inside the enclosure exceeds 80 °C, a warning needs to be given (normally by a label) to the installer identifying this so that the cable can be chosen accordingly.

14.3.5 Conductor insulation and separation

As with increased safety 'e' (Chapter 12) and intrinsic safety 'i' (Chapter 13) there are requirements for separation of uninsulated conductors in air (clearance), for uninsulated conductors across a surface of insulating material (creepage in air), separation of uninsulated conductors across varnished surfaces (creepage under coating), and separation distances through encapsulation where breakdown of such distances could produce incendive sparking either at the point of breakdown or elsewhere. The minimum distances in question are given in Table 14.3. It will be noted that

Table 14.3 Minimum creepage distances, clearances and separations between conductors

Nominal rms supply voltage (U_n) or nominal rms voltage between conductive parts (Notes 1 and 2)		Minimum separations in air, under coating (Notes 3 and 4)			Minimum creepage distances in air at various CTI values (Note 5)			
ac	dc	In air	coated	Encapsulated	CTI 125	CTI 175	CTI 250	CTI 500
V	V	mm	mm	mm	mm	mm	mm	mm
12	15	0.4	0.3	0.13	1.0	1.0	1.0	1.0
30	36	0.8	0.3	0.26	1.0	1.0	1.0	1.0
60	75	1.3	0.43	0.43	1.3	1.3	1.3	1.3
130	160	2.0	1.0	0.66	2.5	2.0	1.7	1.4
250	300	2.0	1.7	0.66	4.0	3.4	2.8	2.3
380	500	2.8	2.6	0.73	6.7	5.1	4.3	3.7
500	600	3.4	3.0	0.9	7.1	6.0	5.1	4.4
660	900	5.0	4.4	1.1	11.0	9.0	7.5	6.5
1000	1200	6.8	5.8	1.7	14.0	12.0	10.0	8.6
3000	N/A	23.0	N/A	N/A	60.0	42.0	35.0	28.0
6000	N/A	45.0	N/A	N/A	N/A	85.0	70.0	55.0
10,000	N/A	75.0	N/A	N/A	N/A	N/A	100.0	80.0

(from BS 6941)

Notes:
1 The highest voltage which can appear between any conductive parts will be used even if, at some points due to voltage multiplication, this can exceed the nominal supply voltage.
2 Actual voltage may exceed nominal values by up to 10% without any necessary increase in the voltage used to apply the table.
3 Sealed values apply to conducting parts covered by a conformal coating. Where they emerge from the conformal coating creepage distances apply, and the coating must have the required CTI in addition to any supporting insulation.
4 Encapsulated values apply where the conductive parts are surrounded with encapsulant to a depth of at least 0.4 mm. Where any conductive parts exit the encapsulation the creepage distance in the table apply and the encapsulant must have the required CTI in addition to any support insulation.
5 The CTI is determined in accordance with BS 5901,[15] notwithstanding the fact that the voltages increase to values exceeding those to which that standard applies

there are no requirements for separation through solid insulation but, in the absence of these, insulation satisfying the separation distance through solid insulation should be used. Table 14.3 follows a similar approach to those in protection concepts 'e' and 'i', being derived from IEC work on minimum separations in various environmental conditions. It was, however, derived by different committees at a different time and although the base derivation criteria were similar, differences will inevitably arise. These will not have an adverse effect on safety as they are minor variations and, a comparison of them with the tables associated with other protection concepts shows clearly that they are in excess of one third of the other distances. This is adequate bearing in mind that this figure represents a countable fault level in intrinsic safety (chapter 13) which is adequate for Zone 2 in the light of the reduced risk of the presence of an explosive atmosphere.

The table in the Standard for Type 'N' (BS 6941) differs from those in other Standards in that it uses different terms but this is only because a different committee produced the requirements and not because there is any difference in the intent. The actual meaning of the terms is as follows.

Creepage

Creepage is the creepage distance across an unprotected insulating surface and is specified as 'Creepage distance in air' in other documents.

Clearance and separation in air

Clearance and separation in air is the minimum direct distance in air between two uninsulated conductive parts and is elsewhere referred to as 'clearance'.

Separation – sealed

This is the minimum distance across an insulating surface where the surface and conductive parts are covered with varnish or similar and is referred to elsewhere as 'creepage under coating'. The covering is in this case referred to as a conformal coating and BS 5917[16] is referred to as controlling it. Reference to IEC 79–15[11], however, shows the intent in that it specifies the use of a single coat of a soft setting medium or two coats of lacquer or varnish. The intent is to ensure that the coating is complete without pinholes. Where uninsulated conductive parts exit the coating, as elsewhere, the creepage in air figures apply and both the coating material and the supporting insulation require to have the necessary CTI.

Separation – encapsulated

This is the distance between two uninsulated conductive parts through encapsulation and is elsewhere known as 'separation distance through casting compound'. The requirement here is for encapsulation to surround both conductive parts to a depth of at least 0.4 mm. This 0.4 mm figure is only of importance up to 500 V, however, as above this distance the separation requirement is for 0.9 mm and the path from both conductive parts to the surface of the encapsulant is only 0.8 mm. The creepage across the surface of the encapsulant cannot, in this case, be added as there is no method specified for this in Type 'N' and the encapsulant depth would need to be enhanced to achieve the necessary separation. There are no specific further reductions for separations through solid insulation and so these requirements will apply to solid insulation also.

Insulation tests between conductors

The requirements of Table 14.3 are not excessively onerous as they may be waived if the electrical insulation between the two conductors (e.g., the supporting printed circuit board, the encapsulant the insulation, etc.) passes the following electric strength test. A voltage of minimum value (1500 + 2U) V rms (either ac or dc as appropriate) should be applied between the two conductive parts for one minute without breakdown of the insulation. This voltage may be applied by increasing the voltage to the necessary level in 10 seconds and then holding it for one minute. Any leakage current should remain stable or fall during the test. Increases are assumed to be a precursor of failure.

This test is a routine test and must be applied to all apparatus where the requirements of Table 14.3 are not complied with. In electronic apparatus items such as transistors and integrated circuits, which would be damaged by the test, need not be installed at the time of testing as the test is to prove the integrity of insulation alone.

Insulation tests between conductors and the frame or earth

In addition, where the apparatus is not intended to be connected to the frame or earth, in all cases – even where the requirements of Table 14.3 are met – the insulation between the electrical circuits and earth must satisfy the following voltage tests.

First, where both the supply voltage to the apparatus and any internal voltages exceed 90 V peak the insulation or separation between earth or the frame and the electrical circuits must not break down when a test voltage of (1000 + 2U) V rms ac or dc as appropriate is applied between them, as before. RF-suppression capacitors must be included in this test and their current, if the test is ac, allowed for in the identification of breakdown.

Second, where the supply voltage to the apparatus is not more than 90 V peak and likewise the internal voltages do not exceed that figure (there are no internal voltage enhancement provisions) the earth or frame test voltage may be reduced to 500 V rms ac or dc as appropriate.

All of the above test voltages are minima and it is not necessary to control the voltage any more than to ensure that it does not exceed +5 per cent of this figure.

14.4 Additional requirements for certain types of non-sparking apparatus

Continuing the theme that the basic requirements for Type 'N' apparatus are normal industrial requirements which would produce a reliable item of equipment, there are only a limited set of additional requirements applied to specific items of apparatus.

14.4.1 Rotating electrical machines

Both BS 6941[8] and IEC 79–15[11] make the initial premiss that the machines must meet basic industrial Standards, the standard in question in the UK being BS 5000, Part 16[9] which details Type 'N' machines and the international Standard being IEC 34[17] which is a more general standard for rotating electrical machines. The IEC document is the more general document leaving the Type 'n' special additions for IEC 79–15[11]. The basic matters which require consideration are such things as the security of fitting of rotor bars, enclosure, etc. In common with Type 'e' machines, the rotor bars are required to be secured in the slots so as to minimize, the possibility of their movement and hence sparking. Similar methods of securing as for Type 'e' machines (e.g., die-cast aluminium, etc.) are proposed as appropriate and the sparking which would be otherwise produced needs, as for Type 'e', to be addressed during both starting and running. Fanhoods are expected to be constructed so as to reduce the risk of damage causing contact with the fans and, in addition to withstanding the impact tests for Type 'N' described earlier, the running clearance between them and the enclosed fan must have a basic value of at least 1 per cent of the fan diameter. There are limits to this in that the clearance must also be at least 1 mm but need not exceed 5 mm.

Type 'N' machines must satisfy the enclosure requirements stated earlier in this chapter but in this case BS 4999[14] is the appropriate Standard used. If the machine is fitted with a terminal box that box must achieve IP54 to the outside world but need only provide IP44 to the interior of the machine as that is already protected by its own enclosure and the outer protection of the terminal box.

Finally, because of the low risk of an explosive atmosphere in Zone 2 the surface temperature classification of the machine may consider running under recognized maximum load only and exclude starting conditions as these are unlikely to coincide with the presence of an explosive atmosphere within the machine which is usually where the maximum temperature occurs. If the machine is for duty cycling where it is regularly started and stopped, such as would occur in a batch process or where it is used for topping up a tank or similar vessel, the argument for excluding the starting conditions for temperature classification is not valid and these conditions will have to be included.

There is not special requirement for t_e time in respect of faults as these are not considered for Type 'n' machines.

14.4.2 Fuse links and fuseholders

In general, rupture of a fuse, provided the element is enclosed, is not considered as an ignition-capable occurrence. Thus provided fuse elements are non-indicating cartridge types, usually sand filled for voltages over 60 V, the arc produced by the element during rupturing can be ignored as a source of ignition as long as the fuse element satisfies the necessary mounting requirements.

Currently, fuse links interrupting voltages below 60 V may be installed in open holders retained by spring end clamps or soldered in position, whereas those operating at more than 60 V need an enclosed holder within the apparatus although it may be accessible from the outside of the apparatus. Obviously fuses below 60 V may be installed in such holders also but this is by choice and is probably only necessary where have access is needed to the fuse from the outside of the enclosure. Where fuse holders are so accessible the normal warnings apply and the enclosures must achieve IP54.

Where several fuses are mounted within a fuse enclosure (an enclosure dedicated to fuses) these rules may not apply but the enclosure itself needs to provide the necessary IP protection and control to prevent fuse extraction live (i.e., interlocking or fastening with a warning label). In such cases diversity may be applied in determination of maximum temperature. This is normally determined with the fuse carrying its rated current as higher currents are considered as abnormal operation but, where several fuses exist the temperature could be further elevated by several fuses carrying this current simultaneously. In cases where this is not likely diversity (e.g., the assumption that not all fuses will carry such current at once) may be applied as long as the user of the apparatus knows on what basis that diversity has been applied so that the apparatus can be used safely.

14.4.3 Fixed luminaires

Fixed luminaires (lighting fittings) are, subject to additional requirements to reduce the risk of sparking and, low pressure sodium lamps are not permitted, as is the case with Type 'e' protection. British Standard BS 4533[10] is called up for certain luminaires in BS 6941[8], as are BS 5042[18] for bayonet lamp holders, BS 6766[19] for screw lampholders, BS 6702[20] for bi-pin lampholders and starter holders, BS 3772[21] for starters and BS 2818[22] and 4782[23] for ballasts. All of these standards cover normal equipment, once again reinforcing the use of good quality industrial equipment in Zone 2. IEC 79–15[11] similarly addresses this by referring to IEC 61[24], IEC 238[25] and IEC 400[26] for lampholders, and IEC 262[27] and IEC 598–1[28] for auxiliary gear. Both standards also address the minimum requirements for safety which may not appear in some of these industrial Standards and cover the important features of these devices which are as follows.

Lampholders

The lampholders need to be effectively non-sparking in normal operation which does not include lamp changing. This leads to specific requirements with which the lampholders need to comply but which may not be requirements in the industrial Standard concerned. The basic requirements are as follows.

1. Screw lampholders must be shown to be sufficiently secure against loosening so that it can be ignored as a possible source of incendive sparking. To this end the requirements are as in Table 12.5 (Chapter 12) which require the lamp to be tightened in the holder with a specific torque, then loosened by 15° after which the removal torque must be at least a specific figure. The tightening and release figures are repeated in Table 14.4. This table applies to the three Standard sizes E14, E27 and E40 but not to the smallest size, E10, where the torque test is not considered necessary and all that is required is that the lamp is tightly fitted. This is because lamps using E10 are normally very small, such as those used in torches, and the problem of loosening by normal vibration is considered less.
2. Bayonet lampholders produce a particular problem in that each contact normally comprises two concentric parts with an internal coil spring to ensure full extension of the lower part (see Fig. 14.1). Current to the lamp is normally passed down a combination of the friction contact between the two concentric parts and the coil spring. This makes the type of connection very vulnerable to dirt in between the two parts or weakening of the spring. One possible method of spring weakening is heating due to the passage of current and to this end there must be some other principal method

Table 14.4 Torque tests for screw lampholders

Lamp cap size	Insertion torque Nm	Minimum removal torque Nm
E10	Note	Note
E14	1.0 ± 0.1	0.3
E27	1.5 ± 0.1	0.5
E40	3.0 ± 0.1	1.0

(from BS/EN 50019)

Note: No test is considered as necessary for this small size of lamp.

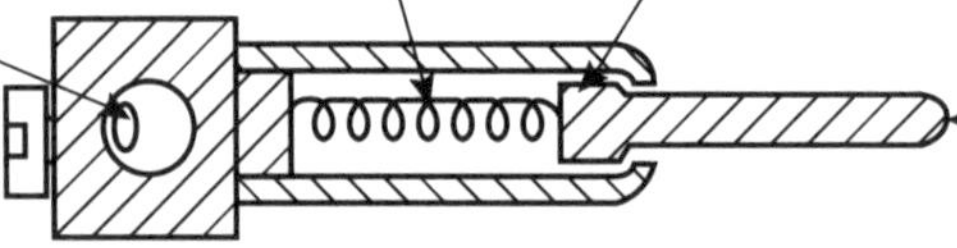

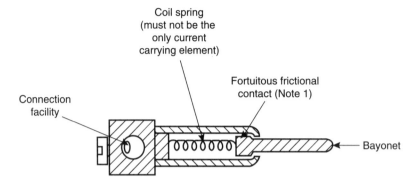

Fig. 14.1 Typical bayonet used in bayonet fitting luminaires. *Notes*: This contact cannot normally be relied upon for transmission of current to the lamp. In addition of the spring, additional conduction elements are required e.g.: (1) A leaf spring inside the outer tube to bias the bayonet and thus ensure pressure connection if this can be achieved while continuing to permit adequate bayonet movement; or (2) A broad connection between the bayonet and the outer tube either inside or outside the tube

of carrying current in addition to the spring and the fortuitous contact between the two parts of the bayonet is not sufficient. There are many ways of doing this, for example, the addition of spring sliding contacts which play no part in extension of the bayonet, and additional flexible connections between the connection facility and the lower part of the bayonet. In general, however, screw lampholders are to be preferred due to the positive connection achieved.

3. For fluorescent tubes and similar lamps the normal bi-pin connection methods are permitted, allowing hot cathode operation. In this case the current to the lamp may be carried by the lateral spring used to apply pressure to the pins when the tube is fitted, but there must be some method of ensuring that the tube pins cannot distort inwards under such pressure, as is possible with many standard holders. To ensure this it is only necessary to have a central insulating boss against which the contacts rest (see Fig. 14.2).

Lamp control gear

Lamp control gear such as that used for fluorescent fittings must also be non-sparking. In the case of Type 'N', switch starters are acceptable provided the switch contacts, normally a discharge tube, are contained in a hermetically sealed enclosure (see later in this chapter) which is afforded additional mechanical protection (e.g., a hermetically sealed envelope in an additional metal or plastic canister complying with BS 3772). As devices which are known to have a regular failure pattern the starters are normally plug in, and the contacts on the base of the starter and in its receptacle must have similar reliability to those used for the tubes. In addition it is not normally acceptable to have the starter rely upon these contacts for

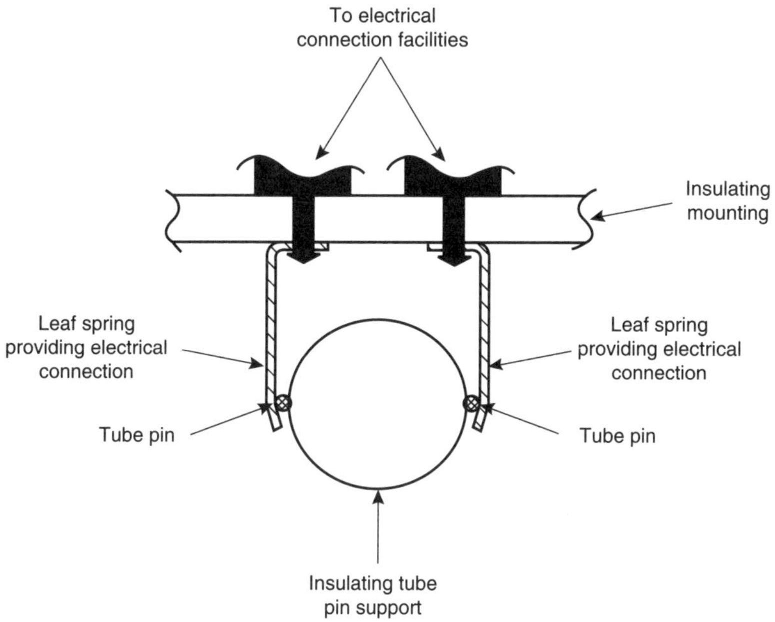

Fig. 14.2 Method of tube pin support provision

its support, and additional support to prevent untoward movement of the starter in situ is necessary. The normal holder ring is usually sufficient for this.

Ballasts (chokes) and similar devices are in this case of normal industrial construction as failure is abnormal. Unlike Type 'e' chokes, however, there is no requirement for prevention of overheating or failure in case of tube failure as the likelihood of this occurring at the same time as an explosive atmosphere is present in Zone 2 is remote. A situation where the choke becomes very hot and is not subject to a failure which causes protection elements to operate, isolating the fitting is not, however, acceptable. Thus if the choke does exceed the temperature classification or the operating limit of its insulation on lamp failure, it must fail in a way which causes safety devices (such as circuit fuses) to operate within a short time. No time is given but any time in excess of say 30 minutes is unlikely to be acceptable.

14.4.4 Portable luminaires and other light sources

Portable luminaires and other light sources, such as those forming parts of other apparatus rather than luminaires, need to comply with the same requirements as those specified above unless they can be shown to be inappropriate (e.g., in the case of a soldered-in indicator lamp lampholder requirements are clearly not appropriate). In addition, in the case of portable luminaires the luminaire must be capable of being dropped four times from a height of 1 m on to a smooth concrete floor without other than superficial damage and, in particular, without the lamp envelope breaking. The conditions under which this drop test is carried out are given in Chapter 8 and are the same as for other protection concepts.

14.4.5 Electronic and low power apparatus

This type of apparatus is specifically identified separately as it normally operated at low voltage and power, comprising typically instrumentation and intelligence transmitting equipment. This type of apparatus is absolved from the necessity to achieve the level of separation of conductive parts either by meeting the creepage or clearance requirements of Table 14.3, or the electrical insulation tests between conducting parts given as alternatives to compliance with that Table (see earlier in this chapter) but not the insulation requirements between circuits and earth or frame provided that it satisfies all of the following three requirements.

1. The apparatus enclosure must be at least IP54 when tested, as described earlier in this chapter, or must be intended for installation in a location which itself provides that protection. If the latter is the case the user of the apparatus needs to be informed of the installation needs and it is not expected that the apparatus enclosure will ever be permitted to reduce to below IP20 in such circumstances.
2. The rated voltage of such apparatus (or the parts of apparatus in question) must not exceed 60 V rms ac or 75 V dc. It follows that higher voltages should not be generated within the apparatus.
3. Provision needs to be made either within the apparatus or by installation specification to prevent the supplies to the apparatus from exceeding the rated values significantly and for any length of time. Where the provision is outside the apparatus its requirements must be made known to the installer by information provided with the apparatus and marking upon it (usually the 'X' mark to draw attention to unusual installation requirements).

As the apparatus is normally non-sparking then transient supply elevations of a minor nature are not expected to cause sparking or overheating and for this reason the apparatus is assessed at its normal maximum supply voltage. The method of preventing excess voltage supply is normally a device such as a zener diode, or combination of zener diodes across the supply with series fusing between the supply and the diodes. The diodes need to have a minimum conduction value, probably 10 per cent higher than the maximum supply voltage and with normal tolerances will allow, transiently, an elevation of around 30 per cent during the rupturing period of the fuse. The energy transmitted into the apparatus during this period, which is milliseconds, is not normally expected to cause problems as in the unlikely event that a spark occurs during this time the possibility of the presence of an explosive atmosphere being coincident in a Zone 2 situation is considered as unlikely.

14.5 Apparatus producing arcs, sparks and/or ignition-capable hot surfaces

As discussed earlier in this chapter the advent of type of protection 'N' was not only to precise the selection requirements for non-sparking apparatus which were historically used for selection for Zone 2 but, in addition, to introduce simplified methods of protection of ignition-capable sparks and hot surfaces produced by apparatus in its normal operation to remove the necessity to use the Zone 1 protection concepts. The techniques used for these simplified methods are similar in concept to the more classic methods developed for Zone 1 with the addition of the possibility being recognized that the explosive atmosphere can be excluded to a sufficient level of confidence for Zone 2, an approach not considered as suitable for Zone 0 and 1.

14.5.1 Enclosed break devices and non-incendive components

These methods of prevention of general ignition by sparking contacts (or for that matter hot surfaces despite the title of the device) are effectively a sort of simplified flameproof construction. There is little difference between their construction but, in the enclosed break device, it is ensured that any explosive atmosphere entering the device is ignited and the protection is in prevention of flame transmission into the surrounding explosive atmosphere. In the non-incendive component no attempt is made to ensure internal ignition and protection may be as for the enclosed break device but, equally, it may be that the contact configuration or surface configuration within the component may quench any incipient flame and prevent effective internal ignition.

Construction

Both types of enclosure may be opened in service and may contain thermoplastic or elastomeric seals. In general these seals must be proof against deterioration and this requires any gaskets containing thermoplastic or elastomeric materials to be preconditioned before any testing is carried out. In the case of gaskets containing thermoplastic materials, this comprises of the placing of the gaskets in an oven at $80\pm2\,^{\circ}C$ for 168 hours (7 days), and in the case of gaskets containing elastomeric materials the placing of the gaskets in a chamber containing pure oxygen at $70\pm2\,^{\circ}C$ at a gauge pressure of $2 \times 10^6\,N/m^2$ for 96 Hours (4 days). In addition, any gaskets which are used to seal covers which are opened in service or which are not protected against or proof against mechanical or other environmental conditions (e.g., exposure to light) must be wholly or partly removed – whichever is considered worst. Partial removal may be worse because it can result in jetting, which will make the transmission of flame more likely and testing is likely to be necessary in both total removal and partial removal (say 1 per cent of the gasket).

Poured seals which are used as permanent seals and not subject to separation in normal service must have a melting point which is at least 20 °C higher than the maximum temperature which the device is expected to reach in service at maximum ambient temperature.

The internal free volume of both enclosed break devices and non-incendive components must not exceed 20 cm^3.

Ratings

There are also limits on the rating of these devices and these are as follows. First, enclosed break devices shall not be rated at voltages exceeding 660 V and which are rated for currents in excess of 15 A.

Second, non-incendive components have similar but lower absolute limits which are 250 V and 15 A. In this case, because of the nature of the device, the circuit feeding any sparking contacts is important as flame quenching is the possible means of protection. They are usable only in particular circuits and testing for ignition must be in circuits typical of those in which the component is intended to be used. For this reason non-incendive components normally appear only as parts of other apparatus and not as apparatus in themselves – unlike enclosed break devices which can more readily stand alone.

Type tests

To execute the necessary type tests the devices are filled and surrounded with the explosive atmosphere specified in Table 14.5.

In the case of enclosed break devices the atmosphere within the enclosure will be ignited by the contacts within it or by the internal hot surface and ignition verified by some means (e.g., thermocouples or ionization detection). The external atmosphere must not be ignited. The test will be repeated three times using renewed explosive atmospheres in each case and the ignition will be by the contacts operating at their maximum rating or the hot surface at its maximum temperature.

In the case of non-incendive components there is no need to confirm internal ignition. The enclosure is filled and surrounded with the explosive

Table 14.5 Test mixtures for flame transmission in enclosed break devices and non-incendive components

Sub-group	Test gas mixture
IIA	6.5 ± 0.5% ethylene in air
IIB	28.2 ± 2% hydrogen in air
IIC	34 ± 2% hydrogen/17 ± 1% oxygen in nitrogen

(*from BS 6941*)

atmosphere as before and the contained hot surface or contacts operated in the most onerous condition in the circuit in which they are used. In the case of contacts they will be preconditioned by being operated 6000 times at a rate of around 6 operations per minute at their rated load (not the circuit load). The contacts are then operated at their maximum circuit load 50 times at around the same rate when the explosive atmosphere is present and ignition of the external explosive atmosphere must not take place. No time criterion is given for hot surfaces but allowing the test to proceed for 10 minutes is acceptable. These tests also must be repeated three times with new explosive atmospheres each time.

The apparatus is, in this case, sub-grouped IIA, IIB or IIC depending upon the test mixture used. A typical use for an enclosed break device is shown in Fig. 14.3 where it is used as an automatic isolator for a screw lampholder. A microswitch which is a typical non-incendive component is shown in Fig. 14.4.

14.5.2 Hermetically sealed devices

Hermetically sealed devices are devices which are permanently sealed by means such as fusion. This type of seal is used in normal equipment for such things as contacts and relays to allow for the production of a controlled atmosphere around contacts to give maximum efficiency and longevity. In Type 'N', however, they can be used to exclude an explosive atmosphere.

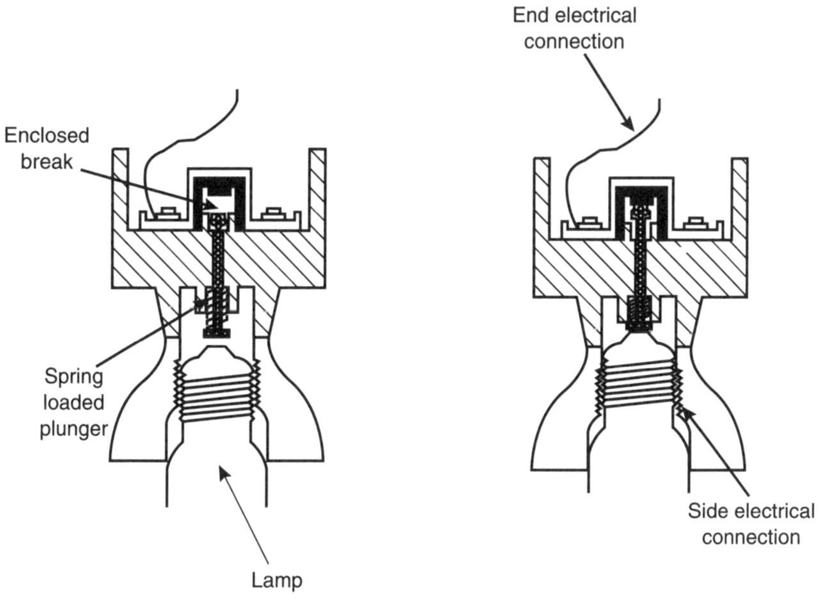

Fig. 14.3 Automatic isolation of lamp on removal using enclosed break/non-incendive component technique

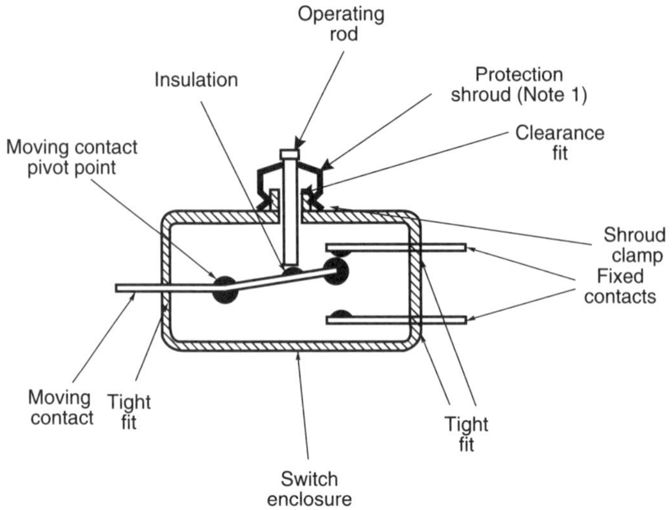

Fig. 14.4 Microswitch using enclosed break/non-incendive component technique. *Note*: The shroud is removed for testing

Construction

Seals are made by such arrangements as glass/metal fusion, welding, brazing or soldering. Seals made using gaskets cannot be termed as hermetic seals. Where hermetic sealing is used the seal must not be damaged in installation of the device in apparatus and must not be damaged by the normally applied impact and, if appropriate, drop tests.

Type testing

Once the seal is made it is not possible to carry out any measurements inside the enclosure and the only test which can be carried out is a leakage test. This can be carried out by placing the device in hot water to expand the internal gas (water at 75 °C to 85 °C is used and the initial apparatus temperature is between 15 °C and 35 °C), or by evacuating the air above the water in which the device is immersed to encourage leaking (in this case the temperature of both test item and water are between 15 °C and 35 °C and the pressure over the water is reduced to an absolute value of $5 \times 10^3\,N/m^2$ absolute).

The differential temperature test is normally for 2 minutes and leakage is observed by noting a single large production of bubbles at the device surface, or a train of bubbles for at least 20 seconds. Normal air release from the surface on initial immersion should be ignored even though it gives similar indications for a short time. In the case of reduced pressure a continuous train of bubbles will be noted until the enclosure reaches the pressure of the air over the liquid.

14.5.3 Sealed devices

Sealed devices are similar in operation to hermetically sealed devices but use sealing gaskets and poured seals, and are often secured together by such things as rivets. Like hermetically sealed enclosures, they are not intended to be opened in service and by the use of such things as rivets or adhesives they are destroyed by opening.

Construction

Sealed devices are limited in size, unlike hermetically sealed devices, to 100 cm^3. Their gaskets are conditioned as for enclosed break devices but in situ and they must be protected against mechanical damage or environmental damage in the same way. Poured seals are also subject to the same limitations.

Type testing

The type tests applied to sealed devices are identical to those for hermetically sealed devices.

14.5.4 Energy limited apparatus and circuits

This technique is very similar to intrinsic safety in that it relies on the limitation of power and energy in the circuit in question to levels that, even if released as a spark or delivered to heating of a surface, will not cause sparks or hot surfaces which are ignition capable. The approach is much more simple.

There are two types of energy limited apparatus: the first type, 'apparatus containing energy limited circuits', is that which is connected to a circuit which contains ignition-capable energy where limitation is within the apparatus where sparking contacts or possible hot surfaces are present; the second type, 'Apparatus for connection to energy limited circuits', is that which is connected to a circuit usually initiated in a non-hazardous area where the entire circuit in the hazardous area – both within and outside the apparatus – does not contain incendive levels of energy.

Construction

Apparatus containing energy limited circuits is fed from a supply which is not energy limited and will be either limited by means described earlier for non-sparking circuits or by the mains. It will normally contain further voltage limiting devices, such as a transformer if mains fed, or zener diodes. Further current limiting by such things as resistors will normally also be present, the objective being to define clearly the power and energy which can be fed to sparking contacts or potentially ignition-capable hot surfaces. In the case of sparking contacts the sparks are always there (unlike sparks caused by faults) and the likelihood of coincidence of a spark and the explosive atmosphere is thus increased. This means that the maximum voltage and current let-through of the limiting devices, in the case of mains with a 10 per cent elevation, become important and form the basis of evaluation of safety for both spark ignition, and hot surface ignition rather than the normal operational limiting circuit parameters. Thus the voltage and current are in all cases based upon the tolerances of the voltage and current limiting components in the apparatus. In many cases these elements will not form a part of the operational circuit and thus, if voltage limiters such as zener diodes are used and their failure is not identified by maloperation of the circuit, they must be duplicated if they protect a sparking contact. This also applies to such things as resistors used in a shunt mode to limit voltage but not to such devices used in series. Where such components are used to suppress inductances their connection to the inductance must be made reliable by placing them as close to it as possible with arrangements to limit the possibility of their becoming disconnected without the simultaneous disconnection of the inductor, unless their disconnection is identified by maloperation of the apparatus.

Apparatus for connection to energy limited circuits may or may not have within it limiting devices to prevent overheating or incendive sparking but, they will be based upon the energy limited source specified for connection to the apparatus. In this case such devices will be predominantly for temperature limitation or for energy limitation in cases where storage within the apparatus can occur, such as included inductors or capacitors.

The important thing here is to specify the maximum open circuit voltage, short circuit current, and power transfer capability required in the circuit to which the apparatus is connected, together with the maximum inductance and capacity (with L/R ration as a possible alternative to inductance) which may be present in that circuit. It is then up to the installer to ensure that these parameters are complied with. This will often mean the apparatus in the non-hazardous area containing voltage and current limitation to a level similar to that required in this type of apparatus.

It must be remembered here that use of the non-incendive circuit approach, where the entire circuit is non-incendive, is intended to allow live working to a similar degree as that for intrinsic safety (see later in this book).

Testing

Testing of non-incendivity is carried out at points where sparking will occur using the spark test apparatus and the same test mixtures as for intrinsic safety (see Chapter 13) but in this case no safety factors are used.

The test gas mixtures and calibration currents for the spark test apparatus are repeated in Tables 14.6 and 14.7, with additional calibration currents for resistive circuits. The presence of resistive calibration currents stems from the historic position in intrinsic safety where it was felt that the difference between inductive calibration and resistive calibration was sufficient to warrant separate calibration for resistive and capacitive circuits to that used for inductive circuits. This difference has now been accepted in intrinsic safety as not significant and only the inductive calibration is used. While it may be expected that the same will be the case in Type 'N' it is not currently so and thus the two different calibration currents still exist. Another difference here is that the test may be carried out with a tin disc in the spark test apparatus rather than the normal cadmium. This gives higher levels of ignition power and energy because it does not have an ignition enhancing effect. It is not permitted for intrinsic safety because of the difficulty of exclusion of cadmium, zinc and magnesium, all of which have this ignition enhancing effect. In Type 'N', however, where the risk is more remote it is concluded that the level of attention to adequately ensure the absence of these materials may be less rigourous and thus possible. Notwithstanding this, however, it is recommended that the cadmium disc (i.e., the more sensitive) test is used where possible.

Assessment of sparking circuits is possible for type 'N' using the curves given in Chapter 13 (Figs. 13.5, 13.6, 13.8 and 13.10). The curves can be used directly as there are no added safety factors as in intrinsic safety.

Table 14.6 Test gases for non-incendive sparking

Sub-group	Test gas
IIA	5.25 ± 0.25% propane in air
IIB	7.8 ± 0.5% ethylene in air
IIC	21 ± 2% hydrogen in air

Table 14.7 Calibration currents for spark test apparatus

Sub-group	Inductive circuits		Resistive circuits	
	Cadmium disc mA	Other disc mA	Cadmium disc A	Other disc A
IIA	100	125	1.0	2.75
IIB	65	100	0.7	2.0
IIC	30	52	0.3	1.65

14.5.5 Restricted breathing enclosures

This is a somewhat unusual type of protection relying not on total sealing but on the limitation of entry and exit of gas (breathing). Historically it has only been used on certain lighting fittings in the UK and has not been considered as acceptable for sparking equipment. In Switzerland, however, where much more use of the technique has been made, quite the reverse is the case. The technique used by the Swiss does not permit hot surfaces and only allows sparking contacts. Its use is much more prevalent, for example it can be applied to large switchboards.

The historic UK approach, which is still current, is the use of restricted breathing for luminaires and its exclusion for sparking contacts. This stems from the view that luminaires are not regularly switched on and off and that, even if some breathing occurs, it is unlikely that anything like an ideal explosive atmosphere will ever exist in the enclosure. For this reason it is considered that the approach is acceptable for Zone 2 and, indeed, the historical use of this approach without problems supports this. While the approach has been considered as suitable for luminaires which are not regularly switched on and off (i.e., not subject to duty cycling) the support for any other use where temperature cycling within the enclosure occurs more regularly does not exist. This is not a problem for the UK because restricted breathing has in the past been restricted to luminaires and this continues to be the case. The following is the situation for restricted breathing as practiced in the UK.

Construction

There are no constructional requirements for restricted breathing enclosures other than that thermoplastic and elastomeric seals are preconditioned, as for those in enclosed break devices, before any type testing is carried out and that they need to be protected against mechanical and environmental damage in the same way. Likewise poured seals are subjected to the same requirements as those in enclosed break devices.

Restricted breathing enclosures are required to have facilities for execution of the restricted breathing test in service and there has, therefore, to be a facility to allow the connection of a test device.

Testing

Type testing for restrictive breathing enclosures is quite simple as it is solely a test of the inward breathing of the enclosure (the outward breathing is not important). The enclosure is reduced in pressure to less than $0.97 \times 10^5\,\mathrm{N/m^2}$ absolute (approximately 0.97 atmospheres) and then the time taken for ingress of air sufficient to change the pressure from 0.97×10^5 to 0.985×10^5 is measured. This time must not be less than three minutes. It is possible to determine this time with an internal overpressure only where it can be shown that the performance of the enclosure is the same for overpressure as for underpressure.

This test may need to be carried out after reclosure of the apparatus, sometimes after each opening, and provision needs to be made in the construction to allow this to be done. Usually this is by having an entry device for a simple evacuating device which can be sealed with a valve or a screw and gasket after testing.

Other approaches to restricted breathing enclosure

The other country which has historically used restricted breathing as a protection concept is Switzerland where the concept was used in a quite different way. Here the concept has been used for equipment which may spark in normal operation, such as switchgear, and it has been limited to apparatus where the internally dissipated power is not sufficient to raise the internal temperature by more than 10 °C. Thus it has not been possible to use it for luminaires. While the basic constructional requirements have not differed greatly the testing has. One of three tests have been applied as follows.

1. A diffusion half-time test is applied whereby carbon dioxide is introduced into the enclosure without raising its pressure until the level of internal carbon dioxide concentration is 25 per cent. The internal concentration of carbon dioxide is then monitored for sufficient time to allow a straight line curve showing reduction of concentration with time to be plotted. This curve is then extrapolated to estimate the time necessary for the internal concentration of carbon dioxide to fall to 12.5 per cent which must not be less than 80 hours. Where the pressure measuring device adds significant volume to the enclosure volume (more than say 10 per cent) then the time given above needs to be multiplied by the total volume divided by the enclosure volume.
2. Alternatively, where the enclosure has a volume of less than 10 litres, it should be raised or lowered (alternatives) to a pressure of $500\,N/m^2$ above or below atmospheric pressure and the reduction in pressure differential measured. The time taken for the difference to fall from $400\,N/m^2$ to $200\,N/m^2$ must be at least 80 seconds in this case. The same multiplication of time as for the carbon dioxide test is applied where the measuring device has a significant volume.
3. A third alternative is to pressurize the enclosure to $400\,N/m^2$ above atmospheric pressure and calculate the volume of air required each hour to maintain that overpressure. That volume, divided by the enclosure volume, should not exceed a value of 0.125.

Use of the concept

As with the UK approach the Swiss approach, as defined in IEC 79–15[11], has been limited to apparatus that is not subject to duty cycling, which can cause significant temperature changes. In addition, the technique in its Swiss/IEC guise is limited to gases and vapours which have restricted breathing factors (s) of less than 20. This factor is related to the boiling point (bp), the molecular weight (m) and the lower explosive limit (LEL) of the gas or vapour in question and is derived from Fig. 14.5. The boiling point is identified on the left-hand side of Fig. 14.5 and the molecular weight on the right. These are then joined by a straight line which creates a point Z on the centre line. The LEL of the gas or vapour is then identified on the right-hand side of Fig. 14.5 and a line drawn to the left-hand side via the point Z on the centre line. The restricted breathing factor can then be read off on the left-hand side.

While this approach to restricted breathing is not currently used in the UK, the imminent production of a European Standard for type of protection 'N' may include it as the approach is in IEC 79–15[11] which will form the basis for the European Standard. The presence of such a European Standard may create a situation where it may become incumbent on the UK to utilize this type of apparatus and for this reason it is included. The safety of such equipment may be called into question but its long use in Switzerland produces no evidence to support any such doubts.

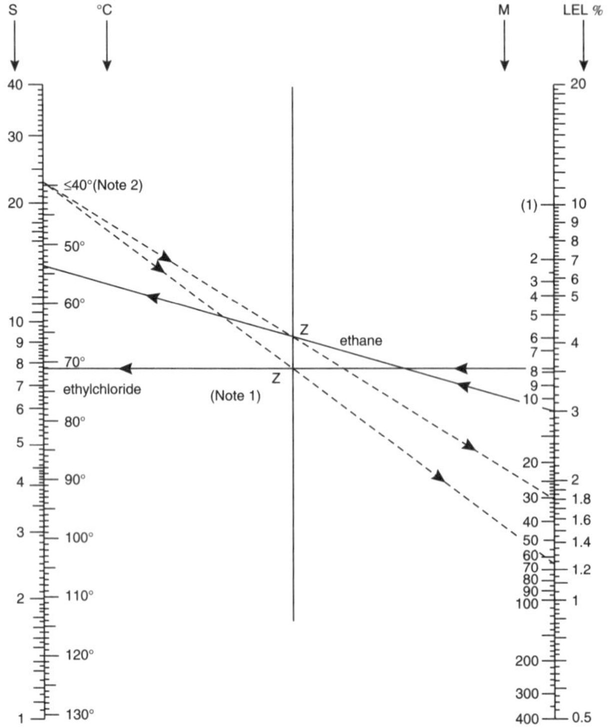

Fig. 14.5 Determination of restricted breathing factor (S). *Notes*: (1) Draw a line between the material boiling point end its molecular weight. This crosses the centre line at Z. Draw a line from the LEL via Z to determine S – the breathing factor. (2) Where boiling temperatures of less then 40 °C occur, 40 °C will be assumed for use of figure

References

1 BS/CP 1003 (1967) Part 3. Division 2 Areas.

2 BS 4137 (1967) Guide to the Selection of Electrical Equipment for Use in Division 2 Areas.

3 BS 5345 Installation and Maintenance of Electrical Apparatus for Use in Potentially Explosive Atmospheres. Part 1 (1976). Basic Requirements for All Parts of the Code.

4 76/117/EEC (1975) Council Directive on the Approximation of the Laws of Member States Concerning electrical Equipment for Use in Potentially Explosive Atmospheres. 18th December.

5 94/9/EC (1994) Directive of the European Parliament and Council on the Approximation of the Laws of Member States Concerning Electrical Equipment for Use in Potentially Explosive Atmospheres. 23rd March.

6 BS 4683 Electrical Apparatus for Explosive Atmospheres. Part 3 (1972). Type of Protection N.

7 IEC International Electrotechnical Commission.

8 BS 6941 (1988) Electrical Apparatus for Explosive Atmospheres with Type of Protection N.

9 BS 5000 Specification for Rotating Electrical Machines of Particular Types for Particular Applications. Part 16 (1972). Rotating Electrical Machines with Type of Protection N.

10 BS 4533 (1976) Luminaires: Part 101, Specification for General Requirements and Tests; Part 102 Particular Requirements: (Section 51) Specification for Luminaires with Type of Protection N.

11 IEC 79–15 Electrical Apparatus for Explosive Gas Atmospheres. Part 15 (1987). Electrical Apparatus With Type of Protection n.

12 CENELEC Comite Europeen de Normalisation Electrique.

13 BS/EN 60529 (1988)	Specification for Classification of Degrees of Protection Provided by Enclosures (replaced BS 5490).
14 BS 4999	General Requirements for Rotating Electrical Machines. Part 105 (1988). Classification of Types of Enclosure.
15 BS 5901 (1980)	Method of Test for Determining the Comparative and Proof Tracking Indices of Solid Insulating Materials under Moist Conditions.
16 BS 5917 (1988) (withdrawn)	Specification for Conformal Coating Material for Use on Printed Circuit Assemblies. This Standard has been replaced by the following: BS/EN 61086–1 (1995); BS/EN 61086–2 (1995); BS/EN 60086–3 (1995).
17 IEC 34	Rotating Electrical Machines. Part 5 (1991). Classification of degrees of protection provided by the enclosures of rotating machines.
18 BS 5042 (1987)	Specification for Lampholders and Starter Holders.
19 BS 6776 (1990) (withdrawn)	Specification for Edison Screw Lampholders: this Standard has been replaced by BS/EN 60238 (1992).
20 BS 6702 (1991) (withdrawn)	Specification for Lampholders for Tubular Fluorescent Lamps and Starter Holders: this Standard has been replaced by BS/EN 60400 (1992).
21 BS 3772 (1980)	Specific for Starters for Fluorescent Lamps.
22 BS 2818 (withdrawn)	Ballasts for Tubular Fluorescent Lamps. This standard has been replaced by the following: BS/EN 60920 (1991); BS/EN 60921 (1991).
23 BS 4782 (1971) (withdrawn)	Specification for Ballasts for Discharge Lamps (Excluding Ballasts for Tubular Fluorescent Lamps). This standard has been replaced by the following: BS/EN 60922 (1991); BS/EN 60923 (1991).
24 IEC 61 (1969)	Lamp Caps and Holders Together with Gauges for Control of Interchangeability and Safety.

25 IEC 238 (1982)	Edison Screw Lampholders
26 IEC 400 (1982)	Lampholders for Tubular Fluorescent Lamps and Starter Holders.
27 IEC 262 (1969)	Ballasts for High Pressure Mercury Vapour Lamps.
28 IEC 598–1	Luminaires. Part 1 (1979). General Requirements and Tests.

— 15 —

Protection concepts for apparatus for dust risks
(BS 6467, Part 1 (1985))
(BS 7535 (1992))

The approach to protection of apparatus for use in the presence of combustible dusts has always been quite different to that for gases and vapours. The fact that dust clouds are clearly visible, producing a high degree of opacity, has created a situation where processing of dusts needs a high degree of control of dust clouds so that work can take place. In addition, the prevention of entry of particulate matter such as dust into the interior of electrical apparatus is relatively easy by the specification of its enclosure, unlike the situation in gases and vapours where this is difficult to achieve and maintain.

Conversely, dust settles unlike gases and vapours and a release leading to a dust cloud will leave a dust layer around the point of release rather than dispersing. This requires a high standard of housekeeping and the consideration of the effects of layers of dust (nominally assumed to be 5 mm of maximum thickness) on surface temperatures of enclosures. This has coloured the approach to use of electrical apparatus in dust risks and led to a situation where the construction of apparatus is based upon the ability to exclude dust, and a less rigorous form of certification control has been applied. The effects of dust layers raising the temperature of enclosures is dealt with in the selection of apparatus and not the construction.

15.1 Situation in respect of standardization

Although the installation of apparatus in dust risk areas has been practiced for very many years, the apparatus was generally selected from industrial ranges of apparatus on the basis of its ability to exclude dust and no formal Standards or Certification/Approval procedures have been present. This changed in 1985 with the publication of BS 6467, Part 1[1] which, for the first time, specified in considerable detail the constructional requirements for apparatus for this type of explosive atmosphere.

BS 6467, Part 1 (1985)[1] specified two types of apparatus: dust tight apparatus; and dust protected apparatus. This reflected the approach at the time which divided hazardous areas where dust was present into two areas, Zone Z and Zone Y, the former being similar in definition to Zone 1 in the case of gases and vapours, and the latter to Zone 2, an approach later confirmed in BS 6467, Part 2[1] in 1988. This approach excluded any consideration of areas such as the interior of dust vessels, which would be Zone 0 in the gas or vapour case, and such Zones have been considered as those in which electrical equipment should not be mounted or only be mounted in exceptional conditions and, in those cases, treated specially. This has not produced too much of a hardship as installations in such Zones where dust is a problem have tended to be rare and often have been such things as thermocouples, resistance thermometers and similar devices, which need only to insert a sealed stainless steel or similar tube into the area. It is upon this basis that the requirements in BS 6467, Part 1 (1985) for 'Apparatus with Protection by Enclosure for Use in the Presence of Combustible Dust' were framed. (The use of the term 'Combustible Dust' is used rather than 'flammable dust' to emphasize that dusts behave differently to gases and vapours).

BS 6467, Part 1[1] effectively considers apparatus protected against the ingress of dust, where dust can enter but not in sufficient quantities to interfere with the operation of apparatus, and dust tight apparatus, where dust is effectively excluded. The reason for the two different levels is to relate to Zone Z where dust tight apparatus is necessary, and Zone Y where only dust protected apparatus is necessary except where the dust is conducting (when no differentiation is made because of the added risk of internal short circuiting by the dust).

In addition to BS 6467, Part 1[1], a further Standard, BS 7535 (1992)[2] exists which gives guidance upon the selection of apparatus to the BS/EN 500 range of Standards (Electrical Apparatus for Potentially Explosive Atmospheres of gas/air, vapour/air or mist/air, see Chapters 7 to 14) for use in the presence of combustible dusts. This Standard actually refers to the European Standards in their first editions (BS 5501 series) due to its age but its criteria are equally relevant to the second editions (BS/EN 500 range). Again, because of its age, it still refers to Zone Z and Y.

As earlier explained in Chapter 6, the situation in regard to area classification for dusts is set to change in a very short time to a three-Zone system similar to that for gases. This is based upon an IEC draft document (IEC 1241–3), which has received approval as a possible new British Standard and identifies the following zones.

Zone 20

Zone 20 is defined as being where dust clouds are normally present, such as the inside of vessels, and is similar in definition to Zone 0 for gases and vapours.

Zone 21

Zone 21 is defined as being where dust clouds are regularly produced, such as loading apertures, and is similar in definition to Zone 1 for gases and vapours.

Zone 22

Zone 22 is defined as being where dust clouds are rare, usually being produced by disturbance of dust layers which have formed despite the high level of housekeeping required in such areas, and is similar in definition to Zone 2 for gases and vapours.

The specific construction requirements for apparatus for dust risks in respect of these Zones do not yet exist, the production of the relevant Standards not yet being complete. There is, however, some guidance in this matter. First Zone 21 can be related to Zone Z and thus apparatus for Zone Z, as previously described, may also be considered as appropriate to Zone 21 and apparatus for Zone Y for Zone 22. This leaves Zone 20 where no national or international approach has historically existed. The problem is not, however, new and in 1973 a particular company Code (RoSPA/ICI[3]), recognizing the ultimate likelihood of a requirement for sophisticated instrumentation in what will be Zone 20, used a three-Zone classification system for dusts. This led to some guidance for intrinsically safe apparatus in Zone 20 appearing in both that code and other documents based upon the use of intrinsically safe apparatus 'ia' contained within an IP6X enclosure to BS/EN 60529[4] (like the situation in gas and vapour risks intrinsically safe apparatus is the only type of equipment likely to be acceptable in such high risk zones because of the constant or nearly constant presence of the explosive atmosphere).

15.2 Basic types of apparatus for use with combustible dusts (apparatus in accordance with BS 6467, Part 1)

The method by which this apparatus is made suitable for use in explosive atmospheres of dust and air is to exclude the dust from within the enclosure. This type of apparatus is, tested to ensure that it does so.

The possibility of decrease in pressure in all enclosures due to temperature changes, either ambient or operational, needs to be recognized and thus all dust-tight enclosures are tested on the basis of reduced internal pressure as defined in the appropriate Standard.

While testing for dust entry is all that is required to satisfy the basic requirements for this type of apparatus, it must be recognized that testing for liquid ingress is also necessary for all outdoor apparatus.

15.2.1 Degrees of enclosure

There are two types of apparatus which are differentiated by their degree of enclosure. These are as follows.

Apparatus with dust tight enclosures

This constitutes apparatus with an enclosure which is so constructed as to exclude all ingress of observable dust particles. This means that the apparatus is dust tight as no visible dust will have entered during the tests for enclosure suitability which includes the enclosure being operated in the dust-test atmosphere at reduced pressure to give dust every opportunity to enter. Such enclosures must be tested for Degree of Protection IP6X in accordance with BS/EN 60529[4] (for older enclosures produced prior to the introduction of BS/EN 60529 the Standard used was BS 5490[5] and for swichgear, which is now included in BS/EN 60529 and therefore does not have a specific unique Standard, BS 5420[6] was historically appropriate). It is notable that even rotating machines must comply with this requirement rather than the requirements of EN 60034, Part 5[7] (produced in the UK as BS 4999, Part 105[8]) which allow variations specifically relating to enclosures of rotating machines and are in normal circumstances considered as sufficient in other areas. For apparatus for outdoor use is a total enclosure integrity package of IP65 is required and this enclosure is considered as necessary for all apparatus used in Zone Z and, in conducting dust situations, apparatus for Zone Y.

Dust-protected enclosures

This is a lower level of enclosure integrity and what is required here is that the enclosure is at least IP5X to BS/EN 60529[4] or the more historic equivalent Standards already quoted. In addition, because of the different intended use such apparatus is restricted to Zone Y and only then acceptable for non-conducting dusts). In addition, enclosures offering IP5X to EN 60034, Part 5[7] (BS 4999, Part 105[8]) are acceptable in these circumstances even though they offer a slightly lower level of protection due to the requirement of normal rotating machines. In this case, however, there is a specification additional to those in the IP Standards quoted above in that the amount of dust entering the enclosure during the test must not exceed the equivalent of 10 gm/m^3 as derived from the mass of dust entering divided by the free volume (after deducting the volume of components and assemblies within the enclosure from the total internal enclosure volume) of the enclosure. This is an approach to defining the criteria for passing the test and reduce the reliance on the opinion of the expert executing the test, and again it must be remembered that the dust level quoted only refers to non-conducting dust. This means an IP54 enclosure for use outdoors.

15.3 Operational requirements

The apparatus may or may not spark within the enclosure as the enclosure constitutes the protection. Thus there is no requirement for energy limitation in a spark or arc but only of limitation of the maximum external surface temperature of the enclosure. The enclosure temperature needs to be determined in the following conditions: first, with the enclosure mounted in the most unfavourable normal mounting position (that which gives the maximum temperature on any part of the surface of the enclosure); second, the supply voltage must be adjusted to any value within its operating tolerance to give the maximum temperature in the above position (where no supply voltage tolerance is quoted it is normal to utilize ±10 per cent).

In the above circumstances the maximum surface temperature of the apparatus must be 10 °C lower than the maximum permitted temperature for any dust cloud or layer in which the apparatus is intended to be used. These permitted temperatures are as follows.

First, the maximum surface temperature of the apparatus enclosure must be not more than two thirds less 10 °C of the ignition temperature of the dust cloud in which the apparatus may operate. (This means, for example, that for a dust with a cloud ignition temperature of 280 °C (sulphur) the maximum surface temperature of the enclosure may not exceed 176 °C {[280 × 2/3] – 10} at the maximum ambient temperature (a surface temperature elevation of 136 °C at an ambient of 40 °C)).

Second, the maximum surface temperature of the apparatus enclosure may not exceed a temperature 85 °C lower than the minimum ignition temperature of a 5 mm dust layer. (This means that for lignite, which has an layer ignition temperature of 225 °C, the maximum enclosure surface temperature permitted will be 140 °C (225 – 75 – 10) or an elevation of 100 °C at an ambient of 40 °C).

The 10 °C margin is normally included in the maximum operating surface temperature specified for apparatus to BS 6467, Part 1[1] and thus it is only necessary to multiply the dust cloud temperature by two thirds and subtract 75 °C from its layer ignition temperature in order to identify the suitability of the apparatus. Where apparatus complying with these requirements is also used in gas and vapour risks and is thus temperature classified, the

Table 15.1 Equivalent minimum dust ignition temperature for gas/vapour temperature classifications

Temperature classification	Minimum acceptable dust ignition temperature			
	Protection concepts 'd' 'e' 'i' 'm' 'o' 'p' and 'q'		Type of protection 'N'('n')	
	Cloud	Layer	Cloud	Layer
T1 (450 °C)	675 °C[1]	525 °C	685 °C[1]	535 °C
T2 (300 °C)	450 °C[1]	375 °C	465 °C[1]	385 °C
T3 (200 °C)	308 °C[1]	280 °C	315 °C[1]	285 °C
T4 (125 °C)	195 °C	205 °C[1]	203 °C	210 °C[1]
T5 (100 °C)	158 °C	180 °C[1]	165 °C	185 °C[1]
T6 (85 °C)	135 °C	165 °C[1]	143 °C	170 °C[1]

Notes: [1]As a dust cloud cannot practically exist without dust layers forming, and dust layers are a result of dust clouds, this figure is predominant in the apparatus selection procedure and should always be used.

10 °C margin is not necessarily taken into account during temperature classification. For all types of protection appropriate to gas or vapour risks with the exception of type of protection 'N' a factor of only 5 °C is used for temperature classes T3–T6 with the 10 °C only being applied to T1 and T2. (For type of protection 'N' no factor at all is used.) Where apparatus which is temperature classified to BS/EN 50014[9] is used in dust situations without change because, in other than surface temperature considerations, it can be shown to satisfy BS 6467, part 1,[1] the permissible usage of the apparatus is shown in Table 15.1.

15.4 Basic constructional requirements

As may be expected, the requirements for the construction of this type of apparatus revolve principally around the needs of the enclosure integrity which have already been dealt with in Section 15.2. There are, however, requirements for physical strength and electrical connection but these are very general and not dissimilar to those applied to apparatus for gas and vapour risks.

15.4.1 Enclosure materials and mechanical strength

Enclosure materials

The basic enclosure material requirement is that it will withstand the environmental and other operating conditions which it may be called upon to deal with in operation. These are mainly a matter of ensuring that the manufacturer's material specification matches chosen use and thus selection criteria. There is, however, a specific requirement to ensure that all enclosure materials are not operated outside their manufacturer's ratings when subjected to a temperature 10 °C higher than the maximum temperature which they will achieve at maximum ambient and in the most onerous service conditions for which they are designed. This is clearly identifiable at the construction stage and is necessary to ensure that enclosure strength and IP-rating can be maintained. This requirement is, of course, no more onerous than those applied to apparatus for gas and vapour risks.

As with enclosures for apparatus for gas and vapour risks, there is a restriction on the magnesium content of any of the externally exposed light metal enclosures or parts thereof to minimize the risk of thermite sparking if the enclosure is struck by an oxidized (rusty) steel item.

A final requirement is that materials must not be combustible or propagate flame if ignited. This is not principally an enclosure requirement as if the enclosure is ignited from outside the source of dust ignition already exists. It is, however, important for both enclosures and all other parts inside the enclosure, as ignition may occur due to electrical fault before the electrical protection operates, and it must be remembered that there is no internal constructional requirement other than normal industrial requirements to prevent such ignition. If it did occur there is a real danger that the elevated temperature may damage the enclosure integrity leading to ignition of any surrounding dust cloud or layer and thus the requirement assumes a greater importance in this context. Methods of demonstrating non-combustibility and prevention of flame transmission are not specifically defined in relation to this particular risk and typical industrial methods of demonstration are acceptable (e.g., BS 2782, BS 6458 and BS 6334 are typical Standards which may be used for this purpose but they are not exclusive and other recognized methods may be used).

Mechanical strength

The mechanical strength of the enclosure is required to be such that it will not be damaged other than superficially by impact and drop tests. These tests are identical to those used for apparatus for gas and vapour risks (see Chapter 8) except that, because the enclosure is all important, the lower level of impact test for enclosures intended for installation only in areas where the risk of mechanical impact is low is not acceptable, the higher figure always being required.

15.4.2 Joints intended to be opened in normal service

Non-gasketted joints

Metal/metal and similar joints in enclosures which do not use compressible gaskets may be used provided that the enclosure may be shown to achieve the desired IP-rating. Such joints have minimum requirements applied to them to ensure that they are repeatable and these are that the joint be close fitting and have a minimum width over which this is achieved, defined as the dust ingress path. No figure is given for close fitting but it is recommended that a maximum separation limit of 0.5 mm be applied with the proviso that the enclosure has to satisfy the necessary IP-rating. This would allow the use of all flameproof enclosures which satisfied the necessary IP test. A minimum joint flatness requirement of at least 6.3 μm be applied for the same reason. Typical joints are shown in Fig. 15.1.

The minimum dust ingress paths (widths) for such joints need to be as follows:

Flat flanged joints	–	5 mm
Spigot joints	–	3 mm
Cylindrical joints	–	3 mm
Conical joints	–	3 mm
Threaded joints	–	5 mm

These joints may not use additional measures such as non-setting sealing compounds to assist in the achievement of the necessary IP-rating but must

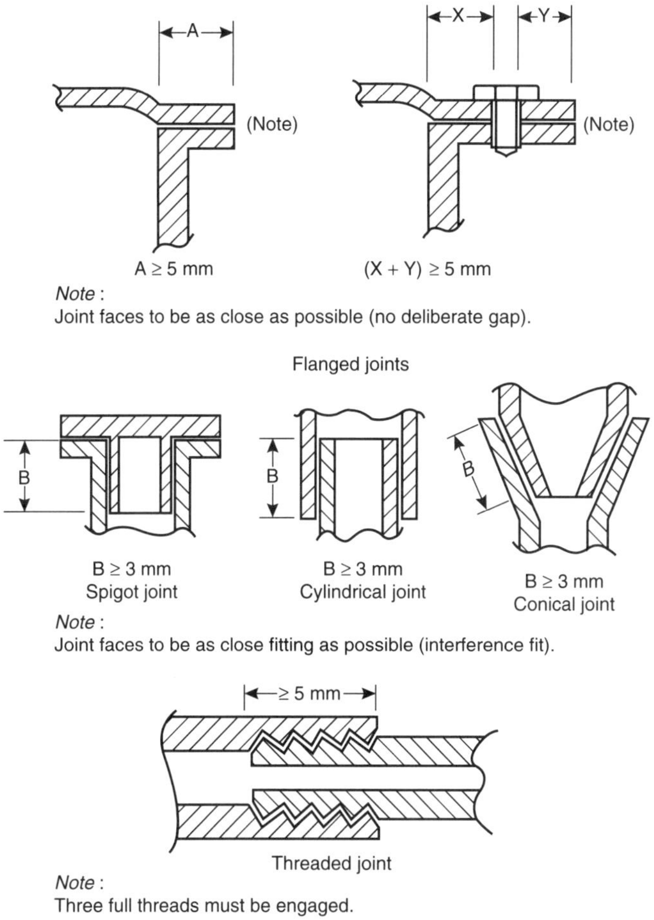

Fig. 15.1 Minimum dimensions for ungasketted joints

achieve the necessary IP-rating 'dry' on the basis of the fit of the two parts of the joint alone.

Threaded joints, in addition to satisfying the length requirements, must have at least three threads fully engaged, whether parallel or taper threads.

It is necessary to identify these joints if they are intended to be opened in normal service in view of their importance to the protection offered by the apparatus. Additionally and particularly it is necessary to identify the fact that no compound is used in their completion. The purchaser of the apparatus must be aware of these matters if the apparatus is to be used safely.

Joints having gaskets and other types of sealing device

Plane joints may use flat gaskets to prevent the ingress of dust into enclosures as shown in Fig. 15.2, provided that the gasket width is at least

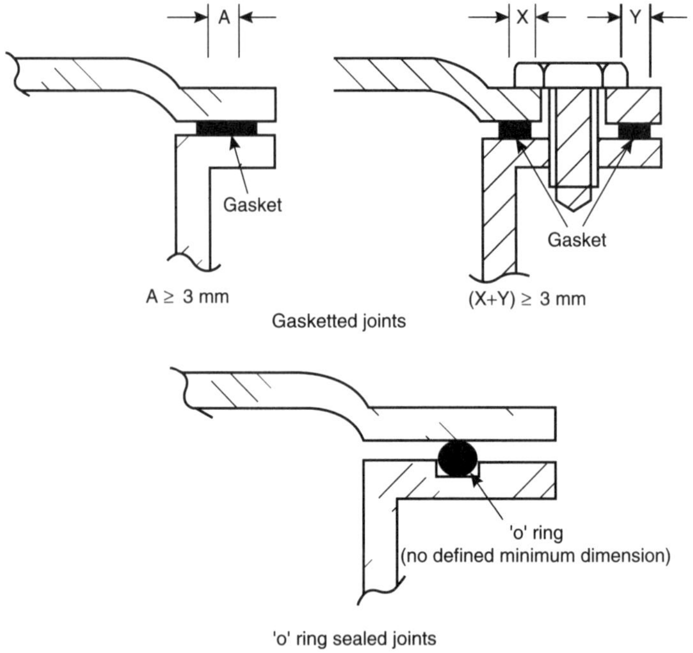

Fig. 15.2 Use of gaskets and 'o' rings. *Note*: Gaskets must be secured to one face of joint and 'o' rings in slots (by adhesive or other means which does not adversely affect sealing of joint)

3 mm. These joints include plain flanged joints and spigot joints where the gasket is in the plane part and thus the spigot ceases to be important. In this case the gaskets must be effectively continuous in that any joints within them need to be bonded together and not just rely on pressure. The gaskets should be fixed to one of the joint parts, possibly with adhesive, to prevent their displacement but their material of construction should be such that they do not stick inadvertently to mating faces. They must also be fabricated of a material which is not damaged by the extremities of their service conditions either by ageing or operation outside their material specification.

Other types of sealing unit, such as 'o' rings, may also be used and in this case securing of the ring to one side of the joint will not be necessary as such rings need to be fitted in recesses which effectively perform the necessary action. Lip seals are also possible where the seal is by a shaped ring at the edge of the joint. Again, these seals are profiled and positively located by their form.

15.4.3 Semi-permanent joints

Joints which form part of an apparatus which is not addressed in normal service and which are seldom opened, need in principal to comply with the foregoing requirements. A relaxation is, however, permitted in the case of flanged joints and threaded joints, whereby the dust path through the joint is reduced to 3 mm provided the joint surfaces are coated with a non-setting sealing compound of adequate specification before assembly. Such non-setting compounds may, unlike the situation in the case of regularly opened joints, be used to assist exclusion of dust in all cases where the joint is seldom opened in service and is flanged, cylindrical conical or a spigot joint and is static.

The basic requirements for such non-setting compounds is that they be chemically and thermally stable, and inert between a temperature 5 °C below the minimum ambient temperature specified for the apparatus and 20 °C above the maximum temperature which they can reach, with the apparatus operated at the maximum ambient temperature in the most adverse supply and mounting conditions. They also need to be impervious to deterioration as a result of the environment (e.g., moisture) or be protected from contact with it.

15.4.4 Spindles and shafts

Spindles and shafts which move or rotate should be sealed against the unacceptable entry of dust by suitable bushings, the fitting of a dust exclusion seal, a labyrinth joint or a combination of these types of device. Simple cylindrical joints are not considered as suitable for this use. In addition, the dust exclusion properties of the joints must be maintained when any grease or oil applied to the joint for operational reasons is absent and the joint relies only on its solid parts for its performance.

No minimum lengths of dust path are specified for such joints and their dimensions are solely affected by their ability to achieve the necessary IP-rating.

15.4.5 Light-transmitting parts

Light-transmitting parts need to be fixed to the enclosure by one of the joint techniques already mentioned or be fixed by cementing or similar methods. Any transparent or translucent material may be used provided it complies with the materials requirements already stated, and securing to the enclosure by cement alone is acceptable provided that the cement adheres to both the light-transmitting part and the enclosure. The assembly including the light-transmitting part needs to achieve the necessary IP-rating and must not be damaged by the impact tests already described. The cements used for cemented light-transmitting part assemblies needs to satisfy the same requirements as those for non-setting sealing compounds already specified (except of course that the cement is required to set). If the light-transmitting part is glass then a thermal shock test of spraying a 1 mm jet of water at 10–15 °C onto the glass when it is at its maximum operating temperature is required.

15.4.6 Fasteners

The fasteners used to secure parts of the enclosure play an important roll in the protection concept. Unless there is a specific additional device to prevent the ingress of dust via their mounting or fixing holes, these should not enter the enclosure and the thickness of metal or other enclosure material between their sides and bottom and the inside of the enclosure needs to be not less than one third of the hole diameter to ensure the enclosure is strong enough to prevent cracking in service.

Hinged lids are acceptable provided that the hinge does not apply the pressure necessary for sealing. A flexible hinge which allows lid movement during tightening of fixings is therefore necessary in such cases. Also, because such movement may allow the displacement of the lid during tightening, locating pins may be necessary.

15.5 Specific additional requirements for particular types of electrical apparatus and connections

As is the case with other protection concepts there are specific requirements concerning connections, cable entry and for specific types of apparatus. These are generally similar to those required for types of apparatus used in gas and vapour risks and may generally be described as those applied to industrial apparatus but with a few additional specifications.

15.5.1 Connection facilities

The requirements for connections to apparatus are very similar to those required for apparatus for gas and vapour risks. This requires the provision of connection facilities (except for apparatus manufactured with a permanently connected cable) which are: accessible and allow effective clamping of incoming cable, connection of conductors without relying on any plastic part in the case of terminals and other connectors which rely on pressure to hold the conductor; have sufficient separation so as to minimize the risk of inadvertent short circuits to the normal industrial degree; and have enclosures which ensure the required IP-rating after fitting and connection of the conductors.

Earth connections are required within the terminal enclosure close to the other circuit connections and, where the enclosure or any accessible part of it is conducting, outside the enclosure also. The internal and external earth connection facilities need to be able to accommodate a conductor of at least the size required by Table 15.2, with a minimum size for the external conductor of 4 mm which is not dissimilar to the specific requirement for apparatus for gas and vapour risks. No external earth connection facility is necessary for an enclosure which is wholly insulating as the objective of this is to bond the enclosure locally to remove any risk of it being at a different

Table 15.2 Required protective conductor cross-sectional area relative to phase conductors

Phase conductor cross-sectional area (mm^2)	Minimum cross-section required for protective conductor (mm^2)
≤ 16	As the phase conductor
>16 but ≤ 35	16
>35	Half of the phase conductor area

potential to the local metalwork. The internal earth connection facility may also be omitted where it has no purpose (e.g., in double insulated apparatus) or where it is specifically not permitted for a particular type of apparatus.

15.5.2 Cable and conduit entries

Where cables or conduits enter the enclosure, the method of entry must be such as to ensure that the enclosure integrity is maintained. This may involve the fitting of washers at the entry point and sealing of the interstices of the cable, particularly where tape bedded cable is used.

Conduits will almost certainly require to have a stopper box fitted close to the point of entry as otherwise the conduit will need to be considered as part of the enclosure.

Cable glands need to clamp the cable sheath or armour to secure the cable and prevent stress on the electrical connections. The requirements here are identical to those for cable entries for apparatus for gas and vapour risks (see Chapter 8), requiring a test on the clamped cable constituting application of a specific tensile stress of specific values for specific times to the clamped cable without any significant movement of the cable. Details for these tests are given in BS/EN 50014[9].

15.5.3 Fuses and switchgear

Enclosures of fuses and remotely operated switchgear, including apparatus with switching contacts, should be interlocked to prevent the enclosure being opened while the apparatus is energized and, in both cases, the interlock needs to be on-load rated. If interlocking is not provided, the enclosure needs to be fitted with a label warning against opening in a hazardous area while the fuses or switchgear enclosed are energized. The term 'remotely operated' is used in relation to switchgear as locally operated switchgear is always assumed to have mechanical interlocking to prevent enclosure opening unless the switchgear is in the isolated position. In the unlikely event that this is not so, then the interlocking or warning requirements apply to locally operated switchgear also.

Disconnectors (isolators) are a particular problem as they are 'off load' devices and are not intended to be operated on-load. These therefore require that an interlock preventing their on-load operation is fitted, or a specific warning against such action is provided.

The interlocking devices used in any circumstance must be such that they cannot be readily defeated by use of such tools as screwdrivers or pliers which are generally carried by personnel. The objective of this is to minimize the risk of mistakes and is a similar requirement to that used in the case of interlocks for apparatus for gas and vapour risks.

15.5.4 Plugs and sockets

As with apparatus for gas and vapour risks, plugs and sockets need to be interlocked to prevent energized separation or, if not interlocked, to be identified by warning as items which must not be so separated. The fixed part of the plug and socket (that forming part of the apparatus) is also required to maintain the IP-rating of the enclosure when the moving part is not present. Again, the interlocking devices, if fitted, must be on-load operable and not defeatable by normally carried tools.

15.5.5 Luminaires and similar apparatus

Apparatus, such as luminaires, where enclosures are more readily opened than is the case for other apparatus, because of the needs of relamping, etc., should also carry a label warning against opening while energized unless they are similarly interlocked. This is necessary as it is normal in standard industrial circumstances to carry out such practices as relamping live and this must not be the case in hazardous areas.

15.6 Apparatus conforming to the protection concepts appropriate to gas, vapour and mist risks

There are large quantities of apparatus designed and often certified/approved for operation in explosive atmospheres of gas, vapour or mist, and air. These are subject to detailed construction requirements which are not dissimilar or inferior to those required for apparatus for use in explosive atmospheres of dust and air. Third-party certification of construction of apparatus for gas/vapour/mist air risks is provided which gives a high degree of confidence in its construction. In addition many hazardous areas are created by both dust/air and gas/vapour/mist/air risks requiring apparatus to be suitable for operational situations as, even though apparatus may be incapable of igniting a dust/air mixture, it may ignite a gas/air mixture which itself may form the source of ignition of the dust/air mixture. For the above reasons (and also economy of design and construction) it is advantageous to utilize one type of apparatus for both risks whether they occur together or separately. For this reason consideration has been given to the suitability of apparatus constructed to the BS/EN 500 range of Standards in relation to BS 6941[10] for use in dust risks with the following results.

15.6.1 Spark ignition

Apparatus used in explosive atmospheres of gas, vapour or mist, and air and in which sparking in either normal or recognized fault conditions occurs, is required to provide protection for sparking by the use of such techniques as intrinsic safety (Chapter 13), flameproof enclosure (Chapter 10) or use of non-incendive techniques (Chapter 14). This is because it is not normally possible to exclude mixtures of gas/vapour/mist and air from enclosures. In the case of dust/air mixtures it is, however, possible to do this and so, provided the enclosure of apparatus is adequate, sparking becomes less of a problem for dusts in general.

15.6.2 Hot surface ignition

Surface temperature classification as carried out for gas/vapour/mist and air risks is not immediately appropriate to dust situations, as it often includes temperatures within the apparatus which are accessible to the gas/vapour/mist and air mixture but not to dusts where the enclosure criteria for dust exclusion are applied. In addition, the factors used in surface temperature classification are different to those applied for the dust risks already explained in this chapter.

The simplest method of selection of gas or vapour risk apparatus for use in dust risks on the basis of Surface Temperature Classification is to use Table 15.1, but it must be recognized that this will often give a very onerous solution because of its consideration of internal temperatures. Alternatively, the apparatus could be tested for maximum external surface temperature and the figure resulting used for selection purposes. In this latter case, however, the 10 °C safety factor explained earlier in this chapter should be used.

15.6.3 Basis of selection of apparatus with protection concepts appropriate to gas/vapour/mist and air risks

As already shown, the basic requirements for apparatus for use in dust risks are almost the same in many cases to those required for apparatus for gas and vapour risks. This means that, with little or no modification, such apparatus may be shown to be suitable for dust risks subject to temperature classification selection as already described.

Oil-immersed apparatus 'o' (Chapter 9)

This type of apparatus will be suitable in the following circumstances.

First, its enclosure must be IP5X or IP6X, depending on the intended Zone of use (IP5X for Zone Y or Zone 22, and IP 6X for Zone Z or Zone 21). While the variation of enclosure integrity for conducting dusts is not appropriate here, there is a risk that some dusts may degrade the oil and in such cases IP6X is always required.

Second, in the case of this protection concept, the surface temperature classification is for the surface of the oil, which is practically equivalent to the enclosure temperature and no advantage can be gained by added surface temperature testing. The maximum surface temperature reached should therefore be the maximum permitted for the surface temperature class given.

Pressurized apparatus 'p' (Chapter 11)

This type of apparatus will be acceptable in the following circumstances.

First, the general requirement for the enclosure is that it satisfies IP6X (for Zone Z or 21) or IP5X (for Zone Y or 22) in circumstances where the pressure is not present. In this case the conducting dust requirement of IP6X in all cases is relevant as consideration is given in the absence of pressurization. Additionally it is necessary to consider the effects of outlets for exhaust of gas in the hazardous area. These need to be considered in the IP-rating, unlike the gas inlets which do not as they will not be exposed to the dust atmosphere.

Second, surface temperature classification will have been carried out on the outer surface of the enclosure and there is no advantage in attempting a determination of external surface temperature. Thus the surface temperature will be assumed to be the maximum permitted for the surface temperature class awarded.

Powder-filled apparatus 'q' (Chapter 9)

This type of apparatus is acceptable in the following circumstances.

First, this type of apparatus should be selected on the basis of the IP-selection criteria (IP6X for Zone Z and 21 and IP5X for Zone Y and 22). Once again, however, it is necessary to have IP6X in all cases where the dust is conducting as, if it enters the enclosure and mixes with the powder, it could adversely affect the operation of the apparatus. There is little likelihood of the dust reacting with the powder as the latter is normally quartz or glass.

Second, surface temperature classification will have been carried out on the surface of the powder, which is effectively the enclosure temperature, and thus no advantage will accrue by measuring enclosure temperature. The surface temperature will, be the maximum temperature permitted by the surface temperature classification awarded.

Flameproof enclosure 'd' (Chapter 10)

This type of apparatus is acceptable in the following circumstances.

First, the choice of flameproof apparatus for use in dust risks is on the basis of enclosure integrity. IP6X is required for Zone Z and 21 and IP5X for Zone Y and 22. For conducting dusts IP6X is always required as entry of dust into the enclosure could give rise to an internal dust explosion, and the performance of the enclosure in such circumstances is not known.

Second, temperature classification of flameproof enclosures is carried out on the enclosure outer surface and no advantage will result from measuring enclosure temperature. The surface temperature is assumed to be the maximum permitted by the surface temperature classification awarded.

Increased safety apparatus 'e' (Chapter 12)

This type of apparatus is acceptable in the following circumstances.

First, increased safety is a technique which relies in part on enclosure integrity and requires an IP54 enclosure, making it normally usable in Zone Y and 22. Increasing its enclosure integrity to a minimum of IP64 will make it suitable for Zone Z an 21. One point to be stressed is that increased safety relies to a significant extent on the protection equipment in its supply, particularly in the case of rotating machines. This is no less true in the case of dust risks and t_e time particularly must be adhered to.

One significant point is that temperature classification is based upon the hottest part of the apparatus, be it within or outside the enclosure. If its temperature classification is found to be too restrictive using Table 15.1 then temperature measurement of the outside of the enclosure may produce significant gains. This is even true of rotating machines when the machine is rotor sensitive (i.e., the rotor temperature decides the surface temperature classification).

Intrinsic safety 'i' (Chapter 13)

Apparatus of this type will be acceptable in the following circumstances but as intrinsic safety does not rely on its enclosure for security then a more flexible approach is possible.

If the intrinsically safe apparatus has an enclosure of IP6X it will be suitable for use in Zone Z or 21 and if it has an enclosure of IP5X for Zone Y or 22 without further consideration. As before, taking this approach the enclosure will need to be IP6X even for Zones Y or 22 if the dust is conducting.

The above approach takes no account of the added security of intrinsic safety in that faults are required before an installation can become ignition capable. This is true whether the installation is 'ia' or 'ib'. In this case, however, there is much to be gained by considering the internal circuits. If the enclosure is not of sufficient integrity then the dust can enter. When, for instance the dust is non-conducting then it will only have the effect of providing a layer over the components in the enclosure. This is unlikely to significantly alter the temperature classification of the apparatus and as, 'without fault', 'with one fault' in the case of 'ib' and with two faults in the case of 'ia', any internal sparking is non-incendive the apparatus should be suitable for Zone Z.

If the dust is conducting then any conducting parts within the apparatus may be assumed to be interconnected unless they are either coated (varnished), encapsulated or insulated. In these circumstances the apparatus should be assessed on this basis and if sparking and hot surfaces can still be shown not to be incendive in conditions of two faults for 'ia' with these additional internal connections, then the equipment remains suitable for Zone Z or 21. Likewise, if the same evaluation is done for 'ib' apparatus it will be suitable for Zone 22 or Zone Y. In conditions of humidity or other situations in which the dust can be assumed to be moist then it should be treated as conducting dust, even if when dry it is non-conducting.

Extending this approach, an item of 'ia' apparatus which satisfies the above requirements for either non-conducting or conducting (or moist) dusts, and which is also enclosed in an IP6X enclosure, has a much higher level of protection than any other of the foregoing equipment. This apparatus should be safely usable in the new Zone 20 for the relevant type of dust for which no other protected equipment is currently available.

Encapsulation 'm' (Chapter 9)

Encapsulated apparatus, by definition, excludes dust to at least IP6X and such apparatus is suitable for Zone Z and 21 (and thus Zone Y and 22) without further consideration. The surface temperature class is based upon the external temperature of the encapsulant and the maximum temperature should normally be taken as the maximum permitted by the surface temperature classification.

It should, however, be noted that the connection facilities for such apparatus will normally utilize alternative protection concepts and their requirements should also be considered.

Apparatus with type of protection 'N' (n) (Chapter 14)

This type of apparatus is normally only acceptable in Zone Y or 22 and only then if it has an enclosure integrity of IP5X for non-conducting dusts and IP6X for conducting dusts. As its surface temperature may be produced on the basis of internal components, measurement of the enclosure temperature may be helpful when the maximum temperature permitted by the surface temperature classification is not acceptable.

References

1 BS 6467 — Electrical Apparatus with Protection by Enclosure for Use in the Presence of Combustible Dust. Part 1, (1985). Specification for Apparatus. Part 2 (1988). Guide to Selection, Installation and Maintenance.

2 BS 7535 (1992) — Guide to the Selection of Apparatus Complying with BS 5501 or BS 6941 in the Presence of Combustible Dust.

3 RoSPA/ICI — Engineering Codes and Regulations, Electrical Equipment in Flammable Atmospheres (1973). Group C (Electrical), Volume 1.5.

4 BS/EN 60529 (1991) — Specification for Degrees of Protection Provided by Enclosure.

5 BS 5490 (1977) (withdrawn) — Specification for Degrees of Protection Provided by Enclosure. This Standard has been replaced by BS/EN 60529 (1992).

6 BS 5420 (1977) (withdrawn) — Specification for Degrees of Enclosure of Switchgear and Control Gear for Voltages up to and including 1000 V ac and 1200 V dc. This Standard has been replaced by BS/EN 60947–1 (1992).

7 EN 60034 — General Requirements for Rotating Electrical Machines. Part 5 (1986). Classification of Degrees of Protection Provided by Enclosures for Rotating Machinery.

8 BS 4999 — General Requirements for Rotating Electrical machines. Part 105 (1988). Classification of Degrees of Protection Provided by Enclosures for Rotating Machinery.

9 BS/EN 50014 (1993) — Electrical Apparatus for Potentially Explosive Atmospheres. General Requirements.

10 BS 6941 (1988) — Electrical Apparatus for Explosive Atmospheres with Type of Protection N.

— 16 —

Other methods of protection and future apparatus requirements

To fully understand the future approach to apparatus for use in explosive atmospheres it is necessary to consider the problems with the present system which is based upon Directive 76/117/EEC[1] and its supplementary Directives. These define the detailed constructional standards with which apparatus must comply to be suitable for formal conformity certification by a 'notified body', as described in earlier chapters. This method of definition effectively restricted the types of equipment which could be used in Zone 0 and 1 as, although the Directive only addressed conformity certification as a method of European market admission, it effectively defined what could be used in those Zones because user industry was unwilling, in the main, to utilize any other type of equipment. This did not apply to Zone 2 as the approach was much more relaxed due to the much lesser risk envisaged.

In the case of Zone 0 and 1, however, the approach led to considerable restriction and inability to deal with technological advance and special circumstances. Accordingly, within a national arena, the UK exploited the protection concept known as special protection 's'. The objective of this concept was to provide a vehicle which would allow formal approval of apparatus which, while not complying (or not complying fully) with any of the standardized protection concepts ('d', 'e', 'i', 'm', 'o', 'p', 'q') achieved the minimum required level of security in respect of ignition capability. The objective of this was not to certify 'near misses' but to allow for advances in technology. The proof of the value of this approach is clear when it is recognized that it has been used for such protection concepts as encapsulation 'm' and devices without measurable flamepaths, such as sinters, before these were included in the relevant protection concept Standard and specifically recognized by the Directive. More recently, the approach has been used to permit bi-pin tubes used in the cold cathode mode in luminaires on the basis of multiple (at least four) connections allowing redundancy, an approach not recognized in increased safety 'e', and to recognize gas detectors measuring oxygen, and similar apparatus where the oxygen concentration of the explosive atmosphere was enhanced and not covered by the standard protection concepts, on the basis of special testing (usually in oxygen enriched atmospheres).

Within the UK, national certification to an agreed set of requirements has been historically available on the same basis as it has been for the more classic approaches to construction. Directive 76/117/EEC[1] attempted to address this problem by introducing the Inspection Certificate which allowed certification of special protection methods. This certificate, however, was noticeably different to the Certificate of Conformity and required, before issue, the agreement of all of the European notified bodies who had the right to perform their own tests at the expense of the manufacturer before granting such approval. The result of these two situations made the Inspection Certificate approach very unattractive and resulted in very few certificates being issued and, resultantly, slow advance in technology in the European scenario. In addition, 76/117/EEC addressed only the gas, vapour and mist scenario, leaving dusts outside European legislation.

In the production of the new Directive 94/9/EC[2] an attempt has been made to overcome both of these problems. The new Directive does not refer to European Standards for definition of construction requirements but includes them as 'essential requirements' within its own text. This allows a much simpler method of addressing European Standards by merely referring to them in the EU Journal[3] as Standards defining constructional requirements which satisfy essential requirements and removes the previous cumbersome Inspection Certificate approach by using Certificates of Conformity in all cases and providing a more rapid acceptance route for technological advance. In addition, apparatus for dust risks is now included together with protective systems, such as those used with pressurized apparatus 'p' which were hitherto not adequately addressed.

The one negative aspect of the new Directive, however, is its requirement for compliance. Under 76/117/EEC[1] use of conforming apparatus was optional, the Directive merely stating that member states could not prevent its import. Directive 94/9/EC[2] is quite different in that it prohibits marketing and putting into use of apparatus not complying with it thereby reducing widely used national flexibility. While it permits the 76/117/EEC approach until the end of June 2003, and hence the use of apparatus subject to a Certificate of Conformity or an Inspection Certificate until that date, the marketing in member states of apparatus which does not conform to 76/117/EEC or 94/9/EC is already in force, having been introduced with the implementation of the new Directive.

16.1 Acceptance of technical requirements

As already stated, the essential requirements for construction of apparatus in order to comply with 94/9/EC are contained within the Directive itself. These are, however, considered as insufficiently detailed to allow construction of apparatus and CENELEC[4] has the mandate to produce Standards which satisfy the 'essential requirements' and contain the required level of detail. This activity is expected to be complete for 'd', 'e', 'i', 'm', 'o', 'p' and 'q' in mid-1997 and for some time later. The situation in regard to 'n' is not quite so difficult as the Directive maintained the lower level of certification formality previously used in Zone 2 equipment.

When produced, these European Standards will be identified in the EU Journal as satisfying 'essential requirements' and any future additions will also follow this route. Thus technological progress is placed clearly in the hands of the technical-standards-making body and a much more rapid route to recognition is made available. How this will ultimately operate is not yet clear but if the approach is positive then a much more flexible situation should emerge.

16.2 Essential requirements

The 'essential requirements', not withstanding their technical impact were, in fact, written by employees of the European Commission taking such advice as they felt necessary. They tend to specify the objectives to be achieved in a general way and leave the technical rules necessary for the achievement of these objectives to others. While this approach is generally reasonable it does throw up some curious anomalies as will be seen later in this chapter.

The requirements apply, unlike those of 76/117/EEC,[1] to both electrical risks and mechanical risks, although implementation in the case of mechanical risks is delayed as there are currently no Standards which can be used to identify detailed requirements. They are divided into three parts:

16.2.1 General requirements

These identify five basic requirements which apparatus must meet:

Principles

The equipment is required to prevent, if possible, any explosive atmosphere being formed by any gas, vapour, mist or dust which it may itself release and prevent, as far as possible, any ignition of an explosive atmosphere formed by is own release or otherwise. Where it cannot do this it is required to contain the explosion as far as possible to prevent damage or injury.

Environmental requirements

The apparatus or protective system (protective systems, such as shut-down systems, are included) is required to be capable of operation without damage or deterioration in the environmental conditions in which it is intended to be used. This is not uniquely an explosive atmosphere requirement but is very important in the explosive atmosphere context; if the apparatus deteriorates excessively then so may its explosion protection elements. Thus any identified problems with its environment must not adversely affect its explosion protection.

Basic construction and use

The apparatus or protective system must be designed and manufactured so that within its specified tolerances, in normal operation and with any expected faults having occurred, and taking account of any required checking and maintenance envisaged by the designer, it does not create a dangerous condition. Dangerous condition in this context means an unacceptable risk of ignition.

Information

Sufficient information must be supplied with the equipment to allow its safe use. Manufacturers may well be required to release sufficient information to permit repair; a level of information which some manufacturers are reluctant to release because of the possibility of copying of designs.

Marking

All apparatus complying with the Directive is required to carry the Community Mark (Fig. 16.1), the Explosion Protection Mark (Fig. 16.2) and a mark to indicate the hazard which it is intended to address (which is 'G' in respect of explosive atmospheres of gas, vapour or mist, and 'D' if it is intended for use in respect of dust risks). This, importantly, represents an extension of the use of the 'Ex' mark (Fig. 16.2) to protective systems as well as protected apparatus. The use of the 'G' and 'D' are also new and may cause some confusion unless clearly identified with the 'Ex' mark.

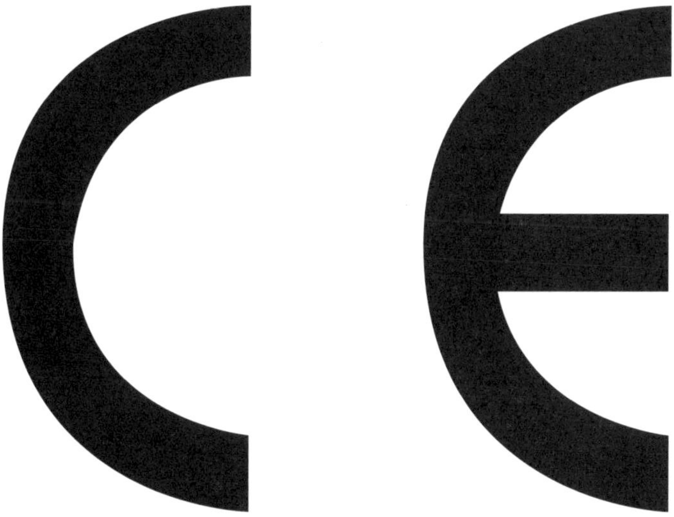

Fig. 16.1 The community mark

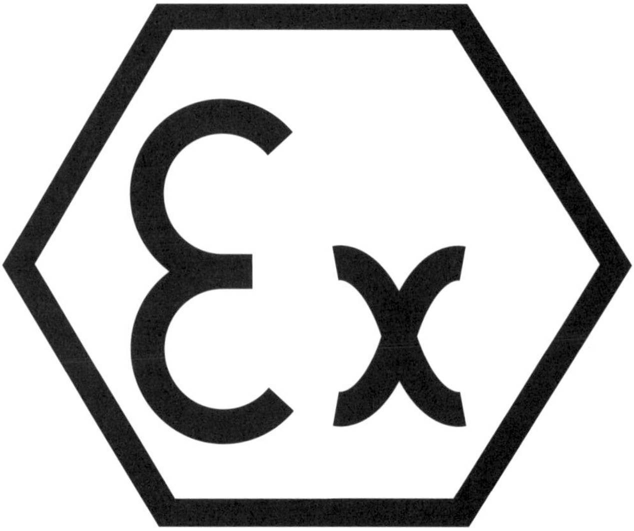

Fig. 16.2 The explosion protection mark

Apparatus and protective systems are also required to be identified by type, serial number and the year of construction, the latter being a requirement not previously applied.

16.2.2 Materials of construction

The 'essential requirements' include basic requirements for the material used in construction in that:

1. They must not themselves trigger off an explosion in any stress applied in use. This requirement identifies the problems which could occur if light metals were used without restriction on outer parts of an enclosure because of the frictional (thermite) sparking risk which certain of these materials exhibit when struck by rusty steel.
2. The material of construction must not be such as to react with any flammable gases, vapours, mists or combustible dusts in a way which would impair explosion protection. The principal problem is likely to be in respect of plastic and elastomeric parts which could be degraded by contact with chemicals and damage enclosure integrity or reduce insulation quality. Any such reaction between any materials of construction and the explosive atmosphere needs to be considered.
3. Material of construction must be stable within the operating tolerances of the apparatus. Instabilities (e.g., the possible corrosion or change of state of materials due to temperature) must be identified and shown not to affect explosion protection or the operation of protective systems.

16.2.3 General design and constructional requirements

The basic requirements for the components used in protected apparatus and protective systems are that they should only be used within their manufacturer's ratings and, in the light of the state of technical knowledge at the time of their construction, they will be capable of performing their duty throughout their projected lifetime. (Apparatus in general use would normally be expected be capable of operating, with a minimum of maintenance, for around ten years).

The Directive goes on to identify requirements for control of leakage from apparatus, allowance for dust layer formation without danger, overloading of equipment, identification of hazards introduced by necessary opening of apparatus, and the control of internal ignitions. In addition it identifies sparks, arcs, surface temperatures, static electricity, and pressure changes as possible ignition sources which need to be guarded against.

The general requirements go on in much the same vane but in all cases identify problems and require that they be guarded against without identifying in detail how this is to be done. Thus the production of Standards and their reference in the EU journal[3] is of great importance as without them it is not possible to have confidence in compliance with the Directive.

16.2.4 Specific requirements for particular types of apparatus and protective systems

In addition to the general requirements which apply to all explosion protected apparatus and protective systems there are additional requirements which apply to specific types of explosion protected apparatus. The delineation is basically by the level of safeguarding applied relating to the intended Zone of use.

Category 1 apparatus and protective systems

Category 1 apparatus and protective systems are, by their requirements, intended for operation in all hazardous areas including Zone 0 if for gas, vapour or mist risks and Zone 20 if for dust risks. No delineation between the two is present in the basic requirement which is: that the apparatus must be protected by at least two independent means of protection such that, when one fails the other remains operative; or that the apparatus must remain non-incendive in both normal operation and with up to two faults applied.

The two-fault criteria is readily recognizable as that used in intrinsic safety (see Chapter 13) but the dual protection approach is new and not has been fully addressed internationally in any technical forum. It thus represents an unknown quantity and one which will require considerable technical consideration before it can be fully implemented. The question as to what is an 'independent method of protection' is a vexed one. Flameproof enclosure 'd' (Chapter 10) and increased safety 'e' (Chapter 12) appear at first glance to be totally independent but on closer inspection there is evidence to suggest that a flameproof enclosure may not be proof against the results of a catastrophic internal electrical fault. Thus if an increased safety apparatus is placed within a flameproof enclosure, the accepted fault in the increased safety apparatus may damage the flameproof enclosure at the same time. While appearing independent, the two protection concepts may not be and may not fulfil the requirements for Category 1 equipment. This shows the importance of producing the technical Standards to be referred to in the EU journal, as any Standard for Category 1 equipment based on independent protection concepts will address these problems in detail.

It is worth noting that until now only intrinsically safe equipment 'ia' has generally been permitted in Zone 0 for gases, vapours and mists, and Zone 20 has only just come into being so there is no precedent. In these circumstances industry has managed very well and it is recommended that electrical equipment, particularly that which is not intrinsically safe, should not be placed in Zone 0 or Zone 20 unless it is absolutely necessary (not just convenient) due to the very high level of risk associated with the continuous, or almost continuous, presence of an explosive atmosphere.

Currently the only type of apparatus which clearly satisfies Category 1 and for which a detailed Standard exists is intrinsic safety of the higher grade 'ia' and this is designed for gas, vapour and mist risks only. An approach which may satisfy the Directive and allow its use in Zone 20 is identified in chapter 15.

The Directive goes on to identify protection against specific hazards but these will need to be more intensively addressed in Standards (in the case of intrinsic safety these have already been identified).

Category 2 apparatus and protective systems

Category 2 apparatus and protective systems are intended by their specification to be installed in Zone 1 and 2 if for gas, vapour or mist application, or for Zone 21 and 22 for dust application. The requirements of the minimum level of protection afforded is that the apparatus must be designed and constructed so that ignition of explosive atmospheres is prevented, even in the event of frequently occurring disturbances or operating faults which normally have to be taken into account.

These requirements are more readily identifiable as those present in all the standard types of protection defined and described in Chapters 9, 10, 11, 12, 13 and 15 and constitute the requirements for the majority of explosion protection concepts currently used.

Category 3 apparatus and protective systems

This category of apparatus and protective system is intended for installation in Zone 2 if for gas, vapour or mist risks and Zone 22 if for dust risks.

The requirement that the apparatus must remain safe in normal operation is well recognized already in type of protection 'N' (Chapter 14) for gas, vapour and dust risks and the concepts described in Chapter 15 for dust risks. The Directive also allows the more flexible certification approach for such equipment.

16.3 Use of apparatus

The fact that the essential requirements are within 94/9/EC, rather than identified by reference to Standards as was hitherto the case, is not intended, as far as can currently be identified, to permit direct measurement of apparatus against the Directive but rather to identify the suitability of the detailed content of technical standards to which the apparatus will then be designed and constructed. It will still probably be acceptable to produce special equipment such as that which would previously be identified by an Inspection Certificate but in the new situation that would receive a Certificate of Conformity. No mechanism is yet defined to gain the acceptance of such special requirements by all the notified bodies but it is expected that it will not be dissimilar to what exists at present in its operation.

References

1 76/117/EEC (1975) Council Directive on the Approximation of the Laws of Member States Concerning Equipment for Use in Potentially Explosive Atmospheres. 18 December.

2 94/9/EC (1994) European Parliament and Council Directive on the approximation of the Laws of Member States Concerning Equipment and Protective Systems for Use in Potentially Explosive Atmospheres. 23 March.

3 EU Journal The Journal of the European communities.

4 CENELEC Centre Européen de Normalization Electriques.

— 17 —

Selection of power supply, apparatus and interconnecting cabling system for both gas/vapour/mist risks and dust risks

Having identified the degree of risk and the various methods by which electrical apparatus and instrumentation may be constructed to address the risk it is now necessary to consider the actual selection of apparatus to address those risks, its installation and associated electrical supplies, and protection, as all of these have an effect on overall security against ignition and resultant explosion. There are three basic matters which need addressing: First, the basic electrical supply to all apparatus in the hazardous area and any other apparatus which may have an influence on security including electrical protection and potential equalization (bonding) requirements; second, the types of apparatus which should be selected for particular risks; and third, the methods of interconnection of apparatus with power sources and any other necessary interconnections with electrical circuits external to the apparatus itself.

17.1 Electrical supply systems

The majority of electrical apparatus in the UK is designed to be fed from a supply whose rated voltage is 240 V rms ac single phase (i.e., phase to neutral) at 50 Hz or, in the case of such things as rotating machines, 415 V rms three phase (i.e., phase/phase) as this is the supply which is normally used throughout the UK. (To come into line with EU Directives this rated voltage is set to change to 230 V but this change is not considered as significant as it is within the tolerance band of the current supply norm.) This supply is derived from a much higher voltage such as 3300, 6600, 11 000 or 33 000 V by step-down transformers as shown in Fig. 17.1.

The normally used system uses only two wires for a single-phase supply (four for a three-phase supply) the neutral or return conductor being combined with the protective (earth) conductor (TN–C–S system[1]–see Fig. 17.1.) This conductor is relied upon to carry both the return current and any fault currents which occur as there is usually no direct conductive connection between any installation and the supply source other than the combined protective and neutral (PEN) conductor which is connected to

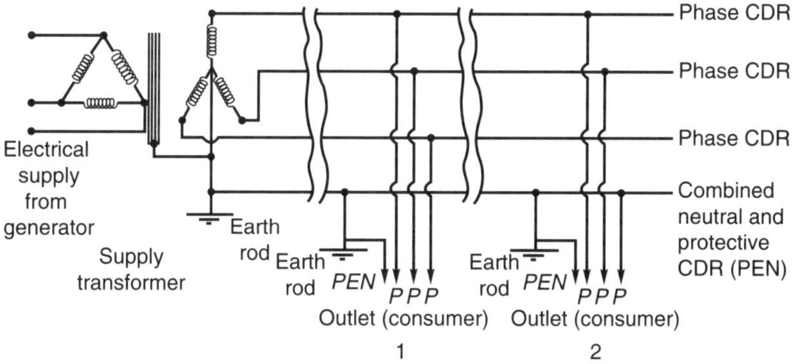

Fig. 17.1 Typical multi-outlet T–N–C–S electricity distribution system. *Note*: All exposed metal is connected to the PEN conductor

earth at the source of supply. To ensure that voltages of local conducting enclosures of electrical equipment are at the same potential as the PEN conductor and any other local conducting surfaces including the ground, the PEN conductor is normally earthed at each user site. This leads to problems in that, if the PEN conductor breaks between sites then any neutral return current will flow into the ground and reappear at the nearest point where the PEN conductor remains connected to the supply source, which is usually the earth connection at a neighbouring user site. This is clearly not acceptable as far as sites with hazardous areas are concerned as it produces a situation where their electrical installations could be invaded by currents from other sites and over which they have no control. For this reason such types of supply should not be used for sites containing hazardous areas and instead a supply using a separate protective conductor (TN–S[1]–Fig. 17.2) connected to the neutral conductor and earthed at the source of supply. The neutral conductor is now no longer earthed at each user point and the failure described previously cannot normally occur.

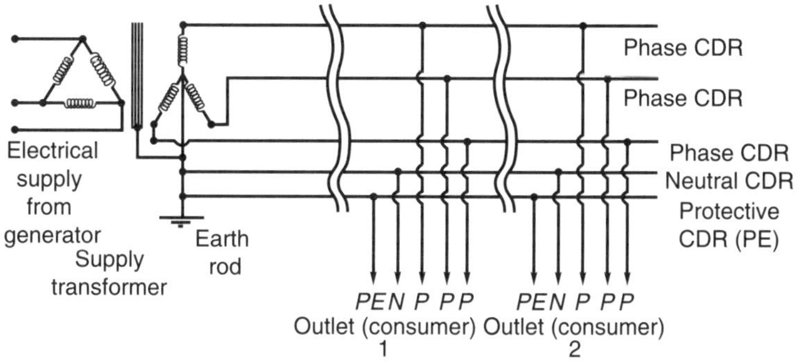

Fig. 17.2 Typical multi-outlet TN–S electricity distribution system. *Note*: All exposed metal is connected to the PE conductor

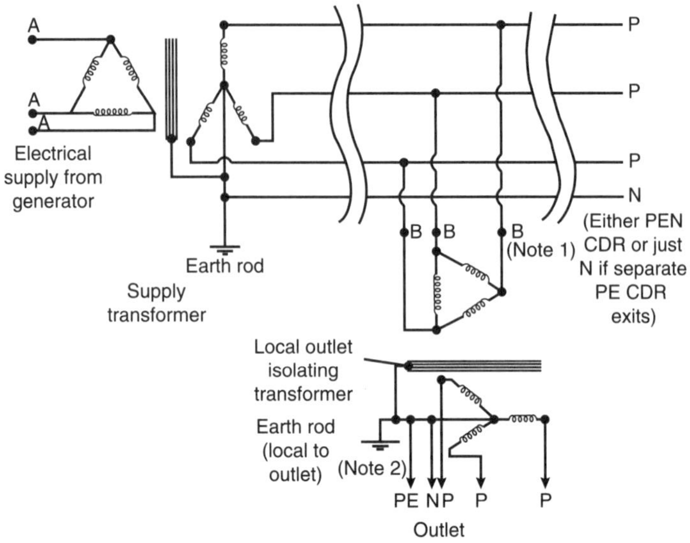

Fig. 17.3 Typical earthing arrangements for installations with explosive atmosphere risks. *Notes*: (1) Points 'B' may be fed directly from power generator if demand is large or if convenient. (2) Earth rod reserved for particular installation

There is still, however, the possibility that failure at other user sites, over which no control can be exercised, could result in current being passed through the ground on to the protective conductor in a hazardous area and thus, in addition to using the TN–S distribution system, it is recommended that supplies to locations where hazardous areas exist are separated from any other supplies, particularly those over which the user in the hazardous area has no control (see Fig. 17.3). On large sites, such as oil refineries or chemical plants, this is easy to achieve as the supply is normally fed to the plant at high voltage and transformed after it arrives, so that galvanic isolation exists between the particular plant and other installations. It is not so easy in the case of small isolated installations, such as pumping stations, as their feed is usually at the normal supply voltage described earlier and is common with other users. In this case it is recommended that a transformer still be fitted to provide galvanic isolation between the supplies used and the incoming supply unless it can be assured that the problem of invasion is not critical. In cases where the supply is only common to the individual user, for example, feeding different parts of the same site, then an analysis may show that additional isolation is not necessary but this will be the exception rather than the rule.

The general requirement which should be applied therefore is that all supplies to apparatus in hazardous areas should have separate return (neutral) and protective (earth) conductors and should be isolated by a transformer from other users of the supply unless those users are under the control of the user in the hazardous area and an evaluation has shown that such a transformer is not necessary.

17.2 Electrical protection

The electrical protection of all supplies to apparatus in hazardous areas (explosive atmospheres) is of fundamental importance. Apparatus protected as described in Chapters 7 to 16 is constructed so as to be unlikely to produce an ignition-capable situation in normal operation or due to fault. It has to be remembered, however, that it is possible that in very rare circumstances it may become ignition capable. When this occurs its duration must be limited so that the chance of an ignition is acceptably low, because of the low likelihood of coincidence, or of the situation arising before routine inspection and maintenance has identified any deterioration which could lead to ignition, and the necessary action taken.

Electrical protection should be set with its operating level as close to the normal operating levels as possible without producing a situation in which nuisance rips become a problem, and should cover overload, short circuit of the supply and earth faults. The electrical protection should be the same whatever the zone of risk but extreme care must be taken in respect of any circuits which enter Zone 0 or 20, due to the fact that the explosive atmosphere is assumed always to be present, and that significant duration of overloads, faults, short circuit faults or earth faults is least acceptable in these circumstances.

In addition to the above, electrical protection/isolation facilities which isolate all phase conductors and the neutral conductor (but not the potential equalization or protective conductor) should be present in non-hazardous areas to permit isolation of circuits entering hazardous areas. The neutral isolation by the switch isolating the phase conductors is recommended but not essential in these circumstances. The minimum requirement is for a separate link in the neutral conductor which may provide manual isolation. Where, however, additional isolation facilities in the hazardous area are required, the isolator must be protected by one of the concepts dealt with in Chapters 7 to 16 and the isolator must isolate the neutral at the same time as the phase conductors. This is because the neutral may be carrying fault current from other sources even when the phase conductors are isolated, and in these circumstances isolating the neutral with a manual link could produce an ignition-capable spark.

High voltage circuits, such as those used for supply of large rotating machines, should be treated in the same way as other supply circuits but isolation is particularly critical here and must be as rapid as possible. Isolation of earth faults is particularly important as it is this type of faults which is most likely to cause unprotected sparking and this isolation must be as near instantaneous as possible.

The foregoing requirements apply to all circuits entering the hazardous area except intrinsically safe circuits (Chapter 13) and non-incendive circuits (Chapter 14) where voltage and current in the circuit is so limited as to prevent ignition-capable sparking, but in these cases the electrical protection requirements generally apply to the apparatus in the non-hazardous area generating those circuits.

17.3 Selection of apparatus

Hazardous areas are a special type of location where, in addition to there being the normal environmental problems, explosive atmospheres can also occur. The basic selection criteria include the following.

1. The enclosure of apparatus must be sufficient to prevent the ingress of liquids and solids to an extent which could impair the operation of the apparatus by causing partial or full short circuits, corrosion or any other deterioration which would decrease the reliability of the apparatus or damage its safety features. For apparatus mounted outdoors this normally means an IP54 enclosure rating.
2. The enclosure of the apparatus and any interior parts necessary to maintain reliable operation, and the protection concept must be proof against chemical attack from the materials present at its location.
3. The rating of the apparatus must be sufficient to cover the operating conditions at its installation point (these ratings are those given by the protection concept which may include safety factors rather than the basic industrial ratings).
4. The apparatus and its enclosure must be sufficiently robust to withstand any mechanical shock from impact, being dropped if portable apparatus, or vibration. The construction requirements cover normal dropping or impact, but not necessarily vibration, and locations where impact is particularly severe.
5. The particular possibility of static formation on apparatus with plastics enclosures must be addressed.
6. The thermite sparking risk must be taken into account when light metals or alloys are used in enclosure of the apparatus. This is only partially taken into account in construction requirements for the apparatus.

Light metal enclosures

Particular care must be taken in the latter case of apparatus with light metal enclosure. The construction Standards for apparatus take account of magnesium content but there is still a residual risk due to the possible presence of aluminium or titanium and this is also present when aluminium sheathed cables are used. The risk principally comes from the possibility of the light metal being struck by oxidized (rusty) ferrous metal, when the resulting spark is often more intense than is the case when such contact is between two ferrous metals or ferrous metal and copper or brass. This results in a significant risk of ignition-capable sparking.

The risk is negligible in Zone 2 as the likelihood of coincidence of spark and explosive atmosphere is so low as to be acceptable. In the case of Zone 22 the same is basically true but here there is the risk that a blow on the light metal enclosure may at the same time cause deposits of dust on the apparatus to form a cloud, producing a coincidence which is not acceptable. In Zone 22, therefore, apparatus with light metal enclosures should not be used if possible but in any event it should be either protected from impact by location or guarding or it should be constructed and mounted in such a way as to preclude dust deposits (e.g., by having no horizontal flat surfaces or by having a cover to prevent dust deposition).

Apparatus with light metal enclosures intended for Zone 1 is not considered to be an unacceptable risk unless it is mounted in a location where the risk of mechanical impact is high, such as near roadways, or where operatives work with tools regularly. In these cases it should be avoided or provided with a guard to prevent impact directly on its enclosure. The requirement for Zone 21 is the same as that above for Zone 22 impact. In this case the dust problem is principally one of clouds rather than layers (as in the case of Zone 22) but the risk of coincidence is no greater.

In the case of Zone 0 and 20 the explosive atmosphere is considered to always be present and no impact is acceptable. Unless freedom from any impact can be guaranteed apparatus with light metal enclosures should not be used in Zone 0 or 20.

17.3.1 Selection in respect of gases, vapours and mists

Apparatus for gas, vapour and mist risks is defined for surface industry as Group II apparatus (Group I apparatus being for underground use in coal mines and other mines where flammable gas may be present). If the apparatus does not produce sparks to which the explosive atmosphere has access (i.e., is protected by pressurization 'p' (Chapter 11), powder filling 'q' (Chapter 9), oil immersion 'o' (Chapter 9), encapsulation 'm' (Chapter 9), increased safety 'e' (Chapter 12) or Type 'N' in its non-sparking context (Chapter 14), selection of Group II apparatus is sufficient, subject to surface temperature considerations.

Ignition by sparks and arcs

Where sparks occur to which the explosive atmosphere does have access they will either be rendered as non-ignition capable using intrinsic safety 'i' (Chapter 13) or the energy limited concept in Type 'N' (Chapter 14) or they will be prevented from causing an explosion even though they are capable of causing an ignition by utilization of the flameproof enclosure concept 'd' (Chapter 10) or non-incendive component concept in Type 'N' (Chapter 14). In these cases the degree of incendivity varies as the ignition capability of gas, vapour, mist and air mixtures varies and this allows variation in the severity of the limitation on apparatus construction and such apparatus is divided into three Sub-Groups IIA, IIB, and IIC, depending upon their ignition capability. Gases and vapours are associated with these sub-divisions to permit choice of the most appropriate according to their ignition performance. It will be remembered that energy limitation, such as used in intrinsic safety and the Type 'N' concept is based upon the use of a test apparatus as shown in Fig. 13.2 in Chapter 13 and the explosion prevention technique used in flameproof enclosure and the Type 'N' concept upon a test apparatus as shown in Fig. 8.1 in Chapter 8. Any particular gas or vapour can be measured in these test devices to determine its Minimum Ignition Current (MIC) which is relevant to ignition capability of the spark and its Maximum Experimental Safe Gap (MESG) which is relevant to the performance of the spark enclosure in preventing transmission of the ignition caused by the spark out of the enclosure. Fortunately these two facets of the performance of a gas or vapour are related and so a common approach is possible. Thus gases, vapours and mists are related to the apparatus subgroup on the following basis of their MIC (normally quoted as a fraction of the MIC of methane) and their MESG (normally quoted in mm) as follows:

Sub-group IIA	MIC > 0.8 MESG > 0.9 mm
Sub-group IIB	MIC ≤ 0.45 and ≥ 0.8 MESG ≤ 0.5 mm and ≥ 0.9 mm
Sub-group IIC	MIC ≥ 0.45 MESG ≥ 0.5 mm

It is normally only necessary to measure one or other of these parameters to define the sub-group with which the gas or vapour is associated unless the parameter measured identifies the gas as being near to the limit as follows:

If the MIC measures between 0.8 and 0.9 then the sub-group is determined by the MESG and is not necessarily IIA.

If the MIC measures between 0.45 and 0.5 then the sub-group is determined by the MESG and is not necessarily IIB.

If the MESG measures between 0.5 and 0.55 then the sub-group is determined by the MIC and is not necessarily IIB.

The above situations are based upon the knowledge of the performance of gases and vapours measured to date and so large is that number that there is confidence that these are the only situations where additional measurements of the other parameter are necessary.

Many gases and vapours have been identified both nationally and internationally to be associated with particular sub-groups by measurement or by assessment on the basis of the similarity of their chemical structures to other, gases and vapours whose associated sub-group has been determined by measurement. These are given in Table 4.3 in Chapter 4. No work on mists formed by liquids below their boiling points has been recorded and it is fair to assume that, because of their greater particle size, they will be less ignitable than vapours formed by the same liquid if it is raised to above its boiling point. The sub-grouping chosen for a mist should therefore be the same as that for the vapour which would be formed if the mist-producing liquid were raised to above its boiling point. While this is probably onerous no relaxation can be made unless it can be shown to be valid by measurement of the ignition temperature of a particular mist with the smallest particle size possible in the particular case, and it is unlikely that this can be reliably done.

The grouping system in the USA which seeks to perform the same function as sub-grouping in Europe is shown in Table 8.1 in Chapter 8. It is different to that used in Europe in that a single letter is used, hydrogen and acetylene are separated and carbon disulphide in not addressed. If USA apparatus is otherwise acceptable the USA grouping system should be used for its selection but, as confusion might result, it is not recommended that such apparatus is used unless all involved in the selection, installation and maintenance of apparatus are fully aware of the system and its relationship with the European system. In any event, the implementation of the new EU Directive 94/9/EC[2] is likely to cause the use of such equipment to be phased out unless it complies with the requirements of European Standards, using the European sub-grouping system.

Ignition by hot surfaces

Apparatus constructed in accordance with all of the protection concepts described in Chapters 7 to 14 is classified as to the maximum temperature reached by any surface to which an explosive atmosphere has access and any resulting ignition would result in an explosion which was not contained by the apparatus. The surface temperature classification system is described in Chapter 8 and apparatus is awarded a temperature class of T1 to T6 in Europe depending upon its maximum surface temperature. Table 4.3 in Chapter 4 specifies the maximum surface temperature class required for apparatus which is intended for use in particular gases and vapours based upon the measured maximum ignition temperature of the gas or vapour. A mist will adopt the same maximum temperature class, as would a vapour formed by raising the temperature of the liquid forming the mist to above its boiling point. Apparatus of a more limiting temperature class may be used in particular gases, vapours and mists as follows:

T6 – only apparatus of T6 classification may be used
T5 – apparatus of T5 and T6 classifications may be used
T4 – apparatus of T4, T5 and T6 classifications may be used
T3 – apparatus of T6, T5, T4 and T3 classifications may be used
T2 – apparatus of T6, T5, T4, T3 and T2 classifications may be used
T1 – apparatus of T6, T5, T4, T3, T2 and T1 classifications may be used

In some circumstances apparatus can be shown to satisfy the requirements of a particular protection concept at ambient temperatures well in excess of the 40 °C ambient normally used for temperature classification (e.g., resistance thermometers, thermocouples). In such cases the temperature classification is sometimes based upon the maximum ambient which is possible and this will be identified by the apparatus supplier. However, a surface temperature classification may be given for an ambient of 40 °C, despite the maximum operating temperature being specified as a higher temperature. In such cases it must be remembered that the temperature classification is based upon the rise of the apparatus above ambient and, for example, T5 apparatus is assumed to have a self elevation of 60 °C if classified at 40 °C. If such apparatus can be safely used at an ambient of 100 °C, therefore, its surface temperature for the purpose of use would be 160 °C (i.e., the equivalent of T3 – two classes more restrictive). Where this occurs the actual temperature class of usage should be derived as follows:

$$T_x = T_c - T_{a1} + T_{a2}$$

where T_x = maximum surface temperature for actual use
T_c = surface temperature classification at T_{a1}
T_{a1} = maximum ambient temperature used for surface temperature classification
T_{a2} = maximum ambient temperature of actual use

It must be stressed that such an approach is only possible where the apparatus satisfies the requirements of the protection concept at T_{a2}.

Apparatus from the USA to current US requirements has a much more complex temperature classification system – T2, T3 and T4 being further sub-divided. If such apparatus is decided to be otherwise suitable for use then it is recommended that the sub-divisions be disregarded (i.e., T2A, T2B, T2C and T2D apparatus should be considered as T2). While, in principle, it is possible to utilize them if the ignition temperature of the gas, vapour or mist is known, their use is likely to cause much confusion and could lead to danger unless it is clearly understood by all concerned in selection, installation and maintenance of apparatus. Likewise apparatus to the historic US system, where surface temperature was not separately identified and was related to the US grouping system, may be technically usable but, its use could cause considerable confusion and should be avoided if possible unless the situation is clearly understood as before. The implementation of the new EU Directive 94/9/EU is likely to require the phasing out of the use of such apparatus in any event unless it complies with European Standards which would require it to use the European surface temperature classification system.

Selection on the basis of certification

At present certification of apparatus is not a legal requirement in the UK for apparatus for use in any zone of risk. Notwithstanding this, however, National Codes (BS 5345, Part 1[3]) strongly recommend certification by a nationally recognized certification body for Zone 0 and 1 and although this recommendation is considerably weaker in relation to Zone 2 it is still present. In the UK there has, historically been a culture of utilizing only certified apparatus in Zone 0 and 1 and mainly certified apparatus in Zone 2. Only in exceptional circumstances, such as the use of special one-off types of apparatus, has this general approach been varied and even then great care has been taken to ensure that an evaluation by people of the expertise of those employed by certification bodies is carried out, and such an evaluation is recommended in BS 5345, Part 1[3]. This situation will be reinforced by the new Directive 94/9/EC[2] which will require such certification for all equipment marketed for Zone 0 and 1 use and by a further Directive on Health and Safety which will impose limits on the use of uncertified apparatus.

It is very wise, therefore, to always use apparatus which has been third-party certified in Zone 0 and 1, except in very special circumstances, and to try to use the same approach in Zone 2 although in this case more flexibility in policy is currently possible. All non-certified apparatus should, however, always be expertly evaluated to ensure that it does not introduce an unacceptable risk.

17.3.2 Selection of apparatus for dust risks

The sparking/non-sparking differentiation does not normally have a place in selection of apparatus for dust risks as protection is normally by exclusion of dust from within enclosures and its exclusion from the proximity of sparking contacts. The criteria, which are given in BS 6467, Part 2[4], are much more simple.

Selection on the basis of enclosure protection

Apparatus for use in explosive atmospheres of dust and air need to comply with the constructional requirement of BS 6467, Part 1[4], their enclosures excluding the explosive atmosphere to the degree necessary as defined in that Standard (IP5X or IP6X) depending upon the intended Zone of use (see later in this chapter). Regardless of the Zone of use, enlosures of IP6X are always required where the dust is a conducting dust. In practice this means that for all normal environments enclosures of IP65 or IP54 will be required depending upon the Zone of use and the type of dust, with lesser second numerals only acceptable where liquid ingress can be discounted (such as in indoor environments which are controlled as to the presence of moisture).

Selection on the basis of external surface temperature

Apparatus to BS 6467, Part 1[4] is given a maximum surface temperature on the basis of the maximum surface temperature which it achieves in tests in accordance with that Standard. Such apparatus may be used with dust layers and clouds as follows: first, with any dust where a layer of 5 mm cannot be ignited by a temperature 75 °C in excess of the maximum surface temperature of the apparatus; and second, with any dust with a minimum cloud ignition ignition temperature of 1.5 times the maximum surface temperature of the apparatus.

Selection of apparatus complying also with requirements for gas and vapour risks

Much work has gone into the production of requirements for apparatus for gas and vapour risks and considerable benefit can be obtained by extending the use of such apparatus into dust risk areas. In addition, many hazardous areas are made hazardous by the presence of explosive atmospheres of both gas and dust, so that apparatus must be suitable for both risks. This is made easy by the fact that many of the strength and other requirements applicable to apparatus for dust risks are very similar to those required for dust risks.

The selection of such apparatus is principally by identifying, in addition to those requirements applied for gas and vapour risks, the integrity of the enclosure as IP5X or IP6X as for apparatus to BS 6467, Part 1[4]. The actual selection requirements in relation to each gas/vapour protection concept are specified in BS 7535[5] and are discussed in detail in Chapter 15.

As already specified there is, unlike the gas/vapour situation, no formal classification system and so each item of apparatus is specified as having a particular maximum surface temperature and that must be compared with the minimum ignition temperature of each dust to demonstrate suitability. Where apparatus is demonstrably suitable for gas and vapour risks and has a surface temperature classification it will normally be possible to take the surface temperature classification as an indication of the surface temperature of the outside of the apparatus (see Chapter 15). However, because the safety factor for temperature classes T3, T4, T5 and T6 is only 5 °C (i.e., the temperature class is based upon a temperature 5 °C higher than the measured maximum surface temperature), rather than 10 °C used in the case of dust risks (see BS 6467, Part 1), the relationship between the temperature class and the minimum dust layer and cloud ignition temperature should be that given in Table 15.1 in chapter 15. This presupposes, of course, that the apparatus is otherwise suitable for dust risks.

Selection on the basis of certification

Unlike the situation in the area of gas, vapour and mist risks there is little history of certification and little certified apparatus is available except for that certified for gas and vapour risks which is also suitable for dust risks. Even in this latter case the certification only extends as far as the suitability for gas and vapour risks leaving any additional requirements for dust risks to be separately assessed. The new Directive 94/9/EC[2] will change all this bringing apparatus for dust risks under the same umbrella as that for gas, vapour and mist risks and requiring certification by a notified body for any such apparatus marketed in the EU for Zone 20 and 21. This will ultimately lead to a certification culture similar to the gas/vapour, mist culture for all dust risk Zones. This cannot happen, however, until European Standards exist for apparatus for dust risks and although these are currently being written it is not likely that any change could become mandatory for some years.

In addition to Standards which existed when the approach to dust risks was initially formed there are Standards for apparatus for dust risks which are much more definitive, containing specific testing to determine suitability. The execution of these tests is likely to require organizations similar to the currently recognized certification bodies for gas and vapour risk equipment and these certification bodies will become more and more involved because of the desire of manufacturers to show clearly that the apparatus is suitable, and the desire of users to have some guarantee of this. Thus certification may be expected to increase rapidly as the preferred route to show suitability, however long the EU Directive takes to implement it, and this is a sensible development.

17.3.3 Selection on the basis of zone of risk

Gas and vapour risks

The three Zones appropriate to gas, vapour and mist risks are Zone 0, Zone 1 and Zone 2 in descending order of severity.

Zone 0

It will be remembered (see Chapter 2) that Zone 0 are very dangerous places indeed, being assumed to have an explosive atmosphere always present. For this reason they are very limited in size and contained in some way as the risk of unauthorized access, with the attendant risk of explosion, is too great. In addition, there is only one of the standard forms of protection suitable for installation in Zone 0 and that is intrinsic safety of the higher category 'ia'. This leads to the following policy which should be used in all cases.

1. No electrical installations should be present in Zone 0 unless a clear requirement can be identified, such as significant optimization benefit or increase in operational safety. Every proposed Zone 0 installation should be carefully examined against these criteria before being implemented so that its use can be defended on secure grounds and personnel are not placed at any additional unnecessary risk.

2. Where the above criteria are satisfied installations should, as far as possible, be intrinsically safe installations of category 'ia'. This should satisfy most requirements as there is much operational history which identifies alternatives to Zone 0 installations for almost all types of electrical installation, save such things as sensors providing operational and safety information. This installation is instrumentation and can almost always be protected by intrinsic safety category 'ia' if it needs to be fitted in Zone 0.

3. Where equipment which cannot be protected by intrinsic safety category 'ia' is to be installed in Zone 0, it is almost certainly by definition

more powerful and potentially more ignition capable. Installations of such apparatus therefore must be much more critically examined. Any such apparatus is normally the subject of an evaluation by a nationally recognized certification body and certification as Type 's' which is specifically identified as having been constructed for Zone 0 use. The amount of apparatus will be very limited and this again supports the argument that Zone 0 installations of such apparatus are rarely necessary. It is recommended that this type of installation only be considered when it is absolutely necessary. Such an installation whose *raison d'etre* was a small increase in economy of operation would be unlikely to be justifiable, whereas one which was important to overall safety would.

Zone 1

In Zone the presence of an explosive atmosphere is expected for less than 10 per cent of the year and, unlike the situation in Zone 0 where an explosive atmosphere is always expected to be present, there is added security in the lower likelihood of coincidence of explosive atmosphere and ignition-capable faults, provided electrical protection of installations is adequate. This situation is recognized in the multiple protection concepts for equipment which exist for Zone 1. While the justification for all electrical installations is still necessary, as even properly protected installations do constitute a slight increase in risk over that which would exist if they were not there, the justification criteria can be eased and economic factors given more weight. It should be remembered, however, that Zone 1 is often very small and with a little thought many installations could be sited in adjacent Zone 2 or non-hazardous areas with little loss of effectiveness. Given that such appraisals have been carried out the following protection concepts are acceptable for Zone 1:

1. Any apparatus suitable for Zone 0 is usually acceptable for Zone 1 also.
2. Intrinsically safe circuits 'ib' (see Chapter 13).
3. Flameproof enclosure 'd' (see Chapter 10).
4. Pressurized apparatus 'p' (see Chapter 11). In this case the action taken on pressure failure is important and normally total isolation of all electrical supplies, whether direct or indirect through information transfer circuits, should occur as soon as the pressurization fails.
5. Powder-filled apparatus 'q' (see Chapter 9). The current edition of BS 5345, Part 1[3] does not recognize this type of apparatus for Zone 1 but the recently published BS/EN 60079[6] which will supersede BS 5345, will remove that restriction.
6. Oil-immersed apparatus 'o' (see Chapter 9). Again the current edition of BS 5345, Part 1 does not recognize this type of apparatus for Zone 1 but the recently published BS/EN 60079–14, which will supersede BS 5345, remove that restriction.
7. Increased safety apparatus 'e' (see Chapter 12).

8. Encapsulated apparatus 'm' (see Chapter 9). This protection concept is not recognized by the current edition of BS 5345, Part 1 as it post dates the production of that document. It is, however, recognized in BS/EN 60079 recently published and which will supersede BS 5345.
9. Apparatus which is certified as Type 's' (having special protection – see Chapter 16) by a nationally recognized certification body.
10. Apparatus which is certified as Type 's' by a Notified European certification body under Directive 76/117/EEC[7] using an inspection certificate.

Zone 2

Zone 2 is the least hazardous of the hazardous areas associated with gas, vapour and mist risks having explosive atmospheres present for no more than 0.1 per cent of the year. The minimum protection of electrical apparatus is reduced and the following are acceptable:

1. Any apparatus acceptable for use in Zone 0 is normally acceptable in Zone 2 also.
2. Any apparatus acceptable for use in Zone 1 is normally acceptable in Zone 2 also.
3. Apparatus with type of protection 'N' (see Chapter 14). A European and International Standard for type of protection 'n' is currently being produced. Apparatus in accordance with this Standard will also normally be acceptable.
4. Industrial apparatus which does not arc or spark and does not produce ignition-capable hot surfaces in normal operation is also acceptable, provided that it has been so evaluated by experts. It is likely that the need for such apparatus will slowly disappear as time progresses and Type 'N' or 'n' apparatus becomes more readily available. It is stressed that if Type 'N' or 'n' apparatus is available the justification for the use of this industrial apparatus is much weaker.

Apparatus for dust risks

Although it is not as clear cut, the division between dust Zones is essentially that between gas and vapour Zones. Similar approaches also exist but it must be remembered that Zone 20, the equivalent of Zone 0, has not historically existed and the approach to installations in this Zone is much more tenuous.

Zone 20

Zone 20, being the Zone in which dust clouds are always or nearly always present, is usually a contained Zone inside dust processing vessels. As with its gas/vapour counterpart (Zone 0) electrical installations should only be placed in Zone 20 when absolutely necessary. The situation is exacerbated here because of the effect of dust entering an enclosure and causing special problems because of its continued presence once inside, and the resultant protection concept of excluding the dust. This means that no electrical apparatus can be effectively protected for use in Zone 20 if its supplies and other electrical connections contain ignition-capable energies. The exception is intrinsic safety where the feeds to the apparatus are not ignition capable but, even here, the presence of dust in the interior, whether it is conducting or not, may cause internal short circuits particularly in damp conditions. Thus the only apparatus which could possibly be used in Zone 20 intrinsically safe circuits category 'ia' (see Chapter 13) where the enclosure is at least IP6X and the circuit is reassessed assuming the possibility of connection between any internal conducting parts which are not coated, encapsulated or insulated.

Zone 21 (Zone Z)

This is the equivalent of Zone 1 and the approach to suitable apparatus is similar but takes into account the problems of settlement particular to dusts. The following apparatus is therefore acceptable:

1. Apparatus suitable for Zone 20 is normally acceptable.
2. Apparatus in accordance with BS 6467, Part 1[4] with an IP6X enclosure (see Chapter 15).
3. Oil-immersed apparatus 'o' (see Chapters 9 and 15), provided its enclosure is at least IP6X.
4. Pressurized apparatus 'p' (see Chapters 11 and 15), provided its enclosure is at least IP6X (excluding purge outlets) in the absence of pressurization. The action taken on pressurization failure should be as that required in Zone 1.
5. Powder-filled apparatus 'q' (see Chapters 9 and 15), provided its enclosure is at least IP6X.
6. Flameproof enclosures 'p' (see Chapters 10 and 15), providing its enclosure is at least IP6X.
7. Increased safety apparatus 'e' (see Chapters 12 and 15), provided its enclosure is at least IP6X.
8. Intrinsically safe circuits of both categories 'ia' and 'ib' (see Chapters 13 and 15), provided their enclosure is at least IP6X or, where this is not so, category 'ia' with reassessment assuming that all conducting parts not coated, encapsulated or insulated are assumed to be capable of interconnection.
9. Encapsulated apparatus 'm' (see Chapter 9). In this case the encapsulant is considered as adequate without the necessity for an IP6X enclosure, although such an enclosure will be necessary for any exposed termination facilities.

Zone 22 (Zone Y)

This again is the least hazardous of the dust-related hazardous areas, being similar in risk to Zone 2. The suitability of apparatus reflects this as follows:

1. Apparatus suitable for Zone 20 is normally suitable for Zone 22 (Zone Y) also.
2. Apparatus suitable for Zone 21 (Zone Z) is normally suitable for Zone 22 (Zone Y) also.
3. Apparatus conforming to BS 6467, Part 1[4] (See Chapter 15) with an enclosure which is at least IP5X, provided that the dust is non-conducting.
4. Oil-immersed apparatus 'o' (see Chapters 9 and 15) with an enclosure of at least IP5X provided the dust is non-conducting and the dust does not cause deterioration of the oil.
5. Pressurized apparatus 'p' (see Chapters 11 and 15), provided the enclosure is IP5X (excluding purge outlets) and the dust is non-conducting. The action taken on pressurization failure should be at least that required in Zone 2.
6. Powder-filled apparatus 'q' (see Chapters 9 and 15), provided the enclosure is at least IP5X and the dust is non-conducting.
7. Flameproof enclosure 'd' (see Chapters 10 and 15), provided its enclosure is at least IP5X and the dust is non-conducting.
8. Increased safety apparatus 'e' (see Chapters 12 and 15), provided its enclosure is at least IP5X and the dust is non-conducting.
9. Intrinsically safe circuits 'ia' or 'ib' (see Chapters 13 and 15), provided the apparatus enclosures are at least IP5X and the dust is non-conducting. Intrinsically safe apparatus 'ib' is also acceptable if the enclosure does not achieve IP5X, provided the apparatus is reassessed assuming that all conducting parts not coated, encapsulated or insulated may be interconnected. This approach is also acceptable for conducting dusts.

17.4 Selection of conduit or cable systems

The cables used for interconnection of apparatus in the hazardous area to that in the non-hazardous area, and different items of apparatus in the hazardous area, are subject to essentially the same requirements whether they are associated with gas/vapour/mist risks or dust risks. Two features of the cable are important, namely its adequacy in respect of electrical stresses (voltage and current flow including temperature elevation resulting) and their adequacy for the environment (heat, cold, moisture, airborne chemicals, etc.). The requirements stated here are appropriate to a normal outside environment but any unusual situations (such as the presence of unusually high concentrations of solvents in the atmosphere, etc.) need to be individually addressed in respect of the materials of construction and siting of cables, the objective being to achieve at least the same level of security as the recommendations given here would achieve in a normal industrial environment.

17.4.1 Zone 0 and Zone 20

The only standard protection concept suitable for Zone 0 and Zone 20 use is intrinsic safety of the higher category 'ia'. This type of protection is based upon the presumption that the energy levels in the hazardous area are non-incendive and thus the requirements for cable and conduit systems are minimal and are only those required in a normal installation where hazardous areas are not present. Likewise, in the event that conduit is used only basic industrial requirements need to be met.

In both cases, however, the need to prevent explosive atmospheres from entering a non-hazardous area via the cable or the conduit needs to be addressed. This will normally require sealing of conduits but will probably require no additional arrangements for cables except where the cable has open interstices or where it is connected to a device, such as a transmitter, which could have an explosive atmosphere at greater than atmospheric pressure within it. Such precautions will normally consist of sealing the cable or conduit or venting them to prevent transmission to any area which would be adversely affected (a non-hazardous area or one of lesser hazard).

In exceptional cases specially protected non-intrinsically safe installations are used where the cable or conduit may carry highly incendive energies and an entirely different approach is needed. Damage or deterioration of the cable or conductors within the conduit may have much more serious results and thus the choice of cables or conduit system becomes much more critical.

Cables

For intrinsically safe circuits there have historically been no minimum requirements save those for multicores which contain more than one intrinsically safe circuit and require each circuit to be in an individual screen (see in Chapter 22). The advent of the proposed BS/EN 60079[6] has, for the first time introduced recommendations for these which state that the cables should not have any conductor or conductor strand of less than 0.1 mm diameter and the insulation must be suitable for 500 V rms ac operation. Because of the necessity of specification of cable inductance and capacitance an overall sheath is also necessary to define the positions of the conductors. It is possible to utilize cables containing more than one intrinsically safe circuit to carry circuits entering Zone 0, but such cables should be such that each circuit is individually contained in a screen which can be connected to the potential equalization (bonding) system to preclude interconnections of circuits (see in Chapter 22). In addition, the cable must contain only 'ia' circuits and the screens must either be insulated from one another or all connected to the potential equalization (bonding) system at the same point and at the same point as the circuits contained within them.

In exceptional cases, where specially protected non-intrinsically safe circuits are installed in Zone 0, the possibility of cable damage releasing incendive energy is much more serious. Here the only real solution is to prevent the external release of such energy and the best way to do this is to ensure that the cable carries the features necessary to minimize such a risk. The basic recommendations for such cables will be:

1. The cable should have thermoplastic or elastomeric insulation (or insulation of material satisfying similar requirements such as the mineral insulation in metal sheathed cables) on their cores sufficient for normal industrial use.
2. The cores should be contained within a bedding of similar material unless the cable is mineral insulated, when the mineral insulation will suffice.
3. The cable should be fitted with a steel wire or braid armouring over its bedding unless it has a continuous metal sheath, such as with metal sheathed mineral insulated cable, to minimize the risk of damage. This also provides a short circuit within the cable in the event of damage which minimizes the risk of arcing or sparking outside the cable before circuit protection operates.
4. All cables including those with continuous metal sheaths should be fitted with an outer polyvinyl chloride (PVC), chlorosulphinated polyethylene (CSP), polychloroprene (PCP), chlorinated polyethylene (CSP) sheath or sheath of similar material to prevent earth faults to the armouring along the cable length and to protect the cable from the environment.

Most Standards for cables protected by armouring for normal industrial use will satisfy these requirements without the application of additional protection concepts.

A new recommendation included in BS/EN 60079-14[6] is that all cables except those used in sand-filled trenches or the like need to be constructed of material which can satisfy the requirements of IEC 332, Part 1[8] insofar as their ability to transmit flame once burning are concerned. While this is not yet included in national recommendations it is wise to address it as this will minimize the risk of transmission of fire around an installation should a fire occur within it.

It is highly unlikely that non-intrinsically safe portable or transportable apparatus will be considered for use in Zone 0 or 20, but in the unlikely event that such use should be considered no relaxation in cable requirements are considered as reasonable and, in addition, the effect of flexing on armouring should be carefully considered to ensure that breakage due to flexing is unlikely.

Conduits

For intrinsically safe circuits the only requirement for conduit is that it should constrain the enclosed conductors so that parameters are definable and that it should be fitted with a stopping device to prevent gases, vapours, mists or dusts from moving from one hazardous area to another or to a non-hazardous area. In addition, each individual intrinsically safe circuit within the conduit should, as in the case of a cable, be enclosed in an individual screen and those screens should satisfy the same requirements as for cable screens.

For other circuits it should be a solid drawn or seam welded conduit in accordance with BS 4568[9] or flexible metal or plastic conduit with heavy mechanical strength classification and an overall plastic sheath (see BS 731, Part 1[10]) to minimize the possibility of damage and prevent ingress of an explosive atmosphere. Such conduit systems are required to be fitted with recognized sealing devices (stopper boxes) where such conduits exit the hazardous area to enter another less hazardous area or a non-hazardous area.

If possible it is wise to fill the conduit with pressurized inert gas or powder or similar filler to prevent the ingress of explosive atmosphere although this is not strictly necessary.

17.4.2 Zone 1 and Zone 21

In Zone 1 and Zone 21 there is a much lower possibility that cables or conduit systems could become damaged in such a way and at such a frequency as to cause a coincidence between ignition-capable sparking and the presence of an explosive atmosphere. Thus in some cases a slightly more relaxed approach is possible. Again, BS/EN 60079–14[6] requires cables not in sand-filled trenches to comply with IEC 332 Part 1[8] for flame transmission.

Cables for non-intrinsically safe installations

The steel wire armoured and steel braided cables described as suitable for use in Zone 0 and 20 are also suitable for use in Zone 1 and 21 for normal installations and particularly for installations where risks of mechanical impact are higher than normal. In normal installation conditions the armouring is less necessary and cables as described for Zone 0 and 20 use, but without the armouring, will be suitable provided the outer sheath is suitable for a standard industrial installation. In addition, cables with a semi-rigid sheath may be used without armouring where the risk of mechanical impact is higher than normal. Standards for normal industrial cables of this type will normally be sufficient to satisfy these requirements.

For portable and transportable apparatus cables of the following types are acceptable for use:

1. Standard or heavy-duty tough rubber sheathed flexible cables;
2. Standard or heavy-duty polychloroprene sheathed flexible cables;
3. Cables of equally robust construction.

In all cases the choice of cables should be determined by the intended use (e.g., where the risk of mechanical damage is high, cables should always be fitted with steel wire or braid armouring and, particularly in the case of flexible cables, heavy-duty cables should be used). While not being necessary in all cases, steel wire or braid armouring is a wise precaution due to its protective value and its containment of faults during operation of protection equipment, and it is normal UK practice to use such cables in hazardous areas unless the cable is very well protected against damage (such as being led in a sand-filled trench). Other precautions may be necessary in certain cases, such as provision of an overall lead sheath, where the cable is likely to be in contact with petroleum products for long periods (such as when it is installed in trenches or buried).

Cables for intrinsically safe circuits

The requirements for these are basically as given for Zones 0 and 20 use. Less well-protected multicores may be used in Zone 1 and 21, however, without the need to consider faults between separate intrinsically safe circuits in the multicore. The minimum requirements for such cables are that conductor strands should not be below 0.1 mm, each conductor should have at least 2 mm of polyethylene or PVC insulation or an equivalent thickness of other types of insulation (e.g., thinner insulation of polytetrafluoroethylene (PTFE) can be shown to be equivalent) which must be capable of withstanding a 500 V rms voltage test and the cable is fixed and protected where mechanical stresses are likely. This type of cable is restricted to intrinsically safe circuits with voltages of less than 60 V peak ac or dc

Any multicore cable not satisfying the requirements above or those for Zone 0 or 20 use is assumed to be capable of causing interconnection between separate intrinsically safe circuits within it, and thus can only be used if an assessment of such interconnections is carried out.

More detailed information on the subject of cables for intrinsically safe circuits is given in Chapter 22.

Conduits

The requirements for conduits in either intrinsically safe or non-intrinsically safe circuits are essentially the same as those for conduit installations in Zone 0 and 20 with the exception that the cores of individual intrinsically safe circuits need not be in individual screens. They must, however, have some form of overall serving to ensure that their inductive and capacitive parameters are clearly known unless these are based upon the maximum separation which can occur in the conduit.

17.4.3 Zone 2 and Zone 22

All cable and conduit systems suitable for Zone 0 and 20 and Zones 1 and 21 will also be suitable for Zone 2 and 22. In addition it must be remembered that the risk in Zone 2 and 22 is much less and, subject to the necessary exclusion of dust, which all cables with a plastic or elastomeric or equivalent overall sheath will meet, the requirements for cables and conduits in Zone 2 and 22 are no more onerous than those which would apply for an industrial installation in a similar situation where explosive atmospheres were not present, except that materials of construction should not transmit flame (IEC 332 Part 1[8]).

References

1 IEE (1991) Regulations for Electrical Installations (16th edition).

2 94/9/EC (1994) Directive of the European Parliament and Council on the Approximation of the Laws of Member States concerning Equipment and Protective Systems for Use in Potentially Explosive Atmospheres 23 March.

3 BS 5345 Selection, Installation and Maintenance of electrical Apparatus for Use in Potentially Explosive Atmospheres (Other than Mining Appications or Explosive Processing and Manufacture): Part 1 (1989). General Recommendations; Part 4 (1977) Installation and Maintenance Requirements for Electrical Apparatus with Type of Protection 'i'. Intrinsically Safe electrical Apparatus and Systems: Part 7 (1979). Installation and Maintenance Requirements for Electrical Apparatus with Type of Protection 'N'.

4 BS 6467 Electrical Apparatus with Protection by Enclosure for Use in the Presence of Combustible Dusts. Part 1 (1985) Specification for Apparatus; Part 2 (1988) Guide to Selection, installation and maintenance.

5 BS 7535 (1992) Guide to the Use of Electrical Apparatus Complying with BS 5501 or BS 6941 in the Presence of Combustible Dust.

6 BS/EN 60079 Electrical Apparatus for Explosive Gas Atmospheres. Part 14 (1997) Electrical Installations in Explosive Gas Atmospheres.

7 76/117/EEC (1975) Council Directive on the Approximation of the Laws of Member States Concerning Electrical Equipment for Use in Potentially Explosive Atmospheres 18 December.

8 IEC 332 Tests on Electric Cables Under Fire Conditions. Part 1 (1993). Test on a Single Vertical Insulated Cable or Wire.

9 BS 4568 Specification for Steel Conduit and Fittings with Metric Threads of ISO Form for Electrical installations. Part 1 (1970). Steel Conduit, Bends and Couplers; Part 2 (1970). Fittings and Components.

10 BS 731 Flexible Steel Conduit for Cable Protection and Flexible Steel Tubing to Enclose Flexible Drives. Part 1 (1952) Flexible Steel Conduit and Adaptors for the Protection of Electric Cable.

— 18 —

Installations in explosive atmospheres of gas, vapour, mist and dust

BS 5345, Part 1 (1989)
BS/EN 60079-14 (1997)
BS 6467, Part 2 (1988)

While much apparatus intended for use in explosive atmospheres is the subject of formal construction Standards and equally formal certification/approval, installation is left largely in the hands of the actual user or their contractor. This is because of the wide variety of differing situations of use which mean that only those with intimate knowledge of a particular process or location have sufficient knowledge to ensure that the installation is suitable for that process or location. Individual installations in particular locations may require variations on normal installation, maintenance and inspection procedures (such as installation of flanged flameproof enclosures which may from time to time require additional weather protection to prevent ingress of liquids or solids present in a particular environment). Thus the only practicable approach is to provide advice for activities such as installation, inspection and maintenance which cover most normal uses, and rely on those who have responsibility for particular sites to implement the recommendations as far as they are appropriate and to justify any deviation from them. Requirements for installation which have mandatory status are possible but will need to be minimal to avoid them having an adverse affect on safety in particular environments.

Accordingly installation, maintenance and inspection are currently dealt with in what are called Codes of Practice which provide recommendations as to what should be done, rather than Standards which contain rigid requirements. In case of regulatory body intervention, however, any deviation from these recommendations will need to be justified and in practice most installations comply with them completely. This situation is set to change in the near future when installation matters will fall within the control of a proposed new EU Directive[1] which is likely to call up a proposed European Standard[2] for installation. This Standard has mandatory requirements for compliance rather than the recommendations in current Codes. These requirements are, however, minimal and thus will need to be augmented by additional measures which will reflect particular situations.

18.1 Standards and Codes

In areas where explosive atmospheres of gas, vapour and mist are present installation, maintenance and inspection recommendations are included in BS 5345[3] and, in areas where explosive atmospheres of dust occur, by BS 6467, Part 2[4]. The current issue of BS 5345 will shortly be replaced by BS/EN 60079[2] which will became the installation Standard of the EU. It should be noted that this document is a Standard not a Code and contains requirements of a mandatory nature, rather than recommendations as is the current situation. For this reason a possible problem exists for the future where variation of installation requirements is currently possible for commercial reasons, or must exist for safety reasons in the case of particular installations, as such variation could be contrary to the requirements in the new Standard. This does not, however, appear at present to be a great problem as the requirements of BS/EN 60079 are considerably more basic than those in BS 5345 and not dissimilar. Thus the present installation practice, together with all the currently used variations, is unlikely to create a conflict and, where it does, any change to accommodate the new document is unlikely to create significant problems. This is because most practical variations will be in the form of additional and not variational requirements, and where this is not so any change required will be of a minor nature. The introduction of BS/EN 60079 will, however, support the more formal approach of the proposed EU Health and Safety Directive[1] in this area.

18.2 Legislation and enforcement

The use of the formal third-party certification/approval tool (which has historically been used as a matter of course in the case of construction of apparatus for use in gas, vapour and mist risks associated with Zone 0 and 1 within the UK) is not a feature of current installation practice in this field within the UK. This is not universally the case in all of the countries of Europe as, for example, in Germany all installations are required to be approved by a *Lander* (State of Federal Germany) registered expert who may be in the employ of the owner of the installation or from a third party, such as the TÜV, an inspection organization in Germany covering a wide range of activities as diverse as explosive atmosphere installations and the German Equivalent of MOT tests for cars.

The law within the UK has historically placed the onus for safety on the owner and operator of the installation and regulation has been achieved by routine visits to operating plant by the regulatory body (the Factory Inspectorate) who have wide powers to apply penalties for failure to achieve necessary standards of operation. Over recent years there has been a significant pressure to change this and produce a much more 'front-end control' operation of safety and this is now being reinforced by the production of a new Directive[1] in the EU, currently in development, which addresses the health and safety of workers in industry where explosive atmospheres can occur.

This Directive addresses installations in explosive atmospheres created by gases, vapours, mists and dusts and, in its draft of 1992 numbered 6430/92 EN, it requires the following actions:

1. Classification of hazardous areas and their indication by signs. (Although area classification is normal in the UK there is currently no legislation specifically requiring area classification, and in specialized cases other means are currently possible. In addition, detailed identification of hazardous areas by signs is not usual in the UK at present).
2. Formal training and appointment of those involved in installation, maintenance and control and written work instructions in all cases. (Again this is a more formal approach to that historically used and, although it will probably make little practical operational difference, it will involve much more formal documentation in respect of personnel and their duties, powers and responsibilities).
3. Inspection of all installations by 'experts' before their use is permitted and the experts must be appointed and approved by the regulatory body (the Factory Inspectorate) for all specific areas in which they operate. (This is a significant formalization of operation as, even though employers are currently required to ensure that employees are competent for what they do and should carry out pre-use inspections, there is likely now to be a legal requirement to do so and the regulatory body will control those who carry out such inspections, even though they may be employed by the owner of a particular plant).

The proposed Directive (6430/92 EN) is likely to be subject to some change before it becomes law but it is clear that, in the future, the practical arrangements in respect of installation will become much more formal than at present and although it will not significantly change the current approach of many organizations, it will introduce a significant further layer of regulation and approval which will move the UK situation to one much more like that used in Germany.

18.3 Basic installation requirements

The following general recommendations apply to all types of apparatus installed in all zones of risk. Their objective is to ensure that apparatus is properly installed and recorded so that its installation is suitable for its location, its location is recorded, and it is installed in a manner which facilitates inspection. It should be noted that the requirements for choice, location and electrical protection apply to cables and conduits which traverse the hazardous area to the same degree that they apply to apparatus installed in the hazardous area and the cables or conduit which supply such apparatus.

18.3.1 Pre-installation checks (electrical ratings and physical location)

Although the ratings of the apparatus have been compared with the requirements at its point of installation during the design stages it is rare that changes do not take place during construction and it must be expected that a few errors will occur during design. To cover the situation where such situations could occur a check should be made that the apparatus chosen is appropriate to the electrical and physical parameters of its point of installation. Typical of the checks which need to be made are:

1. Is the electrical supply appropriate to the apparatus?
2. Does the apparatus sub-grouping, if any, match the actual hazard?
3. Does the temperature classification or maximum external surface temperature satisfy the requirements for the explosive atmosphere concerned. In particular, are there sources of heat in the installation locality which could cause heating of the apparatus and have these been allowed for, or is the location such that restricted ventilation could lead to overheating of the apparatus?
4. Is the location particularly exposed and if so has additional protection been provided to protect the apparatus from mechanical damage?
5. Are the cable glands appropriate to the apparatus enclosure specification (IP-rating) and are suitable blanking plugs fitted to all unused cable entries?
6. When the apparatus is fitted at its planned location is it easily accessible for inspection and are all labels clearly visible?
7. Does the geographical documentation for the area of the plant or location clearly identify the location of the apparatus and its interconnecting cables or conduits? Are records of the detail of the apparatus complete and clear?
8. Is the electrical protection against overload, short circuit and earth fault appropriate to the apparatus? Is it sufficiently sensitive?

18.3.2 General installation recommendations

When installing apparatus the following points should be given particular attention:

1. The apparatus should be firmly fixed at its intended location.
2. Cables should be fitted to cable entries as specified and individual cores in terminal boxes should be crimped where necessary to prevent wandering wire strands causing short circuits.
3. Lengths of leads (cable tails) within terminal boxes should be kept to a minimum consistent with not placing stress on the leads, and the possible future necessity of remaking the end of the lead once.

4. Cable installation should be such that, consistent with not producing a situation where the cable is inadequately fixed or overly subject to damage, there is sufficient slack in the installation to permit total remaking of the cable to the apparatus once.
5. Cables should be fitted on suitably located cable trays (normally located at high level, employing ceilings or upper floors as overhead protection) or in trunks or within the webs of girders to minimize the risk of mechanical damage.
6. Cables with armouring or screens should have an overall insulating sheath which should adequately insulate it from other cables in a trunk or from a metallic cable tray. (In exceptional circumstances such as where only one cable is led in a single trunk this overall sheath may not be necessary if the trunking itself provides the insulation.)
7. Cable and conduit entry to apparatus should be on the side or bottom if there is any chance of the apparatus being subjected to water by rain or hosing, etc. If cable glands or conduit entries are fitted to the top of the enclosure then, unless they are protected from moisture, there will be a build up of moisture around and possibly inside any gland, entry or protective boot which will often ultimately lead to liquid leakage into the apparatus enclosure which could adversely affect the security afforded by the apparatus.
8. Enclosures of conducting material should be securely bonded to any exposed local structural metalwork to prevent sparking if fault currents could otherwise cause a differential potential to exist between them (see the following guidance on earthing and bonding).

18.3.3 Post-installation checks

After installation the apparatus and its interconnecting cables should be inspected to ensure that no damage has occurred during installation, particularly to enclosures and cables, that all earthing and bonding is secure, and that any parts isolated from earth are still so isolated. The best way to do this is by a full (initial) inspection of the installation after completion and before it is energized. The full detail of such an inspection is given in Chapter 21. It will also be necessary to ensure the effectiveness of bonding electrically by measurement and information on this is also given in Chapter 21.

18.3.4 Earthing and bonding (connection to the potential equalization system)

The two activities 'earthing' and 'bonding' (connection to the potential equalization system) refer to two quite different exercises and it is important that their meaning is clearly understood.

Earthing

Earthing refers to the connection of an electrical conductor to earth, usually done with an earth rod, to give an electrical circuit a reference to earth and to allow current to return to its supply source when no direct electrical connection is present, such as is the case with a general three-phase supply to a site. The electrical return connection is, in such cases, via the ground (see Fig. 18.1) but, because of the fact that as the current leaves the earth rod, the dimensions of the ground (which is acting as a conductor) increase rapidly causing a fast reduction in return path resistance. A considerable voltage gradient may occur close to the earth rod causing significant voltage differences in short distances (see Fig. 18.2). Because of this the return of any fault current from an apparatus fault via the earth alone is not acceptable in hazardous areas because the potential differentials occurring could cause other conducting elements in a given small area to achieve very different voltages, resulting in an unacceptable risk of incendive sparking and possibly electric shock.

Bonding (connection to the potential equalization system)

The term bonding is really a shortened form of 'equipotential bonding' and refers to the activity of connecting, for example, apparatus enclosures to the point of system earth connection by designated conductors to ensure return of fault currents efficiently to their source, and interconnecting conducting parts to ensure that, as far as possible, the voltages between them are not significant. It has a separate function to the process of earthing, and connections between the two (other than at the point of supply system earthing) is not always necessary for apparatus protection against its own faults. The two will, however, have many accidental connections, such as those produced by the necessity for bonding of earthed metallic parts.

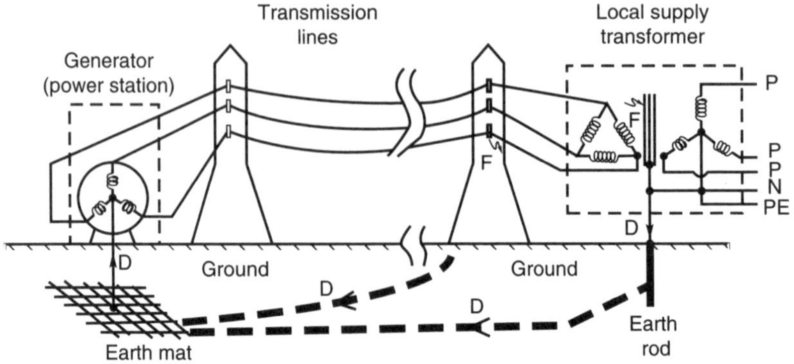

Fig. 18.1 Typical fault current return via the ground (earth)

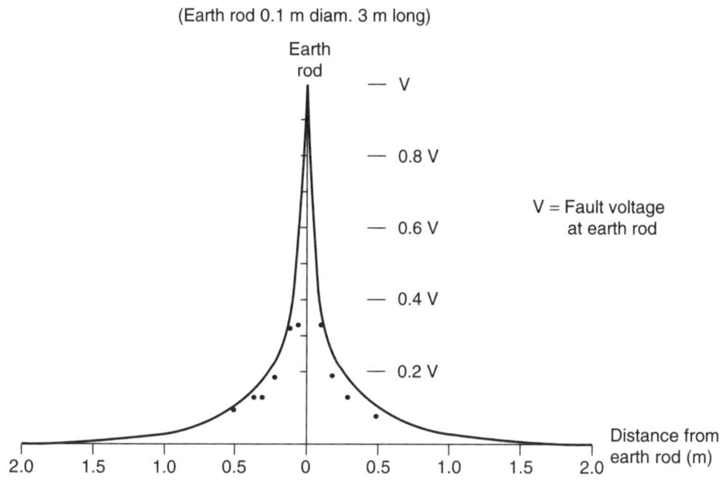

Fig. 18.2 Typical potential gradient at earth rod site

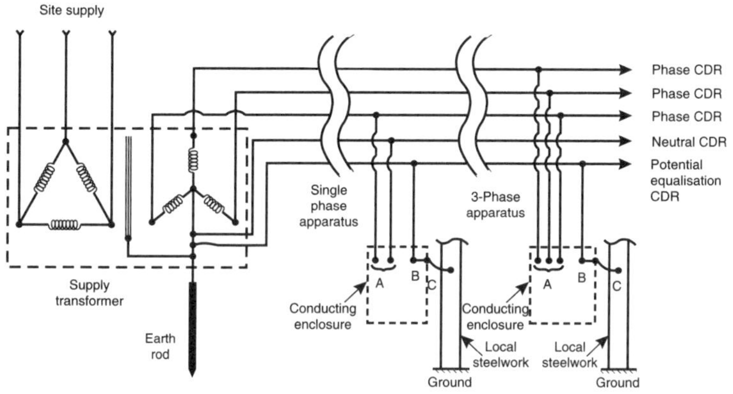

A = Electrical supply connections
B = Connection of PE conductor to internal 'earth' terminal (cable armouring may perform this function)
C = Connection of external 'earth' terminal to local steelwork (normally by conductor but may be by enclosure fixing bolts)

Fig. 18.3 Typical plant bonding system

The two operations are even then quite distinguishable one from another. Bonding for assurance that protection operates and bonding to ensure that all local conductive parts are at a similar potential are shown in Fig. 18.3.

18.3.5 Application of earthing

Formal earthing at a particular location containing hazardous areas is normally limited to the provision of an earth connection to provide a return path for fault current from the primary of the supply transformer (discussed in Chapter 17) to the supply source which is usually the power station or a main distribution station. This connection is achieved by the provision of an earth rod or mat at the location of the transformer and the conduction requirements for such earths are those which would apply even if hazardous areas did not exist. The quality of this rod or mat connection to earth should, however, be such as to ensure that the majority of the fault current flows in it and not the structural steelwork of the plant or building which will also be connected to earth via its construction (e.g., by being concreted into the ground) and connected by such things as apparatus enclosures to the equipotential bonding system which is connected to the transformer secondary star point.

18.3.6 Application of bonding (potential equalization)

The primary need in sites containing hazardous areas is to minimize the difference in voltage which can occur between separate exposed conducting parts (such as enclosures and structural steelwork) so that interconnection of the two via a piece of metal or a human being cannot generate ignition-capable arcs or sparks, and to ensure that any faults which occur between enclosed circuits and metal parts (such as chassis and enclosures) cause swift disconnection of supplies.

To achieve this any conducting apparatus chassis, enclosures and other parts not forming parts of the electrical circuit, but to which electrical conductors and components of the apparatus may, in fault conditions, be connected, need to be firmly and reliably connected to the protective conductor. From earlier chapters it will be remembered that an internal terminal is provided for this purpose and the protective conductor which is connected to the main power supply earth should be connected to this. While it is recommended that a protective conductor should be included in the apparatus supply cable it is accepted that the steel wire or braid armouring of a cable and similar electrically conducting sheaths, such as the copper sheath of mineral insulated cable (but not screening as this is considered as subject to damage causing disconnection), may, perform this function if its connection can be adequately guaranteed.

In the case of conduits, a properly installed solid drawn or seam welded rigid conduit may also perform the function of protective conductor if, in its installation, the effects of corrosion at its joints has been considered and action taken to minimize this risk. (Flexible conduits may not, however, perform this function as their reliability is considered as inferior in this regard.) The armouring or conduit should fulfil the following conditions.

1. It should have a resistance per unit length of not less than the following:
   - The same as the largest of the supply conductors in the cable up to conductors of cross section 16 mm^2

- 16 mm^2 where the largest supply conductor within the cable in the cable exceeds 16 mm^2 but does not exceed 35 mm^2
- A conductor of the same material as the conductors within the cable but half the cross-sectional area of the largest supply conductor within the cable where this exceeds 35 mm^2

2. The armouring or conduit should be terminated at both ends in an appropriate gland or by other appropriate means, giving secure electrical contact to the armouring or conduit and providing facilities for a secure connection to the internal earth terminal. A typical acceptable gland for armoured cables is shown in Fig. 18.4 and it clamps both the armouring and the outer sheath of the cable to prevent the ingress of moisture which

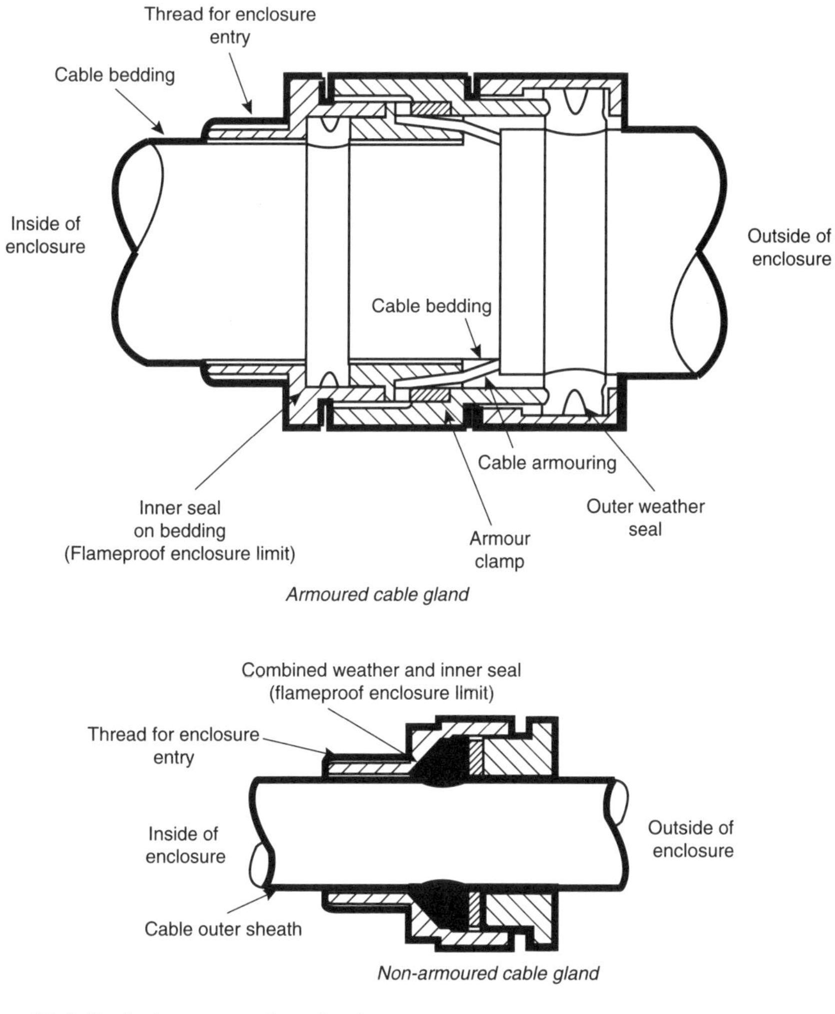

Fig. 18.4 Typical compression glands

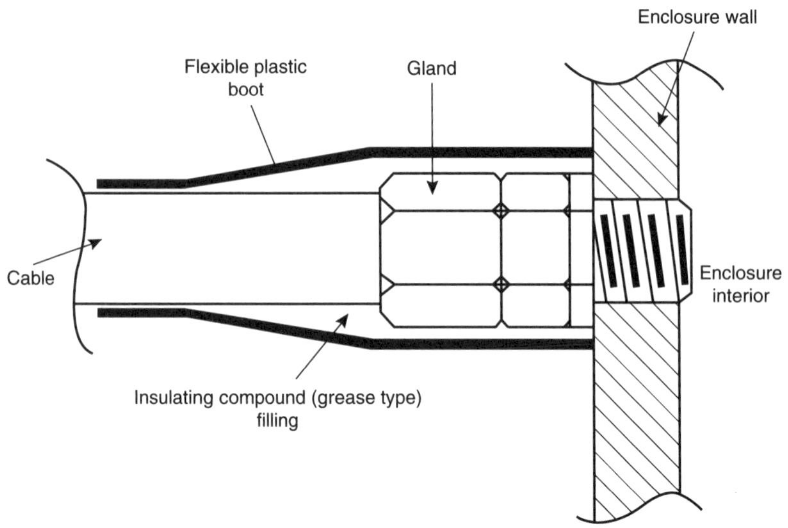

Fig. 18.5 Typical protective gland boot

could cause corrosion and loss of electrical connection. Such glands are often covered with a grease-filled boot (see Fig. 18.5) but, if this is done, regular inspection is necessary to ensure that the grease has not flowed out leaving the boot empty or partially so. If this occurs the boot can have a deleterious effect in harbouring moisture and aiding corrosion.

3. The gland or termination method used should be connected to the metalwork in question if it is fitted through a clearance hole by using a serrated conducting washer and eyelet tag on the rear of the fixing from which a conductor of the requisite size should be fed to the internal earth terminal (see Fig. 18.6.) Only in cases where the gland or conduit is screwed into the enclosure wall with more than five threads engaged can the connection between the gland and enclosure be considered as satisfactory without these additional precautions and, even in such cases, the additional lead may be necessary if the installed environment is particularly hostile such as in the offshore situation.

In addition, all exposed metalwork on apparatus such as enclosures and the like needs to be firmly and reliably connected to the local exposed structural and other non-electrical conducting materials such as steelwork, etc. From previous chapters it will be remembered that apparatus is required to have both an internal and an external earth connection facility and this is the reason for the external facility. Concern in respect of hazardous areas is that, if the local metalwork, such as structural steelwork, adopts a voltage significantly different to the enclosure of apparatus which is connected to the potential equalization or protective conductor, any event such as intervention of personnel or connection of the two by accidental conducting items could cause an incendive arc or spark.

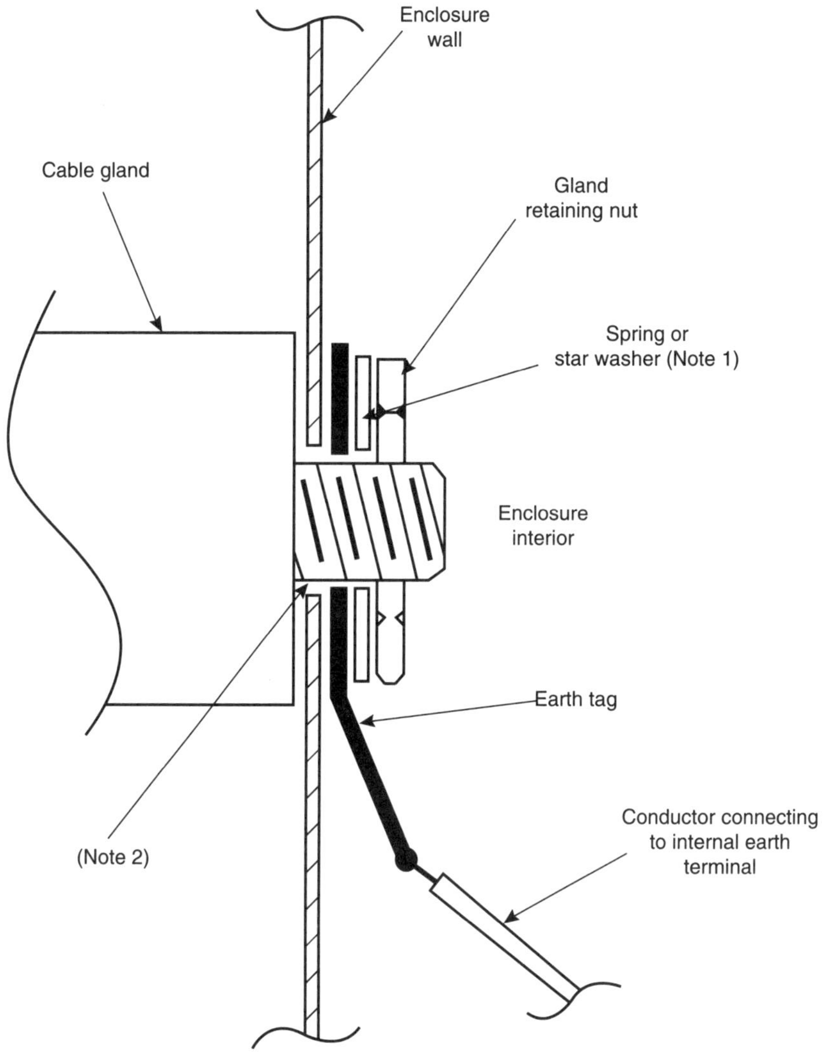

Fig. 18.6 Using armouring as PE connection to internal earth terminal. *Notes*: (1) Where the weather sealing necessitates a sealing washer between the gland and outer enclosure wall or where the enclosure is plastic, a spring washer is always necessary to allow for resilience and cold flow. (2) Where gland is screwed into metal enclosure and 5 or more threads are engaged, the conductor connection to internal earth terminal may not be necessary

By connection of all metalwork or other conducting materials which may adopt different potentials to apparatus enclosures, which are in their turn connected to the potential equalization system, significant differential potentials are minimized. While the mere bolting of apparatus to structural metalwork may satisfy this requirement it is not felt to be sufficient in general, and a deliberate wire connection between the external earth terminal of the apparatus and local conducting parts is felt to be the normal minimum requirement. This poses problems because of the nature of conductors, for example, local steelwork and it is necessary to ensure, by use of serrated washers or similar components which bite into the structural metalwork, that a good connection exists (see Fig. 18.7).

In addition, all steelwork and other conducting parts of a plant or building should be firmly bonded together to prevent any discharges between separate conducting parts of the construction.

18.3.7 Electrical isolation

As already specified in Chapter 17, all installations in hazardous areas need quick-acting isolation which protects against overload, short circuit and earth fault. All protective devices must be 'quick acting' in that no in-built delay is acceptable as this could prolong incendive sparking in case of fault and significantly increase the risk of ignition. This requirement is particularly important in Zone 0 or 20 where the explosive atmosphere is always assumed to be present.

Normal fuses and circuit breakers (which will operate within 20–30 milliseconds with faults at prospective currents of 20 times their rating

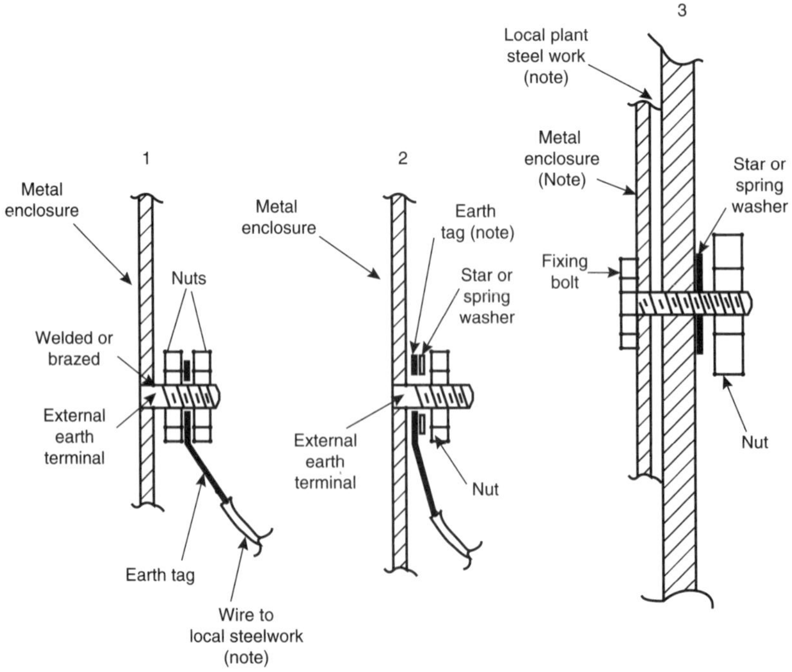

Fig. 18.7 Typical methods of local bonding. *Note*: Where connection is made using enclosure outer surface and/or local steel work, (2 and 3) surfaces should be cleaned of paint and corrosion before connection is made

or more) are usually sufficient. Fuses are preferred as, due to the increase in their resistance which occurs during their pre-arcing period, the fault let-through energy is less than with normal circuit breakers. Such devices will normally also operate within two hours at 1.6 times their rated current but will not operate a current significantly less than that even though such currents are above their rating. For this reason the fuse or circuit breaker should be rated as close to the normal apparatus current as possible and the manufacturers will give advice upon the recommended ratings for protective devices for their apparatus.

Because of the fact that the electrical apparatus is installed in explosive atmospheres it is not considered as acceptable to use electrical protection devices which automatically reset as, if a fault is indeed present, the reclosure of such devices would provide an ignition-capable incident.

Apart from the manual means of isolation of apparatus provided in the non-hazardous area to allow isolation for maintenance, etc., emergency switch-off facilities need to be provided for all apparatus located in a given hazardous area (location). The objective of such facilities is to ensure isolation of all electrical supplies to a particular hazardous area in cases of emergency (such as a major release of flammable materials in the case of a catastrophic accident, or to ensure the supply of flammable material is stopped in case of fire in a given area where the driving force for delivery of such fuel is therein and thus cannot be readily accessed). This emergency facility is normally manual but is in the form of an emergency button or switch so that one operation can isolate many items of apparatus. There is an automatic element in that the operation of the emergency switch or button must be recognized by circuits which rapidly operate automatically all of the individual means of isolation for each individual circuit. It is possible that some items of apparatus need to remain powered in such circumstances to, for example, assist in removal of flammable material from the area or to ensure continuity of fire-fighting supplies. In such cases these particular circuits should not be included in the emergency isolation system but have individual emergency isolation facilities.

The location of all emergency isolation facilities should be carefully considered to ensure that they are always accessible and this may mean their installation remote from the particular location or their being repeated at more than one point to ensure access to them is never blocked by the emergency situation which necessitates them.

Rotating machines

In existing codes of practice there are no specific variations on this recommendation in general but in BS/EN 60079[2] a specific variation is included for all rotating machines which cannot withstand their on-load starting current without overheating or becoming faulty. This requirement is that the machine must be fed from a supply which has a protective device which will operate within two hours at currents which exceed the maximum rated operating current on full load by 20 per cent or more.

Rotating machines powered by three-phase supplies are also required by BS/EN 60079–14 and by BS 5345[3] to have electrical protection against loss of a single phase (single phasing) which could cause excessive heating in the machine due to rotational problems.

Transformers

BS/EN 60079[2] also identifies transformers needing to be provided with overload protection similar to that provided for rotating machines unless the transformer can itself withstand a short circuit of its secondary winding without exceeding the temperature rating of its insulation, in which case the more normal level of protection is admissible. Overload of transformers can also be ignored if the installation is such that overload due to external loads is not considered possible.

18.3.8 Conduit and cable installation

The possibility of cables or conduits providing means of transmission of flammable materials between hazardous areas of different severity, and hazardous areas and non-hazardous areas needs to be considered.

In the case of conduits, because of the open interior of the conduit, this must always be considered as a possibility and a suitable sealing 'stopper'

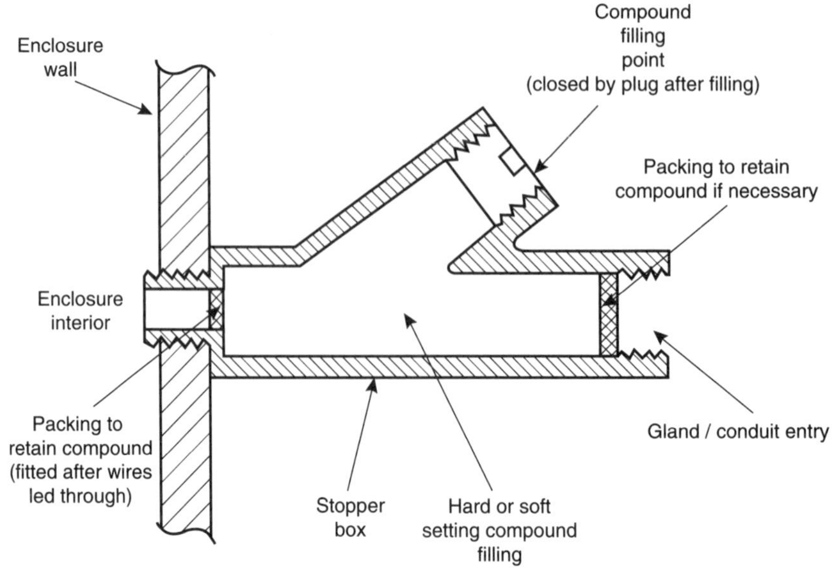

Fig. 18.8 Stopper box

box needs to be fitted to conduit installations in such cases at boundary points (see Fig. 18.8) wherever conduit is used. Cables offer more resistance to such fluid transmission and normally need no such stopping element if no significant pressure exists between the ends of the cable. Where a significant pressure may exist, for example, when a cable is terminated in apparatus into which flammable material under pressure is also fed and there is a possibility of leakage of this material pressurizing the enclosure, consideration must be given to interstice transmission. In such cases an extruded bedded cable with solid non-hygroscopic fillers which enters via a compression gland will usually provide sufficient sealing, but a tape bedded cable or one with no fillers or hollow fillers may not. In this latter case sufficient sealing can normally be achieved by utilization of sealing compound at the cable branching point which is normally the interior exit of the gland (see Fig. 18.9). A sealing type gland as used in flameproof enclosures (see later in this chapter) may also be used for this purpose.

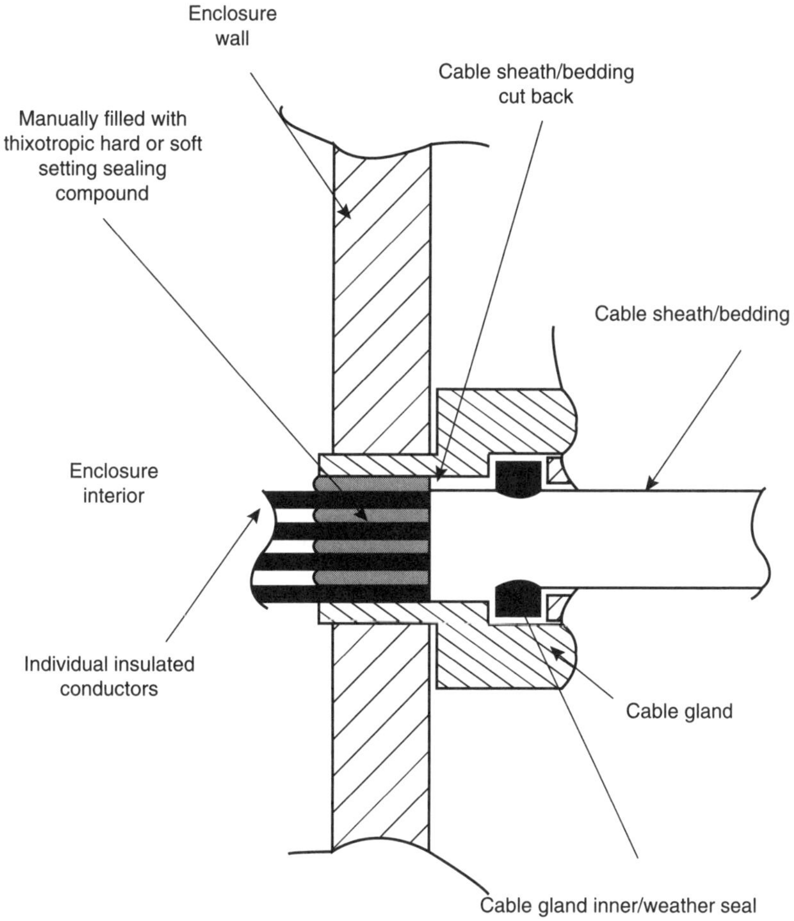

Fig. 18.9 Fluid transmission prevention with compound

In addition, the passage of cables or conduits may introduce possible routes for transmission of flammables from one area to another through walls, etc., which separate different areas of risk. Conduits may be sealed into walls by normal cementing as they are rigid and can form part of the rigid wall structure. This is not the case in respect of cables which are more flexible. The easiest method of dealing with this problem in the case of walls is by the use of a sandbox (see Fig. 18.10) through which cables may pass without the risk of flammable passage also. These have the advantage of a very high level of flexibility allowing for additional installations and modifications without change. Gland plates using the outer parts of compression glands (see Fig. 18.11) are also acceptable but they must take account of cold flow which can, in the case of some insulation, be a problem, and they may be less flexible.

Where cables or conduits traverse between different areas in trenches the most effective way of prevention of transmission is by filling the trench with sand, but here the sand bar must be long enough to give confidence of sealing or have some sand retention arrangements (see Fig. 18.12) as there is the possibility of sand migration.

There is also the problem of accidental connection between cable armouring or conduits with extraneous constructional metalwork such as cable trays, etc. In the case of a conduit, which is rigid, this is not a problem and provided care is taken to ensure the quality of bonding at each fixing point (e.g., where the conduit is supported by a saddle) and the conduit does not come into accidental contact with other metalwork at other than fixing points after installation, no further action is necessary. Where there is armouring, screening, and a flexible conduit this is not, however, the case and precautions need to be taken to prevent accidental connection. An overall insulating sheath will be sufficient, for permanently installed cables and flexible conduits where no unusually high level of mechanical

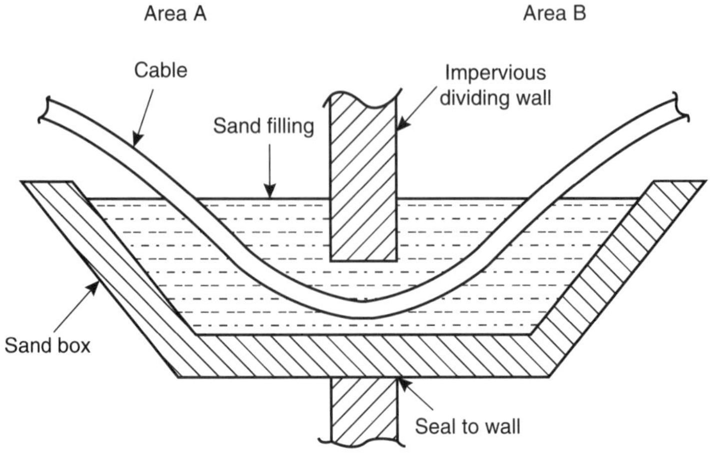

Fig. 18.10 Typical sandbox separation of areas

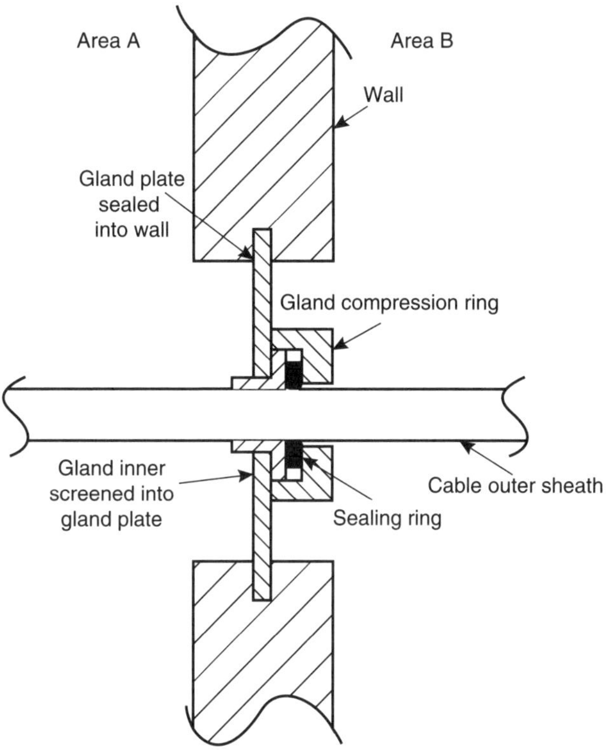

Fig. 18.11 Area segregation using gland plates

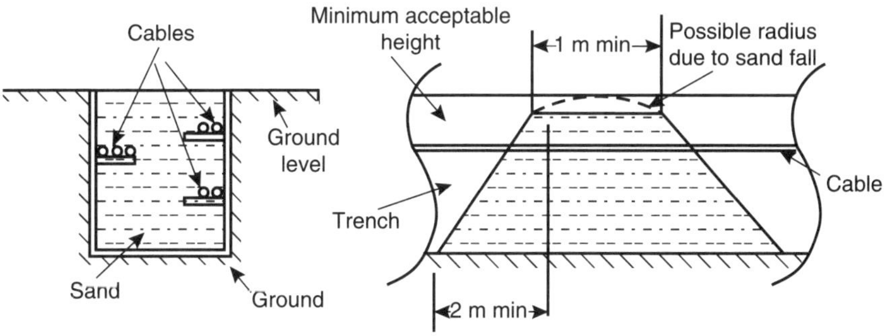

Fig. 18.12 Typical sand barrier in trench

or environmental danger is present but where risk of damage is high, additional protection may be needed for the cable or flexible conduit.

Joints in conductors of cables or those in conduits should be avoided as far as possible, but where they are necessary they should be executed in an appropriately protected junction box or encapsulating type of connection device by compression connectors, screw connectors, welding or brazing, and there should be no mechanical stresses on the terminated conductors. Soldering is also acceptable provided the conductors themselves are mechanically secured together by a means other than the solder which then only has the effect of providing the necessary electrical connection.

18.4 Additional requirements or relaxations for particular protection concepts

There are other considerations which need to be taken into account for particular protection concepts which may take the form of additional recommendations as in the case of increased safety apparatus 'e', or relaxations as in the case of type of protection 'N' ('n'). These are discussed in this section of Chapter 18 with the exception of pressurization 'p' which is widely used for rooms and analyser houses and is thus dealt with in Chapter 19, and intrinsic safety 'i' which is very different in that it works by energy limitation instead of circuit protection and is dealt with in Chapter 20.

18.4.1 Flameproof electrical apparatus 'd'

Flameproof electrical apparatus installation is currently covered in BS 5345 part 3[3] but this is now being replaced with BS/EN 60079[2]. Because of its particular method of operation there are specific additional recommendations including those concerning weatherproofing, cabling and glanding, and siting which need to be observed.

Entry devices

Where flameproof enclosures are connected via conduit systems these systems need to comply with the requirements already stated in this chapter. In addition, flexible conduit systems should not be used in Zone 0 or 1, and the use of any conduit systems in outdoor areas should be minimized because of the effect of normal outdoor environmental conditions on the conduit and its joints. To further provide security all conduit couplers should be screwed couplers (running couplers should not be used), and parallel threaded couplings and terminations should be fitted with locking nuts to ensure security. The fact that the conduits can also transmit any ignition within a flameproof enclosure requires the use of a stopper box (such as that described in Fig. 18.8) at each entry into a the enclosure, and must be no more than 4.5 cms from the entry point to prevent flame transmission.

BS 31,[5] BS 4568[6] and IEC 614[7] give additional information on the types of conduit and conduit fittings appropriate.

Where entry is via cables the situation is more complex as the type of cable is important and the following should be considered. First, the termination of mineral insulated cables usually includes the use of a compound-filled termination device through which only the individual cores of the cable protrude (see Fig. 18.13). This gland provides the necessary stopping action between the enclosure and the cable but, in its entry into the enclosure, the normal flamepaths need to be observed. Fig. 18.13 shows the possible flamepaths in a normal mineral insulated cable gland which must comply with the flameproof requirements (see Chapter 10), and glands for this use normally require certification or approval (as does the apparatus itself).

Second, where thermoplastic or elastomeric cables with extruded bedding and solid non-hygroscopic fillers are used, so that when the cable is compressed it forms an effectively solid cross-section, then normal compression glands can be fitted provided their threads and general

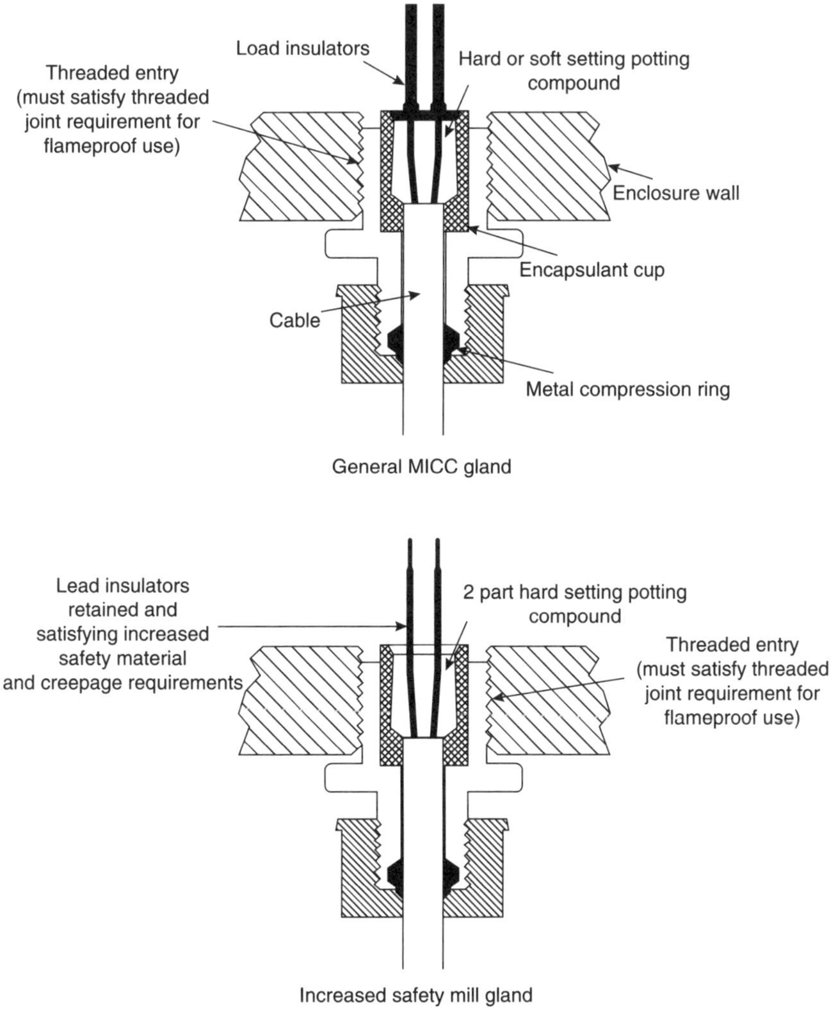

Fig. 18.13 Glands for mineral insulated cables

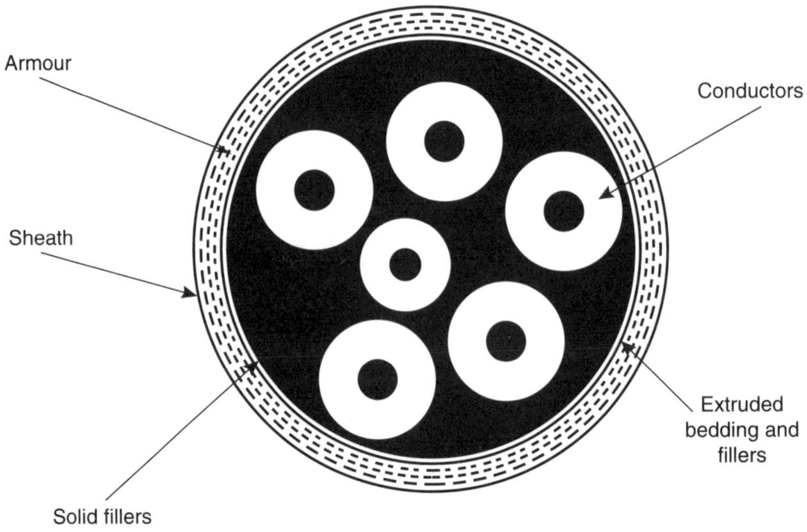

Fig. 18.14 Extruded bedded cable

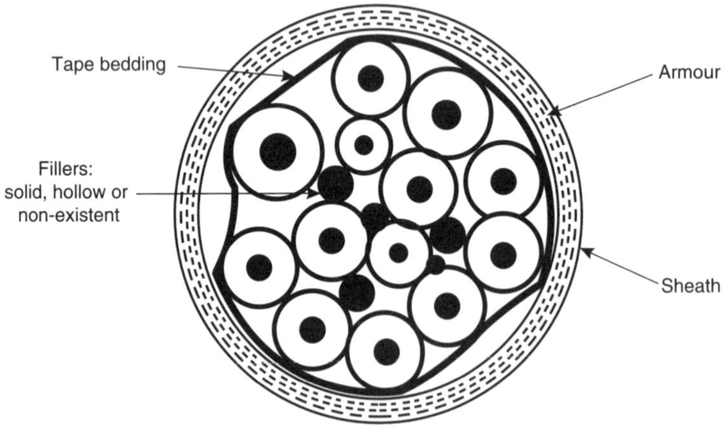

Fig. 18.15 Tape bedded cable

assembly satisfy the requirements for flamepaths in Chapter 10. A typical gland is shown in Fig. 18.4 and a typical cable in Fig. 18.14.

Third, for other cables (such as tape bedded cables – see Fig. 18.15) it must be assumed that there is the possibility of flame transmission down the cable which would negate the effectiveness of the enclosure and this must be prevented. A gland using a compound seal is shown in Fig. 18.16.

The foregoing information on the choice of cable terminations for cables in flameproof enclosures is synopsized in Table 18.1.

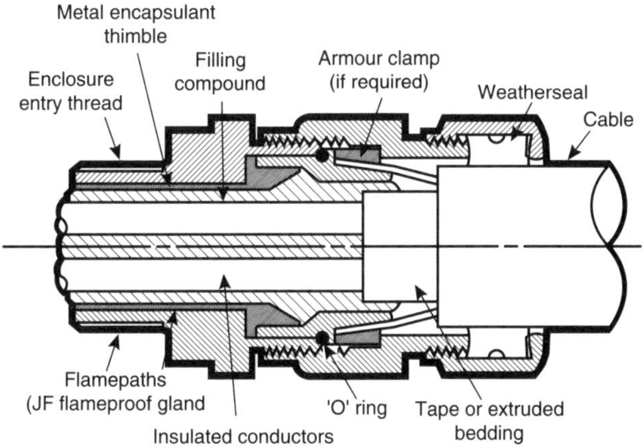

Fig. 18.16 Typical compound filled gland

Table 18.1 Choice of termination glands for cables used in flameproof enclosures

Is the apparatus certified with integral entry devices?	Yes	No	No	No	No	No	No	No
Is the cable mineral insulated?	N/A	Yes	No	No	No	No	No	No
Is the cable extruded bedded with non-hygroscopic fillers?	N/A	N/A	No	Yes	Yes	Yes	Yes	Yes
Does the enclosure contain an ignition source?	N/A	N/A	N/A	Yes	Yes	No	Yes	Yes
Is the risk associated with sub-group IIC	N/A	N/A	N/A	Yes	No	N/A	No	No
Is installation in Zone 1 (not Zone 2)?	N/A	N/A	N/A	N/A	Yes	N/A	No	Yes
Is the enclosure free volume greater than two litres?	N/A	N/A	N/A	N/A	Yes	N/A	N/A	No
SOLUTION	A	B	C	C	C	D	D	D

Notes:

A Use the cable specified in the apparatus certification or approval as appropriate for such use and no other.

B Use glands for mineral insulated cable which have also been certified or approved for use with flameproof enclosures. (mineral insulated cable has solid interstices by its very construction.)

C Use a compound-filled stopper box (Fig. 18.8) or a certified or approved flameproof gland containing a compound seal (Fig. 18.16).

D Use a certified or approved flameproof compression gland (see Fig. 18.4).

Siting/obstructions

The siting of flameproof enclosures is especially important from the point of view of the performance of the flamepaths in the case of an internal ignition. Experiments have shown that if an external obstruction is placed in close proximity to a flamepath it disturbs the flame profile and can cause flame transmission into the external atmosphere in extreme circumstances. To avoid this it is necessary to ensure that no obstructions are in the proximity of flamepaths after installation (e.g., metal supports, other enclosures, cable trays, etc.). The minimum distances which such obstructions must achieve as separation from the outer flamepath edge (including the plane part of spigot joints) is given in Table 18.2 and care should be taken to achieve these in all cases.

Table 18.2 Minimum separation between outer edge of flameproof enclosure flamepath assembly and any external solid obstruction

Apparatus sub-group to which the enclosure is certified	Minimum distance from flamepath to external obstruction (mm)
IIA	10
IIB	30
IIC	40

(from BS/EN 50018)

It is not necessary to take account of any obstructions which form a part of the enclosure itself as these will already have been considered in the testing process associated with certification or approval.

Weatherproofing

By their very nature, flamepaths cannot have gaskets within them and thus any weatherproofing needs to be outside the flamepath. In the case of spigot joints the fitting of gaskets outside the flamepath in the plane part of the joint is usually provided for and covered by enclosure certification or approval. For plane flanged joints, etc., however, it is not so easy to ensure weatherproofing and, although this is sometimes achieved by the use of an 'o' ring in a recess outside the joint but in the flange itself, this is not a popular approach as it requires considerable care in closing the joint because if the ring is not correctly seated it can cause the final gap in the flamepath to be enlarged. Because of this most available flanged enclosures have no deliberate weatherproofing by design and it is necessary to apply this on site where necessary. There are two ways to do this.

Applying grease to the faces of the flanges prior to closing the joint can produce the necessary weatherproofing with relative ease but such greases can adversely affect the flameproof properties by preventing full closure of the joint, resulting in enlarged gaps through which flame could pass. Thus any grease used must flow relatively freely to ensure this does not happen. Free flow of this type is contrary to the longevity of the weatherproofing provided as the grease will migrate over time. A compromise is necessary to accept a grease which is fluid enough not to adversely affect the flamepath dimensions and yet viscous enough not to migrate at too high a rate. This has led to the acceptance of certain greases as suitable and the principal ones currently used are:

Any light petroleum grease
Any silicon grease
Hylomar (Marston Lubricants)
Moly-Paul (Anti-seize compound – K. S. Paul)
Kopr Cote (Jet Lube)
Coppergrease (Chemodex Products)
TS–6 Plastic Jointing Compound (Vecom)
Ensis Compound 356 (Shell)

Many of these greases and compounds particularly those with trade names identified by a manufacturers name in brackets, have been tested to demonstrate their suitability. However, the use of greases will require specific regular inspection to ensure migration has not occurred if the weatherproofing is necessary for operation, as it will be also for flameproof purposes.

A further, and older, technique is to tape the flanges with a suitable non-setting tape such as Denso tape. The problem here is that in doing this an obstruction is being introduced the outer edge of the flamepath and this can, as already mentioned, cause problems. Experimentation has, however, shown that it is acceptable to tape in certain circumstances with appropriate tape, provided that the tape consists of only one layer with around 2.5 mm minimum overlap to prevent jetting at the tape join and that this tape is evenly applied. In these circumstances the following situations are acceptable as, even though the taping decreases the safety factor of the gap against flame transmission, some safety factor still exists and thus the action of taping as described above is generally acceptable providing no special factors exist and the following limitations are applied to any taping activity:

IIC enclosures

No taping is permitted under any circumstances as taping applied as specified has been shown to produce a situation where flame transmission can occur.

IIB enclosures

Taping as described above is acceptable provided the design maximum design gap of the enclosure is less than 0.1 mm. (This is approximately half of the maximum gap permitted for IIB enclosures – see Chapter 10).

IIA enclosures

All enclosures used in areas associated with sub-group IIA including those certified for use in sub-groups IIB and IIC may be taped as described above. IIC enclosures used in areas where the risk is associated with sub-group IIB are also acceptable in these circumstances.

Apparatus to mixed standards

In the UK there is a long history of the use of flameproof enclosure, and apparatus to four Standards is still available (BS 229[8], BS 4683, Part 2[9], BS 5501, Part 5[10] and BS/EN 50018[14]). While the requirements of BS 5501 Part 5 and BS/EN 50018 do not vary greatly in principle there are some differences and, in the case of the older standards, the differences are even greater. The basic principal differences associated with installation are as follows:

BS 229[8]

This Standard did not permit 'direct' entry and so cable/conductor terminations were always made in terminal boxes. Thus termination in enclosures with normally sparking contacts or hot surfaces did not occur and did not have to be allowed for. In its later modifications the Standard did, permit threaded entries (a procedure not permitted in earlier apparatus which required a special entry with a cylindrical flamepath). The length of threads was, considerably greater than is the case with modern apparatus, which means that the normal glands used for current Standards are not acceptable. A comparison is given in Table 18.3. In addition, no temperature classification was given in certification or approval documents for these enclosures and so installation requires consideration of maximum surface temperatures.

BS 4683 Part 3[9]

This Standard did accept direct entry and so the requirements given in Table 18.1 apply. In addition, the requirements for thread engagement for glands and conduit differ from those currently used and current glands may not be suitable. A comparison of requirements is given in Table 18.3.

Although flameproof apparatus to the older Standards is still acceptable in many circumstances, it must be remembered that they are unique to the UK and only apparatus to BS 5501 Part 5[10] and BS/EN 50018[14] are

Table 18.3 Required thread engagement for cable and conduit entries

Type of enclosure	Thread engagement					
	Length (mm)			Number of threads		
(See Notes 1, 2, 3 and 4)	BS 229	BS 4683	BS 5501 BS/EN 50018	BS 229	BS 4683	BS 5501 BS/EN 50018
IIA enclosures with free volume <100 cm^3	18	8.0	5	N/S	5	5
IIA enclosures with free volume >100 cm^3	18	8.0	8	N/S	5	5
IIB enclosures with free volume <100 cm^3	18	8.0	5	N/S	5	5
IIB enclosures with free volume >100 cm^3	18	8.0	8	N/S	5	5
IIC enclosures with free volume <100 cm^3	18	9.5	5	N/S	6	5
IIC enclosures with free volume >100 cm^3	18	12.5	8	N/S	8	5

(The thread engagement specified is the same in the case of conduit or cable entries.)

Notes:

1 In BS 229 no number of engaged threads is specified (N/S) and the figures are valid for both taper and parallel threads. The thread lengths are also only valid for diameters up to 25 mm.

2 Again, in BS 4683, Part 2 the thread lengths and number of engaged threads was the same for both taper and parallel threads.

3 In the case of BS 5501, Part 2 and BS/EN 50018 taper threads were not included in these requirements but instead have their own requirements which are that each half of the joint must have six threads, the cone angles must be the same, the pitch of thread must not exceed 0.9 mm and the thread type must be defined.

acceptable in Europe. This situation is also only temporary as when the latest Directive 94/9/EC[12] becomes effective it will not be legal to market such apparatus. For this reason it is recommended that for all new installations apparatus to BS 5501, Part 5 or BS/EN 50018 be chosen.

Special requirements

Recently it has become more and more common to produce variable speed drive using invertors to provide various frequencies to rotating machines in order to vary their speed. The use of invertors with their less ideal waveform and the effects of frequency on the efficiency of the machine combine to produce a situation where the power dissipation in the machine may exceed that which would occur if it were fed from normal mains supplies. The ideal situation is to have the machine surface temperature classified with its supplies from the intended invertor, thus giving a certified temperature classification applicable to variable speed use. This is not always possible, however, and can be very restrictive in application.

This problem has been addressed in the draft of BS/EN 60079[2] and advantage has been taken of the fact that only the enclosure outer surface is relevant where surface temperature classification is concerned in the case of flameproof apparatus. Accordingly it is noted that if the internal winding temperatures can be monitored by embedded thermal detectors the machine can be isolated if its temperature rises to a level which is likely to cause its surface temperature classification, specified at normal mains frequency, to be exceeded. It is, therefore, acceptable to utilize rotating machines that are surface temperature classified at normal mains frequency in variable speed installations, provided that they are fitted with such thermal detectors and have control systems which switch off the machine if internal temperature rises to a level which may cause the external surface temperature to rise unacceptably. It should be noted that the approach is only applicable to the flameproof elements of the machine and if, for example, it has an increased safety 'e' terminal box (a common combination) that must be dealt with as for other increased safety apparatus because voltage spikes are also a feature of many invertors and these must not damage the insulation of the terminal box nor cause heating within it due to their presence.

18.4.2 Increased safety apparatus 'e'

The installation and maintenance of increased safety apparatus is currently dealt with in BS 5345, Part 6[1] but this Code of Practice will soon be replaced by BS/EN 60079. Because this protection concept relies on the operation of the apparatus as designed and the absence of faults, its installation and operation is subject to particular limitations particularly in the case of rotating machines.

Enclosure integrity

This type of protection depends to a large degree on the integrity of its enclosure being sufficient for the environment in which it is installed as, if moisture, solids or solvents enter, for example, they could damage or by-pass insulation and cause incendive sparking or surfaces to become hotter than envisaged by the certification/approval. Thus great care should be taken in installation to ensure that in normal cases the location is not more onerous than one affected by the normal environment. Places where hosing down may be necessary, where solvents or moisture can fall on the enclosure (the latter more onerously than would be the case in a rainstorm) or where a build-up of solids such as dust can occur, should be avoided unless the enclosure of the apparatus has a degree of protection appropriate – higher than IP54. In this context some increased safety apparatus has an enclosure of less protection than IP54 (or IP44 for wholly insulated conductors). Such apparatus is identified by special marking. Typical of such apparatus are increased safety rotating machines for use indoors in clean environments. Where these are used the environment must be carefully monitored to ensure that it remains clean and no build-up of such things as dust occur at the location.

It is also important to ensure that entry devices maintain the integrity of the enclosure and to this end cable glands and conduit entries will normally be fitted with a plastic or elastomeric washer to maintain the rating of the enclosure. A thread alone will often achieve this requirement if it complies with the advice given in Chapter 17 but, as there is no problem such as could occur with washers reducing thread engagement in flameproof enclosures, the use of a washer is probably the easiest way of achievement of enclosure integrity and does not require the careful monitoring of thread engagement.

Termination

Termination is also important as terminations must, in the case of increased safety, be effectively non-sparking. It is essential to ensure that conductors are properly terminated and, in particular, that more than one conductor is not terminated in a terminal not intended to terminate more than one conductor. Most terminals used are only intended to terminate one conductor and thus the effective way to do this is to only design for one conductor to be terminated in one terminal, and to treat multi-conductor terminations as abnormal and needing special consideration.

Rotating machines

As previously stated (see Chapter 12) rotating machines need special attention to ensure that they do not exceed their surface temperature classification or the maximum safe operating temperature of their stator insulation during starting or in such situations as locked rotor conditions which may occur if the equipment which they drive siezes. The hottest part of an increased safety machine is normally (although not always) its rotor which reaches a higher temperature than its stator (these are called rotor sensitive machines). In a few unusual circumstances this may not be so and the machine in such circumstances is called a stator sensitive machine. Such machines are, however, unusual. In addition, the performance of increased safety machines is inferior to their industrial counterparts because constructional requirements (e.g., the running stator/rotor clearances required to give the necessary low likelihood of stator/rotor clashes) mean that the machine will have greater losses, generate more heat, and be less efficient.

In general a rotor temperature of more than 300 °C is not permissible for an increased safety machine because the rotor stability will deteriorate above this temperature. Therefore, in practice most increased safety motors will have a temperature classification of T2 or better. In addition the temperature limitations on such motors will have further limitations because of the limit on operating temperature of the stator insulation which is generally imposed by the temperature class of the insulation. This must not be exceeded as the insulation would deteriorate at higher temperatures causing fault liability to increase unacceptably. The limiting temperatures for the various grades of insulation are higher during the protection operating period in the shut-down cycle than in normal operation and Table 18.4 shows this relationship.

Table 18.4 Permissible maximum temperature rises for winding insulation in rotating machines

	Class of insulating material				
	A	E	B	F	H
Limiting temperature					
– rated service	90 °C	105 °C	110 °C	130 °C	155 °C
– during shut-down	160 °C	175 °C	185 °C	210 °C	235 °C
Limiting temperature rise (40 °C ambient)					
– Rated service	50 °C	65 °C	70 °C	90 °C	115 °C
– During shut-down	120 °C	135 °C	145 °C	170 °C	195 °C

Notes:
1 These winding temperatures are measured by the winding resistance method and will be higher than those which might be found using a thermometer which will not be as accurate.
2 The temperature rise figures given are based upon the motor operating at the normal maximum ambient temperature of 40 °C. If the motor is used in higher ambients the temperature rise tolerable will be less (e.g., for class A insulation at a maximum ambient of 60 °C the permissible temperature rise will be reduced to 30 °C during normal service and 100 °C during shut-down.

The protection devices for the machine must therefore ensure that the machine is isolated from its electrical supplies before: the maximum operating temperature of its rotor is exceeded (normally 300 °C); and the maximum operating temperature of its stator insulation in the shut-down condition is exceeded (see Table 18.4); and before any part of the machine exceeds the maximum temperature permitted for its surface temperature classification (normally 5 °C less than the class limit as nearly all machines will be T3 or better, but where the stator can actually reach 300 °C, 10 °C as the resultant surface temperature classification will be T2).

Table 18.4 indicates the maximum temperature which insulation may reach in the machine stator during shut-down conditions, and if the stator is the limiting feature this will mean a surface temperature classification of T4 for insulation classes A, E and B, but T3 for insulation classes F and H. In these cases, care is necessary to ensure that the motor protection clears the machine from the supply before the limiting temperature (not the surface temperature classification maximum) is reached because if the machine temperature exceeds this the reliability is prejudiced and ignition-capable faults become unacceptably likely. This is also true of normal operation where the continuous operating temperature of the machine stator must not exceed the maximum specified in Table 18.4.

The majority of machines, particularly of the smaller type widely used in industry, do not have embedded thermal detectors in their stators and instead are given a t_e time by the manufacturer. This will define the time taken for the machine to reach its limiting temperature when fed with its starting current with a locked rotor. This takes the form of a curve showing the maximum permissible t_e time for varying ratios of starting current (I_a) to maximum on-load operating current (I_n) (see Fig. 18.17) and allows the user to ensure that the protection mechanisms satisfy this curve by isolating the electrical supplies to the machine before these internal temperatures are reached. All of the internal temperatures in the machine will have been taken into account in the determination of t_e time.

Machines which utilize this function to control isolation are normally protected by using inverse time delay protective devices matched to the t_e time so that disconnection will occur before the defined t_e time specified in the curve for the I_a/I_n ratio achieved in the particular installation.

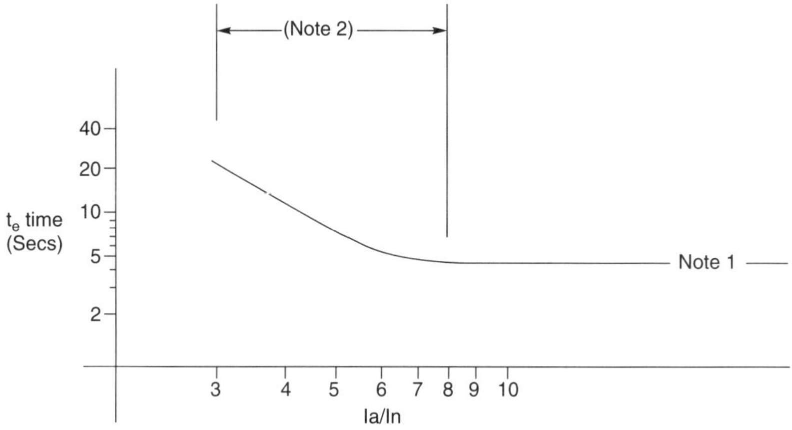

Fig. 18.17 Typical t_e time curve. *Notes*: (1) t_e times of less than 5_S are not permitted. Thus Ia/In of >8 is not permitted. (2) Normal range of t_e quotation is Ia/In ratio of 3–8

The protective devices for this use normally take the form of inverse time delay overload protective devices which are required to clear in time frames defined earlier in this chapter (i.e., while not operating within two hours at an overload current of 105 per cent they must operate within two hours at overload currents in excess of 120 per cent). In addition, these devices, when used for increased safety machines, must isolate the machine within the t_e time specified for the starting current achieved in the particular situation. Although the tripping time of such devices will vary in respect of overload current it is recommended that the tripping curve is essentially asymptotic as near above 105 per cent maximum operating current (full load current) as possible, giving tripping times close to the t_e time in all such circumstances.

Overload protection devices which have nominal tripping times of 80 per cent of the t_e time should be chosen to allow for tolerances and drifts which occur in service.

Overload protection devices should monitor all three phases of a three-phase machine and protect against single phasing (where one phase of the machine becomes open circuit) as, although in the case of star-connected stators the machine will stop, the current which then flows will in total be less than if all three phases were connected, which could otherwise cause tripping problems. There is a particular problem with delta-connected three-phase machines in this regard in that, if one-phase open circuits, the machine may continue to rotate and may even be restarted unlike the situation in the case of its star-connected counterpart. To overcome this and ensure that the machine is isolated before limiting temperatures are reached in phase-failure conditions in delta-connected machines (single phasing) it is normally sufficient to additionally ensure that the protection device will clear within the t_e time produced by a current ratio using a figure of 0.87 I_a instead of I_a itself. Again a nominal figure of 80 per cent should be used for device selection.

The foregoing assumes that the machine is at maximum permissible operating temperature when the overload or failure occurs, and the overload protection is in the condition which would occur if those machine operating conditions existed. Thus If a previous failure had occurred and the machine had not had sufficient time to cool to the maximum permissible operating temperature before being restarted, this type of protection device may not afford the necessary protection. In such cases this type of motor protection is not acceptable and machines installed where this situation occurs by necessity or accidentally should not be protected in this way. They should have embedded temperature sensors in the stator so that isolation is controlled by temperature rise and occurs before the stator temperature rises to a value which would mean that the motor exceeded its temperature classification, or the maximum operating temperature values for its stator or rotor. These devices are normally thermistors.

All machines consume larger currents than their full load operating current during starting and there is the possibility of tripping during starting if the starting time is too long. There is normally no problem if the starting time is shorter than the t_e time and, in most cases, where it is shorter than 1.7 times the t_e time. This is because the machine is cold when it starts and more heating is necessary. In addition, the current falls as speed increases and this produces a longer tripping time from cold for the protective device. If, however, the starting time exceeds the t_e time by more than 1.7 it will again be necessary, in winding, to use temperature sensors to control tripping so that starting can be achieved.

In general terms, where arduous (on full load) starting or duty cycling are the norm, it is always preferable in winding to use temperature sensors to control tripping in preference to devices which utilize t_e time.

Increased safety machines are sometimes fed from invertor devices to allow variable speed operation. Unlike flameproof motors, safety in this case is achieved by the control of such things as temperatures in the motors themselves, and because the waveforms of invertors vary giving variable heat dissipation in the machine, safety can only be guaranteed if the performance of the combination of motor and invertor is known. Thus increased safety machines can only be used with invertors with which they have been tested as a combination and shown to satisfy increased safety requirements.

18.4.3 Type 'N' apparatus

Such installations are covered in BS 5345, Part 7[3]. Because of the lower risk of the presence of an explosive atmosphere, installation requirements are less onerous than those for other protection concepts and are essentially those which would be required for a normal industrial situation. Attention needs to be paid, however, to location and termination of cables to minimize the risk of sparking due to damage or poor jointing procedures, and care needs to be taken to ensure that enclosure integrity is maintained after entry of cables via glands and conduits.

18.4.4 Other types of protection

Installation of other types of protected apparatus is covered in other parts of BS 5345 and, for dusts, in BS 6467[4]. There are few variations from general installation requirements but those Standards should be consulted in all cases.

18.4.5 Particular problems

In some cases there is a need to maintain electrical apparatus in operation as to isolate it would lead directly or indirectly to a non-electrical danger, such as a poisoning risk or catastrophe. In such circumstances it may be argued that disconnection could not be permitted even if apparatus protection failed. This is a difficult problem to address as by leaving the apparatus energized one is merely substituting one risk for another. The design of the process should ensure that such an eventuality does not occur as the danger of a major explosion (such as that occurring at Flixborough) is just as unacceptable as is the risk of a major release of a toxic chemical. The problem should be approached from the following direction.

Zone 0 and 20

There is no circumstance where it can be justified to leave energized an electrical installation which has become ignition capable. This is normally not a problem as only intrinsic safety is used in Zone 0 and 20 but it may be relevant in some special circumstances.

Zone 1 and 21

There is a reduced risk of the presence of an explosive atmosphere and, as a result, it may be possible to relax the approach. It is still not acceptable to have protected apparatus remain energized after it becomes ignition capable if the release of explosive atmosphere is a result of the same malfunction, but if the two are separate it is possible to leave the apparatus operational if an immediate alarm is sounded and there is a clearly detailed action plan to remove the hazardous material and then isolate the apparatus immediately on such an alarm. This approach is still of lower integrity than normally acceptable and can only be invoked where design cannot preclude such a situation, and where the operation can be fully justified even in these circumstances. Commercial justification alone is not expected to be sufficient.

Zone 2 and 22

The approach here should be the same as in Zone 1 and 21.

18.5 Heating tapes

Heating tapes (electrical conductors which are used for resistance heating) and cartridge heaters are used widely in areas where explosive atmospheres may occur. These devices are required to have a type of protection appropriate to the area in which they are installed. The requirements for design of electrical heating units/cables their system design and installation are given in BS 6351[13] and this Standard should be read in detail before any electric heating is installed. As far as hazardous areas are concerned the following recommendations will ensure a suitable installation (taken together with BS 6351[13]).

1. All heating devices should be selected as having a protection concept appropriate to their Zone of risk in accordance with BS 5345[3] or BS 6467[4] to ensure that they are suitable for the risk of explosion involved.

2. Cartridge heaters, such as those used in electrical machines, and similar devices to prevent condensation should form part of the apparatus itself or, if this is not possible, should not adversely affect the protection of such apparatus. Special care is necessary in respect of electrical isolation for maintenance to ensure the heater is isolated in addition to the apparatus, particularly as the heater may be required to be energized when the apparatus is not in use.

3. No electrical surface heating should be applied in Zone 0 or 20.

4. Where electrical surface heating of any type is used in hazardous areas it should be temperature classified, taking account of the maximum temperature required to be reached by the element which it is heating (e.g., pipe) as the heater will adopt a temperature higher than this.

5. Surface temperature classification should always be guaranteed by over-temperature trips which are separate from any temperature control elements. This is true even with so-called self-limiting heating tapes.

6. Heating cables and tapes should not be fitted to items which are removed regularly for maintenance, and cartridge heaters in position defining jigs should be used in such circumstances where heating is required to ensure that the design conditions can be regularly repeated.

7. Heating cables and tapes used in Zone 1 or 21 should always be metal or braid sheathed to ensure rapid isolation in case of fault, and the metal sheath or braid should be insulated from any uninsulated metalwork as for cable armouring. While such metal or braid covering is not necessary in Zone 2 or 22, earth fault protection should be of the same type as for Zone 1.

8. Heating units and cables in all hazardous areas should be fitted with sensitive earth fault protection which has a rating of at least 300 mA and preferably 30 mA. This protection needs to operate within 5 seconds at its rated operating point (300 mA or 30 mA) but at 0.15 seconds at 5 times this figure. While protective devices of greater than 30 mA operating currents are permitted, the 30 mA figure should be adhered to unless it results in an unacceptable level of nuisance tripping and re-design of the system cannot resolve that problem. Increases in operating current are only acceptable to a level which will remove this problem and in no case may the increase produce levels above 300 mA. It must be recognized that even low current earth faults may produce potentially ignition-capable sparking and thus their current level and duration should be as low as possible with the figures here considered as maxima.

9. In addition to temperature limitation protective devices and earth fault protective devices, heating elements and tapes should always have overcurrent protection by fuses or similar devices whose rated current is as close to the maximum heater or heating tape operating current as possible.

References

1 Directive (6430/92 EN) (draft) — Proposal for a Council Directive Concerning Minimum Requirements for Improving the Safety and Health Protection for Workers in Potentially Explosive atmospheres.

2 BS/EN 60079 (96/209563) (draft) — Electrical Apparatus for Explosive Gas Atmospheres. Part 14. Electrical Installations in Explosive Gas Atmospheres (other than mines). (1997)

3 BS 5345 — Selection, Installation and Maintenance of Electrical Apparatus for Use in Potentially Explosive Atmospheres (other than mining applications or explosive processing or manufacture): Part 1 (1989). General Recommendations; Part 3 (1979). Installation and Maintenance Requirements for Electrical Apparatus with Type of Protection 'd'. Flameproof Enclosure; Part 6 (1978). Installation and Maintenance Requirements for Electrical Apparatus with Type of Protection 'e'. Increased Safety; Part 7 (1979). Installation and Maintenance Requirements for Electrical Apparatus with Type of Protection 'n'; Part 8 (1980). Installation and Maintenance Requirements for Electrical Apparatus with Type of Protection 's'. Special Protection.

4 BS 6467 — Electrical Apparatus with Protection By Enclosure for Use in the Presence of Combustible Dusts. Part 2 (1988). Guide to Selection, Installation and Maintenance.

5 BS 31 (1940) — Specification. Steel Conduit and Fittings for Electrical Wiring.

6 BS 4568 — Specification for Steel Conduit and Fittings with Metric Threads of ISO Form for Electrical Installations: Part 1 (1970). Steel Conduit, Bends and Couplers; Part 2 (1970). Fittings Components.

7 IEC 614 — Specification for Conduits for Electrical Installations. Part 2 (1982). Particular

	Specifications for Conduits, Section One, Metal Conduits; Part 5 (1992). Particular Specifications for conduits, Section 5, Flexible Conduits.
8 BS 229 (1957)	Flameproof Enclosure of Electrical Apparatus.
9 BS 4683	Electrical Apparatus for Explosive Atmospheres: Part 1 (1971). Classification of Maximum Surface Temperatures; Part 2 (1971). The Construction and Testing of Flameproof Enclosures of Electrical Apparatus. Part 3 (1972). Type of Protection 'N'; Part 4 (1973). Type of Protection 'e'.
10 BS 5501	Electrical Apparatus for Potentially Explosive Atmospheres. Part 1 (1977). General Requirements. Part 5 (1977). Flameproof Enclosure 'd'.
11 BS/EN 50014 (1993)	Electrical Apparatus for Potentially Explosive Atmospheres. General Requirements.
12 94/9/EC	Directive of the European Parliament and the Council on the Approximation of the Laws of Member States concerning Equipment and Protective Systems Intended for Use in Potentially Explosive Atmospheres.
13 BS 6351	Electric surface Heating: Part 1 (1983). Specification for Electric Surface Heating Devices; Part 2 (1983). Guide to the Design of Electric Surface Heating Systems; Part 3 (1983). Code of Practice for the Installation, Testing and Maintenance of Electric Surface Heating Systems.
14 BS/EN 50018 (1995)	Electrical Apparatus for potentially Explosive Atmospheres. Flameproof Enclosures 'd'.

19

Installation of pressurized apparatus and other uses of the pressurization technique

BS 5345, Part 5 (1983)
BS/EN 50016 (1995)
BS/EN 60079-14 (1997)

The technique of pressurization has been in use for almost as long as the classic flameproof enclosure technique but until the advent of European Standards it was always applied in an *ad hoc* manner, being referred to in a Code of Practice but not having detailed requirements as a formal protection concept. This is not surprising as the technique relies upon external intervention by inputting a pressurization medium (inert gas or air) into the apparatus from an external source and monitoring it with external monitors which operate external protective apparatus. Its use was, therefore, mainly for rooms and apparatus where other protection concepts were not possible. While this was a UK view it was not necessarily shared in other countries: the USA, for example, having the technique described in detail in the National Electrical Code[1]. Likewise, in some other countries in Europe the technique was much more formally identified.

When discussions began in CENELEC[2] for the development of the EN 500 range of Standards to cover all of the recognized protection concepts, pressurization was one of the techniques in the list to be discussed. The development of North Sea oil also produced requirements for apparatus for use in hazardous areas which were effectively only solvable economically by pressurization, which added further impetus to the technique, as did the rapid expansion of complex analytical instrumentation following the exploitation of the transistor. These facts led to a recognition that pressurization was a technique which should rank with all of the other formal techniques, such as flameproof enclosure and intrinsic safety. Thus interest quickened in the production of a European Standard for the technique. In addition, a UK entrepreneur recognized the potential of the technique and in exploiting it produced the result that much of the initial practical development and application of the technique was carried out in the UK.

19.1 Standards for pressurization

The first Standard was BS 5501 Part 3 (1977)[3] which was the UK text of EN 50016[4] (the first European Standard on the technique), but this only covered apparatus which neither had any flammable atmosphere deliberately introduced into it, nor any possibility of people inside it. In these circumstances pressurization was normally derived from a compressed air or compressed inert gas source as a matter of convenience, although there was no reason why, if it had it been more convenient, a fan-driven system, using a fan blowing air or gas into an enclosure via a duct, should not have been used (indeed such systems were common for rooms which were outside the scope of the Standard but were pressurized in accordance with BS 5345, Part 5[5]).

The second edition of the European Standard which appeared in the UK as BS/EN 50016 in 1996 partially corrected this in that it included apparatus with flammable material fed into the enclosure so that the technique could be used for such things as analysers. This Standard, however, still does not include enclosures into which people go, whether they have flammable materials piped into them or not.

19.2 Certification/approval

The current situation in respect of pressurization is therefore as follows.

Enclosures without entry of flammables

Apparatus enclosures of such things as switchgear, motors, display units and instruments, and larger enclosures containing several such items may be certified/approved in accordance with BS/EN 50016[4] provided entry of people is not possible. Enclosures such as control rooms, workshops or other large enclosures or buildings, where provision for human access is provided cannot be certified/approved (other than possibly as specially protected 's') as no Standard exists. It should be noted, however, that the UK National Code of Practice, BS 5345, Part 5[5] gives guidance on the application of the technique to such places. The replacement Standard for BS 5345, Part 5 (BS/EN 60079[6]) shortly to be published, limits itself, to pressurized apparatus 'p' and thus to apparatus complying with BS/EN 50016 which does not include this type of room or enclosure.

Enclosures with entry of flammables

Apparatus with flammable entry, such as chromatographs and other analysers, can be certified/approved provided there is no possibility of human entry into the apparatus or, if the apparatus is large enough for such entry, entry is prevented. The appropriate Standard in this case is, again, BS/EN 50016[4]. Buildings and other enclosures with flammable entry, such as analyser houses, laboratories sited in hazardous areas and similar locations where personnel need access, are not covered by any apparatus Standard and thus cannot be certified/approved, except possibly as specially protected 's'. They are, covered in BS 5345, Part 5[5] but its proposed replacement, BS/EN 60079[6] limits itself to pressurized apparatus 'p' and thus to apparatus complying with BS/EN 50016 which excludes this type of building.

19.3 Basic installation approach

All pressurized enclosures, however pressurized, need to be installed taking account of the general installation recommendations given in Chapter 18.

Unpressurized situations

In addition to the general installation requirements it should be noted that such enclosures are sometimes left unpressurized with the electrical circuits inside them de-energized. Thus the overpressure inside the enclosure when it is pressurized cannot be relied on to exclude the external environment as it will not be present at such times. The enclosure needs to have a level of security when no pressurization is present so that such things as moisture and dust are adequately excluded. Even though the internal circuits are isolated once these elements have penetrated the enclosure, they may cause problems when re-energization takes place and adversely affect safety features. This would mean, for example, that an enclosure mounted outdoors would need to be at least IP54 with no pressurization. This integrity need not extend to pressure outlets from the enclosure but they must be designed to prevent ingress of moisture and dust by configuration rather than by enclosure.

Purge and pressurization inlets and outlets need also to be designed so that when there is no pressurization they do not admit an external explosive atmosphere any more readily than the remainder of the enclosure.

These necessities may involve the fitting of flaps over the outlets but it is less likely that attention is required in respect of the inlets because of their configuration (they are normally sealed and only connected to closed ducting or piping).

Electrical isolation

Automatic isolation provisions for use when pressurization fails need to isolate all electrical circuits entering the enclosure, unless those circuits are otherwise made safe for use in explosive atmospheres (e.g., by being intrinsically safe). It should be noted that circuits fed into the enclosure as intrinsically safe may not be so when the pressurized apparatus is energized, and installation must take account of this.

19.4 Pressurization arrangements

There are three principal methods of pressurization: static pressurization; pressurization with leakage compensation; and pressurization with continuous dilution. Tables 19.1 and 19.2 summarize the possible uses of these various pressurization media.

Static pressurization

Static pressurization is only usable where there is no possibility of the release of flammable material within the enclosure (i.e., where any flammable material fed into the enclosure is infallibly contained within a further enclosure within the pressurized enclosure). Static pressurization does not need

Table 19.1 Possible utilization of pressurization with leakage compensation

	No people and no flammable release	People and no flammable release	No people but flammable release	People and flammable release
Compressed air	Yes	No[2]	No	No[2]
Compressed inert gas	Yes	No[1]	Yes	No[1]
Fan-driven air	Yes	No[2]	No	No[2]

Notes:
1 Because of the asphyxiation risk it is not possible to utilize inert gas in respect of any enclosures into which people go.
2 The technique of pressurization with leakage compensation is not acceptable for enclosures into which people go.

Table 19.2 Possible utilization of pressurization with continuous dilution

	No people and no flammable release	People and no flammable release	No people but flammable release	People and flammable release
Compressed air	Yes	N/R[1]	Yes/No[2]	N/R[1]
Compressed inert gas	Yes	No[3]	Yes	No[3]
Fan-driven air	Yes	Yes	Yes/No[2]	Yes/No[2]

Notes:
1 Compressed air is not recommended for any enclosure into which people go.
2 Air in any form is only permissible when the flammable release is controlled so that it can be diluted within the enclosure to below its lower explosive limit.
3 Inert gas is not permitted in enclosures into which people go.

any supply of protective gas in the hazardous area as it is charged in a non-hazardous area and then sealed before being taken into a hazardous area. This type of apparatus is normally charged with protective gas, which must be inert gas, to a pressure such that its pressure loss in service does not create a problem. Its pressurization requirements will be specified in its certification/approval documents but are not directly relevant to its installation. Thus apparatus with static pressurization should be installed in accordance with the general installation requirements in Chapter 18, and its pressure failure sensing devices treated as described Section 19.5.

Pressurization with leakage compensation

Pressurization with leakage compensation using air is normally only possible when there is no release of flammable material within the enclosure and no normal access for personnel. This removes the necessity to have a continuous flow of protective gas through the enclosure. The reason for its prohibition in the case of the presence of personnel is the possibility of the build-up of poisonous or asphyxiant gases within the enclosure if it is not regularly swept with clean air.

Pressurization with leakage compensation using inert gas is acceptable in circumstances where the use of air is acceptable and, in addition, when there is the possibility of release of a flammable material within the enclosure as, although it may not dilute such a release, it removes the oxygen which has a similar effect. Obviously the use of inert gas where people may enter the enclosure is not acceptable.

Pressurization with continuous dilution

Where releases occur within the enclosure the use of pressurization with continuous dilution by air, rather than leakage compensation, is more normally used as it allows for dilution of the flammable atmosphere to below its lower explosive limit within the enclosure and thus prevents ignition or the release of an explosive atmosphere from the enclosure. It is only possible to do this, however, when the release is controlled so that dilution can be assured and where this is not so then recourse has to be made to the use of inert gas. The presence of people is acceptable when the dilution medium is air, subject to the other properties of any release being acceptable for personnel access, but in the case where inert gas is used such access is, of course, not acceptable.

Enclosure overpressure

In all cases the minimum overpressure acceptable to ensure that no flammable materials enter from the surrounding atmosphere is $50\,N/m^2$ and in specific circumstances (e.g., where the enclosure is subjected to high winds with unusual regularity) the minimum required pressure may be higher to ensure security against entry of external atmosphere. In all cases protective devices need to be fitted to identify situations where the pressure falls below the specified minimum level.

An enclosure pressurized from compressed air or with an possible internal release of flammable gas or vapour at high pressure may, in fault conditions, exceed its permissible maximum pressure. This must also be identified by pressure monitoring devices.

Spark arresters

Where pressurization uses continuous flow of protective gas the outlet aperture of the enclosure remains open after the purging period and thus is open when the internal circuits are energized. It is possible that in normal or fault conditions arcs or sparks may be produced in the enclosure and the products of these may exit down the ducting and initiate an ignition. To prevent this spark arresters are sometimes fitted in the exit ducting. The normal approach to these depends upon the zone of installation and the type of assemblies within the pressurized enclosure. Table 19.3 defines the situations where spark arresters are necessary.

Table 19.3 Necessity for fitment of spark arrester on purge exit

Purge exhaust Location (Zone)	Pressurized apparatus producing arcs or sparks in normal service	Pressurized apparatus not producing arcs or sparks in normal service
Non-hazardous area	Spark arrester not required	Spark arrester not required
Zone 2	Fit spark arrester	Spark arrester not required
Zone 1	Fit spark arrester	Fit spark arrester
Zone 0	Not an acceptable area for purge exhaust	Not an acceptable area for purge exhaust

It should be noted that apparatus defined as producing ignition-capable sparks or hot particles in normal operation is not limited to apparatus with type of protection 'N' but also includes any other apparatus which satisfies the requirement, provided it is of normal industrial quality so the faults are at an acceptably low level in common with the acceptance criteria for apparatus other than Type 'N' apparatus in Zone 2 (see BS 5345, Part 1[5]).

19.4.1 Pressurization with leakage compensation using air

Pressurization with leakage compensation using air is not permitted in any situation where flammable material is released either normally or in fault conditions from the enclosed apparatus or its connections. It is also not recommended for use in enclosures where people may enter because of the possibility of a build-up of toxic or asphyxiant gas within the enclosure during service.

Where pressurization with leakage compensation using air is the chosen approach it is usual in small enclosures to utilize compressed air from a plant supply or cylinders. The certification/approval documentation for particular enclosures will identify the minimum flowrate of air and purge time necessary before energization and this must be adhered to as a minimum.

The volume of the inlet piping after the pressure reducing valve (which will need to be fitted if compressed air is used) plus the total volume of any exhaust ducting must be taken into account in the purging cycle and the purge time lengthened to allow for this extra volume. It is normally only necessary to ensure that the purge air volume is that specified by the certification/approval documents for the enclosure plus five times the volume of the ducting and piping (see BS 5345, Part 5). Thus the minimum time allowed for purging needs to be:

$$t_t = t_{enc} + t_p + t_d$$

where t_t = total required purge time
t_{enc} = time specified for purge of the enclosure
t_p = time required to pass five times its volume of air through inlet piping at minimum specified purge rate
t_d = time required to pass five times its volume of air through exhaust ducting at minimum specified purge rate

It is often not necessary to make any allowance for the volume of the air supply pipework when compressed air is used as this is normally very small in comparison with the volume of the enclosure. The criteria applicable in this case is that where five times the volume of the inlet piping is less than 10 per cent of the free volume of the enclosure no addition should normally be necessary. In addition, no allowance is usually made for the high pressure part of the piping as the high pressure is such that, if any gas ingressed during pressure shut-down it would only form a small part of the gas in the pipe when repressurization takes place (for a $10 \times 10^5\,N/m^2$ air supply the gas in the pipe would constitute only around 10 per cent of the mixture in the high pressure piping as it is only likely to enter at atmospheric pressure).

The flammable release at the purge exhaust will only be produced by the flammable material which may have entered from the surrounding atmosphere before the enclosure has been purged, and this will constitute only a small amount of explosive atmosphere (for example, an enclosure which together with its inlet piping and exhaust ducting has a total volume of 5 litres is not likely to produce a hazardous area of a radius of more than 10 cm). The exhaust may therefore be either in the local hazardous area as it will not in such cases affect area classification, or in a non-hazardous area. If it is in a non-hazardous area its siting should be such that the small volume of explosive atmosphere produced during purging is not likely to be ignited by any electrical equipment, and this is normally achieved by siting it at a high level (as is done in petrol stations).

For larger enclosures, such as large rotating machines and instrumentation cabinets, it may be costly to utilize compressed air due to the purge quantities necessary and, in such cases, it is often better to utilize a system where air is fed into the enclosure from a duct which is connected to the exhaust of a fan. This approach has the advantage that, because the pressure generating capability of the pressurization system is low, it is much less likely that an unacceptable overpressure will occur in the enclosure.

In this approach the air drawn into the fan should be from a non-hazardous area which often means that ducting lengths are long and, because of the low pressure involved, large diameter ducting is normally necessary. This gives a ducting volume which will be more significant in relation to the enclosure volume than is usually the case with the use of compressed air. In these circumstances it is likely that the purge airflow required to clear the enclosure (based upon the calculation already described) with the inlet piping volume replaced by the inlet ducting volume (which will be much larger) and thus the purge time will be considerably extended over that which is specified for the enclosure itself.

Where fan-driven systems are used the fan itself may be mounted at the enclosure entry or at the non-hazardous-area end of the ducting. The non-hazardous-area end is the preferred location as this will ensure the ducting is all above atmospheric pressure thus preventing the ingress of flammable material from the hazardous areas through which it passes. If the fan is at the enclosure end of the ducting the converse is true and the ducting will be at less than atmospheric pressure. In this case the integrity of the ducting becomes much more important and a high level of assurance that it will not leak is necessary. Figure 19.1 shows typical arrangements for the purging and pressurization of an enclosure using both compressed air and fan-provided air. It will be noted that the pressure in the enclosure and all inlet and exhaust ducting should not fall below 50 N/m^2 which is considered as the minimum permissible pressure below which safety cannot be assured.

In this case, unlike that which occurs in the highly pressurized small bore pipes used for pressurization from a source of compressed air, the flowrate of air down the inlet ducting must be maintained during the purging cycle at a rate which assures turbulent flow. If this is not the case the ducting may not be effectively scavenged. The boundary which effectively defines the start of turbulent flow and the cessation of streamline or laminar flow is usually accepted, within pipes and ducts, as the flow which would produce a reynolds number (R_e) of 4000 or above. (The reynolds number is

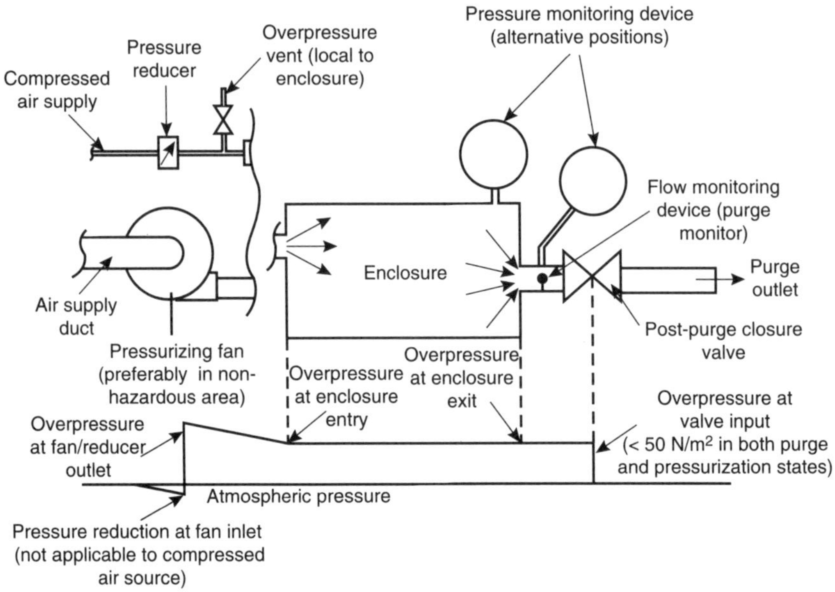

Fig. 19.1 Typical arrangements for pressurization with leakage compensation with pressure profile

a dimensionless factor which defines the degree of turbulence). This allows a calculation of flow velocity required from the following equation:

$$v = (R_e \times \delta)/(d \times \sigma) \qquad m/s$$

where v = air velocity — m/s
R_e = reynolds number — –
δ = absolute viscosity — Ns/m^2
d = diameter of duct — m
σ = density — kg/m^3

With rotating machines within pressurized enclosures there is often a circulation of air for cooling purposes produced by the motor fan. The inlet pressure to this fan occasionally may be below atmospheric pressure but in these circumstances the enclosure must be arranged so that the fan inlet does not cause the pressure at the inside walls of the enclosure to fall below the 50 N/m^2 required for pressurization (see Fig. 19.2).

19.4.2 Pressurization with leakage compensation using inert gas

Inert gas may be used in all situations where pressurization with leakage compensation using air is possible. In addition, it may be used in enclosures where an internal release of flammable material is possible provided that any release occurs in abnormal circumstances only (e.g., is not a deliberate

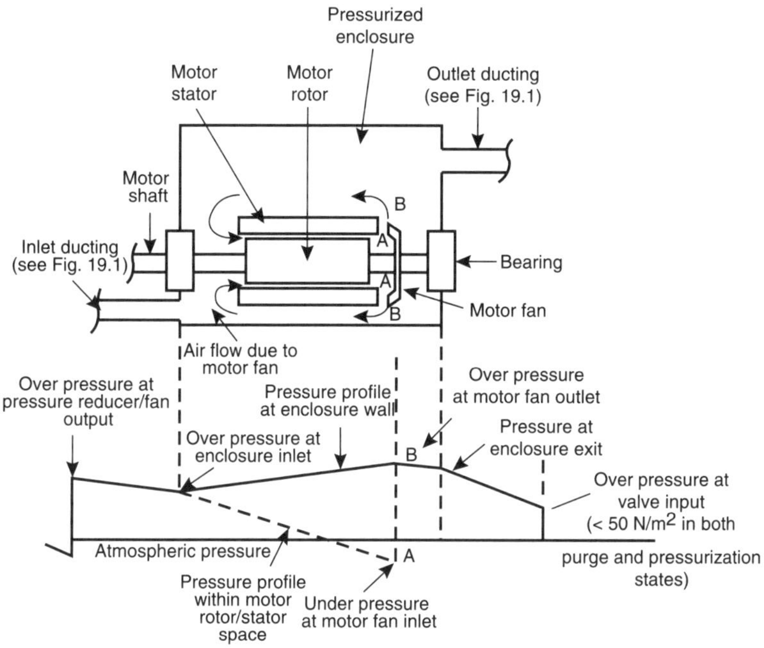

Fig. 19.2 Pressurization profile of rotating electrical machine. *Note*: Purge/ pressurization and monitoring arrangements are as shown in Fig. 19.1

release which occurs during the normal operational functioning of the apparatus). The release itself must not contain more than 2 per cent oxygen by volume in the gas or vapour which is present at the point of release and the amount of such material released can be controlled such that it can be assumed to be a 'limited release' (a release of flammable gas or vapour which can be quantified – see BS/EN 60079). This will mean that the flammable material inside the containment from which release occurs will be in the form of a gas or vapour and will permit calculation of the gas or vapour leak rate. This would not be possible in the case of liquid release due to the problem of definition of the vaporization rate from the liquid.

Pressurization with leakage compensation using inert gas cannot be used where the release of flammable material inside the enclosure is a part of the normal function of the enclosed apparatus and/or not definably restricted so that its flowrate cannot be defined making the release an 'unlimited release' (one where the rate of release cannot be readily defined – see BS/EN 60079). Such situations usually occur when the release is of liquid as the amount of vapour released is then related to the rate of vaporization and is more difficult to define. It is also not permitted when the oxygen concentration in the released gas or vapour exceeds 2 per cent by volume and in such cases pressurization with continuous flow of protective gas should be used (see Sections 19.3.3 and 19.3.4).

In addition, pressurization with leakage compensation is not permissible (where there may be any internal release of flammable material which is so unstable as to be capable of exothermic reaction) when little or no oxygen is present. Typical of these latter materials is acetylene which contains highly unstable chemical bonding in its molecules and can effectively explode in the absence of oxygen.

A liquid build-up in the enclosure cannot be tolerated and suitable draining facilities need to be provided to remove the liquid from the enclosure and dispose of it in a protected drain or blow egg or some similar facility.

In some cases liquid release will contain dissolved oxygen which may be seen as a complication. Where this occurs the only possible problem is the amount of oxygen which may be liberated at the point of release due to immediate vaporization of a flammable liquid (for instance by significant pressure reduction on release). This must also be less than 2 per cent of the gas phase.

When inert gas is used as the pressurization medium it is treated exactly as would be the case with air in that the pre-pressurization purge must be sufficient to clear all the atmosphere existing in both the enclosure and any ducting at the outset. This means that it must produce at least five gas changes in both and must also satisfy the requirements of flowrate and volume/time specified in any certification/approval documentation.

19.4.3 Pressurization with continuous dilution using air

In this approach a continuous flow of air is passed through the enclosure after purging. The purge to remove any explosive atmosphere initially existing within the enclosure may be at a higher flowrate than the ensuing continuous airflow, or may be the same the decision being made on grounds of economy provided that the flow is sufficient to dilute any internal release to the required level (see Fig. 19.3). The air for purging and the ensuing continuous flow may be from a compressed air source or a fan-driven system, although because of the usage it is normally more economic to utilize fan-driven systems.

This type of pressurization is suitable for enclosures into which people enter if it is pressurized with a fan-driven system, but not if fed from compressed air sources as it is possible that in fault conditions considerable pressure could exist within the enclosure, or in error a supply of inert gas could be connected to the enclosure. It is also suitable for those situations where a limited release of flammable material occurs in normal service or occurs abnormally (see Section 19.3.2). It is not, however suitable where an unlimited release of flammable material occurs (see Section 19.3.2), be it in normal service or abnormally. People may also enter enclosures where limited releases occur provided the pressurization is produced by a fan-driven system and such personnel are not able to compromise the dilution area (the area in which the flammable gas, vapour or mist is being diluted but has not yet reached the final maximum acceptable level – see Fig. 19.4). The toxicity of flammable materials usually prohibits this, however, as the

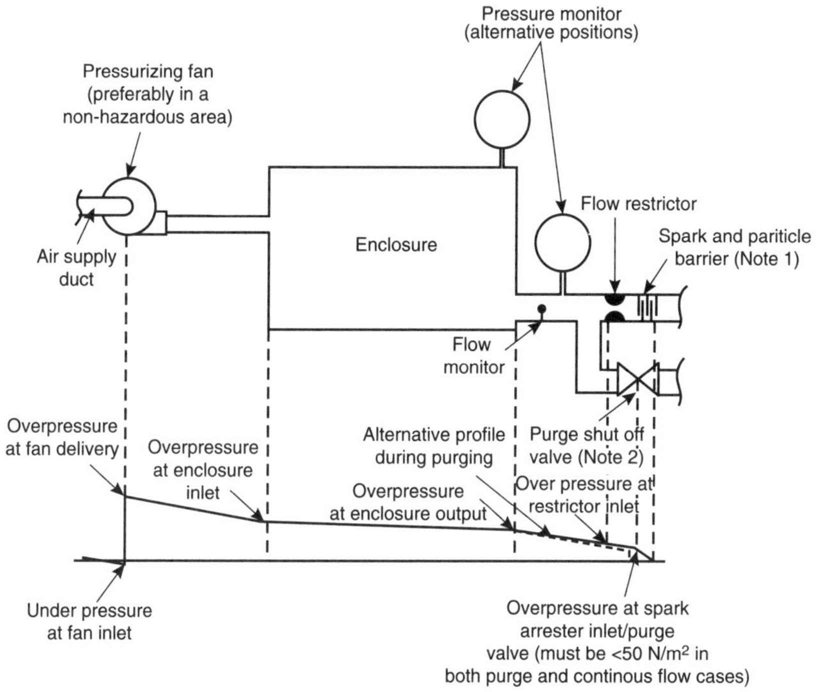

Fig. 19.3 Typical system for pressurization with continuous flow of protective gas. *Notes*: (1) Only necessary as defined in text. (2) Alternative exit route only necessary when purge flow is greater than continuous flow

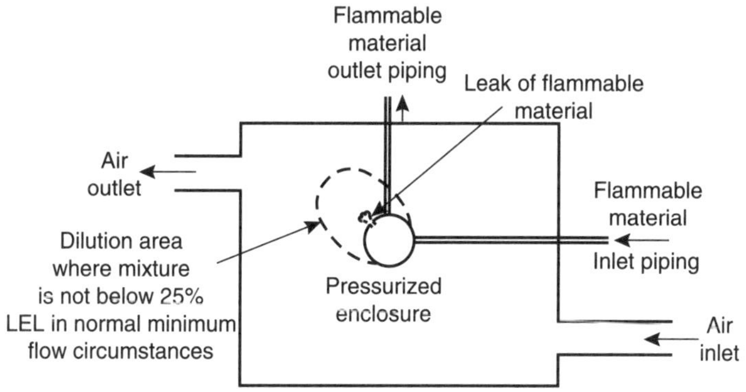

Fig. 19.4 Example of dilution area

threshold level for toxic reasons is very much smaller than the acceptable level for explosion safety reasons.

The initial purge of these enclosures needs to achieve the same requirements as for an air-fed leakage compensation system in that it must effectively sweep the enclosure and any ducting (in the case of fan-driven systems) of flammable gases, vapours or mists which may have entered while the enclosure was out of use with the pressurization isolated. The ensuing continuous flow of air has to be sufficient to dilute any internal release to less than 25 per cent of its lower explosive limit in all but the dilution area (see Fig. 19.4).

This approach to pressurization is not acceptable where an unlimited release is possible in either normal service or abnormally as it is not possible to ensure the necessary dilution required at or close to the point of release.

The pressure in the enclosure and any associated ducts must be maintained at more than 50 N/m^2 in both the purge and continuous flow conditions to ensure that no external atmosphere can access the enclosure, and enclosures should be fitted with protection against overpressure monitoring devices particularly if the pressurization is by compressed air.

19.4.4 Pressurization with continuous dilution using inert gas

This approach may be used where there is no release of flammable material into the enclosure, where there is a limited release of flammable material in either normal service or in abnormal circumstances, and where there is an unlimited release of flammable material (although in this latter case any release must not occur in normal service). Obviously, people may not enter such enclosures because of the risk of asphyxiation.

Where any release occurs within the enclosure it must be noted that it will be transmitted to the surrounding atmosphere by the continuous flow of gas and thus may have a significant effect on the area classification of the surrounding area unless precautions are taken, such as feeding it into a vent or scrubbing system.

Again it is not possible to utilize pressurization with continuous flow of inert gas where any normal or abnormal release is of the more unstable gases, such as acetylene where the upper explosive limit exceeds 80 per cent as so little oxygen is necessary to cause an explosion that safety cannot be guaranteed, even with the use of inert gas (acetylene will explode with no effective oxygen presence).

The approach in this case is similar to the approach using air in that a pre-purge is necessary to ensure that the enclosure is swept of any flammable material which may have entered during the time when it has been out of use, and the minimum overpressure should exceed 50 N/m^2, both during the purging time and after in the pressurized situation. After purging the dilution situation is, however, different. There is no limit on the oxygen in the gas or vapour mixture at the point of release but the dilution rate must be sufficient to ensure that the oxygen content of the atmosphere within the enclosure is less than 2 per cent everywhere except in the dilution area (see Fig. 19.4). Clearly the dilution area should not include the exhaust ducting. This 2 per cent figure is based upon the gas/vapour/oxygen mixture at the point of release which, in the case of liquid release, will be determined by such things as the immediate vaporization due to a change in pressure, and the vapour pressure of the liquid itself. Again a build-up of liquid in the enclosure cannot be tolerated and suitable draining arrangements need to be made.

19.5 Safety devices and procedures

The safety devices to protect against continued operation in the face of loss of pressurization, loss of gas/airflow, or overpressure of the enclosure may be fitted to the enclosure by the manufacturer or merely specified by the manufacturer in the certification/approval documents in which case it is for the user to supply the devices. The use of these safety devices depends upon the particular use of the pressurized apparatus and although the necessary control systems may be supplied by the manufacturer as part of the apparatus such systems will have facilities to provide the correct level of response in all cases. However, in apparatus which is certified/approved in accordance with BS/EN 50016[4] the manufacturer is primarily responsible for assuring that the devices and systems used are acceptable in that they do not reduce the level of security of the system.

The devices used need to be of adequate reliability and there are currently no specific constructional standards. The devices should be of the quality generally used for safety related systems, should be of good industrial quality and of high reliability, and should fail as safely as far as possible (e.g., the general mode of failure of the flow monitor should be to low flow, etc.). A European Standard, EN 954, covering the safety related parts of control systems is in preparation and when published will be the appropriate Standard for determination of the quality standard for the pressurization control systems.

The manufacturer's responsibility is normally satisfied as follows, although a purge and pressurization system can be purchased complete from a supplier which simplifies the situation.

19.5.1 Manufacturer provision of control devices and systems

The manufacturer is responsible for the provision of all of the hardware to achieve the following and for the programme by which it operates.

1. The isolation facilities for power supplies and any other electrical connections to the apparatus which are not otherwise made suitable for the hazardous area of installation (e.g., by use of another protection concept) when the enclosure is not pressurized, except where a time is allowed between pressure failure and shut-down, and provision to ensure that reconnection is not possible until after a purge cycle.
2. The control system which identifies failure of pressurization and of purge flow during the purge cycle.

3. The recognition by the control system of overpressure and isolation of the electrical supplies and connections, while at the same time its venting of the enclosure to prevent damage (particularly important in the case of pressurization with compressed air or inert gas).
4. It is normally not possible for the manufacturer to define the ducting used in all installations but where this happens there must also be a specified maximum overpressure, and this overpressure must be monitored to allow action to be taken if the overpressure is exceeded.
5. The manufacturer is responsible for provision of purge time control provision with variability to permit adjustment to take account of additional time necessary to purge the ducting.

The user is then responsible for:

1. Calculating the additional amount of inert gas or air necessary to purge the inlet piping or ducting and adding this to the purge time setting.
2. The provision of appropriate ducting unless this has been provided by the manufacturer. This ducting must be capable of withstanding the necessary overpressure.
3. The provision of secondary devices, such as secondary electrical shutdown systems, where these are not provided with the apparatus supplied by the manufacturer.

19.5.2 Manufacturer provision of control devices only

The responsibilities of the manufacturer are as follows:

1. Provision of a purge flow rate monitoring device.
2. Provision of an enclosure minimum overpressure monitoring device (where this is in the enclosure and the exhaust ducting has significant volume, a second device needs to be provided by the user for the exit ducting).
3. Provision of a maximum overpressure monitoring device if necessary. This is usually only necessary where compressed inert gas or air is used as the pressurization gas.
4. Provision of a variable timer to permit the user to allow the purge time necessary for the pressurized enclosure, its inlet piping or ducting, and its outlet ducting.
5. Provision of the necessary information to allow the user to use the pressurized enclosure. In this case the purge procedure and timing need to be supplied, together with information on the electrical circuits which need to be isolated when the enclosure is not pressurized.

The user then is responsible for:

All other devices such as the actuators which provide alarms and shut-down and the pressure detectors which monitor overpressure and underpressure in the ducting.

19.5.3 Manufacturer provision of control information only

In this case it is only necessary for the manufacturer to provide the necessary information to allow the user to select and construct the necessary monitors and control system. This information must include (as a minimum):

1. Minimum level of overpressure necessary in both enclosure and ducting during both purge and normal service.
2. Maximum level of overpressure permissible in both enclosure and ducting during purge and normal service.
3. Minimum required flow of protective gas/air for purging and leakage compensation or continuous flow.

Table 19.4 Typical information on pressurization control requirements provided by enclosure manufacturer

	Minimum over-pressure exceeded		Maximum over-pressure exceeded		Purge flow exceeded		Purge time exceeded	
	No	Yes	No	Yes	No	Yes	No	Yes
Initial state before Purging commences	X		X		X		X	
Minimum conditions For purge timing to start (Notes 1 and 2)		X	X			X	X	
Minimum conditions for normal operation to start (Electrical Apparatus to be Energized) (Notes 2, 3 and 4)		X	X			X		X

Notes:
1 If at any time during the purge the flowrate or minimum overpressure fall below the limit specified, the purge cycle must return to its start.
2 If at any time the maximum overpressure limit is exceeded, the purge cycle or pressurization system should return to the initial state.
3 If when the enclosure is in normal operation the pressure or continuous flow of protective gas falls below the specified minimum the enclosure must return to its initial state

4. Details of electrical circuits which need to be isolated when pressurization is not present.
5. Sequence chart for pressurization system control (see Table 19.4).

19.6 Purge gas and operation of control system (gas, vapour and mist risks)

19.6.1 Gases used

The gas used for pressurization should be normal air or its fabricated compressed equivalent (e.g., cylinders of 21 per cent oxygen in nitrogen) or inert gas containing less than 0.1 per cent oxygen. For the purposes of temperature classification the temperature of these gases should be not exceed 40 °C or any other ambient temperature which is specified for the apparatus in accordance with BS/EN 50014[7].

19.6.2 Basic operation of pressurization system

The basic operation of the pressurization control system is to ensure that there is sufficient pressure and flow of protective gas at all times and that if this is not so, or the enclosure reaches a pressure above that for which it is designed, then alarms are provided to alert personnel and any necessary shut-down actions are taken. The basic cycle is given in Table 19.4.

Initial state

The enclosure must initially be isolated from all electrical circuits which are not otherwise explosion protected and this includes such things as outputs from, or inputs to, the pressurized apparatus which may be provided for such things as intelligence transfer or control of apparatus operation. This is usually done by isolating relays or by making these circuits intrinsically safe. In the latter case it should be noted that while intrinsic safety need not be maintained while the pressurized apparatus is energized its intrinsic safety features must not be damaged by this situation (for instance by back feeding currents to barrier devices and causing damage to their safety components), and such circuits will need to be separated from other intrinsically safe circuits and non-intrinsically safe circuits.

Initial purging

The protective gas flow should be established at a rate at least equivalent to the minimum flow required by the certification/approval documentation. In addition, the pressure inside the enclosure and its ducting must be established to be above the $50\,N/m^2$ minimum and below the maximum acceptable pressure specified for the enclosure. The purge timing may begin when all of these conditions are met.

If during the purge time the flow of protective gas falls below the minimum figure specified, the flow detection device should initiate a cessation of purge and purging should not again begin until the purge criteria are re-established. The purge timing should then begin again from zero. Likewise if the pressure in the enclosure falls below the minimum specified figure or rises above the maximum permitted overpressure the purge should be shut down and restarted only when the correct conditions have been re-established. Additionally, in the case of overpressurization of the enclosure or ducting, the enclosure (and, if necessary, the ducting separately) should be vented or its supply of gas removed to prevent damage.

The electrical circuits within the enclosure must remain isolated from all supplies and other unprotected electrical circuits (circuits not otherwise explosion protected) during this purge period.

Normal operation

When the purge has been completed and the time delay relay or other timing device indicates this to be so then, provided the flow and pressure conditions remain within those acceptable, the outlet of the enclosure is closed (in the case of pressurization with leakage compensation) or reduced in size (in the case of pressurization with continuous flow of protective gas). At this time provided the internal pressure remains within its limits and, in the case of continuous flow, the flowrate is above the minimum specified for normal operation, the electrical circuits within the enclosure may be energized and the other energized intelligence connected circuits (such as control and intelligence transmission circuits which were isolated) may be reconnected.

Actions on faults in the system

If the pressure inside the enclosure falls below the minimum of $50\,N/m^2$ or the flow, in the case of enclosures with continuous flow of protective gas, falls below its acceptable minimum, the monitoring devices should identify this.

In all cases (both where the enclosure does not have flammable materials fed into it and where it does have limited normal and any abnormal release) the action required on this identification is given in Table 19.5. The alarm-only requirement for apparatus suitable for Zone 2 without isolation refers only to Zone 2 compatible apparatus (i.e., Type 'N' apparatus and suitably selected industrial non-sparking apparatus) and not to all non-sparking apparatus. It is also only of limited term and if the pressurization cannot be restored in a short time (say four hours) then isolation must take place. In this case it can be automatic or manual rather than automatic only as is the case with immediate isolation requirements.

Table 19.5 Alarm and shut-down requirements for pressurized enclosures without internal releases

Classification of area of installation	Enclosure contains apparatus Suitable for use in Zone 2 without pressurization	Enclosure contains apparatus not suitable for use in Zone 2 without pressurization
Zone 1	Alarm (Note)	Alarm and isolation
Zone 2	No action	Alarm (Note)

Note: Only valid in the short term. If situation persists then isolation will be required.

Where it is not possible to isolate apparatus in situations where isolation (either immediately or delayed) is necessary it is not acceptable to waive this requirement. Thus some more reliable pressurization method, such as the use of main and standby pressurization supplies, must be used with isolation not necessary unless both supplies fail. If this is not possible then the technique of pressurization is not possible.

19.7 Multiple enclosures

There is nothing in principal to prevent several enclosures from being pressurized from the same source provided that no action in respect of any one of the enclosures results in any other enclosures in the group exceeding any of the pressure/flow requirements applied to them. This normally precludes serial connection of enclosures and is subject to the following requirements:

1. Opening of any door or cover in any one of the enclosures is preceded by manual or automatic isolation of that particular enclosure. (It is recommended that this action be automatic wherever it is possible, usually executed by a switch which senses the opening of the door as soon as opening is started thus ensuring isolation occurs before the door is fully open). If there is residual heat in the enclosure it will be marked with the minimum time before which opening can commence and in such circumstances isolation will need to be manual.
2. The pressures and flow rates in the other enclosures in the group are not affected to the extent that they exceed the appropriate limits and their parameters continue to be monitored effectively.
3. When any enclosure in the group has been de-pressurized it must go through its entire purge cycle after pressurization is restored and before the electrical equipment enclosed is re-energized and other unprotected electrical circuits reconnected.

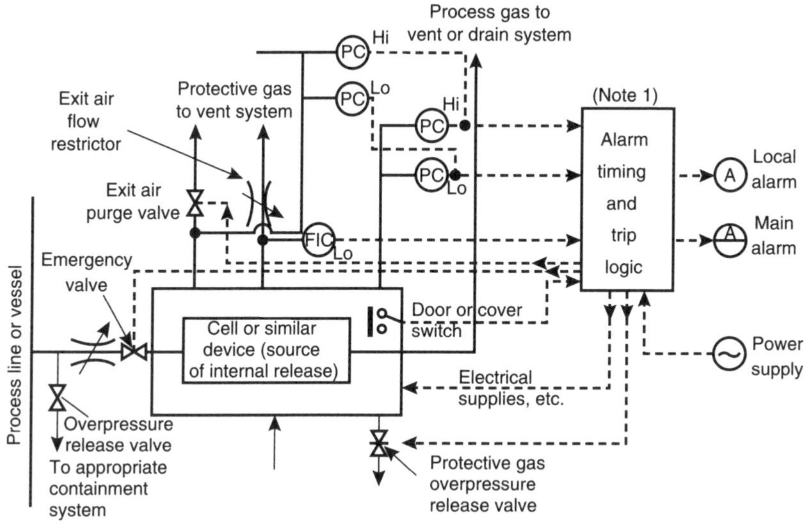

PC(Hi) = High pressure switch (alternative positions shown)
PC(Lo) = Low pressure switch (alternative positions shown)
FIC(Lo) = Low flow switch

Fig. 19.5 Typical pressurization control system. *Notes*: (1) The control unit should be mounted in a non-hazardous area or suitable for potentially explosive atmospheres (e.g., flameproof). (2) All electrical switches and electrically operated valves to be suitable for hazardous areas (e.g., flameproof or intrinsically safe).

19.8 Typical pressurization control system

A typical pressurization control system is shown in Fig. 19.5. It will be noted that the flow monitor device needs to be in the exhaust duct or very close thereto to ensure that it monitors the flow leaving the enclosure. Where the exhaust ducting is long it needs to be close to the valve which closes after purging or the restrictor which controls operational flow to ensure that it identifies leakage in the ducting. Likewise, the low pressure indicator needs to identify the pressurization of the exhaust duct as well as the enclosure where the latter is long.

19.9 Pressurized enclosures in dust risks

Installations should comply with the requirements applied to gas/vapour risk areas installations in Zone 21 and with requirements for installations in Zone 1, and those for Zone 22 with Zone 2 requirements. In addition the ducting used in any installation must ensure that, although the enclosure may not remain IP6X (for Zone 21) or IP5X for (Zone 22) after pressure failure when the ducting is no longer pressurized closures are present which effectively prevent the ingress of dust by closure of outlet apertures. The ducts themselves must, with the exception of their outlets, satisfy these enclosure integrity requirements.

Table 19.6 Alarm and shut-down requirements for enclosures with internal sources of release

Internal release description	Enclosure is in Zone 1 and contains:		Enclosure is in Zone 2 and contains:	
	Zone 2 Protected	Non-protected	Zone 2 Protected	Non-protected
No normal release and limited abnormal release	Alarm (Note)	Alarm and isolate	No action	Alarm (Note)
No normal release and unlimited abnormal release	Alarm (Note)	Alarm and Isolate	No action	Alarm (Note)
Limited normal and abnormal release	alarm (Note)	Alarm and isolate	Alarm (Note)	Alarm and isolate
Limited normal release and unlimited abnormal release	Alarm (Note)	Alarm and isolate	Alarm (Note)	Alarm and isolate

Note: Although it is permitted to maintain the apparatus energized this is a short term relaxation only and if the pressurization is not quickly reinstated isolation is also, necessary particularly where normal releases occur

19.10 Analyser houses

Analyser Houses have become very common over the last decade or so. These are small, usually prefabricated, buildings into which several instruments and analysers are fitted and which are regularly accessed by personnel. They are common where more sophisticated analytical processes are carried out, requiring apparatus which is not necessarily appropriate to outdoor mounting. Analyser houses are pressurized to prevent any external explosive atmosphere from entering the house thus permitting the use of normal electrical apparatus. They also, however, normally have flammable materials fed into analysers within them and these constitute internal sources of release, and can have an effect on the external hazardous area by release of explosive atmosphere into that area. There are three considerations:

1. Purging and subsequent pressurization of the analyser house to exclude external explosive atmospheres.
2. Purging and subsequent pressurization of the analyser house or the analysers within it to dilute the release of flammable atmospheres within the analyser house or analysers therein.
3. Purging and pressurization of the analyser house to ensure that it is safe for personnel to enter.

19.10.1 Pressurization considerations

Exclusion of external atmosphere

For the purposes of external atmosphere, exclusion is only necessary to follow the procedures for a pressurized enclosure without internal sources of release. As people may enter this enclosure, however, pressurization with inert gas is not permitted and thus air must be used. Likewise, it is preferable to use a fan system rather than compressed air and to utilize a continuous flow of air rather than leakage compensation. The continuous flow to satisfy this requirement will normally be five times the analyser house volume as in other cases (see BS 5345, Part 5[5]).

Dilution of internal sources of release

The instruments within the analyser house may release flammable material into the house normally or in fault conditions. This may be liquid or gas/vapour/mist.

In the case of liquid it is necessary to provide a drain which removes the liquid from the house expeditiously to a collection point such as a blow egg, and this provides a further aperture as far as pressurization is concerned which exhausts gas and vapour to the external atmosphere unless exit is via a closed lute which prevents this.

The releases of flammable gases, vapour or mists released within the analyser house must be diluted to 25 per cent of their lower explosive limit in all but the dilution areas within the analyser house. These dilution areas need to be small so that people are not likely to enter them and must not include any electrical apparatus except that which is protected appropriately for use in an explosive atmosphere of the appropriate Zone in the absence of pressurization. (This means that for a normal release only intrinsically safe apparatus may be used in the dilution area, and for abnormal release only apparatus suitable for Zone 1 use). Entry of feeds of flammable gases or vapours must thus be restricted to as low a pressure as possible, and pressures of less than $5 \times 10^4\,N/m^2$ maximum are recommended to reduce the volume of any leaks. Likewise, the same maximum pressures for liquid lines inside the house are recommended both to reduce leakage and to prevent mists forming. Where fast sample loops are necessary to reduce sampling times for both liquids and gases/vapours these should terminate outside the analyser house, and inputs to the house in all cases should have pressure relief facilities if their pressure could rise above the values recommended above. Flow restrictors should also be provided where necessary to limit the flow into the analyser house and hence the release in fault conditions.

Where flammable material in the form of gas or vapour is deliberately released as a function of the apparatus into which it is fed, it should preferably be exhausted outside the house taking account of its effect on external area classification. If this is not possible then the apparatus should be separately pressurized with air within the house so that any release into the house is normally non-explosive.

It is very difficult to make the airflow through the house to dilute areas of any normal or abnormal release sufficiently small without producing an airflow which is uncomfortable to personnel. A release of ethylene, for example, at a rate of $0.015\,m^3/m$ (250 ml/s) would require an airflow of $6\,m^3/m$ to dilute it to 25 per cent of the lower explosive limit of ethylene at the exhaust of the house (based on the equations in Chapter 4 for an aperture of $10^{-6}\,m^3$ and a pressure of $5 \times 10^4\,kg/m^2$). In the case of an analyser house the dilution needs to take place in the small area of the house where the leak occurs to ensure the remainder of the house is gas free. This would require significant airflow to ensure dilution in that small distance. This often conflicts with the normal expectation that air movement velocities in excess of 0.5 m/s are not acceptable indoors which would militate against the level of airflow required in some circumstances. Where this occurs a possible solution is to provide airflow outlets close to the sources of release of sufficient velocity to cause rapid dilution. As the air expands into the analyser house the flow velocity rapidly reduces to an acceptable level. Another variation is to provide such local outlets but also provide local extract so that releases are diluted and removed from the analyser house locally to the point of release. This latter approach must be treated with caution as the overall level of operating pressure in the house still needs to be greater than $50\,N/m^2$.

One point which is helpful is that the airflow required inside the analyser house is not likely to need a velocity of anything like the velocity required in outdoor situations to achieve rapid dilution as the airflow is controlled and directed and not random.

The basic method of calculating local airflows, should this route be taken, is given in BS 5345, Part 5 which gives a method for pressurized apparatus with an internal source of release. This method is not suitable for calculation of the total airflow necessary within the house, as the analyser house, will be much larger than the enclosure of an item of apparatus in relation to the volume of released gas and thus the dilution performance would not be the same. If, however, the air provision is local to the leak it will be more relevant.

$$Q = F \times (A/100) \times (100/LEL) \times S \qquad m^3/s$$

where Q = airflow needed $\quad m^3/s$

F = maximum release rate $\quad m^3/s$

A = percentage of gas in release (where the release is not a mixture of gases this is 100) — %
LEL = lower explosive limit — %v/v
S = safety factor (See BS/EN 60079–14) — 4

As already stated, this calculation should be carried out for each component of the released gas mixture and the results added together to give the necessary local gas flowrate. It must be remembered that, in addition to these local air inputs, there must still be an overall input to the analyser house to ensure that it is effectively purged before any electrical apparatus is energized in common with all other pressurized apparatus.

Although toxic matters are not within the scope of this book it is worthy of note here that the use of the above formula using the maximum acceptable gas level for toxic risks, instead of the lower explosive limit, will often ensure proper dilution of toxic elements in any release. This is important in view of the personnel access although this must be proved in each case by test or assessment.

There are two approaches to provision of proof that analyser houses are suitable for their use. The first approach is to carry out dilution tests similar to those carried out for pressurized apparatus with internal release with the normal airflow passing through the house and, by doing this, show that dilution takes place in an acceptably small area which includes no electrical apparatus and is not one where personnel are expected to be present. Certification/approval is currently optional in this case and a route exists whereby the user can, by evidence obtained from similar analyser houses, assess the suitability of the airflow in the analyser house without the need for testing. In such circumstances, it should be ensured that the evidence of similar situations is complete and relevant. The use of the equation detailed above may well form part of such an assessment although the actual positioning of the air duct in each case is important. It should be as close to the source of release as possible and direct its flow away from electrical apparatus in the immediate vicinity and from areas where personnel may be present.

The second method is to divide the house into two sections, one of which contains the sources of release and the other the majority of the electrical equipment. Personnel would then only have normal access to the part of the house with the majority of the electrical equipment. The airflow in the other part could then be much higher or the few electrical circuits in that part protected for use in explosive atmospheres. Typical approaches to analyser house construction are shown in Fig. 19.6 and 19.7.

Personnel protection

The toxic threshold level of many if not most of the flammable gases and vapours which occur in industry is very much lower than their lower

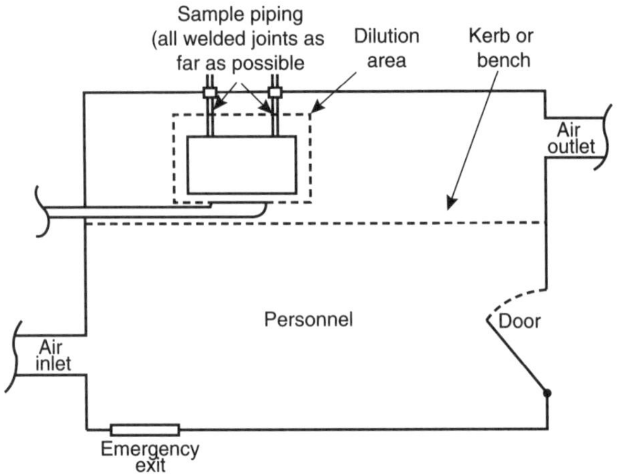

Fig. 19.6 One-part analyser house

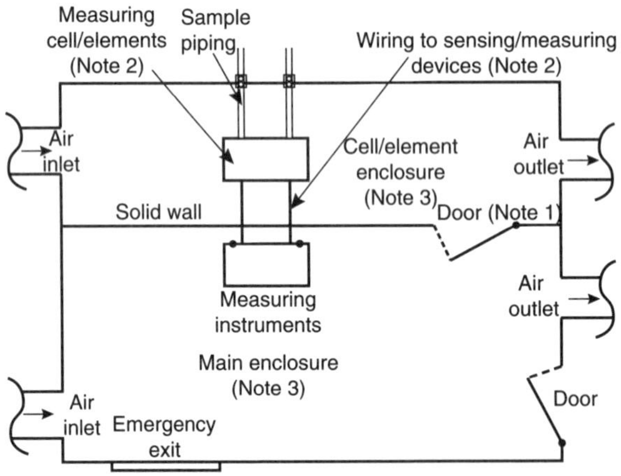

Fig. 19.7 Two-part analyser house. *Notes*: (1) This door must be gastight and secured closed so that normal access is not possible. (2) Wiring and sensing devices must be otherwise protected (e.g., flameproof) if they enter the dilution area. If this is the case, pressurization is not necessary in this part of the house unless personnel require access. (3) The pressure in this part of the house must always be higher by 50 N/m^2 than that of the other part

explosive limit. If the gases and vapours released are toxic then the approach should be to apply the criteria which would be necessary in any other indoor situation where toxic risks occur. These can be applied alongside the protection against explosion risks but should not dilute them. If it is not possible to apply both then an alternative solution should be adopted. As already stated, it may be possible to cover the toxic risk by using the local airflow to dilute the toxic gas/vapour to below its occupational exposure limit[9] by using the calculation already described.

19.10.2 Analyser house construction and protection

It is not really relevant to test analyser houses in the same way as other pressurized apparatus although the same criteria apply in that they should be sufficiently strong to prevent damage in service and must provide the appropriate degree of protection by enclosure required for the risk at their point of installation with the pressurization off. (IP54 for normal outdoor situations rising to IP65 for such areas where dust risks occur). This does not, of course, include the air outlet but it should be fitted with some device to ensure that moisture or dust cannot enter when pressurization is off.

Analyser houses additionally require local alarms to ensure that personnel inside know if the airflow or pressure falls below the acceptable minimum but require a delay of around one or two minutes before electrical shut-down to permit people to enter and leave as pressure in the analyser house and flow in the exit ducting will fall at such times. An override is necessary to allow maintenance work but this should be secure to ensure it cannot be inadvertently used.

The problem of personnel being trapped in the analyser house also needs attention and an emergency exit such as a second door or kick-out panel, should be fitted at the end of the house remote from the normal door. To avoid operational problems it is recommended that the second exit be such that it cannot be used in normal service and both exits should be fitted with alarms which identify when they are open. Lighting which is protected by another protection concept needs to be provided for emergencies as does some secure form of protected communication.

Because of the internal release the interior of the analyser house should be considered as Zone 1 in respect of all electrical apparatus installed within it and remain energized when no airflow is present, and all apparatus not so protected must be isolated when airflow fails (with the delay already identified as necessary) even if the enclosure is installed in Zone 2 or 22. A typical electrical installation is shown in Fig. 19.8.

19.11 Pressurized rooms

Pressurization is sometimes used for such things as control rooms where no internal source of release occurs. These are not enclosure in the sense of 'pressurized enclosures' but the protection technique is similar. The basic requirements for strength, keeping out the dust and environment apply and, in this case, special attention is necessary to ensure that no excessive leaks occur at such points as windows and cable inlets. Because such rooms are usually very important to the operation of a plant it is not normally possible to isolate all electrical equipment therein if the pressurization fails. This leads to a main and stand-by pressurization system being necessary to give a very high integrity to the pressurization, together with the need for an airlock at points of entry to minimize the risk of ingress even if both pressurization systems fail. Utilization of both of these precautions is

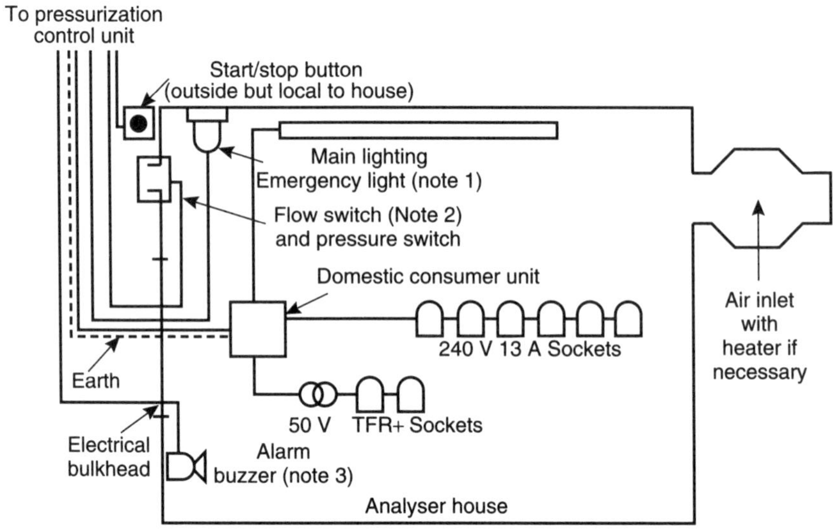

Fig. 19.8 Typical analyser house electrical installation. *Notes*: (1) The emergency light must remain on when pressurization fails and when main electrical supplies fail. It must be fed from a separate supply and explosion protected (e.g., flameproof). (2) Pressure and flow switches must be explosion protected (e.g., flameproof or intrinsically safe). (3) Alarm buzzer must be explosion protected (e.g flameproof or intrinsically safe)

not intended to allow continuous use of the room without pressurization, but to allow it to remain in operation long enough to allow a controlled shut-down of the plant to be undertaken if the pressurization cannot be re-applied within a short time (e.g., four hours). The use of such a room without pressurization should be limited to as short a time as possible (probably not longer than one day) and access should be restricted as far as possible during that time. Entry points should have warning notices to alert personnel to the fact that the doors must be kept closed and should be fitted with alarms which sound if a door is deliberately propped or inadvertently left open. The alarm need not sound during the period of normal entry.

Initial purging to remove any internal flammables before start-up is again necessary and should be at least long enough to allow five times the room volume in air to flow through the room. Pressure detectors and flow detectors similar in position and operation to those in analyser houses should be fitted.

References

1 NEC — National Electrical Code (US). Chapter 5 'Special Occupancies', Article 500, hazardous (Classified) Locations.

2 CENELEC — Centre Européen de Normalization Electrique

3 BS 5501	Electrical Apparatus for Potentially Explosive Atmospheres. Part 1 (1977). General Requirements. Part 3 (1977). Pressurized Apparatus 'p'.
4 BS/EN 50016 (1995)	Electrical Apparatus for Potentially Explosive Atmospheres. Pressurized Apparatus 'p'.
5 BS 5345	Selection, Installation and Maintenance of Electrical Apparatus for Use in Potentially Explosive Atmospheres (other than mining applications or explosive processing and manufacture). Part 1 (1989). General recommendations. Part 5 (1983). Installation and Maintenance Requirements for Electrical Apparatus Protected by Pressurization 'p' and by Continuous Dilution, and for Pressurized Rooms.
6 BS/EN 60079	Electrical Apparatus for Explosive Gas Atmospheres. Part 14 (1997) Electrical Installations in Explosive Gas Atmospheres other than mines)
7 BS/EN 50014 (1993)	Electrical Apparatus for Potentially Explosive Atmospheres. General Requirements.
8 RoSPA/ICI	Engineering Codes and Regulations, Electrical Installations in Flammable Atmospheres (1973). Group C (Electrical) Volume 1.5.
9 EH 40	Guidance note from the Health and Safety Executive. Occupational Exposure Limits. (Updated Regularly).

— 20 —

Installation of intrinsically safe apparatus/associated apparatus and intrinsically safe systems 'i'

BS 5345, Part 4 (1977)

BS/EN 60079–14 (1997)

Intrinsic safety is very different to the other protection concepts in that it does not operate by prevention of the release of ignition-capable energy, the prevention of access of the explosive atmosphere to such releases, or the control of the ignitions which result when such releases occur, but by the prevention of ignition-capable energy from entering the hazardous area and control of energy stored in the hazardous area by electrical components which can store energy, such as inductors and capacitors. Thus release of energy in the form of arcs or sparks in an explosive atmosphere is permitted and this feature dictates the installation practice together with the fact that some intrinsically safe installations are permitted in Zone 0 (and probably in Zone 20 – see Chapter 15).

Intrinsically safe installations are also normally based upon instrumentation rather than electrical bases. A result of this is that in many, if not all, use is made of multicore cables which carry more than one intrinsically safe circuit, the installation splitting into individual cables to supply individual circuits in a particular location at each end of the multicore. Figure 20.1 shows the typical way in which instrumentation systems are installed and this also applies to intrinsically safe circuits.

These attributes require the following features of any installation to be carefully considered.

1. Any invasion of the intrinsically safe circuit by energy from other intrinsically safe circuits or non-intrinsically safe circuits may add energy to a particular circuit and hence may make any release of energy ignition capable. Thus separation of intrinsically safe circuits from other circuits is an important consideration whether those circuits are intrinsically safe or non-intrinsically safe.

2. When fault currents are flowing in earth and bonding conductors are in conditions of electrical fault, different parts of a potential equalization systems may be at different voltages. Although these differences are not large and have little effect in the case of installations with other protection

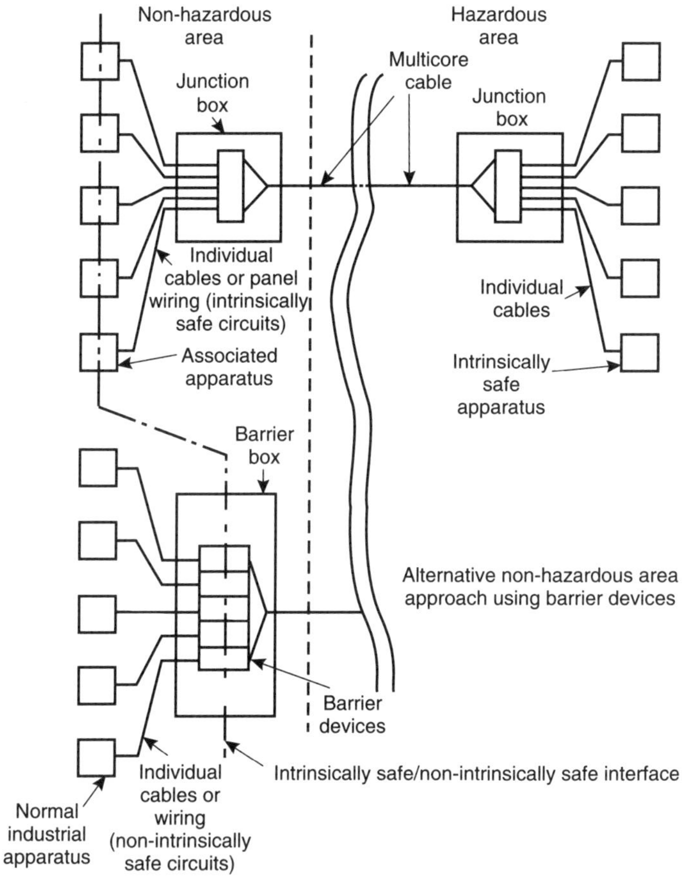

Fig. 20.1 Basic multicore cable intrinsically safe installation

concepts, they may be significant if added to the potential of an intrinsically safe circuit and thus installations must take this situation into account.

3. The energy storage capability of certified/approved apparatus is defined and its safety can be determined. Any energy stored in interconnecting cables can add to the total and thus cable construction is more important in this regard than in respect of non-intrinsically safe installations.

4. Intrinsically safe installations in Zone 0 (and where possible in Zone 20) achieve a much higher level of integrity than those in Zones of lower risk. The effects of this must be taken into account for installations in Zone 0.

20.1 Standards and Codes

Due to its unique approach, the division between construction and installation in intrinsic safety is not as clear as is the case for other protection concepts in that installation matters, such as choice of cable and termination, also impinge upon apparatus and system design. Some information, particularly that in the intrinsically safe system Standard, is also installation information (e.g., the choice of type of cable – A, B, C or D – is a matter for intrinsically safe system design where a system is certified/approved and also is a matter for installation where a system is produced on the basis of the parameters of certified/approved apparatus and is not itself certified). While the basic installation is currently in the Code of Practice, BS 5345, Part 4[1] (now being replaced by BS/EN 60079[2]), relevant information also appears in the apparatus construction Standard BS/EN 50020[3], and its predecessor, BS 5501, Part 7 Part 9[4].

20.2 Basic installation requirements

As with other protection concepts, apparatus should be installed where it is accessible and its labels are clearly visible to facilitate inspection. Also, not withstanding that physical damage will not result in the release of ignition-capable energy, it should be remembered that the construction Standards do not include any enclosure strength requirements and thus, to ensure that reliable operation is achieved, locations should be such that mechanical damage is unlikely unless apparatus with a suitably rugged enclosure has been chosen (see Chapter 17). Also the possibility of hostile environments for which the apparatus is not designed should be taken into account. It is true that most manufacturers will enclose intrinsically safe apparatus for normal outdoor location but it must be remembered that the tests associated with certification/approval do not usually confirm this. In addition, much associated apparatus is designed for indoor use in a control room or similar.

Mains powered associated apparatus should also be fitted with appropriate short circuit overcurrent and mains/earth fault protection to ensure that if a fault occurs in the part of the apparatus where the mains is present, continuous arcing or heating which could adversely affect the intrinsically safe circuit does not occur.

The use of barrier devices either of the shunt zener diode type or of more complex types, some of which offer galvanic isolation between their inputs or outputs, is now very common and the majority of installations use such devices. Barrier devices which do not provide galvanic isolation (e.g., shunt zener diode barriers) are currently in the majority and, unless precautions are taken, the use of such devices can cause danger by providing unplanned connections to the potential equalization system and thus the possibility of invasion of the intrinsically safe circuits. Where such devices are used, and where any other associated apparatus not providing galvanic isolation from the mains supplies is used, the apparatus to which their non-hazardous area terminals are connected must provide such isolation. It is sufficient that any mains fed apparatus connected to their non-hazardous area terminals be fed from the mains via a double wound transformer (not an auto transformer), and the primary of that transformer be appropriately fused (fused as would be required in normal industrial use).

20.3 Cables, conduits and conductors

Cables and interconnecting conductors used within conduits should be chosen in accordance with the requirements set out in Chapters 13 and 17, with particular consideration given to the reactance parameters of the cable or the conductors and their possible heating due to current in the circuit. For new plants these factors will probably have been covered in the design phase where the cables and conductors were initially selected, but in the case of modifications this may not be so as existing multicore routes, for example, may be used for economy. An installation check is necessary to ensure errors have not occurred in either case.

Intrinsically safe and non-intrinsically safe circuits must not be connected to conductors in the same cable except in exceptional circumstances. (It is noted that it is, for example, possible to use an intrinsically-safe circuit to monitor a plug and socket so that if they are separated the non-intrinsically safe circuits within them are isolated before the pins part. This is dealt with later in this chapter but the intrinsically safe circuit in this case must not be mixed with other intrinsically safe circuits.).

20.3.1 Conductor temperature

The conductors of cables and those led in conduit are no different to those inside apparatus and the conductor size (including the screen size if one is fitted) should satisfy the requirements for conductors within apparatus (see Table 20.1)

Table 20.1 Field wiring surface temperature classification

Conductor nominal diameter (mm)	Conductor nominal cross-sectional area (mm^2)	Maximum permissible current in Amps for temperature classification of:		
		T1–T4	T5	T6
0.035	0.000962	N/A	N/A	N/A
0.05	0.00196	N/A	N/A	N/A
0.1	0.00785	2.1	1.9	1.7
0.2	0.0314	3.7	3.3	3.0
0.35	0.0962	6.4	5.6	5.0
0.5	0.196	7.7	6.9	6.7

Notes:

1 N/A because conductors of less than 0.1 mm diameter should not be used in intrinsically safe circuits because they are not considered sufficiently robust to have the necessary integrity.

2 Conductors made up of several strands are only acceptable if no strand is less than 0.1 mm diameter for the same reason, even though their total equivalent cross-sectional area may exceed 0.00785 mm^2.

20.3.2 Inductance and capacitance

The cable or conductor arrangement will have been selected to ensure that its energy storage capability does not adversely affect intrinsic safety and this normally involves inductance/resistance ratio and capacitance. (Inductance itself is normally not used as a selection parameter except where the inductance/resistance ratio acceptable in the circuit is so low as not to be usable with standard conductor configurations such as can be the case in high current circuits.) The capacitance between the circuit conductors may be based upon failures between the causing of interconnection of conductors as this increases capacitance and hence stored energy, rather than reducing stored energy as is normally the case with inductance because of current division. (This is normally only a problem in circuits using screens, using more than two conductors or led through multicore cables which are subject to fault – see Chapter 13). Experiments have shown that the multi-conductor configuration does not lead to a directly additive situation and the capacitance of typical multi-conductor situations approximates to the figures given in Table 20.2.

Table 20.2 Effect on capacitance of interconnection of conductors in multi-core cables

Number of conductors interconnected	Screen fitted/not fitted	Amount by which the capacitance between any two cores should be multiplied
None	Not fitted	1.0
None	Fitted	2.0 (note)
2	Not fitted	1.5
2	Fitted	2.5 (note)
3	Not fitted	2.5
3	Fitted	3.0 (note)

Note: 1 The screen is assumed to be deliberately connected to one side of the circuit which is the normal situation.

Where conduit systems are used it is not possible to use separate insulated conductors as is normally the case unless the inductance, inductance/resistance ratio, and capacitance of the circuit can be defined in the worst case because of the possible movement of conductors within the conduit. It is normally necessary to ensure that the conductors are secured together to guarantee their respective positions and to fit a screen which can be connected to the potential equalization system to negate the influence of the conduit if it is metallic. Any screen used for this purpose must, be insulated to withstand a test voltage of 500 V rms.

Intrinsically safe circuits and non-intrinsically safe circuits must not be contained within the same conduit.

20.3.3 Cable installation

Cables containing intrinsically safe circuits should be installed to minimize the risk of damage. Although failure of a cable which contains only one intrinsically safe circuit does not directly cause ignition-capable sparking its interconnection with local structural steel, for example, can result in invasion. Thus the precautions normally taken with industrial installations in areas of similar mechanical and environmental risk are appropriate. If the risk of mechanical intervention is high, consideration should be given to using armoured or metal sheathed cable to minimize the risk of damage.

In particular multicore cables of Type 'B' (see Chapter 13) require special precautions to be taken to prevent physical damage as they will contain more than one intrinsically safe circuit, with separation only by conductor insulation.

In order to avoid invasion, cables containing intrinsically safe circuits preferably should not be mounted on the same cable tray or in the same cable duct as those for non-intrinsically safe circuits, unless at least one of the types of cable is steel wire or braid armoured or is metal sheathed. If this is not the case then where they are led in the same ducting or on the same tray, the ducting or tray should be fitted with a divider which effectively divides the two types of cable (see Fig. 20.2). This divider should be rigid, robust and, if conducting, be fitted in such a way that it makes good contact with the local structural metalwork and hence the bonding (potential equalization) system.

When cables containing intrinsically safe circuits are fitted in the proximity of other conductors and cables which contain non-intrinsically safe

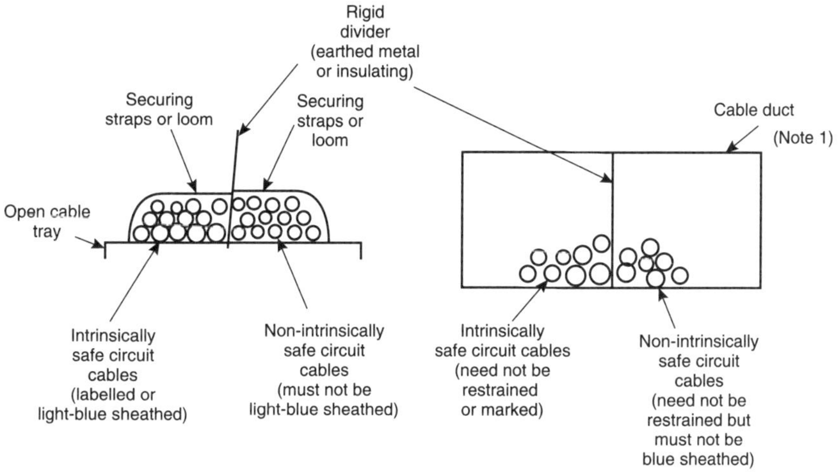

Fig. 20.2 Cable tray and ducting containing mixed cables. *Note*: As the intrinsically safe circuit cables are not necessarily marked or light-blue sheathed then such marking on colouring is necessary on the part of the duct containing intrinsically safe circuit cables

circuits, the possibility of induction of energy from those circuits into the intrinsically safe circuits needs to be considered as in extreme cases it could adversely affect intrinsic safety. This is only likely to be a problem when intrinsically safe circuit cables are led parallel to and, in close proximity with, single conductor cables carrying high currents parallel to high voltage overhead power lines.

20.3.4 Conduit installation

All conduits are subject to the normal installation requirements for conduits (see Chapter 18). The possibility of induction, while being less with conduits, must still be considered in the cases identified in Section 20.3.3.

20.3.5 Marking of cables, cable bundles, cable trays, or ducts and conduits

There are currently no specific requirements in the UK for marking of cables, cable bundles or conduits containing intrinsically safe circuits although, in BS/EN 50020, marking of connection facilities in certified/approved apparatus is required. It is, however, wise to mark cables, cable bundles and conduits in some way to ensure that the security achieved in initial installation is not later compromised by, for example, mixing of unarmoured intrinsically safe and non-intrinsically safe cables on the same tray or in the same duct, or pulling non-intrinsically safe conductors into conduits containing intrinsically safe circuit conductors. BS/EN 60079–14[2] for the first time sets out minimum marking requirements. These requirements are minimum and it is recommended that the following procedure, which is slightly more onerous, be followed.

1. Individual cables should be marked unless their installation makes it obvious that they contain intrinsically safe circuits, for example, where they are in a cable tray or duct or a clearly defined part thereof, which is clearly marked (see 2).
2. Cable trays or ducts or parts thereof, which are reserved for intrinsically safe circuit cables only, should be clearly marked if the cables within them are not marked.
3. Points on conduit systems at which conductors may be drawn into the conduit, such as junction boxes, should be marked to prevent non-intrinsically safe circuit conductors from being drawn into the conduit.

Marking may be by label or colour coding or by equally effective means. It should be noted, however, that connection facilities within certified/approved intrinsically safe and associated apparatus will be marked by the colour light blue if a colour code is used, and thus where colour coding of cables, cable trays or conduits or parts thereof and conduits is used for this purpose then the same colour (light blue) should always be used. It is necessary to ensure that no other cables have sheath colouring of light blue (e.g., thermocouple cable) where sheath colour coding is used to identify intrinsically safe circuit cables. Where the colour coding is used for tray/ducting or conduits, other cables can be light blue although this is not ideal as it could cause confusion.

20.3.6 Additional requirements for Zone 0 (and Zone 20 where appropriate)

Notwithstanding Chapter 13 intrinsically safe circuits entering Zone 0 (or where appropriate Zone 20) should only be fed down Type 9 multicore cables containing more than one intrinsically safe circuit where all intrinsically safe circuits within the cable are category 'ia' (see Chapter 13). (Category 'ib' circuits are only intrinsically safe with one fault and thus, with more faults must be considered as non-intrinsically safe, which means that with two faults the circuits could operate in a way which could damage the cable).

Intrinsically safe circuits may be fed down such multicore cables where the circuits within the cable and its screens are connected to the potential equalization system at the same point, or each screen within the cable is insulated from all other screens with insulation capable of withstanding a test voltage of 500 V rms (this means that the total insulation between screens should be capable of withstanding a test voltage of 1000 V rms). (If the screens can become interconnected and are earthed at different points it is possible to invade the enclosed circuits with any current which flows when the two points on the potential equalization system are at different potentials as may be the case in fault conditions).

20.4 Conductor terminations

In intrinsically safe installations, particularly where multicore cables are used, it is common to find uncertified junction boxes in installations rather, than the case in other protection concepts where any such box would need certification/approval because its content would be ignition capable if sparking occurred. Junction boxes in intrinsically safe installations are used to allow individual distribution of circuits where several are included in the same cable and in individual circuits where advantage can be identified (e.g., in cases where certified/approved apparatus has a flying lead rather than terminals and thus no termination provision, where the terminals in the certified/approved apparatus are in the same enclosure as the electrical components and it is considered this constitutes an unacceptable risk of damage in the particular installation, and where it is considered as advantageous to have a local isolation facility outside the apparatus or its terminal box). In these cases it is necessary to ensure that the terminal box satisfies those construction requirements appropriate which would be applied if it were certified/approved and the duty here falls upon the user.

20.4.1 Terminal construction

The terminals used in such boxes need to be constructed so that the clearance, creepage and distance through encapsulant or solid insulation satisfy the requirements for intrinsic safety (see Tables 13.8, 13.9 and 13.10 in Chapter 13). In addition, to minimize the possibility of inadvertent earths due to stray strands of terminated conductors touching other circuits or earth, the minimum distances between the point of termination and earth, and between the point of termination and other circuits need to satisfy the requirements shown in Fig. 20.3.

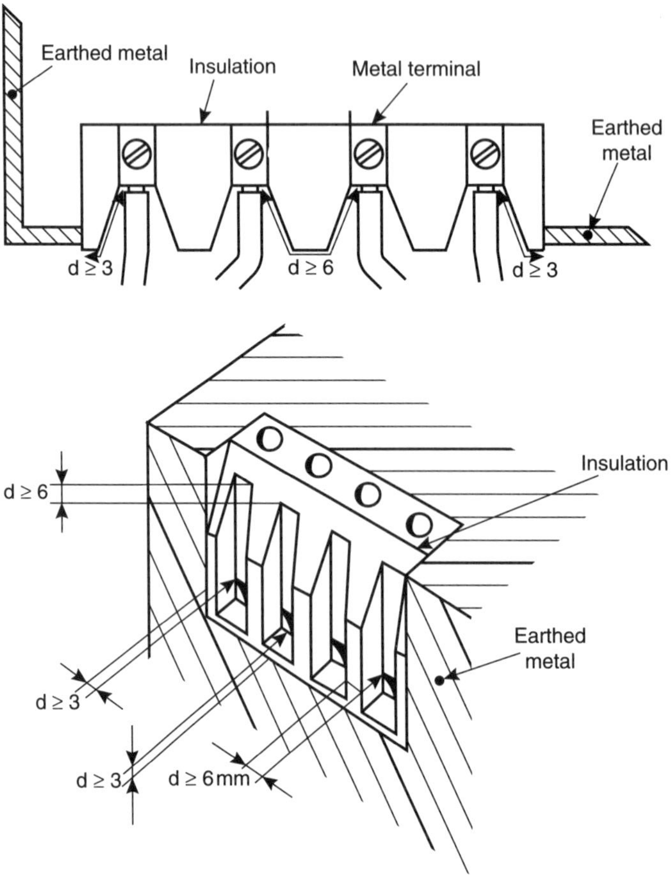

Fig. 20.3 Terminal construction

It should be noted that in BS 5345, Part 4 the separation from earthed metal was 4 mm rising to 6 mm at circuit voltage above 90 V peak and up to 374 V peak. This was to take account of the minimum figures in Tables 13.8, 13.9 and 13.10 which require clearances of 4 mm at 90 V peak and 6 mm at 375 V peak. Such a precaution is not necessary as the clearance figure is determined by the tables where they exceed the clearances given in Fig. 20.3, as the Fig. 20.3 clearances are only to give minimum dimensions for physical reasons rather than electrical ones as is the case with the tables.

Terminals in junction boxes also need to give confidence in the quality of connection. This means that the method of clamping the conductors needs to ensure adequate clamping of all conductor strands and of not damaging them in doing so. While a normal screw terminal will satisfy this requirement where the conductor ends are fitted with a crimped ferrule to prevent direct pressure on the conductor (see Fig. 20.4), the action of the screw when it directly impinges on a conductor, particularly a stranded conductor, is such that effective clamping cannot be guaranteed and possible damage to the conductor or its strands cannot be ignored. The normal terminal used for a single conductor is shown in Fig. 20.5 and for multiple termination in Fig. 20.6.

The use of terminals can be summed up as follows. First, terminals where the screw impinges directly on the conductor are only permissible for conductors fitted with a ferrule, whether they are single conductors or multistranded conductors (see Fig. 20.4). In addition, only one such ferruled conductor may normally be terminated in such a terminal.

Second, terminals of the type shown in Fig. 20.5 may be used for a single conductor with or without ferrule, whether it is a single conductor or a multi-strand conductor. Only one such conductor should be terminated in a terminal of this type.

Third, terminals of the type shown in Fig. 20.6 are specifically designed to allow termination of more than one conductor, whether it is a single conductor or multi-strand conductor. Conductors with or without ferrule

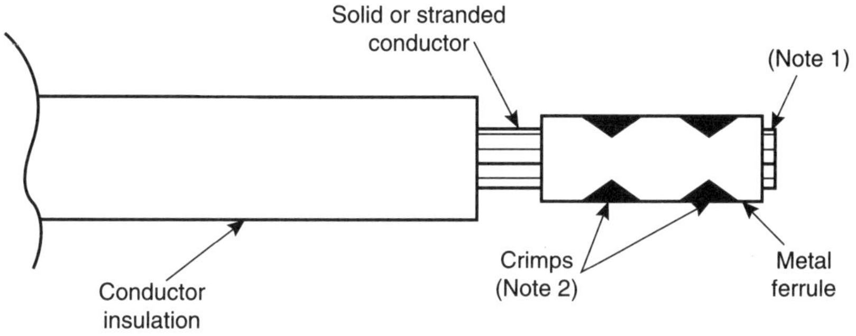

Fig. 20.4 Conductor crimping. *Notes*: (1) Conductor must exit the ferrule but must be cut off as close to the ferrule as possible. (2) Two *Independent* crimping points are necessary to ensure reliable crimping and electrical connection

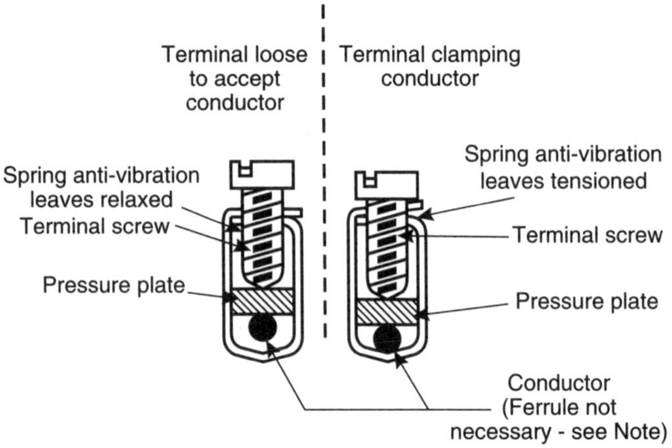

Fig. 20.5 Typical terminal for termination of a single conductor. *Note*: If the pressure plate were omitted a ferrule would be necessary on the conductor

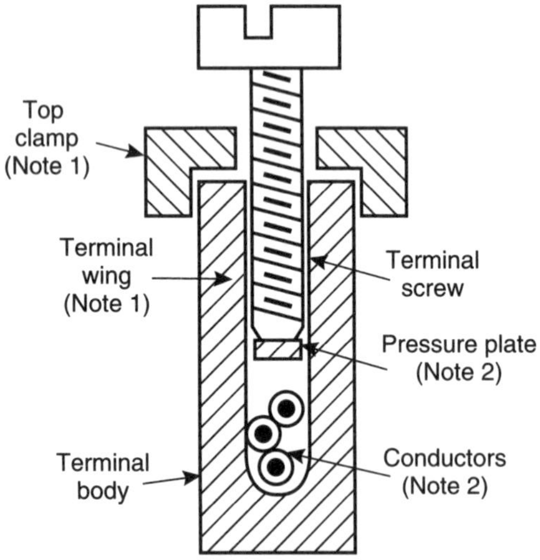

Fig. 20.6 Typical terminal for multi conductor termination. *Notes*: (1) Vibration security is achieved by slight spreading of wings, until retained by top clamp, on tightening. (2) Conductors should be fitted with ferrules even if a pressure plate is present

may be terminated provided the maximum number specified by the terminal manufacturer is not exceeded.

Notwithstanding the above it is always best to use a ferrule with multi-stranded conductors if possible as it gives the opportunity to identify the crimping of all strands in the multi-stranded conductor before termination takes place.

It is also necessary to ensure that terminals are secure against loosening, particularly in the case of multi-circuit junction boxes as loose wires could cause interconnection between circuits or inadvertent earths. Most normal terminals achieve the necessary integrity in this regard but the practice is to use terminals which satisfy the requirements of increased safety 'e' (see Chapter 12) to ensure this. These terminals are not normally certified/approved as such, but use the same forms of construction and are readily available. Most ranges of these also have the possibility of interconnection of terminals by shorting bars which allow termination of more than one conductor at a single electrical point without the necessity of using terminals as described in Fig. 20.6.

20.4.2 Assemblies of terminals (junction and barrier boxes)

In the hazardous area terminal boxes can only contain intrinsically safe circuits when mounted in a hazardous area unless their configuration is certified/approved to another protection concept suitable for the hazardous area of installation (e.g., flameproof enclosure 'd' or increased safety 'e'). In such cases not only must the box comply with the protection concept in question, but the segregation of intrinsically safe circuit wiring and non-intrinsically safe circuit wiring must comply with the separation requirements which are necessary when they are mounted in a non-hazardous area.

Where only intrinsically safe circuit conductors are present the outer sheath of the conductor is usually removed as soon as the cable enters the box, and conductors inside the box are then usually loomed together or fitted inside trunking to give security as they will not move much even if they become disconnected. Figure 20.7 shows a typical arrangement for such boxes. The screens are usually led through the box without being connected to the potential equalization system in such boxes, either by being gathered on a conducting bar or by use of additional terminals (although this latter is difficult where multicore cables with an overall screen only are concerned). It is necessary to exercise extreme care when this is done as the screens are not connected to the potential equalization system and should be capable of withstanding a 500 V rms test. As testing in hazardous areas is often difficult, the physical arrangements for the screen are important and may require its sleeving to prevent inadvertent connections. If a connection to the potential equalization system is intended and possible then all of the screens intended to be connected should be gathered on a conducting bar, and the bar should be connected to the potential equalization system with an insulated conductor which has a level of insulation capable of withstanding a 500 V rms test which gives a connection resistance not exceeding 1 Ω.

The above constructional specifications also apply to junction boxes which contain both intrinsically safe and non-intrinsically safe terminations. While this should be avoided as far as possible where it becomes necessary the best way is to divide the box into two compartments (as shown in Fig. 20.8). The

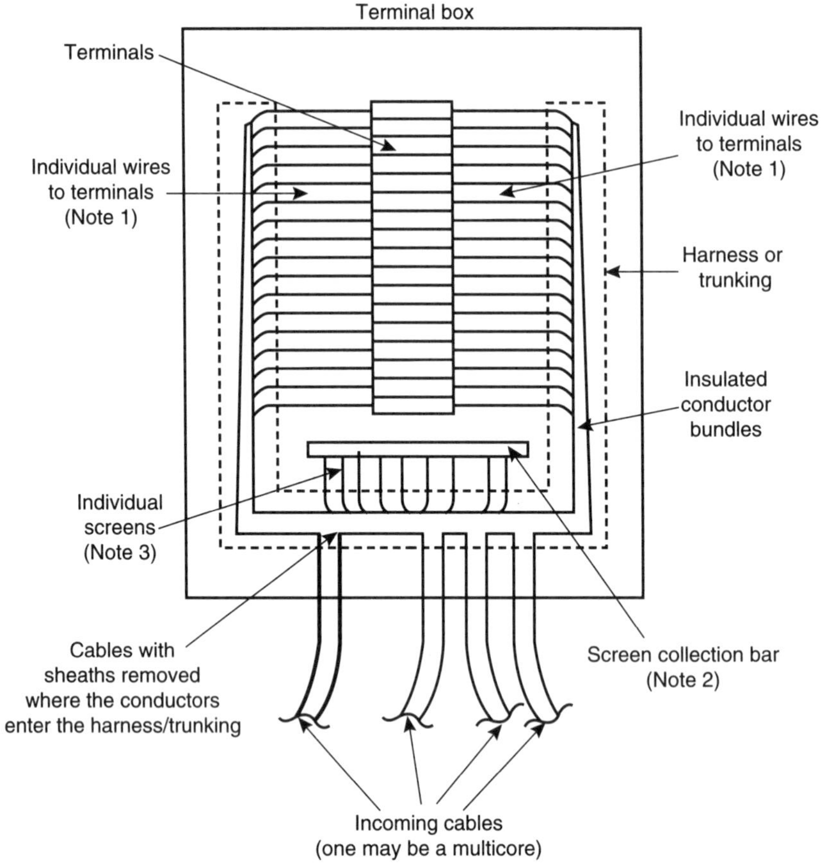

Fig. 20.7 Typical junction box containing only intrinsically safe circuits. *Notes* (1) The wires are insulated up to the terminal. (2) Where screens are connected to the potential equalization system (bonded) at the same point they may be collected on a conducting bar which is insulated from the enclosure. (3) Where individual screens are connected to the potential equalization system (bonded) at different points one to another, they may not be connected to a common bar but shall be sleeved with insulation and fed through terminals as other conductors

partition in this case needs to be the same as would be required in associated apparatus (see Chapter 13) in that it should extend to within 1.5 mm of the enclosure walls and is sufficiently robust. As before, this normally means a metal partition of at least 0.45 mm minimum thickness firmly connected to the potential equalization system or an insulated barrier 0.9 mm thick. If the material used can be easily distorted by manual pressure at these thicknesses they should be increased until it gives confidence that normal termination activities will not cause significant distortion. As there are non-intrinsically safe circuits in this situation it is important that the connection to the potential equalization (bonding) system is not combined with that for the screen of intrinsically safe cables (see Section 20.5 of this chapter).

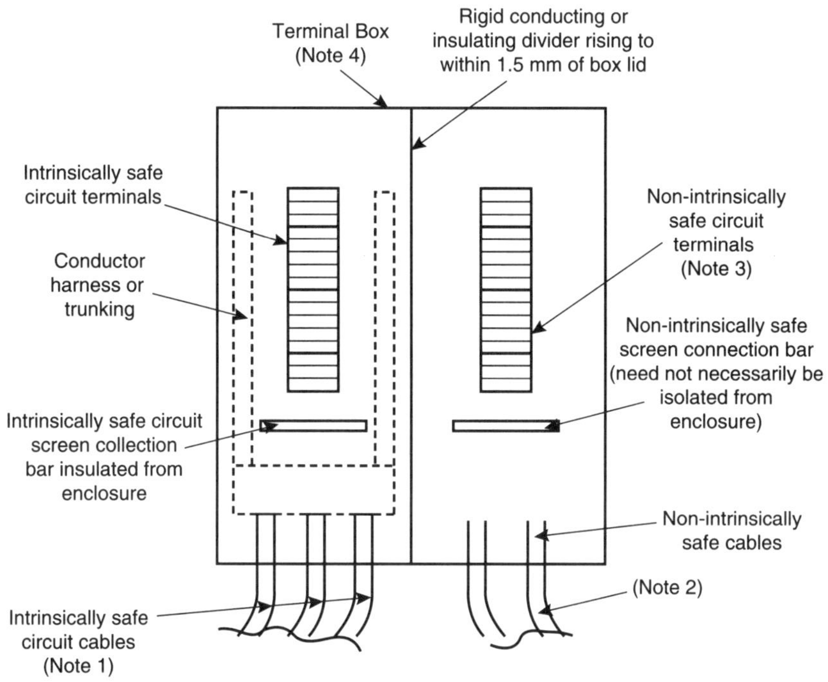

Fig. 20.8 Mixed circuit box with divider. *Notes*: (1) These cables should be fed to dedicated intrinsically safe cable trays/ducts. (2) Non-intrinsically safe circuit cables should be kept separate from intrinsically safe circuit cables. (3) Installation of non-intrinsically safe circuit cable must comply with the protection concept appropriate or industrial practice. (4) Box construction (as far as is appropriate to non-intrinsically safe circuit cables) must comply with industrial requirements. Where it is hazardous area mounted it must satisfy a relevant protection concept (e.g., Ex d or Ex e) as far as non-intrinsically safe terminations are concerned

If such partitions are not present the configuration should be as shown in Fig. 20.9. The termination points of the conductors and screens of the intrinsically safe and non-intrinsically safe circuits are separated by a clearance of at least 50 mm measured through air between them around any rigid insulating or metal partitions present. In this case, insulating rather than metal partitions are to be preferred unless the metal partition is firmly connected to the potential equalization system.

As previously stated, cable harness or trunking for the intrinsically safe circuit conductors and screens is always necessary to prevent excessive movement, but in the case where there is no partition such harness or trunking becomes necessary for the non-intrinsically safe circuit conductors and screens to prevent movement lessening separation from intrinsically safe counterparts.

A particular application of the mixed junction box is the one where it is used for the fitting of barrier devices and thus becomes the intrinsically safe interface of several intrinsically safe systems. This is shown in Fig. 20.10.

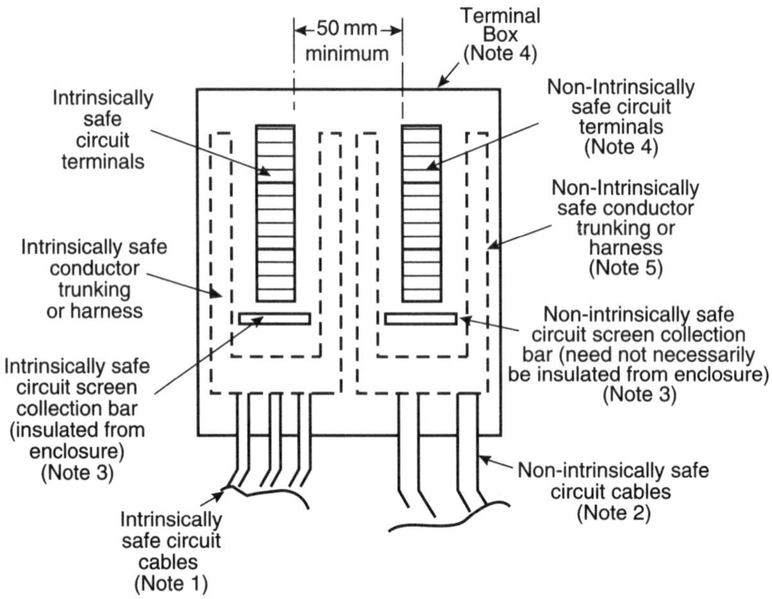

Fig. 20.9 Mixed circuit box without a divider. *Notes*: (1) These cables should be fed to dedicated intrinsically safe cable trays/ducts. (2) Non-intrinsically safe circuit cables should be kept separate from intrinsically safe circuit cables. (3) If the non-intrinsically safe circuit screen collection bar is not deliberately connected to the potential equalization system (possibly via the enclosure) it must be 50 mm from the intrinsically safe circuit screen collection box and the intrinsically safe circuit terminals. (4) Box and non-intrinsically safe parts must comply with industrial requirements if mounted in a non-hazardous area, but if hazardous area mounted must satisfy the requirements of an appropriate protection concept (e.g., Ex d or Ex e). (5) Non-intrinsically safe conductors must be in a restraining harness or trunk, and if a harness, then separation from a harness containing intrinsically safe conductors should be at least in accordance with the requirements of BS/EN 50020 (3 mm minimum is suggested)

Terminal and barrier boxes for general use should be IP54, particularly if used outside, and should be robust to allow for rough handling. This is, of course, not necessary when the terminals or barriers are mounted within a control room or similar, and even a box is not strictly necessary here if the location is protected from the environment and interference by the configuration of the building. It is recommended, however, that a terminal or barrier box should be used in all but the most exceptional of circumstances as otherwise the degree of personnel control necessary to avoid danger will be very high and is unlikely to be maintained over a long period.

It is slightly less usual, but sometimes necessary, to create a junction box where the intrinsically safe system is composite whereby the voltage limitation is in one item of apparatus and the current limiting circuits in another, which is the case with some alarm and public address systems. This involves three types of wiring in the box as follows:

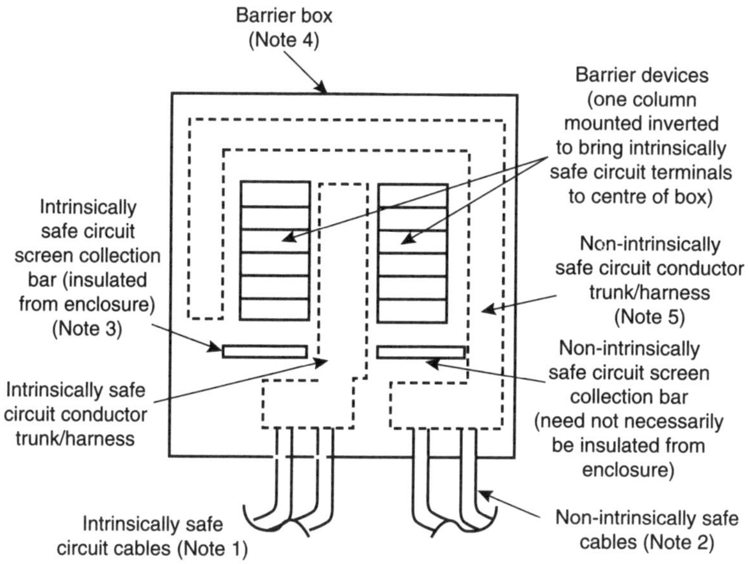

Fig. 20.10 Barrier box arrangement. *Notes*: (1) These cables should be fed to a dedicated intrinsically safe cable tray/duct. (2) Non-intrinsically safe circuit cables should be kept separate from intrinsically safe circuit cables. (3) If the non-intrinsically safe circuit screen collection bar is not deliberately connected to the potential equalization system (possibly via the enclosure) it must be at least 50 mm from the intrinsically safe circuit screen collection bar and the intrinsically safe circuit barrier terminals. (4) The box construction and arrangements must be the same as those for a mixed terminal box without partition (see Fig. 20.9). (5) Non-intrinsically safe circuit conductors must be treated as in Fig. 20.9

1. non-intrinsically safe circuit wiring;
2. wiring where the voltage is sufficiently controlled to satisfy the requirements of intrinsic safety but there is no current limiting and so this is not intrinsically safe circuit wiring;
3. intrinsically safe circuit wiring.

Where all three types of wiring occur they need to be kept apart and the voltage controlled wiring must be separated from the intrinsically safe circuit wiring as though it were non-intrinsically safe circuit wiring and, in addition, it must be separated from the non-intrinsically safe circuit wiring as though it were intrinsically safe circuit wiring.

20.5 Earthing and bonding (connection to the potential equalization system)

Any metal enclosures of items of apparatus in an intrinsically safe system should be connected to the local steelwork and the potential equalization (bonding) system in the same way as above, as are the enclosures of apparatus using all other protection concepts. Likewise, armouring applied to the cables of intrinsically safe systems, metal cable sheaths and conduits should be similarly treated (see Chapter 18).

Connections between the intrinsically safe circuit and any screens used on cables need to be treated quite differently. Because sparking at terminals and elsewhere in the installation is permitted within the concept of intrinsic safety, the emphasis moves from security of connection to prevention of multiple connections to the potential equalization system as, during power faults, the potential at different parts of the potential equalization system may vary from one another. If this is the case and if there is more than one connection between the intrinsically safe system and the potential equalization system a difference in voltage between the two may add to the voltage of the intrinsically safe system which may then spark incendively in normal operation or in fault conditions. Figure 20.11 shows the situation which could occur if an intrinsically safe circuit, connected to the potential equalization at its source, is connected in such a way that fault currents occurring in other electrical circuits cause elevation of the point of connection by even a small voltage. That voltage will be added to the voltage of the intrinsically safe circuit and if a fault to the potential equalization system occurs elsewhere in the circuit where no elevation is present then sparking could be incendive. This is most important at

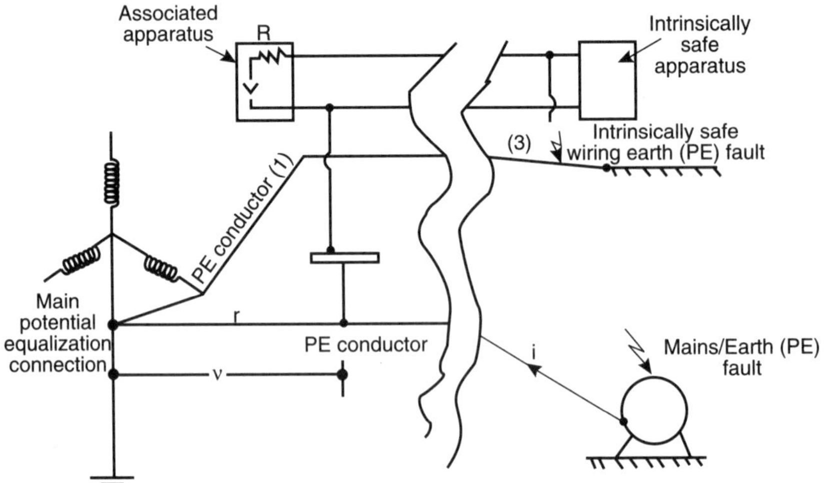

Fig. 20.11 Effect of voltage variation in potential equalization system. *Notes*: (1) i = Electrical fault current, v = Potential difference between point of connection of intrinsically safe circuit to PE conductor and main earth reference point due to '*i*' and the PE conductor resistance '*r*'. (2) The Earth (PE conductor) potential at the point where the earth (PE) fault occurs in the intrinsically safe circuit wiring is equal to the potential at the main connection. (3) Current in I/S fault is (V + v)/R. This may be ignition capable due to the addition of v

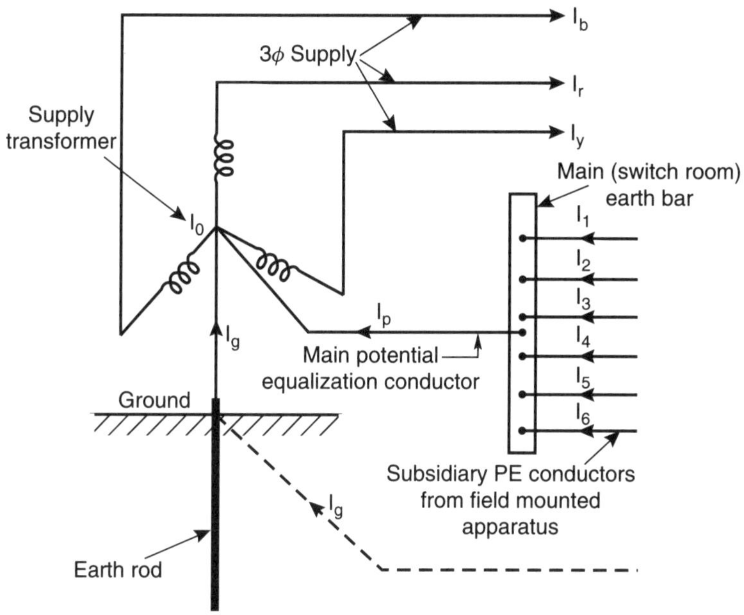

I_p = Leakage and fault currents from field mounted equipment
$= I_1 + I_2 + I_3 + I_4 + I_5 + I_6$

I_g = Leakage and fault ground currents from field mounted equipment

$I_r + I_y + I_b$ = Supply currents

I_0 = Current at transformer star point
$= 0 \quad (I_r + I_y + I_b + I_g + I_p = 0)$

Fig. 20.12 Current flows at supply transformer.

the source end of the system as this is where all return currents congregate, including fault currents, and thus elevation is much more likely. Figure 20.12 shows the general configuration of current flow in the electrical installation.

The base criteria for intrinsically safe circuits are therefore as follows.

1. They should preferably be isolated from the potential equalization system subject to a high resistance connection (say 0.5–1.0 MΩ) to prevent accrual of charge due to static electricity generation.
2. They should be connected to the potential equalization system in one place only and elsewhere insulated from that system with insulation capable of withstanding a 500 V rms insulation test.
3. The point of connection to the potential equalization system, if one exists, must be one where the potential of the system is most likely to be at a similar voltage to the generality of the potential equalization system and hence the involved structural metalwork and ground.

20.5.1 Typical Zone 1 and Zone 21 intrinsically safe circuits with bonding connection in the non-hazardous area

The most general type of intrinsically safe system is one where there is, in fact, a necessity of a circuit earth, and thus typical of the circuit described in 2 in the list on the previous page. This offers considerable financial advantages over the type of circuit described in 1 and, if properly installed, is satisfactory for use in Zone 1 and 21. (The Zone 0 and 20 situation will be described in Section 20.5.5 of this chapter). This circuit will normally have up to three items requiring connection to the potential equalization system, all of them being in the associated apparatus. These are normally the enclosure, a screen in the mains transformer, and the intrinsically safe circuit.

The enclosure

The enclosure is often of metal and if so it needs to be earthed to ensure operation of circuit protection devices in case of fault and to ensure personnel protection from electric shock. It will be normally be mounted on a steel structure which will also mount other electrical apparatus, including such things as lighting and non-intrinsically safe control, indicating and switching apparatus, including the non-intrinsically safe parts of the associated apparatus which could themselves generate considerable fault currents. Thus it will be subject to fault currents from all of the apparatus mounted on it and, because of this needs to be connected to the potential equalization (bonding) system in order to ensure that electrical protection operates and to remove the risk of electric shock. This connection will, however, have many different currents flowing in it due to the multiplicity of apparatus with which it is in contact (see Fig. 20.13).

The intrinsically safe circuit interface

This is often a transformer (see Fig. 20.13) which forms the interface, providing the primary voltage control for the intrinsically safe circuit is likely to be fitted with a screen between the windings feeding the intrinsically safe circuits and other windings, and this will carry current if a fault occurs within the transformer as its objective is to ensure that the transformer protection operates before any breakthrough of the screen occurs. The transformer core will be bonded to the general potential equalization system, usually via the apparatus case, and if the screen is bonded to the core then its connection is already defined. If this is not the case then the screen will satisfy the basic insulation requirements for associated apparatus and it should still be so bonded as its objective is to divert primary current from the intrinsically safe circuit. The intrinsically safe circuit will be connected to the secondary of the transformer and will almost always be connected to the potential equalization system to prevent

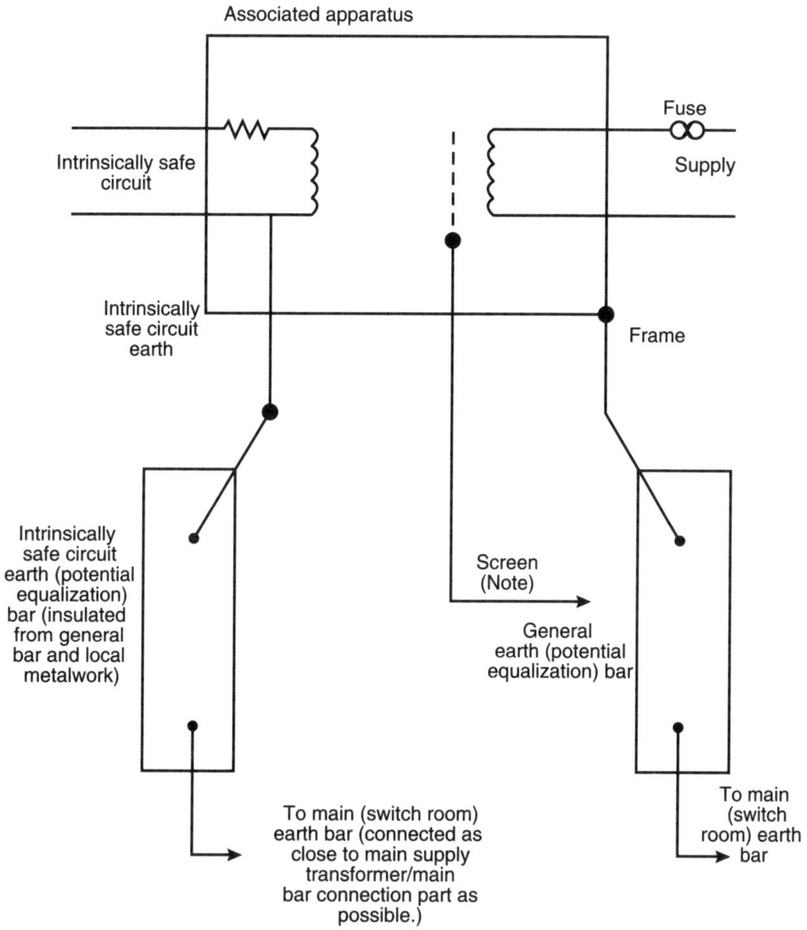

Fig. 20.13 Typical associated apparatus potential equalization (earthing) system. *Note* The screen may be connected instead to the intrinsically safe circuit earth bar but the above connection is preferred.

noise causing operational problems and, as most circuits are basically asymmetrical, to prevent current limiting devices being short circuited by earth faults (see Fig. 20.14). This connection is very important as it is to the intrinsically safe circuit itself and connection to the general potential equalization system together with the transformer screen and the enclosure is normally not acceptable due to the fault currents which could flow. The ideal is to directly connect to the main supply transformer star point as this is the point where fault currents equalize and no voltage elevation occurs. It is not usually possible to achieve connection to the transformer itself but experience has shown that the main earth bar in the principal switchroom is adequate and that is where the connection is normally made. This is the connection used in other cases where the intrinsically safe circuit is directly involved, such as circuits using shunt zener diode safety barriers.

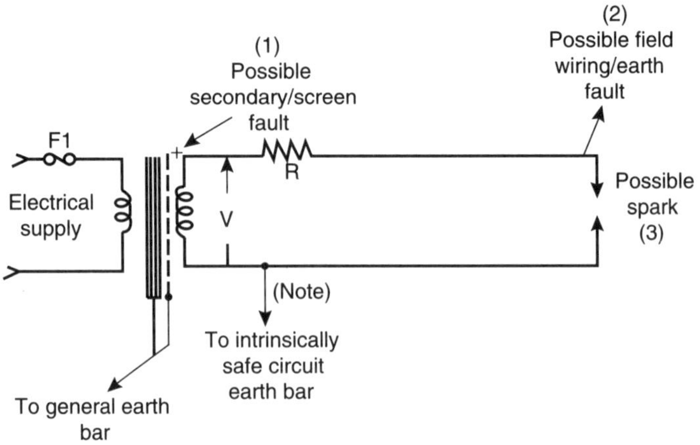

Fig. 20.14 Use of intrinsically safe circuit potential equalization (earth) connection. *Notes*: Without this connection faults (1) and (2) would short circuit *R* and the spark (3) would be ignition capable. With this connection fault (2) has no effect and fault (1) causes rupture of *F*1 by short circuiting secondary. Thus the spark is never ignition capable

The desired situation is achieved by producing two large earth bars, one for general connections to the potential equalization system and a second for the protected (or clean) earth required for intrinsically safe circuits. It is necessary for the latter to be carefully insulated from local steelwork and other conducting items connected to the potential equalization system up to the point where it deliberately connects to that system so that it cannot be invaded by spurious currents flowing in such conducting parts. It is also required to provide a path which will ensure that the total resistance of connection from the circuit to the main point of connection to the potential equalization system (switch room earth bar) is less than 1 Ω. In order to provide sufficient mechanical strength, the conductor used for the connection needs to be of a cross-sectional area of 4 mm^2 or more.

All other parts of the intrinsically safe circuit must remain insulated from the potential equalization system including enclosures and local structural steelwork except for situations where radio interference suppression capacitors are fitted. These connect directly between the circuit and the enclosure and/or potential equalization system. Fortunately they are there to suppress high frequencies and have a significant impedance at 50 Hz, the frequency of the mains which provided the major risk. BS/EN 50020[3] permits a leakage current of 5 mA to flow in the tests which it requires for insulation of intrinsically safe circuits and this equates to RFI capacitors of total value up to around 40 000 μF (that is all of the capacitors in parallel). While RFI capacitors are usually fitted at the manufacturing stage there appears to be little objection to fitting them later as 'simple apparatus' provided they satisfy the requirements of BS/EN 50020[3] and the above requirements.

Barrier installations are unusual in that they usually contain a barrier enclosure containing several intrinsically safe circuits and non-intrinsically safe circuits. The configuration is shown in Fig. 20.10 and needs no further explanation. The problem, however, is that to test the insulated connecting lead which connects the barrier bar to the main potential equalization system would mean isolating several intrinsically safe circuits rather than one as is usually the case. This problem can be overcome by using two parallel connections, each capable of satisfying the connection requirements. Thus one can be disconnected for testing without interfering with the operation of the circuits in question.

20.5.2 Typical Zone 1 and Zone 21 intrinsically safe circuits with bonding connection in the hazardous area

In some cases it is necessary for the potential equalization connection to be in the hazardous area for operational reasons. A typical case is one where thermocouples need to be welded on to a conducting item whose temperature is to be measured and this type of connection is necessary to achieve the required accuracy. The welded-on thermocouple also provides a connection to the potential equalization system via the item in question and no other connection is permissible other than a high resistance connection for the purposes of RFI suppression for instance.

The most simple way of dealing with this problem is to utilize a barrier device which provides galvanic isolation in the non-hazardous area but this will leave a long cable run necessary to transfer the very small thermocouple signal. Possibly a better way of providing a more normal intrinsically safe circuit configuration, as well as being operationally more sensible, is to use a galvanically separating signal conditioner local to the thermocouple itself. This allows a normal zener barrier device to be installed in the non-hazardous area as the interface and earthing to appear more normal. The effect of these two options are shown in Fig. 20.15.

20.5.3 Typical Zone 1 and Zone 21 circuits with bonding connection at more than one point

This type of circuit is becoming less necessary as galvanic isolation techniques become more available and the circuit can now be divided into two circuits if necessary, so that multiple connections no longer occur commonly. Historically, however, they were much more common and several such circuits were certified and remain in use. Typical of such circuits are such things as pH probes and dissolved oxygen probes.

The approach in such cases is to bond both ends of the circuit with a robust bonding conductor in order to try to minimize any potential difference between the potential equalization system at each end of the circuit where the earth connections exist. To further ensure this to be the case the length of the bonding conductor was required not to exceed 100 m which effectively meant that the two ends of the system could not be

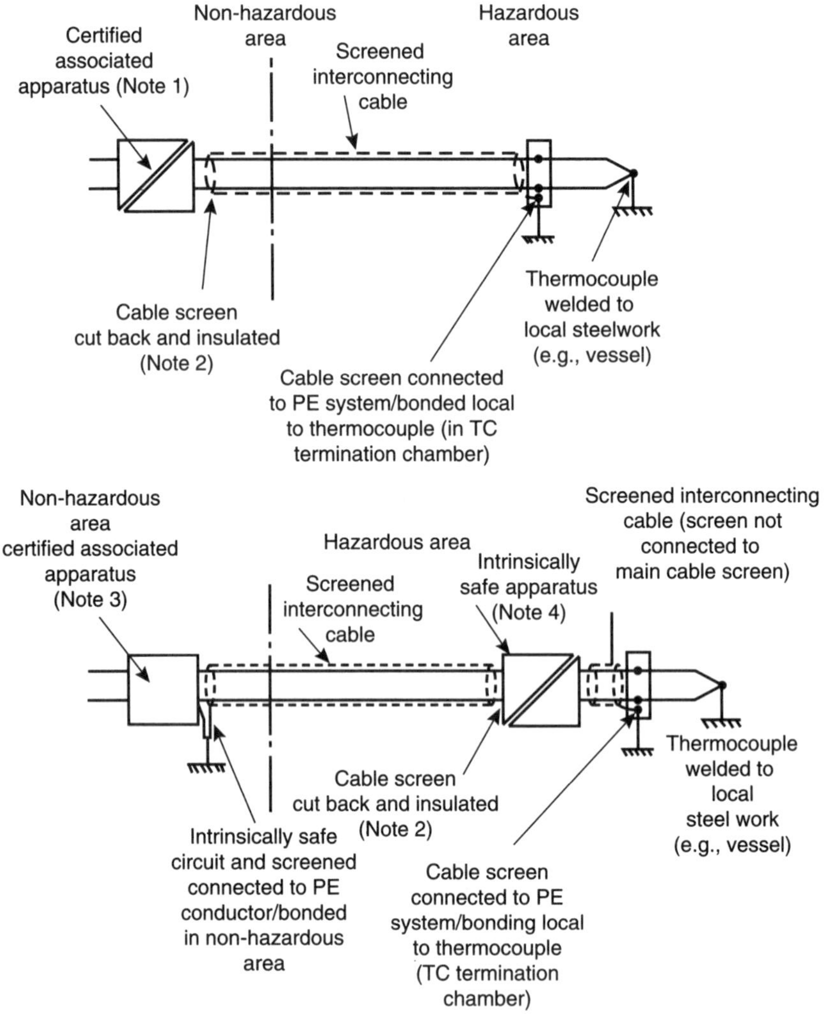

Fig. 20.15 Intrinsically safe circuit bonded in the hazardous area. *Notes*: (1) Associated apparatus must provide full galvanic, isolation (2) Cable screen must be continuous (if two lengths of cable are used screens must be connected together) and connected to PE system/earth only local to the thermocouple (3) Associated apparatus need not provide full galvanic isolation (4) Intrinsically safe apparatus must provide full galvanic isolation

more than around 60 m apart as cable is not routed as the crow flies. It is not clear if it is the proximity of the two parts of the system which assists in the achievement of intrinsic safety or the bonding action of the conductor. The approach did, however, appear to be acceptable and was often used. The wider availability of galvanically isolating circuit elements, such as galvanically isolating barriers and transmitters, has now made this

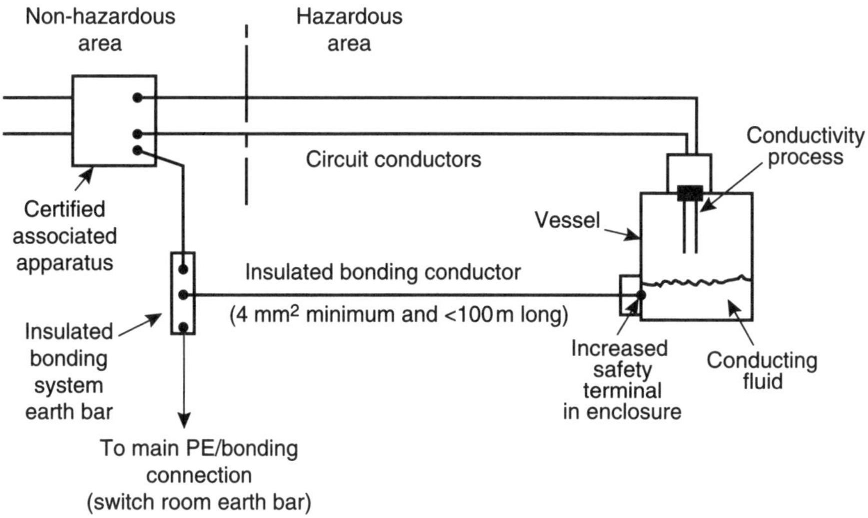

Fig. 20.16 Circuit with more than one operational earth

approach less necessary and it is recommended, that the galvanic isolation approach described in Section 20.5.2 be used wherever it is available.

A typical bonded circuit is shown in Fig. 20.16. It is wise to separate the potential equalization/bonding system for such circuits from that of normal one connection circuits by using a separate collection bar and connection to the main potential equalization system connection point (switch room earth bar). This is considered as particularly important when electrical apparatus with significant fault current capability is installed near the hazardous area end of this type of circuit.

The bonding conductor approach is not recommended for use in any 'ia' circuit which enters Zone 0 or 20 because of the possible currents which may flow in the bonding conductor during electrical faults in or near the hazardous-area end of the installation, and their danger in respect of an area where explosive atmosphere is always or regularly present.

20.5.4 Bonding and insulation of screens for intrinsically safe circuits

The connection of the screens in cables containing intrinsically safe circuits has already been touched on and the basic requirements are as follows.

1. The screen on the cable containing a single intrinsically safe circuit or the overall screen on a Type B multicore cable (see Chapter 13) containing more than one intrinsically safe circuit must be connected to the potential equalization system at the same point as the circuit or circuits, and insulated from the potential equalization system elsewhere when the screen is applied directly over the conductors without consideration of the cable

bedding (see Option a of Fig. 20.17). This means that all circuits in Type B multicore cables (see Chapter 13) of this construction must be earthed at the same point.

2. The screen of a cable including an overall screen on a Type B multicore cable which is fitted over bedding (see Option b of Fig. 20.17), where the bedding satisfies the same requirements as specified for the conductor, insulation may be earthed at a point different to the contained circuits provided that the cable, be it an individual circuit cable or a Type B multicore cable, is installed in the manner required for security against interconnection of circuits in Type B multicore cables (see Section 20.3.3).

3. Where a Type A multicore cable, containing more than one intrinsically safe circuit with screens satisfying the requirements of (2) above, has insulation fitted over each individual screen, which satisfies the insulation requirements specified for conductor insulation, and the cable installation satisfies the installation requirements for security against interconnection of circuits

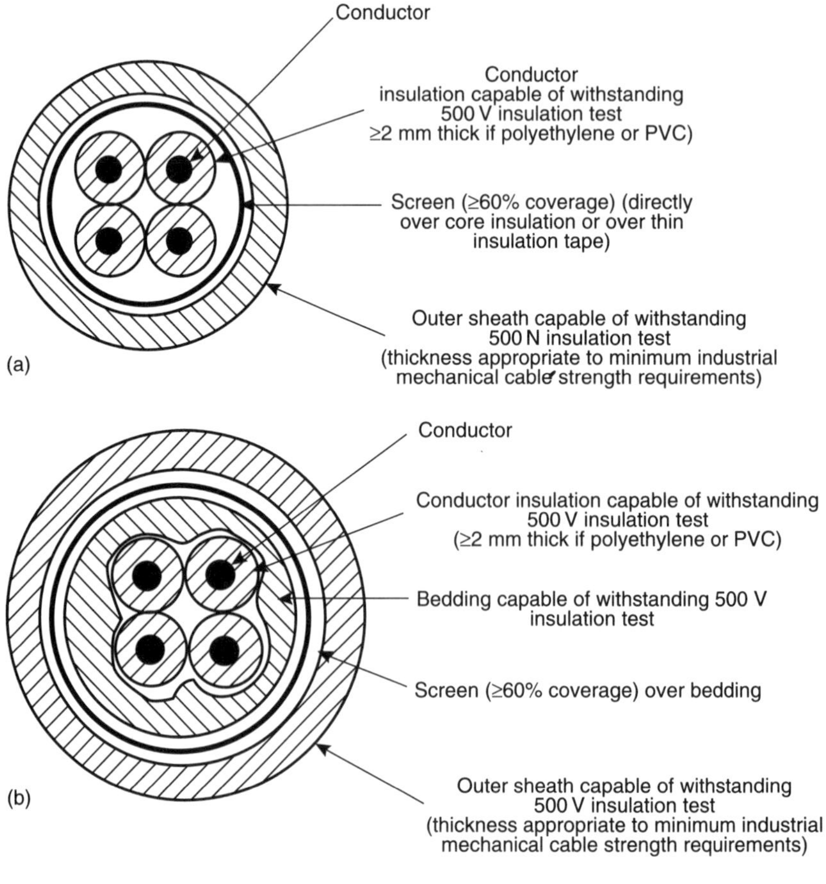

Fig. 20.17 (a) Type 'B' multicore cable without bedding and overall screen, (b) Type 'B' multicore cable with bedding and overall screen

in Type B cables (see Section 20.3.3), the circuits and screens within the cable may be earthed in any combination as follows:

1. Each circuit should be earthed at the same point as its individual screen.
2. The circuits in the cable may all be connected to the potential equalization system at the same or different points.
3. The individual screens may be all connected to the potential equalization system at the same point or different points but should still be connected at the same points as their individual circuits.
4. Where an additional overall screen is fitted the individual screens and the overall screen must all be connected to the potential equalization system at the same point, unless the overall screen is fitted over bedding which satisfies the insulation requirements for conductor insulation when they may be so connected at different points and at points different from the point of connection of the overall screen.

In some cases, for example, in some high frequency applications or where a screen is high resistance, it may be necessary to connect the screen to the potential equalization system at more than one point. This cannot be done directly but may be done by producing a dedicated bonding conductor to which the screen is connected at several points, and then connecting that conductor to the potential equalization system at the point where the screen would otherwise have been connected. This requires that the conductor in question be insulated from all local conducting parts throughout its route, except where the single intended connection is made. To achieve this and to ensure sufficient mechanical strength the conductor used should have a cross section of at least 4 mm^2 and its insulation must be sufficient to withstand a test voltage of 500 V. Figure 20.18 shows the approach which needs to be adopted in such cases.

20.5.5 Typical Zone 0 and Zone 20 intrinsically safe circuits

Zone 0 or Zone 20 circuits are circuits intended for installations in areas where the explosive atmosphere is always assumed present and additional care needs to be taken to ensure that the circuits are secure. This requires that additional precautions be taken.

Only 'ia' circuits (see Chapter 13) may enter Zones 0 or 20 as 'ib' circuits (see Chapter 13) are not considered to have a high enough level of security against becoming a source of ignition.

Use of multicore cables

When 'ia' circuits entering a Zone 0 or 20 are fed in multicore cables all circuits in the cable must be 'ia'. This is because 'ib' circuits, due to

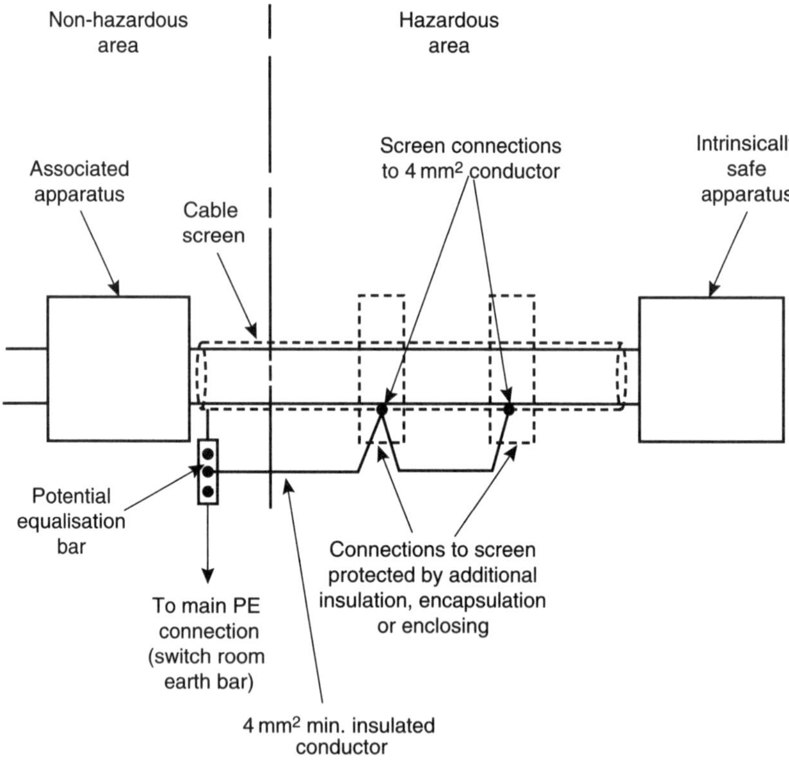

Fig. 20.18 Multiple screen connection

their lower level of security, have to be considered as non-intrinsically safe circuits as far as Zone 0 or 20 are concerned and thus their presence in such multicore cables is not acceptable. Likewise, Type B multicore cables are not acceptable for circuits which enter Zone 0 or 20 unless the combination of circuits in the multicore are intrinsically safe to 'ia' levels even when interconnected. Again, this is because of the lower level of security against fault of Type B cables even when properly installed. Type C and D multicore cables must be also be treated in this way.

Circuits without galvanic isolation

Circuits which do not have galvanic isolation, either in the associated apparatus or in intrinsically safe apparatus placed in the circuit outside the Zone 0 or Zone 20, should only be used where the part of the circuit in the Zone 0 or 20 is exceptionally well protected. Typically this would be where metal sheathed thermocouples or resistance thermometers are led into Zone 0 or 20 through glands so that their terminals are in a less hazardous area, and where the thermocouple or resistance element is insulated from the metal sheath. Figure 20.19 shows the types of circuit referred to.

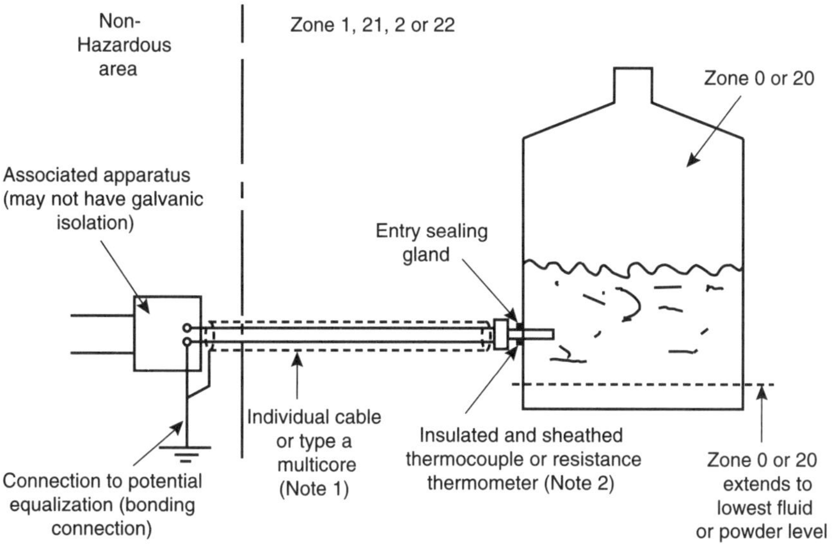

Fig. 20.19 'ia' circuit for Zone 0 or Zone 20 without galvanic isolation. *Notes*: (1) Multicore may contain only 'ia' circuits. (2) Electrical circuit inside sheath must be fully insulated and sheath must be high integrity (e.g., welded metal sheath)

Circuits with galvanic isolation which are fully insulated in the hazardous area

The circuits used may have galvanic isolation and any deliberate connection to the potential equalization system may be at the point where the circuit enters the Zone 0 or 20 or in the non-hazardous area. This type of approach is only acceptable where the apparatus in the hazardous area is fully insulated, for example, in ultrasonic level detectors, etc. Figure 20.20 shows the approach for this type of circuit.

Circuits with galvanic isolation which are not effectively insulated in the hazardous area

Where insulation in the hazardous area cannot be guaranteed, any deliberate connection to the potential equalization system must be local to the Zone 0 or Zone 20. This does not mean inside such a Zone as such connections would be hard to monitor but they should be at the Zone interface. The structure and electrical bonding inside the Zone 0 or 20 should be sufficiently good to give confidence that differential voltages are unlikely to occur within it. In addition, there should be no powerful electrical apparatus near the Zone 0 or 20 which would, in fault conditions, pass large currents through the potential equalization system as such currents could lead to differential potentials in the potential equalization system and could

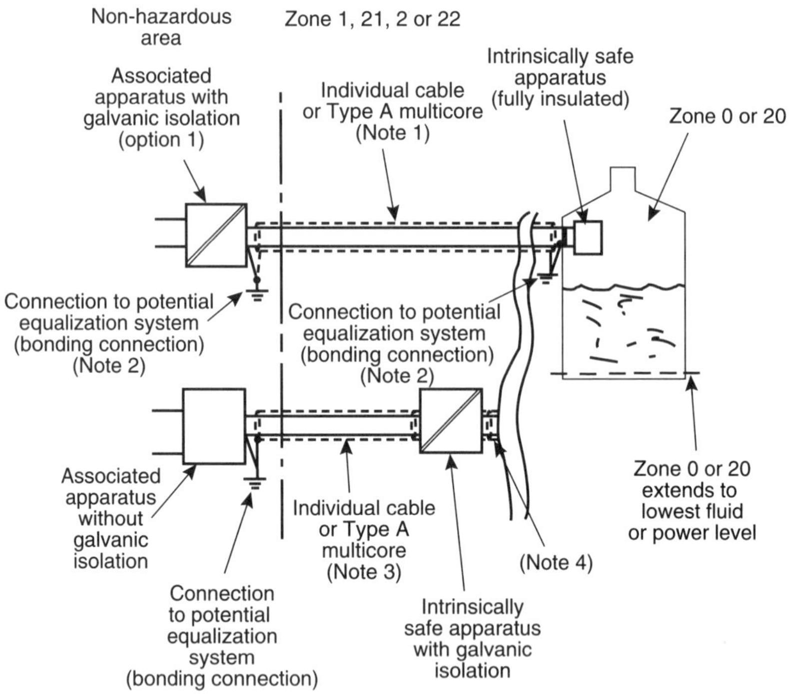

Fig. 20.20 Two options for insulated circuits in Zone 0 or Zone 20 with galvanic isolation. *Notes*: (1) Multicore may contain only 'ia' circuits. (2) The circuit and screen may, in principle, be connected to the potential equalization system (bonded) at either end but not both. (3) Multicore may contain only 'ia' circuits unless intrinsically safe apparatus with isolation maintains intrinsic safety with 'ib' circuit faults in the cable. (4) Connection of screen (and circuit if necessary) to potential equalization system should be at Zone 0 or 20 interface

lead to invasion of the intrinsically safe circuit. Typical of this type of circuit is the conductivity probe or dissolved oxygen cell. Figure 20.21 shows a typical circuit of this type.

Lightning protection for Zone 0 or Zone 20 circuits

The risk of potential elevation by the direct or indirect effects of lightning are a problem with all intrinsically safe circuits. While in Zones 1 or 21 and less hazardous areas this is only likely to be a problem in very exposed circuits, in the case of circuits entering Zone 0 or 20 it becomes a more significant problem because of the increased likelihood of coincidence of such a situation with the presence of an explosive atmosphere. For this reason, wherever the circuit is sufficiently exposed to make this situation possible (even where the cables of the intrinsically safe system are only led outside the structure of a plant or building for a short distance and

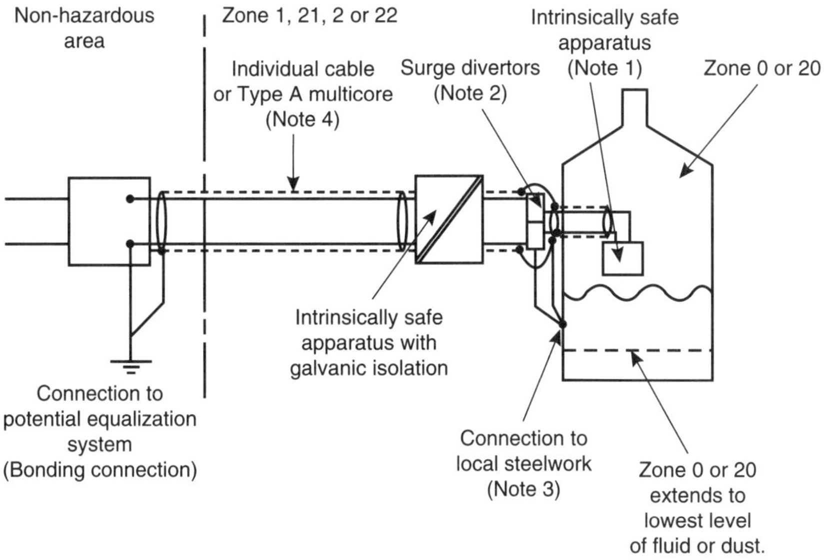

Fig. 20.21 Typical circuit for Zone 0 or 20 apparatus without effective insulation and possible installation of surge diverters. *Notes*: (1) Apparatus may not be effectively isolated (2) Surge diverters only necessary where atmospheric electricity is a problem. If fitted must be as close to Zone 0 or 20 entry as possible (3) Connection to local steelwork also provides connection to PE system (bonding connection) via steelwork (4) Cable may only contain 'ia' circuits unless intrinsically safe apparatus maintains isolation with 'ib' circuits

there is no higher conducting structure which would preferentially attract any atmospheric electricity), surge diverters should be fitted to all of the conductors of the circuit not connected to the potential equalization system as close to the Zone 0 or 20 as possible, but outside it, and bonded to the local structure (see Fig. 20.21).

20.5.6 Special circuits

It is not normally recommended that intrinsically safe circuits share an enclosure with non-intrinsically safe circuits unless the enclosure is effectively divided into two, or the separation of the two types of circuit otherwise satisfies the requirements of BS/EN 50020[3]. There are, however, situations where separation is not possible and even though the separation is as required by BS/EN 50020 the possibility of power faults damaging the intrinsic safety of the arrangement is too high to be ignored. Typical among these is the situation where an increased safety motor is fitted with temperature sensors embedded in its stator winding and, because it is in a hazardous area, the circuits connected to the temperature sensors are required to be intrinsically safe circuits.

Two precautions are required in such cases. First, the installation in the machine of the temperature sensing devices must satisfy the constructional requirements of BS/EN 50020, including the separation requirements for components, wiring and terminations from non-intrinsically safe circuits for the maximum supply voltage of the machine. (The use of separate terminal boxes for the machine and the temperature monitoring devices is recommended, but if not possible the machine terminations should be in a separate inner part of the terminal box with its own cover and incoming cable routing arranged to keep the two types of cable separate).

Second, and notwithstanding the above, the intrinsically safe circuits used for this purpose should be separated from other intrinsically safe circuits and any connection to the potential equalization system (bonding connection) necessary should go directly to the main connection point (switch room earth bar) which should be fully insulated elsewhere. This is because, although ignition-capable faults in increased safety machines are sufficiently rare to make the machines acceptable for Zone 1 or 21, they can be sufficiently severe to cause damage to these intrinsically safe circuits despite their satisfying BS/EN 50020.

A similar situation exists with pilot circuits which have their origin in mining installations but are not limited to such installations. These are intrinsically safe circuits used to prevent energization of plug and socket assemblies unless they are fully assembled. The plug or socket contains an intrinsically safe circuit which will become disconnected if an attempt to remove the plug is made before the other plug/socket contacts separate, or the protection concept (e.g., flameproof enclosure) is compromised, thus allowing automatic isolation of power supplies and preventing ignition-capable sparks. While this is a safety feature it often places the intrinsically safe circuit in the same cable as power circuits and in a position where it can be compromised.

Again a special approach is necessary. First, the cable should be constructed in such a way that the intrinsically safe circuit is contained in a cable in a screen which separates it reliably from the power circuits (the screen must be sufficiently strong to prevent rupture in the case where the power circuits fail to the screen). The power circuits need to be fitted with quick-acting electrical protection to allow for such failures.

Second, the intrinsically safe conductors within the screen and the connection facilities must satisfy the requirements of BS/EN 50020 for the maximum voltage of the power circuits.

Third, and notwithstanding the foregoing, the intrinsically safe circuits must be kept separate from other intrinsically safe circuits as, in the case of the increased safety machine, a severe failure in the cable could adversely affect other intrinsically safe circuits.

References

1 BS 5345 Selection, Installation and Maintenance of Electrical Apparatus for Use in Potentially Explosive

Atmospheres (other than Mining Applications or Explosive Processing or Manufacture. Part 1 (1989). General Recommendations. Part 4 (1977). Installation and Maintenance Requirements for Electrical Apparatus with Type of Protection 'i' Intrinsically Safe Apparatus and Systems.

2 BS/EN 60079 Electrical Apparatus for Explosive Gas Atmospheres. Part 14 (1997). Electrical Installations in Explosive Gas Atmospheres (Other Than Mines).

3 BS/EN 50014 (1993) Electrical Apparatus for Potentially Explosive Atmospheres. General Requirements. See also, BS/EN 50020 (1995). Electrical Apparatus for Potentially Explosive Atmospheres. Intrinsic Safety 'i'.

4 BS 5501 Electrical Apparatus for Potentially Explosive Atmospheres: Part 1 (1977) General Requirements; Part 7 (1977) Intrinsic Safety 'i': Part 9 (1982). Intrinsically Safe Electrical Systems 'i'.

— 21 —

Documentation, inspection, test and maintenance of explosion protected apparatus, systems and installations

The features which provide explosion protection in electrical apparatus do not in many cases form parts necessary for satisfactory operation of installations (e.g., flameproof enclosure, pressurization, additional components necessary to achieve intrinsic safety, etc.). Thus in most cases there is no warning of failure of these features and the apparatus may continue to operate while having faults which make it ignition capable. For this reason a formal and exhaustive inspection procedure, backed by detailed testing and maintenance procedures, is necessary.

21.1 Documentation

The security of a factory, location, plant or area where an explosive atmosphere can occur is heavily dependent upon the electrical installations therein. For this reason all installations must be fully documented and this documentation must be made available to those concerned with the operation, maintenance and inspection of the installations to ensure that they are aware of the detail of the safety features of the installation. Such information should be comprehensive and should include among other information of a more particular nature:

1. Appropriate area classification drawings showing the zone of the hazardous area where all parts of all electrical installations are located, the sub-grouping of all gases, vapours and mists present, and the ignition temperature of any gases, vapours, mists and dusts.
2. Certificates/approval documents for all items of certified/approved apparatus, the sub-grouping and surface temperature classification awarded, and any information necessary to highlight any special installation requirements included in the certificate/approval for a particular installation.
3. Sub-grouping, if appropriate, and maximum surface temperature information on all non-certified apparatus included in the installation, full justification for its use and any special installation requirements necessary.

4. Details of the specific type of interconnecting cabling required, and the electrical protection devices and settings specified for the installation.
5. Any specific additional information, such as purging requirements and shut-down features for pressurized apparatus and its control gear, and multicore cables for intrinsically safe installations, etc.

All of this information will be necessary to prepare any inspection schedules and plan testing and maintenance activities.

21.2 Detailed inspection requirements

There are three types of inspection which can be used and these are as follows:

1. Initial inspection, which is a fully detailed inspection and is necessary after initial installation or replacement of apparatus before the installation is energized or re-energized.

2. Routine inspection, which is essentially as detailed as the initial inspection but may utilize sampling techniques where appropriate. This inspection normally requires isolation of the installations being inspected for at least part of the inspection procedure. As it is detailed it will use the same criteria as the initial inspection in most cases.

3. Visual inspection, which is a more cursory inspection looking for obvious external problems, such as corrosion or damage, and which will not normally require isolation of the installation unless any potential problems are identified when it should trigger a detailed inspection of the installation or part of the installation in question, carried out on the basis of the initial inspection criteria.

21.2.1 Initial inspection

The initial inspection is intended to ensure that an installation satisfies its design criteria and is suitable for its location of installation at the outset. It must be carried out on all installations after they are completed and before they are energized. How this is done will vary as the conditions vary.

For a new plant, factory or location, or extensions of these, it is better to carry out the initial inspection of the installations together as near to the commissioning date as possible but before the energization of the location takes place, or flammable materials are brought to site. This makes the work easier as the locations are not hazardous areas at the time of inspection, but also is more likely to pick up damage or changes inadvertently made after completion of the installation and which often occur when later installations are carried out.

The initial inspection for all types of explosion protected installation should include the following listed items but may include additional items where particular installations require features which make them necessary. The basis on which such a judgement would be made is that if an installation feature is considered necessary for explosion protection purposes (e.g., a special guard where the risk of mechanical damage is unusually high) then it must form part of all inspection procedures.

1. The apparatus should be of a protection concept appropriate to its Zone of installation. This is normally identified by information on the apparatus label.
2. The apparatus should be of a sub-group (if the protection concept is subject to sub-grouping) appropriate to the expected explosive atmosphere. This is normally identified by information on the apparatus label.
3. The apparatus should be of a surface temperature class appropriate to the expected explosive atmosphere. This is normally identified by information on the apparatus label.
4. The apparatus carries the correct circuit (installation) identification. All installed apparatus must be uniquely identified to permit identification of the correct selection and installation information at a later date. This constitutes the inspection of individual installation labelling against its design requirement.
5. There is no evidence of damage or corrosion on the outside of the enclosure and no undue accumulation of dust or dirt. This is a visual inspection carried out from the outside of the enclosure to identify deterioration of the enclosure or accumulation of materials which could harbour corrosion agents.
6. There is no undue accumulation of dust or corrosion inside the enclosure, gaskets are undamaged and all electrical connections are tight including earth connections. This is an internal inspection and requires apparatus to be isolated from its source of supply and have its cover removed. Tools are necessary for tightness inspection.
7. Lamps are of correct rating and type. This is an internal inspection and consists of an examination of the markings of all lamps to ensure they are the ones identified on certificates/approvals. This usually requires the removal of covers and the apparatus must be isolated for the inspection.
8. There are no signs of deterioration of encapsulating materials in enclosures and stopper and cable boxes and stopper and cable boxes are properly filled as specified. This is a visual inspection inside enclosures and requires removal of the enclosure cover. In the case of stopper and cable boxes removal of the filling plug to ensure that the filling is present and appears intact is sufficient, as further inspection in these might be counterproductive in damaging the box. This is an internal inspection requiring the removal of covers and the apparatus must be isolated.

9. Motor air gaps and other running clearance are correct. This may be either an external or internal inspection depending upon machine construction. It seeks to identify undue wear or distortion due to damage-causing changes in rotor/stator clearances or fan clearances. Where it is necessary to remove covers exposing live terminals, etc., the machine must be isolated for this.
10. There are no unauthorized modifications. This is a visual inspection which may be both external and internal and is seeking signs of modification. Where it is internal the apparatus must be isolated before the enclosure cover is removed.
11. Bolts glands and stoppers are tight. This is an external examination in which enclosure retaining bolts, glands, stoppers, external earth connections, etc., are checked for tightness using tools as necessary. If inspection (4.) is carried out this inspection will follow that.
12. Connections to the potential equalization system (bonding connections) are undamaged and secure and earthing conductors are likewise undamaged and secure. This is an external inspection of all bonding and earthing conductors together with a check that all bonding and earthing connections, including those which also form enclosure fixings, are tight and the areas around them are clean and free from corrosion.
13. Any external guards around apparatus or cable trays or ducts or conduits are present and undamaged. This is an external inspection and is a physical inspection of any special guards which are fitted to protect apparatus or cables and conduits.
14. Electrical protection is satisfactory. This is a visual inspection of such things as fuses, circuit breakers, and similar devices, but may require opening of fuse and switch cabinets mainly in the non-hazardous area. Isolation is not always necessary but where the physical inspection is carried out with fuses or switches energized only suitably qualified personnel may carry out the inspection, and the devices must be labelled in such a way that it is not necessary to touch or move them or use such things as mirrors which require close access be used. Where these close access techniques have to be used then isolation becomes necessary.
15. External protection applied to apparatus to prevent corrosion is present and undamaged. This is an external inspection to ensure that any applications intended to provide environmental protection are in place and have not been damaged. Greases applied to joints and gaskets, tape and gland boots are typical of what is included.
16. Cables and conduits are undamaged. This is an external physical inspection of cables, conduits, trays and ducts to ensure that no damage has occurred to sheaths, etc. Where cables are led underground in sand-filled trenches or through sandboxes it is not necessary to remove the sand unless there is evidence of disturbance which cannot be accounted for by construction, modification or maintenance activities.

The above initial inspections will need to be augmented by specific additional inspections which will be particular to the protection concept in question. These will include the following:

Flameproof enclosure

1. Enclosures, fixing bolts, enclosure glasses and any glass/metal seals show no external damage. This is an external inspection to identify any damage to enclosures or glasses and glass/metal seals which form part of the flameproof enclosure and to ensure that gaps are not unduly obstructed by paint or dirt. It is also intended to ensure that bolts of the correct tensile specification are used. These can be identified by the head marking usually applied to identify bolt quality.
2. There are no unacceptable external obstructions to flamepaths. This is an examination of the site surrounding a flameproof enclosure to ensure that there are no external obstructions to the flamepaths which are not a part of the enclosure, within the specified minimum distances (See Chapter 10).
3. Cable glands and stopper boxes are of the correct type. This is an external inspection to identify, by their marking, that cable glands and stopper boxes are of the correct type.
4. Flange gap dimensions are correct. This is a check with feeler gauges to ensure that flange gaps have not opened to above their maximum permissible size. The feeler gauge used should be equal to the maximum specified gap (which may be different from the maximum permissible gap specified for the particular sub-group – see Chapter 10) plus 0.05 mm. This addition is to ensure that enclosures are not rejected when the gaps only equal the maximum specified gap. It should be noted that there is no necessity to ensure that the gap exceeds a specified minimum as no specified minimum exists. Cylindrical gaps and spigot joints cannot be easily measured in the field due to their configuration. They are not, however, as easily distorted as flange gaps and this checking procedure is not normally necessary.
5. Flamepaths and internal parts of glasses and glass/metal seals are undamaged. The flanges and internal parts of glass mountings and glass/metal seals should be examined for damage or corrosion effects. This is an internal inspection requiring the removal of covers and the apparatus must be isolated before they are removed.

Intrinsically safe installations

1. There are no unauthorized connections to the potential equalization (bonding) system. This is an internal inspection but because the circuits are intrinsically safe isolation is not required unless there are non-intrinsically safe circuits in the same enclosure at voltages which constitute an electric shock risk, or the apparatus is associated apparatus.

Particular attention should be paid to multi-circuit junction boxes containing several intrinsically safe circuits.

2. Segregation is maintained in multi-circuit junction boxes. This is an internal inspection but isolation is not necessary unless the box contains non-intrinsically safe circuits at potentials which constitute an electric shock risk. Segregation between intrinsically safe and non-intrinsically safe circuits should be maintained in the way specified in Chapter 20 to the levels specified in Chapter 13.
3. Barrier devices are of the correct type and correctly mounted. This is an internal inspection of barrier boxes but isolation is only necessary when the box contains non-intrinsically safe circuits at voltages which constitute an electric shock risk. Barrier labels should be inspected to ensure that the correct barriers are fitted, the correct mounting of barriers should be confirmed (if they are incorrectly mounted this will be obvious usually by the fact that they will be asymmetrical about their mounting), and segregation of conductors should be verified. The correct connection of the potential equalization (bonding/earth) bar and its isolation from the enclosure are important and should be checked.
4. Cables are correctly segregated and conduits do not contain both intrinsically safe and non-intrinsically safe circuits. This is an external inspection and it should normally confirm that intrinsically safe circuit cables are on different trays or in different ducts to non-intrinsically safe circuit cables or, where they are not, this is by design and the non-intrinsically safe circuit cables are armoured. Conduits should also be checked to ensure that the conductors led in them do not feed both types of circuit.

Pressurized enclosures

1. Inlet and exit ducting is undamaged. This is an external inspection and is intended to ensure that there is no damage to the ducting which could cause gas leakage into or out of the ducting as this could contaminate the enclosure or exhaust area dependent upon the operating system.
2. Pressurizing gas supplies are free from contamination. This is an external inspection to ensure that air inlets are not close to any exhausts which could contaminate the pressurization supply or, if the supply is from a cylinder or compressed air, there is no exhaust near to the compressor inlet or the cylinder is that specified if the supply is from a cylinder.
3. The pressurizing and flow monitoring devices are operating properly. This may not involve opening the enclosure but will involve shutting off the pressurizing gas to ensure that the supplies trip at the pressure and flow specified.
4. The pressure and flow of pressurizing gas is adequate. The enclosure pressure should be monitored to ensure that it is as specified and, likewise, the flow out of the enclosure. The pre-energization purge period should also be checked.

Oil-immersed and powder-filled apparatus

1. The oil seals and powder retention covers are in good condition. This is a physical examination of the sealing arrangements which retain the powder or oil and may or may not involve removal of covers, but if it does and electrical conductors are exposed, then prior isolation is necessary.
2. There is no leakage of oil or powder. In the case of oil this can be ascertained by observation of the sight glass, but in the case of powder filling it is achieved by looking for signs of powder-filling material, either outside the apparatus or inside the parts of the apparatus outside the powder containment. If, in the latter case, electrical conductors are exposed then isolation is necessary.

Initial inspections should also be carried out whenever installations are modified or repaired, or when the classification of hazardous areas or the sub-groups of gases, vapours or mists changes, or the ignition temperature of gases, vapours, mists or dusts changes. The initial inspection in such circumstance is limited to that necessary to ensure that the change or repair does not adversely affect safety.

21.2.2 Inspection after apparatus repair

The repaired apparatus and its installation should be fully inspected against the appropriate construction or installation drawings to ensure that the repair has not changed the apparatus in a way which contravenes its certification/approval, and its re-installation has not changed the installation in a way which contravenes its installation requirements.

21.2.3 Inspection after change in area classification, sub-group or surface temperature classification

Inspection should ensure that the installations are still appropriate. The protection concept of the apparatus, its sub-grouping (if any), and its surface temperature classification or declared maximum surface temperature should be checked to see they are still appropriate.

21.2.4 Routine inspection

Routine inspections are intended to identify deterioration of installations due to environmental and operating conditions and unauthorized modifications (authorized modifications should automatically trigger an initial inspection of the affected parts of the overall installation). Their frequency will vary from site to site depending upon the frequency of changes at that site, the degree of maintenance and modification control exercised and the severity of the environment.

The types of deterioration which should be looked for during a routine inspection includes the following:

1. Deterioration of enclosures, fixings and cable entries due to corrosion.
2. Undue accumulations of dust and dirt particularly on the outside of the enclosure and on cable trays, etc. as these could harbour corrosive liquids and solvents.
3. Physical damage to enclosures and cables or conduits.
4. Loose enclosure fixings, glands, stoppers, etc., and damaged or deteriorating gaskets which could reduce the protection against the environment by the installation.
5. Excessive vibration at the point of installation which could cause deterioration of connections, etc.
6. Condition of bearings which could cause rubbing and overheating.
7. Leakage of oil or powder from apparatus protected in this way which would indicate that the protection was deteriorating.
8. Leakage of oil from apparatus with moving parts.
9. Malfunction of relays and protective devices which are used to ensure safety.
10. Loose electrical connections particularly connections to the eqipotential bonding system.
11. Unauthorized changes, such as changes in fuse values or lamps.

It is recommended that for a new installation the first routine inspection should be within six months of commissioning, and thereafter the frequency reduced on the basis of the nature and number of the faults found. The following is suggested as the criterion:

1. If the faults found during inspection of installations in Zone 1, 21, 2 and 22 are in excess of 0.1 per cent of the total individual inspected items the inspection frequency is too low and should be increased.
2. If more than 0.01 per cent of the total faults found during inspections in Zone 1, 21, 2 and 22 render the apparatus immediately ignition capable and allow the explosive atmosphere ready access (e.g., breakage rather than cracking of a window in an enclosure in which normally sparking or hot apparatus is fitted, or loose and sparking terminations) then the inspection frequency is too low and should be increased.
3. If the fault level in Zone 1, 21, 2 and 22 remains above 0.1 per cent of all faults and 0.01 per cent of faults rendering the installation immediately ignition capable, even when a routine inspection is carried out every six months, then modification of the installation is necessary to overcome the problem.

4. Inspection of installations in Zone 0 and 20 or of intrinsically safe systems which ultimately enter Zone 0 or 20 are required to reveal a much higher level of integrity as the explosive atmosphere is assumed always to be present. The acceptable fault level in such cases should be at least two orders of magnitude higher for general faults (less than 0.001 per cent) and faults making the installation immediately ignition capable are not acceptable at any frequency. Routine inspection should be such as to identify problems before they reach this stage.
5. If the ultimate routine inspection frequency is in excess of six months, a visual inspection (see Section 21.2.3) should be undertaken every six months.
6. The maximum period between inspections, even when no faults are repeatedly found, must not exceed four years.

In carrying out routine inspections the installation should be disturbed as little as possible, and the inspection should, as far as possible, be carried out externally. This is likely to be more possible as experience of the installations increases than in the initial stages, and so it is likely that more disturbance will be necessary in the earlier life of an installation than after experience of its operation, or experience of the operation of similar installations in similar environments has been gained. If this cannot be shown it may be that the installation should be changed to produce that result. The situation to be aimed for is that the principal parts of all inspections should be external, with only sample internal inspections where the sample needed to ensure confidence is not more than 10 per cent of all installations at a given site. The sample should, of course, be chosen to ensure that particular problems previously identified are adequately covered and that the samples used cover all of the local conditions and types of installation as far as possible.

The routine inspections should generally be based upon the items identified for initial inspection as shown in the following list. A further objective in designing inspections should be to seek, as far as possible, to ensure that internal inspections are all done on the same samples of apparatus, minimizing the number of items of apparatus which have to be disturbed. The list of routine inspections should be chosen from the following, depending upon experience of this or similar installations:

1. All installations should be inspected by viewing the label.
2. Inspection is only necessary on a sample of installations and is by label.
3. Inspection is only necessary on a sample of installations and is by label.
4. Inspection is only necessary on a sample of installations and is by label.
5. All parts of the installation should be inspected externally.
6. Only sample inspection is necessary.
7. All parts of the installation should be inspected externally but it is only necessary to inspect a sample internally.

8. Both external and internal inspection need only be carried out on a sample.
9. Only a sample inspection is necessary.
10. Only a sample inspection is necessary.
11. All parts of the installation should be externally inspected.
12. Only a sample inspection is necessary.
13. All parts of the installation should be inspected externally.
14. Only a sample inspection is necessary.
15. All parts of the installation should be inspected externally.
16. All parts of the installation should be inspected externally.

Flameproof enclosure

1. All parts of the installation should be inspected externally.
2. All parts of the installation should be inspected externally.
3. Only a sample inspection is necessary.
4. Only a sample inspection is necessary
5. Only a sample inspection is necessary.

Intrinsically safe installations

1. Only a sample inspection is necessary.
2. Only a sample inspection is necessary.
3. Only a sample inspection is necessary.
4. Only a sample inspection is necessary.

Pressurized enclosures

1. All parts of the installation should be inspected externally.
2. All parts of the installation should be inspected externally.
3. Only a sample inspection is necessary.
4. All parts of the installation should be inspected externally

Oil-immersed and powder-filled apparatus

1. All parts of the installation should be inspected externally.
2. All parts of the installation should be inspected externally. Only a sample internal inspection is necessary.

21.2.5 Visual inspection

This type of inspection is only necessary when routine inspections are at intervals exceeding six months and do not involve the opening of the enclosure or the use of any tools. They should include all those items of the initial inspection which can be executed without opening the apparatus and with a minimum use of tools. Again taking the list of items used for initial inspection, the following represent the minimum for visual inspection:

1. All installations inspected by label.
10. Sample external inspection only.
11. All installations inspected.
12. Sample external inspection only.
13. All installations inspected.
15. All installations inspected.
16. All installations inspected.

Flameproof enclosure

1. All installations inspected.
2. All installations inspected.

Intrinsically safe installations

4. Sample external inspection only.

Pressurized enclosures

2. All installations inspected.

Oil-immersed and powder-filled apparatus

1. All installations inspected.
2. All installations inspected externally.

21.2.6 Inspection procedures

It is clear that inspection installation by installation is not usually economic as installations, particularly intrinsically safe installations, traverse more than one physical location. The appropriate way forward is to identify all parts of all installations in a particular location and inspect them together. This requires that installation information be re-divided by location, rather than individual electrical installation, and some arrangement is necessary to ensure that all parts of each installation be identified as having been inspected. In addition, positive reporting is necessary as it must be possible to prove that all parts of an installation have been inspected and found either faulty or in order. Negative reporting would not identify inspection of parts where no faults were found. The basis of a good inspection system is as follows.

First, each area of a particular site should have sheets detailing all parts of all electrical installations in the area with the inspections necessary on them.

Second, A system of recording that each inspection on each part of each installation should be produced so that the inspector can easily record the inspection. It is possibly advantageous if only inspections where no faults are found be so recorded, and faults separately recorded. This record cannot then be completed until all faults have been rectified and a successful subsequent inspection recorded.

Third, After the records are complete there should be a procedure which relates all inspection sheets to individual installations, so that it can be shown that all installations have been fully inspected and faults rectified.

21.3 Testing

Electrical testing of installations is a problem in installations in explosive atmospheres as not only can measuring instruments designed to measure such things as voltage and current cause sparking by their application, but more sophisticated measuring instruments (such as meggers) introduce their own power supplies into the installation thus causing further potential danger. For this reason electrical testing should not be carried out on any installation which is within or enters a hazardous area where physical examination can reliably confirm the freedom from fault of an item. Even electrical test apparatus which can be shown not to be ignition capable (such as a current-limited megger) can, when connected to an installation, become ignition capable due to such things as cable inductance, capacitance etc.

In respect of test equipment, the general approach must be that applied to portable apparatus. No item of test apparatus should be taken into any hazardous area unless it is not self powered or, where it is self powered, it is provided with a protection concept appropriate to the hazardous area in question, or its power source is removed (i.e., a normal test multimeter has a battery which should be removed if it is to be taken into a hazardous area unless the multimeter is provided with a protection concept appropriate to the hazardous area in question).

21.3.1 Necessary testing

Where testing is necessary in a hazardous area, or on installations accessing such areas, it should as far as possible be limited to the following:

1. Monitoring of voltages and currents using non-powered test apparatus.
2. Measurement of insulation resistance.
3. Measurement of earth loop impedance and the resistance of connections to the potential equalization (bonding) system.
4. Earth Electrode resistance measurement.

Voltage and current monitoring

The measurement of these parameters should preferably be carried out on the circuits in the non-hazardous areas. If hazardous area measurement is necessary, the instruments used for measuring these parameters should not have their own source of power if they are to be used in a hazardous area, which will often limit them to galvanometer type instruments.

The ideal situation is one in which all of the hazardous areas affected by a particular test can be shown by test to be free of explosive atmosphere for the duration of the test, and a certificate has been issued to confirm this by the appropriate plant control personnel or where the necessary testing can be carried out before flammable materials are brought on to the plant. In such circumstances testing may be as for any other industrial installation, provided the test will not damage the installation (in the case of intrinsically safe or non-incendive installations, high voltage or current testing could damage safety components which would not be apparent in operation). Even in these circumstances it is necessary to exercise care if any test instruments are self powered as they should not be transported to the testing site via other locations to which the certificate to confirm a non-explosive atmosphere does not apply, unless their batteries have been removed or they can be shown to be suitably protected.

Where it is not possible to confirm a non-explosive atmosphere the tests should be of as short a duration as possible and be carried out as follows:

Non-hazardous area tests

1. The installation should be fully in accordance with its certification/approval in the hazardous area, in that all covers should be properly fitted and other protection concept elements of the physical installation in operation.
2. The measurement should then be made on the circuit in the non-hazardous area by applying the test meter in the supply lines or across them as required. The test instrument may be self powered insofar as its own operation is concerned, but should not be able to supply significant voltage or current to the circuit being tested. Isolation is only necessary to protect against electric shock in these circumstances.

Hazardous area testing

1. It is necessary to take the test instrument into a hazardous area and it must therefore be non-self powered or be suitably protected by a protection concept suitable for the hazardous area into which it is taken.
2. The installation being tested should then be isolated and the test meter firmly connected to the test points (the use of test probes, which are merely pressed on to the test point, is not acceptable). The installation should then be returned, as far as is possible, to its normal condition (covers replaced if possible, etc.) and re-energized to allow the measurement.

3. The installation should then be de-energized before removal of the test leads.
4. Care should be taken to ensure that any stored charge is allowed to dissipate before connection or disconnection of the test apparatus (some specialist test apparatus has a special discharge contact inside it which is in a flameproof enclosure to permit safe dissipation of charge).

Insulation resistance and conductivity testing

Insulation resistance and conductivity testing usually uses a high voltage or high current tester in order to break down any insulation which is failing or to destroy fine wire connections maintaining conductivity, and thus recognizes failures not so readily recognized by low voltage or low current testers, such as normal ohmmeters. However, there is the possibility of incendive sparking produced by the use of high voltage or high current. While this problem cannot be totally removed, the following procedure will minimize the risk and it has to be remembered that the test instrument is of much lower power capability than the circuit being tested, and its use is likely to be beneficial when set against the leaving of the circuit until actual breakdown or failure takes place. The following procedure is designed to limit the adverse effect of such testing.

As with voltage and current measurement, the first approach is to confirm by formal test and certification that no explosive atmosphere exists in any hazardous area affected by the test at the time of testing. On new plant this is relatively easy if the tests are conducted before any flammable materials are brought on to the plant or site, but more difficult thereafter, particularly as this type of test may interact with installations other than that being tested. Also, the transport of the test apparatus is difficult if it passes through areas not covered by the testing certification and the apparatus needs to be de-energized during such transport by the removal of batteries, etc.

Testing procedures should rely on low voltage test apparatus as far as possible and to this end the approach to testing should be as follows:

1. Initial test of insulation resistance or conductivity should be made using a high voltage or high current tester, and recorded.
2. At the same time the insulation resistance or conductivity should be measured using a low voltage test instrument and recorded with the high voltage or high current figure.
3. Routine insulation resistance and conductivity testing should be carried out with the same low voltage testing device and the results compared with the initial test result using the same device.
4. Only where comparison of results shows differences which indicate changes should the high voltage or high current test be repeated.

Testing should be done as far as is possible from a non-hazardous area and the actual testing procedure should be as follows:

1. When testing from a non-hazardous area, the procedures adopted should be as those adopted for voltage and current measurement, but in this case such tests should not be carried out on intrinsically safe installations unless an individual evaluation has shown that no damage to safety components would result.

2. When testing from a hazardous area, the procedures should be those adopted for voltage and current measurement, and high voltage or high current tests should not be carried out on intrinsically safe installations unless an individual evaluation has shown that no damage will occur.

Any testing should be, as previously stated, only carried out when physical inspection cannot give the required confidence, and when carried out should be arranged in conjunction with physical examination using the same sampling procedures to minimize the amount of testing carried out. More detail on testing procedures is given in BS 5345[1].

21.4 Maintenance of explosion protected apparatus

There is considerable scope for the creation of danger in carrying out maintenance of explosion protected apparatus as simple changes, such as the change of a gasket or a component, can destroy the protection concept applied to an item of apparatus, and maintenance should therefore be undertaken with extreme care.

One method of dealing with apparatus which can be repaired is to return it to the manufacturer who will have all the necessary documentation and necessary test equipment to carry out the repair, demonstrate that the repaired apparatus conforms to the requirements of its certificate/approval and give a guarantee to that effect which can usually be relied upon. This is not always possible or preferable, however, for a variety of reasons and the owner of the apparatus or a sub-contract repairer is often considered as more suitable. If this option chosen the repairer must have all the necessary documentation to define the apparatus (usually defined in the schedules to the certificate/approval document) which will typically include:

1. The technical specification.
2. A full set of construction drawings as specified in the Certificate/Approval.
3. Any necessary dismantling/assembly instructions.
4. Details of any recommendations from the manufacturer on repair/overhaul of the apparatus
5. Any other relevant information such as IP rating and any special conditions of use which could affect the approach to maintenance.

The sub-contract repairer must also have all of the test equipment necessary to demonstrate compliance of the apparatus with its certification/approval documents after the repair. This particularly applies where the certificate/approval requires routine manufacturing tests as these will have to be applied after any repair.

Finally, the repairer should have staff with the necessary competence and knowledge to carry out the repair which will normally include knowledge of the protection concept in question.

21.4.1 General maintenance

In general maintenance functions will be limited to replacing components with direct replacements supplied by the apparatus manufacturer, or guaranteed to be identical to those damaged. Typical of these are covers of flameproof enclosures, transformers in intrinsically safe or associated apparatus, etc. In some cases the component will be a standard electrical component not unique to the apparatus in question, such as a resistor or a terminal. In these cases several manufacturers may make similar components and these may be used provided:

1. Their electrical parameters are essentially the same.
2. Their physical size is essentially the same.
3. Their materials and mode of construction is essentially the same.
4. Their physical strength is essentially the same.

This is not intended to allow the manufacture of alternative covers or mounting brackets, etc., but merely to allow an alternative selection of series manufactured equivalents where appropriate and where they exist. Such things as relays, bearings, encapsulated assemblies, gaskets (other than 'o'-rings), glass, plastics, other materials whose dimensional faculties are not dimensionally stable, and similar devices are only usually repairable by direct replacement of like components.

There are, however, other facets of apparatus which may be repaired and principle among these are the following:

1. It is possible for repairers to identify failed windings or parts thereof and replace them with windings of sensibly similar wires and construction. This is not possible with windings of increased safety apparatus and similar windings in the Type 'N' concept as these are so fundamental to the protection concept that they can only be replaced by identically installed identical windings, and this usually results in their being only repairable by the manufacturer or the manufacturer's duly authorized agent.

2. Metal Spraying of rotating shafts is possible where the wear on the shaft, together with the machining of the metal sprayed shaft to produce the original diameter, is not sufficient to significantly weaken the shaft. This technique is not acceptable for large diameter shafts (those in excess of 2.5 cm approximately) and the material sprayed must be chemically compatible with the original shaft.

3. Where wear is a problem electroplating is also a possible method of replacing the loss due to wear but once again it is necessary to ensure that the wear has not significantly adversely affected strength. (BS 4641[3] gives details of plating procedures for chromium plating and BS 4758[3] for nickel plating.)

4. Worn shafts may also be sleeved provided the sleeve is an interference fit and the reduction in diameter of the sleeved shaft necessary to accept the sleeve does not significantly reduce the strength of the shaft or, if it does, the strength is still adequate for the duty for which it is present.

5. Enclosures and other parts of explosion protected apparatus may be repaired by welding or brazing provided the choice used is compatible with the material of the enclosure (e.g., brazing is normally only compatible with non-ferrous materials), and the execution ensures adequate preparation to ensure that strength is not significantly reduced and blowholes do not occur. It should also be noted that both of these techniques generates considerable heat and this must not damage other features or components relevant to the protection concept nor produce such things as stress cracks in the welded or brazed component.

6. The technique of metal (nickel or alloy) stitching for fractured or cracked cast enclosures or covers is acceptable provided the casting has a thickness such that the strength of the enclosure or lid after stitching is not significantly reduced (reduced to below the level necessary to ensure continued protection).

7. The re-machining of worn surfaces is possible provided that the re-machined part is not weakened to such an extent that the protection concept or operation is compromised and, is cases such as flameproof enclosure, the resultant surface satisfies the requirements of the protection concept.

8. Threaded holes may be repaired, if the threads are damaged, by oversize drilling and retapping or the insertion of a proprietary thread insert provided that, in the case of flameproof enclosure, the flange widths or thickness of metal on the inside of the holes continues to satisfy the requirements of the protection concept. For other protection concepts plugging and redrilling at the same place or elsewhere are also acceptable provided the strength is not so reduced as to affect the protection concept or operation.

Temporary repairs should be avoided and if they are considered to be necessary should only be carried out if they do not adversely influence the protection concept in the time frame for which they are intended to cover. There is no question of leaving temporary repairs in place for more than 24 hours.

No modifications should be carried out unless the justification for the modification shows that it does not adversely affect the protection concept.

It must be stressed that as soon as an apparatus is repaired or modified the responsibility for the safety of that apparatus passes from the original manufacturer to the person and organization carrying out the modification or repair.

References

1 BS 5345 Selection, Installation and Maintenance of Electrical Apparatus for Use in Potentially Explosive Atmospheres (other than mining applications or explosive processing and manufacture): Part 1 (1989). General Recommendations: Part 3 (1979). Installation and Maintenance Requirements for Electrical Apparatus with Type of Protection 'd'. Flameproof Enclosure; Part 4 (1977). Installation and Maintenance Requirements for Electrical Apparatus with Type of Protection 'i'. Intrinsically Safe Apparatus and Systems; Part 5 (1983). Installation and Maintenance Requirements for Electrical Apparatus Protected by Pressurization 'p' and by Continuous Dilution, and for Pressurized Rooms; Part 6 (1978). Installation and Maintenance Requirements for Electrical Apparatus with Type of Protection 'e'. Increased Safety; Part 7 (1979). Installation and Maintenance Requirements for Electrical Apparatus with Type of Protection 'N'; Part 8 (1980). Installation and Maintenance Requirements for Electrical Apparatus with Type of Protection 's'. Special Protection.

2 BS 4641 (1986) Method of specifying electroplated coatings of chromium for engineering purposes.

3 BS 4758 (1986) Method of specifying electroplated coatings of nickel for engineering purposes.

— 22 —

Radio frequency radiation and static electricity

BS 5958, Part 1 (1980) and Part 2 (1983)

BS 6656 (1986)

Most plants, factories and similar installations are to a some degree at risk from either radio frequency radiation issuing from transmitters which cover their area, and static electricity in its many forms (one of which is lightning). These are only indirectly related to problems associated with the installation and use of electrical apparatus in explosive atmospheres, with the exception of portable transceivers, mobile telephones and similar devices, and are thus not the direct concern of this book. They do, however, constitute sources of ignition from electrical energy and thus need attention.

As they are all specialized fields insofar as their methods of producing, storing and dissipating energy are concerned only limited guidance will be given here and it is essential that the documents referred to in this chapter are studied carefully and expert guidance sought as necessary.

22.1 Basic situation

Static electricity is normally generated by process related activities, such as spraying of liquids or powders or cleaning, and is thus totally within the control of the operator in that the production situations are those used in process or operation, apart from lightning production and discharge which are normally natural phenomena. Thus, with the exception of lightning against which only protective methods are possible, plant and factory operators can apply measures to limit the build up of static electricity and remove the potential problem.

The effect of the reception of radio frequency radiation by plant or building structures is, again, normally only controllable by measures to screen or reduce the efficiency of such structures, or to prevent incendive discharge from them as the transmission is not normally within the control of the plant or factory operator. In this case, however, an additional tool exists when a person or organization seeks to construct a transmitter because it is their duty under the Health and Safety at Work Act[1] to ensure that any existing sites with hazardous areas in the vicinity of their transmitter are not put at risk by its construction. Likewise, it is the duty of a person or organization constructing any plant or other premises, which contain hazardous areas, in the locality of an existing transmitter to take precautions to ensure that the people who may be affected by the plant or premises are not put at risk. They must take measures to prevent the collection and discharge of radio frequency from causing an explosion. This does not deal effectively with current situations where both plant or premises containing hazardous areas and transmitters already exist. In such cases, while it could be argued that the one which was there is in the right this is not a really effective solution and any problem should be resolved by cooperation.

Portable (hand-held) transceivers, mobile telephones and similar devices are normally not a problem as they have such limited transmission capability that they are unlikely to cause any ignitions unless they are operated in or close to hazardous areas. Their selection and use will be in the hands of the person or organization which operates the plant or premises and who have control over the access to the site and thus can exclude such devices or require them to be de-energized while on the site.

The foregoing situation in the case of portable (hand-held) devices does not apply to mobile installations, such as those fitted in vehicles, and these may, in some circumstances, have the power capability to cause ignitions of explosive atmospheres even when not in the control of the site operator but are nonetheless close to the site. In these circumstances the only practical situation is for the site operator to construct his plant or installation to ensure, as far as is possible, that such mobile transceivers are not a problem. This will be done based upon knowledge of the likely frequencies and maximum power outputs of such transceivers as it is unreasonable to expect vehicle operators to exercise sufficient control to stop vehicles (and this includes aircraft) from approaching the site.

22.2 Static electricity including lightning

Static electricity is created by the detachment of electrons from one material and their transference to another, which is normally achieved by the dissipation of physical energy. This energy is usually created when rapid movement and separation of two materials occurs. Typical of the methods by which static electricity can be generated are cleaning of insulating plastics with dry cloths, high pressure liquid jets (particularly where the released liquid forms droplets), gas jets, and the transport of dusts as fluids. The energy produced in any of these ways is determined by the physical energy applied in the creation of the charge, the capacitance of the charged element to earth or any other point where discharge may take place, and the voltage at which the insulation between the two elements will break down. This often means that the stored energy on an item or surface due to static generation may be ignition capable. Breakdown can occur when the voltage of the charged part reaches breakdown voltage, but is more usually caused by movement (such as when moving liquid particles impinge on earthed surfaces, or when conducting parts, which are earthed, move and touch or come close to charged surfaces). A typical movement which causes discharge is the intervention of a human being, as is evinced by the electric shocks often received by people who walk on artificial fibre carpets and then touch earthed metal.

The ideal is to prevent static charge and this can be done in many cases but, where it cannot, arrangements should be made to dissipate it outside a hazardous area or, where this is not easily possible, to exclude air from the area of discharge so that ignition cannot take place.

22.2.1 Dealing with static charge

Detailed consideration to the handling of static electricity is contained in BS 5958[2] which should be consulted in all cases.

Road tankers

Where road tankers are used it is possible to utilize conducting tyres which, while still being of high resistance, slowly dissipate any static charge generated as soon as the vehicle stops. As a further safeguard, in cases where it cannot be guaranteed that anti-static tyres are used, the tanker could be connected to the potential equalization system (earth) before it enters any hazardous area or the area should be declared free from explosive atmosphere at the time the tanker enters and the tanker can then be connected to the potential equalization system (earth) in the tanker bay. The former is, of course, preferred.

Discharge or loading of the tanker should not then be a problem provided that, if the liquid is not conducting, the filling hose is conducting and firmly bonded to the tanker and plant and the filling is done from the bottom of the tank. Filling from the top, even with conducting liquids, is not recommended unless the filling hose outlet is beneath the surface of the liquid in the tank as otherwise the production of charged droplets is possible and these will discharge as soon as they reach the liquid surface. Filling should always be carried out at low velocity as this minimizes the production of static.

Storage tanks and process vessels

Gases, liquids and powders automatically transferred between vessels during process operations can also generate static if conditions are right. For this reason no gas, liquid or powder identified as a possible static risk, due to its low conductivity or because it can be divided into isolated droplets, etc., should be transferred between vessels at a rate which will cause significant static build-up. If this is not possible, no transfer should take place in the presence of air or oxygen. Again, bottom loading and discharging in flooded lines is to be preferred.

Loading and unloading from/to drums, down chutes, etc

Where filling of liquids, powders and the like is performed manually down chutes or directly from drums or transport from a process vessel, the chute or drum should be bonded to the receiving or supplying plant before any loading takes place to ensure that no static charge exists on the non-fixed part (usually the drum and/or chute).

Tank cleaning

The activity of cleaning the inside of tanks is not compatible with the objective of prevention of static build-up in that the cleaning liquid must be delivered at high velocity to create the necessary cleaning action. If this is the case the only possible solution is to exclude air or oxygen during the cleaning process and as long thereafter as is possible. It is important to recognize that droplets could collect on insulating materials inside the tank and then drop later to the bottom of the tank causing sparking. If this possibility is recognized the tank will need to exclude air or oxygen at all times or the source of continued charge must be removed.

22.2.2 Dealing with lightning

Lightning is a form of static electricity and normally results from very significant energies stored normally in clouds in the atmosphere being discharged by arcs to ground or conducting parts connected to ground. The energy released is always sufficient to cause an ignition of an explosive atmosphere if the arc is in a hazardous area. BS 6651[3] details the methods of protection of structures against lightning and should be consulted for all structures associated with hazardous areas.

The ideal approach is to create a situation using deliberate lightning conductors where necessary which minimizes the effect of a lightning strike on the structure itself so that significant currents do not flow around the parts of the structure in hazardous areas as, in such cases, side flashes at such things as steel structural joints, which are not properly bonded together, could cause ignition. This cannot, however, be a complete protection and the potential equalization (bonding) system is of great importance from this point of view. It must effectively bond together all conducting parts of the structure, the apparatus cases and the parts of the electrical circuits which are connected to the system to minimize the risk of significantly different voltages appearing between different parts.

Where dedicated lightning conductors are used these should be connected to earth outside a hazardous area and should be bonded to the potential equalization system in such a way that differential voltages on that system are minimized. This will usually mean that structural stanchions will need to be properly bonded and earthed with rods.

High level vents which vent explosive atmospheres or flammable materials which create explosive atmospheres close to the vent need careful consideration in that if they are struck by lightning then immediate ignition will occur. One method is to inject inert gas or steam into the vent so that the flammable material cannot form an explosive atmosphere at or near the vent, but this may be expensive and the alternative of using a scrubbing system may be preferable.

22.3 Ignition by radio frequency radiation

In addition to the electrical installations in a given area there is a further danger that conducting parts of its construction (e.g., plant steelwork or steel frames of buildings) may act as aerials and collect energy from any radio frequency radiation field in which they exist. This energy can then be released as a spark or arc by failure of an insulated gap (e.g., an insulated flange joint), or by activities such as separating of flanges and disconnecting of conductors whose containing cables form part of an inadvertent aerial. The recognition of this problem came to the fore in the early 1980s after incidents in Europe and results in the production of a British Standard BS 6656[4] (first issued in 1986 and extensively revised in 1991). The subject is very complex and thus BS 6656 should always be consulted in consideration of this potential problem. There are, however, certain basic facts which can assist in considering this type of danger.

22.3.1 Basic safety assessment

The first step in the safety assessment is to identify a basic threshold above which there will be an ignition risk. Provided the transmit power of any transmitter which can be identified close to the hazardous area, is less than the threshold there can be no risk. A survey of all known transmitters in the UK produced in BS 6656[4] shows that the maximum vulnerable zone within which an ignition risk could occur due to transmissions is as shown in Table 22.1. As it is unlikely that transmitters of greater power or more dangerous configuration are likely to be constructed this gives the first yardstick. (If there is doubt in respect of any transmitter found in a survey of the local area, but outside the distances in Table 22.1, then the transmitter can be compared with the list in BS 6656 and if it cannot be compared with any transmitter in the list then it must be individually assessed). The first criteria are thus:

Table 22.1 Limit vulnerable distances

Type of transmission	Maximum vulnerable Zone		
	Sub-group IIA (Note 1)	Sub-group IIB (Note 1)	Sub-group IIC (Note 1)
Low frequency and very low frequency broadcast and radio beacons (150–530 kHz)	4.5 km	5.5 km	7.5 km
Medium frequency broadcast and communication (530 kHz–1.6 MHz)	11.5 km	14.5 km	17.5 km
High frequency broadcast and communications	9.0 km	11.0 km	14.0 km
Amateur radio (fixed and mobile (see Note 2) (1.8 MHz–430 MHz)	0.75 km	1.0 km	1.1 km
Very high frequency and ultra high frequency fixed and mobile (see Note 3) (87 MHz–2.7 GHz)	0.2 km	0.25 km	0.3 km
Tropospheric scatter transmissions (0.9 GHz–2 GHz)	1.0 km	1.2 km	1.5 km
Civil and military radar (220 MHz–14 GHz)	0.5 km	1.5 km	3.0 km

Notes:
1 These are the sub-groups against which apparatus is chosen for use in a particular hazardous area (BS/EN 60079–10).
2 Citizens band radio is strictly limited in transmit capability and thus does not produce a problem.
3 FM and television broadcast transmitter aerials are designed to give a constant field strength of less than 1 V/m outside the transmitter area and thus do not create a problem – see Fig. 22.2.

1. If no transmitters are present in a radius around the hazardous area of the distance specified in Table 22.1 then no hazard exists – subject to 2. below.

2. If no transmitters exist in the locality (say within a radius of 60 km) hazard exists. (If a transmitter does exist within 60 km and is of a configuration so significantly different to those recorded in BS 6656, such that it is expected to have a greater vulnerable distance, then it must of course be individually evaluated to identify its possibility of producing a dangerous situation).

The figure of 60 km is used because it is the seaward vulnerable distance of the Orford Ness transmitter operating at 648 and 1296 kHz (the most sensitive area for ignition risk – see Fig. 22.2 which is extracted from BS 6656). This has both high power and a directional aerial, together with passage over water which gives a higher vulnerable zone. It is felt that the likelihood of a higher risk situation existing is thus very low.

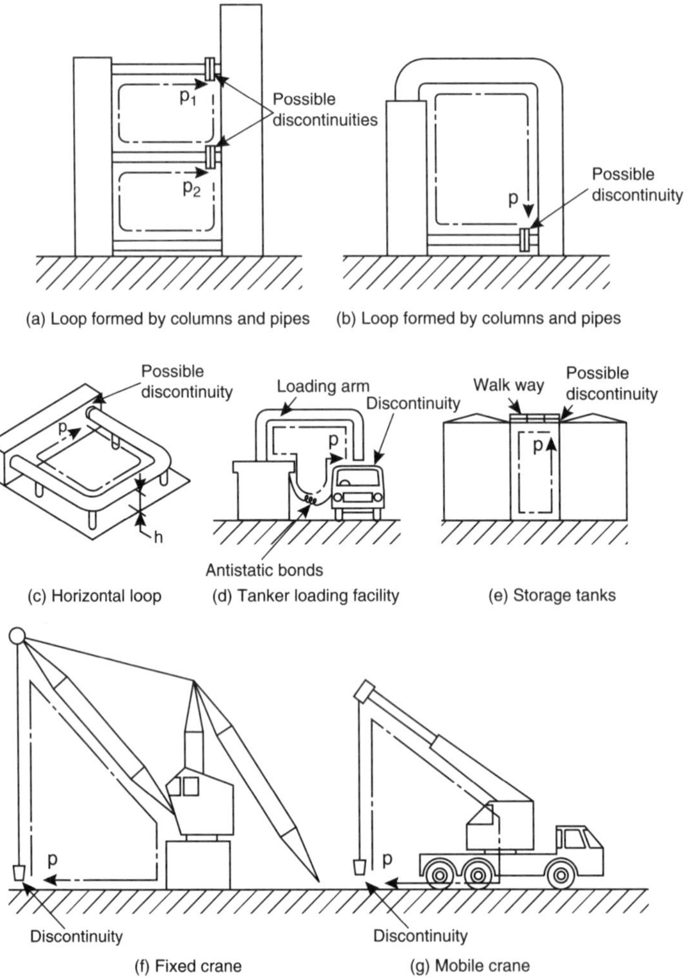

Fig. 22.1 Typical accidental loops (aerials) (from BS 6656). p = the internal perimeter of the loop, h = the height of the loop

Where transmitters are found within the vulnerable zones or are used in the site itself (e.g., portable and transportable transceivers or mobile telephones) their transmitted power or energy can be identified, and it is known that for continuous wave transmitters the transmit power must be in excess of that specified in Table 22.2 if they are to constitute any risk. Table 22.2 also identifies the equivalent energy of the transmission which is that required to be delivered to the flame kernel in the critical time, which is also specified in Table 22.2. Where the transmitter is a pulse transmitter, such as a radar transmitter, then different conditions apply as the energy is supplied to the flame kernel in pulses rather than continuously. This is less efficient and more energy is required and the threshold for this situation is shown in Table 22.3 (also extracted from BS 6656).

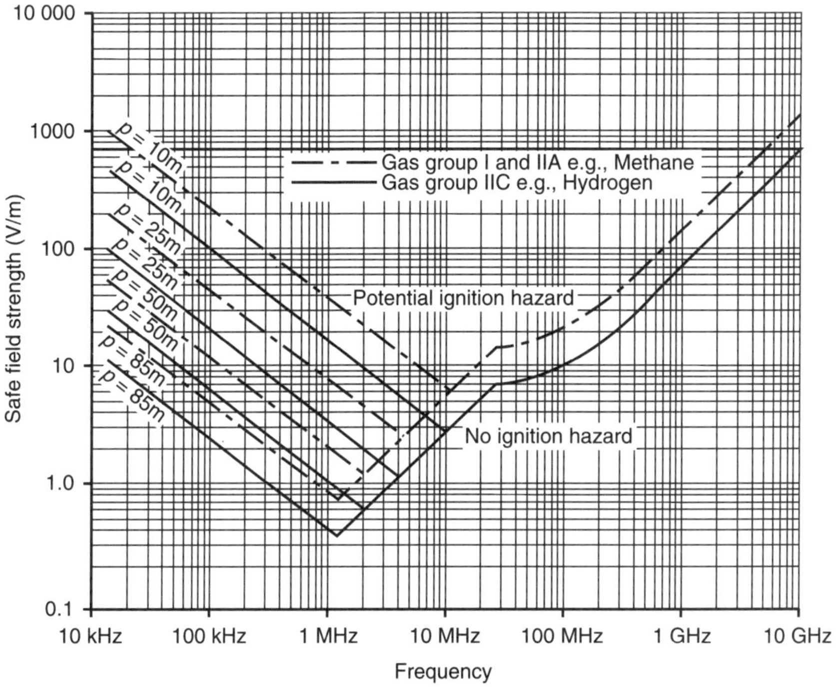

Fig. 22.2 Threshold field strength/frequency (from BS 6656)

Table 22.2 Maximum safe power thresholds for fixed plant (and cranes)

Apparatus sub-group	Threshold power
IIA	8 W – Averaged over any 100 μs period (800 μJ) (see Note 1)
IIB	4 W – Averaged over any 100 μs period (400 μJ) (see Note 1)
IIC	2 W – Averaged over any 20 μs period (40 μJ)

Notes:

1 The ignition sensitivity of cranes is greater (possibly because of the fact that they can be shown to be more efficient structures than fixed plant and they readily form variable loops) and this means that for sub-group IIA the ignition power is reduced to 6 W (600 μJ) and for IIB, 3.5 ,W (350 μJ).

2 The times quoted are ignition times and the energy must be imparted in that time or ignition will not result.

Table 22.3 Maximum safe energy thresholds for radar pulses

Apparatus sub-group	Ignition energy threshold
IIA	7000 μJ
IIB	1000 μJ
IIC	200 μJ

Note: It will be noted that the energies quoted here are significantly larger than is the case for continuous transmissions. This is probably due to both the aerial extraction capability and the effective take up of energy by the flame kernel being affected by the fact that the energy is provided by a very short pulse duration (typically $<10\,\mu s$).

This gives a second criterion as follows:

3. Where transmitters are used on the site, either in or close to the hazardous area or where transmitters are identified within the Vulnerable Zones specified in Table 22.1, then, provided their transmit power (if they are a continuous wave transmitter) or energy (if they are a pulse transmitter) is less than the limiting values in Table 22.2 or 22.3 they do not constitute a hazard.

If multiple transmissions are present the problem becomes more difficult in that the aerial can extract energy from all transmissions present. Figure 22.3 shows an approximate general relationship between the power which can be extracted from an accidental aerial at any field strength (Extractable Power) and that which can be extracted when the field strength is at the ignition threshold against the ratio of the actual field strength to the threshold, field strength. In addition, Fig. 22.4 (which is extracted from BS 6656) shows the multiple of the threshold power used to add extractable powers when one of the available transmissions matches the aerial tuning. Thus if a particular site has more than one incident radio frequency field, a basis for first approximation of any resultant danger can be derived as follows:

4. If no incident field is greater than 1 per cent of the threshold field derived from Fig. 22.2 the transmission can be ignored.

5. Where multiple fields are present then the extractable power as a fraction of the threshold extractable power for a resonant aerial can be derived from Fig. 22.3 for each field after which (6) can be applied.

6. The extractable powers for each field can be adjusted for non-resonance by assuming that the aerial is resonant at one of the frequencies involved

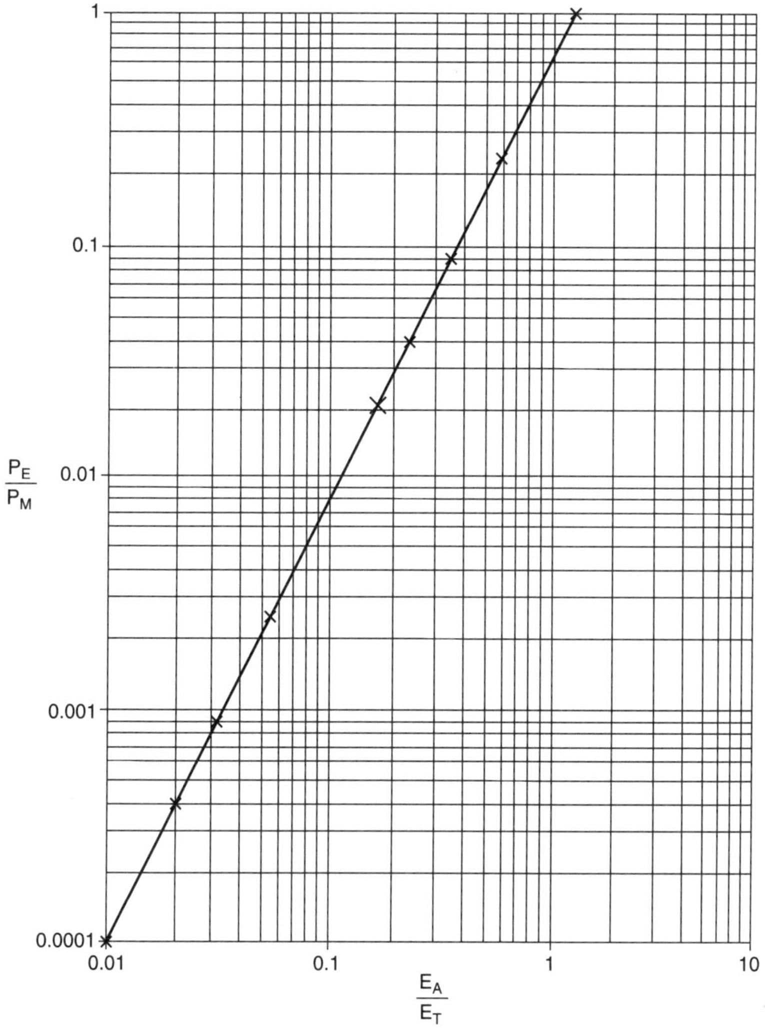

$\frac{P_E}{P_M}$ = Actual extractable power/extractable power at ignition threshold

$\frac{E_A}{E_T}$ = Actual field strength/field strength at ignition threshold

Fig. 22.3 Extractable power vs field strength

and added. This is then repeated assuming each of the frequencies is resonant in turn and repeating the calculation. The results in each case are added and if the fractional power, in any case, approaches one then further investigation will be necessary.

The foregoing are approaches which will give basic information on the incendivity of arcs and sparks due to incident radio frequency fields. If there is any doubt then BS 6656 should be consulted in detail.

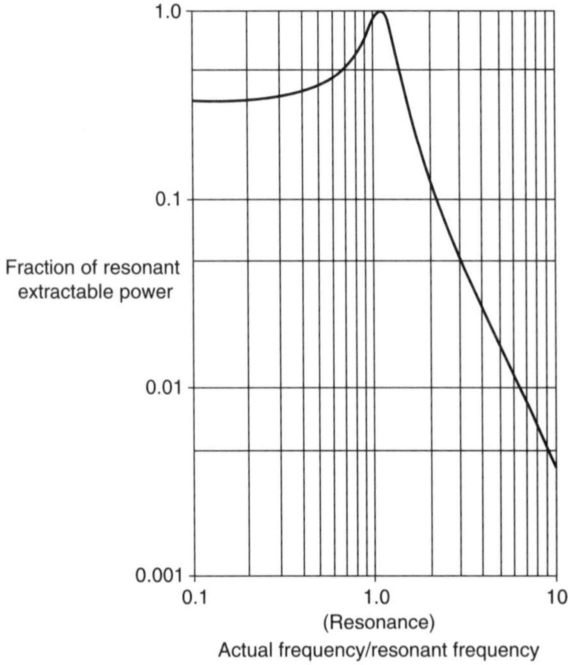

Fig. 22.4 Extractable power capability (from BS 6656)

22.3.2 Dealing with the hazard

Where a transmitter is already in existence when a plant or factory is constructed or where both are in existence already and no consideration has been given to the potential problem, possibly because both predate BS 6656, the only real solution if the transmitter cannot be moved or made directional is to screen the plant, or reduce the efficiency of structures as aerials, or the prevention of sparking.

Prevention of sparking

Sparking occurs where there is a discontinuity in structures associated with the inadvertent aerial and if such discontinuities can be prevented or properly insulated to prevent breakdown, the ignition problem can be reduced to an acceptable level.

The use of deliberate bonding conductors between any two parts between which the connection is not secure, such as insulated flanges or normal flanges where they are being opened for maintenance, will prevent incendive sparking provided the bond is of sufficiently low electrical resistance. While significant currents may flow in the bonding conductor it will, in such cases, prevent the production of significant voltages between the two parts and hence prevent sparking. Such bonds should be short (BS 6656 recommends no longer than 1 per cent of the transmission wavelength) and secure. Bonding to the ground or potential equalization system is not recommended as not only will this introduce currents into that system but the actual length of the bond between the two parts is likely to be longer than would be the case for direct bonding, and may not be definable.

Where bonding is not practicable (bonding being the preferred solution), typically in cases where moving parts are involved and they can come into contact either by chance or by design but bonding would restrict their movement, insulation placed between them to prevent discharge is a possible method of prevention of ignition. The insulation needs, however, to be sufficiently physically robust to prevent damage and undue wear, and must be effective at radio frequencies.

Reduction of aerial efficiency

At the frequencies where the maximum problem occurs (below 30 MHz) loop aerials are much more sensitive than mono or dipole aerials and are likely to be a limiting factor. It is known that when loop perimeters are less than half the transmission wavelength, aerial efficiency reduces radically (e.g., if it is reduced to one quarter of the wavelength then extractable power is reduced by a factor of 11). Thus where a problem is identified loops can be reduced in size by division using conductors to break up the loop. These conductors should be rigid and positioned so as to present a smaller loop or loops to the field.

De-tuning of an aerial

When all else fails it may be possible to reduce the extractable power by the connection of reactive components (e.g., capacitors across the spark gap) to de-tune the aerial. Such connections should be secure and the reactive components of high reliability.

References

1 HSW Act — Health and Safety at Work Act 1974.

2 BS 5958 — Control of Undesirable Static Electricity. Part 1 (1980). General Requirements. Part 2 (1983). Code of Practice for Control of Static Electricity.

3 BS 6651 (1986) — Code of Practice for the Protection of Structures against Lightening.

4 BS 6656 (1986) — The Prevention of Inadvertent Ignition of Flammable Atmospheres by Radio Frequency Radiation.

Glossary

There are many terms used in this field which have specialist meanings. Often these are defined in more than one Standard or Code and the definitions vary in detail but not in meaning. The following should not be taken as strict definitions but as conveying the meaning of the terms within the explosion hazard field.

Abnormal operation outside the normal performance of the apparatus but which recognizes faults, including those which occur only rarely (does not include catastrophic failures).

Analyser house a pressurized enclosure or building into which personnel have routine access which also contains one or more items of apparatus into which flammable materials are fed. When mixed with air at atmospheric pressure and ambient temperature these materials are capable of producing an explosive atmosphere. Releases may or may not occur inside the enclosure or room.

Apparatus (electrical) items applied in whole or in part for the utilization of electrical energy normally comprising an assembly of electrical components or circuits contained within a single enclosure. Some small portable items of apparatus, for example portable transceivers, may be contained in more than one enclosure (the transceiver and its separate microphone) but the enclosures in such cases will be closely coupled.

Approved body (certification) a certification body approved by a member state or associate state of the European Community and notified by that state to the European Community as competent to issue certificates of conformity and inspection certificates

Associated apparatus apparatus which contains both intrinsically safe circuits and non-intrinsically safe circuits which is so constructed that the non-intrinsically safe circuits cannot adversely affect the intrinsically safe circuits.

Battery an assembly of electrochemical cells.

Battery capacity the quantity of electricity or electrical charge which a fully charged battery can deliver under specified conditions.

Breathing device an integral or separable part of a flameproof enclosure designed to permit exchange between the atmosphere inside the enclosure and the surrounding atmosphere.

Bushing an insulating device carrying one or more conductors through an internal or external wall of an enclosure.

Cable entry a device permitting the introduction of one or more electric (and fibre-optic) cables into an apparatus without adversely affecting the protection concept applied to the apparatus.

Cell an electrochemical system capable of storing, in chemical form, electrical energy received and which can give it back by reconversion.

Certification/approval the confirmation, by a recognized third-party expert body, that apparatus or systems are properly explosion protected.

Certificate of conformity a certificate, issued by an approved body, attesting the conformity of apparatus and systems with the essential requirements contained in EU Directive 94/9/EC or with the Standards associated with EU Directive 76/117/EEC.

Clamping device an element of a cable entry for the prevention of tension or torsion in the cable being transmitted to the connections.

Classified area an area in which an explosive atmosphere of gas, vapour, mist and/or dust cloud in mixture with air may exist, or in which a dust layer may be present in such quantities as to require special precautions for the construction and use of apparatus in order to prevent an explosion.

Clearance the shortest distance in air measured between two uninsulated conductive parts.

Combustible dust a dust which, when mixed with air in certain proportions, will form an explosive atmosphere.

Compound a thermosetting, thermoplastic or elastomeric material, with or without fillers and additives, which solidify after their application. Solidification may result in a rigid or flexible solid.

Compression element an element of a cable entry acting on a sealing ring to enable effective sealing of the entry.

Conduit entry a means of introducing conduit into an apparatus without producing adverse effects on the protection concept applied.

Container (cell) a container for the plates and electrolyte of a cell which is impervious to attack by that electrolyte.

Container (battery) an enclosure constructed to contain an already contained cell or assembly of such cells within an apparatus.

Containment system a part of an apparatus used to contain a flammable material within an enclosure. Such a device or assembly may or may not constitute a source of release.

Continuous operating temperature the maximum temperature reached by an apparatus at the maximum ambient temperature for which it is designed with the most onerous operating conditions envisaged in its design or use.

Creepage distance the shortest distance between two uninsulated conducting parts measured across the surface of an insulating material. The conductors and insulating material may be exposed to the air or totally covered with insulating varnish.

Degree of protection (of enclosure) a numerical classification preceded by the symbol 'IP' which identifies the protection afforded by the enclosure against personnel access, the ingress of solid foreign bodies including dust and the ingress of liquids but not gases, vapours or mists.

Dilution the continuous supply of protective gas at a rate sufficient to ensure that the mixture of flammable gas, vapour or mist and air inside an enclosure is continuously maintained at a value outside its explosive limits.

Dilution area an area in the vicinity of a source of release where the concentration of flammable gas, vapour or mist and air is within its explosive limits.

Distance (through casting compound or insulation) the shortest distance between two conductors measured through the casting compound or insulation.

Door or cover a part of an enclosure which is intended to be removed in service but which is important to the protection concept applied to the apparatus. Such parts are normally fixed by screws, bolts studs and nuts or fixings of similar security.

Draining device an integral or separable part of an enclosure designed to permit water, formed by condensation, or liquids, resulting from internal leakage, to escape without adversely affecting the protection concept applied.

Dust small solid particles which settle under their own weight but are small enough to remain in suspension for some time.

Dust protected enclosure an enclosure which does not totally exclude dust but which prevents its entry in quantities such as to interfere with the operation of the enclosed apparatus. (IP5X is normally quoted as the degree of enclosure protection necessary).

Dust tight enclosure an enclosure which excludes the entry of observable quantities of dust particles. (IP6X is normally quoted as the degree of enclosure necessary).

Embedding the process of completely encasing electrical devices by pouring compound over them in a mould which is removed after the compound solidifies.

Encapsulation the process of applying a compound which, after solidification, encloses the apparatus.

Encapsulation 'm' a protection concept where the parts of apparatus which could ignite an explosive atmosphere are enclosed in a compound in such a way as to prevent such ignition.

Encapsulated device a device which may contain voids but which is so constructed that it is totally immersed in compound and the explosive atmosphere cannot gain access.

Energy limitation a concept applied to circuits to ensure that no arc or spark produced in specified conditions is capable of causing an ignition of a specified explosive atmosphere

European committees technical Standards writing committees set up by CENELEC to produce European Standards.

European Standards Standards produced by CENELEC technical committees (normally prefaced BS/EN in the UK).

Ex cable entry a cable entry tested separately from the apparatus in which it is intended to be used but certified as apparatus so that it can be used with other certified apparatus without further certification.

Ex component a part of apparatus for potentially explosive atmospheres or a module (other than an Ex cable entry) which is not intended to be used alone and requires further certification when used in explosion protected apparatus (Certificates for such components are normally suffixed 'U').

Explosion protection (explosion protected apparatus) the measures applied to apparatus to ensure that it is incapable of igniting an explosive atmosphere.

Explosive atmosphere a mixture of flammable gas, vapour, mist or dust, or a combination of these, with air under atmospheric conditions where, after ignition, combustion spreads throughout the mixture.

Explosive limits the limits (upper and lower), usually by volume percentage, of a flammable material with air (or in special circumstances with oxygen) in specified conditions (normally ambient temperature and pressure) outside which combustion will not be achieved.

Explosive mixture a mixture of flammable material with air or oxygen which will burn. Such mixtures are often used for testing of explosion protected apparatus.

Extractable power the power measured in a resistive load connected across a discontinuity in a structure which is acting as a receiving aerial.

Fault a defect of any component, separation, insulation, connection or enclosure upon which a protection concept relies.

Fuse rating the current and voltage rating given to a fuse by its manufacturer.

Filling material quartz or glass particles used for filling apparatus in protection concept powder filling 'q'.

Flameproof enclosure 'd' a protection concept in which parts which can ignite an explosive atmosphere are placed in an enclosure which can withstand the pressure of an internal explosion of a specified explosive atmosphere without damage, and which will not transmit the explosion to the surrounding atmosphere.

Flameproof joint a place where corresponding surfaces of two parts of an enclosure come together and prevent the transmission of an internal explosion.

Flammable gas, vapour or mist a gas, vapour or mist which when mixed with air is appropriate proportions will form an explosive atmosphere.

Flammable material a material which may be a flammable gas, vapour or mist or may be a gas, vapour, mist, liquid or solid material which can give off by evaporation or decomposition a flammable gas, vapour or mist.

Flashpoint the minimum temperature at which sufficient gas or vapour is given off from a flammable liquid (flammable material) to create an explosive atmosphere with air.

Flameproof gap the gap which occurs between two parts of a flameproof enclosure and prevents flame transmission. This has a maximum value which varies according to the flammable atmosphere used which is normally referred to as the maximum experimental safe gap (MESG).

Grade of release this is the measure of the likelihood of release of flammable material in a given area which is graded as Zone 0, 1 or 2 in descending order of likelihood for releases of gas, vapour, mist or liquid and Zone 20, 21 or 22 for dusts.

Hazardous area an area in which an explosive atmosphere is present, or may be expected to be present from time to time, in sufficient quantities to require the use of explosion protected apparatus.

Hermetically sealed device a device, sealed against the ingress of an explosive atmosphere, in which the seal is effected by fusion (e.g., soldering, brazing, welding or glass, glass/metal fusion).

Increased safety 'e' a protection concept in which additional measures are applied so as to give increased security against the possibility of excessive temperatures and of the occurrence of arcs or sparks inside or on the external parts of apparatus which does not arc or spark in normal operation.

Ignition capable apparatus apparatus which in normal operation constitutes a source of ignition for a specified explosive atmosphere.

Ignition temperature the lowest temperature of a surface which will ignite a specified explosive gas atmosphere.

Initial starting current (I_a) the highest rms value of current absorbed by an ac motor when at rest or by an ac magnet with its armature clamped in the position of maximum air gap.

Insulating barrier electrical insulating material between terminals, conductors or groups of cells where it subdivides a battery.

Intercell connector a conductor connected between the cells of a battery and forming part of its construction.

Infallible component, separation, connection or assembly a component, separation, connection or assembly which is not likely to become defective in service in a way as to invalidate intrinsic safety.

Infallible containment a system of containment of flammable gas, vapour, liquid or dust which is of such integrity that the possibility of leakage can be ignored.

Inspection certificate a certificate issued in accordance with Directive 76/117/EEC by an approved body confirming that although apparatus does not conform to one of the recognized protection concepts it is of equivalent safety.

Internal wiring wiring and electrical connections which are made within the apparatus by its manufacturer.

International Standard a Standard published by either the International Standards Organization (ISO) or the International Electrotechnical Commission (IEC).

Intrinsic safety 'i' a protection concept in which the power and energy in a circuit in a hazardous area is limited in both normal operation and fault conditions to below that which will ignite a specified explosive atmosphere.

Intrinsically safe apparatus apparatus in which all of the circuits are intrinsically safe circuits.

Intrinsically safe circuit a circuit in which any spark or thermal effect produced in normal operation and fault conditions recognized by the protection concept is not capable of causing ignition of a given explosive mixture.

Intrinsically safe system an assembly of items of apparatus in which the circuits or parts of circuits including interconnections intended for use in an explosive atmosphere are intrinsically safe circuits.

Latent heat of vaporization the amount of heat which has to be added to a defined quantity of liquid at its boiling point to effect a change of state to vapour.

Limited release a release of flammable gas or vapour the maximum rate of which can be predicted.

Lower explosive limit (LEL) the volume ratio of flammable gas in air below which an explosive atmosphere will not be formed.

Maximum surface temperature the maximum temperature which is attained in service under the most arduous conditions and taking account of tolerances by any part of the apparatus which could cause ignition.

Maximum service temperature the highest value of temperature in which the apparatus is intended to operate.

Minimum igniting current the minimum current flowing in resistive or specific inductive circuits which will, if released as an arc or spark, cause ignition of a prescribed explosive atmosphere.

Minimum igniting voltage the minimum voltage appearing across a specific capacitive circuit which will cause an arc or spark on short circuit of such energy as to ignite a prescribed explosive atmosphere.

National certificate a certificate issued by a nationally recognized third-party expert body confirming that an apparatus or system complies with a recognized National Standard.

National Standard a Standard which is nationally accepted but has no European or international status.

Non-hazardous area areas not designated as hazardous areas.

Non-countable fault a fault which occurs in parts of apparatus not conforming to the constructional requirements of the protection concept.

Non-incendive component a component with sparking contacts which are not themselves ignition capable, or with sparking contacts or ignition-capable hot surfaces which are enclosed such that ignition of the surrounding atmosphere is prevented under specific operating conditions.

Normal operation operation of a process or apparatus within its normally accepted reliability criteria including failures which occur so regularly as to be included in those criteria.

Oil immersion 'o' a protection concept where the apparatus or parts of it are immersed in a protective liquid so that any explosive atmosphere at the surface of the liquid or its containment cannot be ignited.

Operating rod a part used for the transmission of control movements which may be both rotary and linear.

Portable apparatus apparatus which can be moved whilst in operation or can be easily moved from one place to another between operational periods.

Potentially explosive atmosphere an atmosphere which can become an explosive from time to time (the danger is a potential rather than continuous one).

Potting an embedding process in which the mould remains attached to the embedded devices after the encapsulant has set.

Powder filling 'q' a protection concept in which parts of the apparatus capable of igniting an explosive atmosphere are surrounded by a solid (powder) filling material so that an ignition of the surrounding atmosphere is prevented.

Pressure piling the result of ignition, in a compartment or subdivision of a flameproof enclosure, of a gas mixture precompressed for example due to a primary ignition in another compartment or subdivision.

Pressurization 'p' the technique of application of a protective gas to an enclosure in order to prevent the formation of an explosive atmosphere in the enclosure by maintaining overpressure inside. This may be done by static pressurization where the enclosure is pressurized and sealed, by maintaining a supply of protective gas to the enclosure to accommodate leakage, or by maintaining a continuous flow of protective gas through the enclosure.

Protection concept (type of protection) the specific measures applied to apparatus or systems to prevent the ignition of an explosive atmosphere.

Protective gas air or inert gas used in the protection concept of pressurization.

Protective liquid mineral oil or other similar liquid complying with the requirements of protection concept oil immersion 'o'.

Purging the passing of a quantity of air or inert gas through an enclosure to remove any explosive atmosphere prior to the pressurization of the enclosure.

Rated dynamic current (I_{dyn}) the peak value of current whose dynamic effect can be withstood by apparatus without damage.

Rated short time thermal current (I_{th}) the rms value of current required to heat up a conductor from the temperature reached in rated service at maximum ambient temperature to the limiting temperature.

Rated value a quantity value assigned, usually by the manufacturer, for a specific operating condition of a component, device or apparatus.

Rating a set of rated values and operating conditions.

Resistance heating device part of a resistance heating unit, comprising one or more heating resistors, typically composed of metallic conductors or an electrically conductive compound suitably insulated and protected.

Resistance heating unit apparatus comprising one or more resistance heating devices associated with devices to ensure that the limiting temperature is not exceeded.

Sealed device a device which is so constructed that it cannot be opened during normal service and is effectively sealed to prevent the ingress of explosive atmosphere (it may include gaskets, etc.).

Sealed gas-tight cell or battery a cell or battery which remains closed and does not release gas or liquid when operated within the limits of charge or temperature specified by the manufacturer.

Sealed valve-regulated cell or battery a cell or battery which is closed under normal conditions but which has an arrangement which allows the escape of gas if the internal pressure exceeds a predetermined value.

Sealing ring a ring used in a cable or conduit entry to ensure the sealing between the cable or conduit and the entry.

Self-limiting characteristic the Characteristic of a resistance heating device where the thermal output at its rated voltage decreases as the temperature of its surroundings increases.

Shaft a part of circular cross-section used for the transmission of rotary movement.

Short circuit current (I_{sc}) maximum value of short circuit current to which the apparatus may be subjected in service.

Simple apparatus an electrical component, device or assembly of components of simple construction with well-defined electrical parameters.

Source of release (hazard) a point or location from which a flammable gas, vapour, mist or combustible dust may be released into the atmosphere such that an explosive atmosphere could be formed.

Special fasteners devices used to secure an enclosure or other part of explosion protected apparatus so as to give added confidence in its security.

Starting current ration (I_a/I_n) the ratio between the initial starting current I_a of a rotating machine at rest and its rated current (I_n0 when running at full load.

Stopper box a device designed to restrict the flow of gas or liquid between an apparatus and a conduit or cable.

Surface temperature classification a classification system used to categorize apparatus as to the maximum unprotected temperature achieved in service.

Temperature range the range of temperature within which a component, device or compound will retain its properties.

Type of protection 'N' ('n') a protection concept applied to apparatus such that, in normal operation, it is not capable of igniting a surrounding explosive atmosphere and a fault capable of causing ignition is unlikely to occur.

Unlimited release a release of flammable gas, vapour or mist or combustible dust the maximum flowrate of which cannot be predicted (this includes liquid releases above their flashpoints).

Upper explosive limit the volume ratio of flammable gas or vapour in air above which an explosive atmosphere will not be formed.

Vulnerable Zone the region surrounding an radio frequency transmitter in which a potential ignition hazard could arise within any hazardous area.

Working voltage the highest rms value of the ac or dc voltage which may occur (locally) across any insulation at rated supply voltage in both normal operating and open circuit conditions (neglecting transients).

Index